Mandy Arala

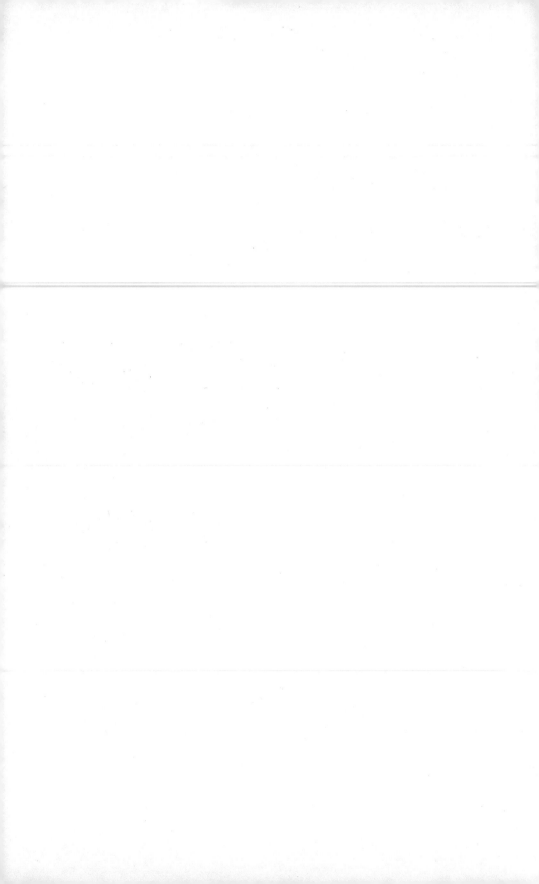

Synopsis of
Paediatrics

Dedicated to Ruth, Sheva, Gideon and Rafi, simultaneously my most solicitous supporters and severest critics, and Shay who tended the wick before going off to bed.

Synopsis of
Paediatrics

Alex Habel MB ChB, FRCP
Consultant Paediatrician, West Middlesex University Hospital, Isleworth, Middlesex, UK

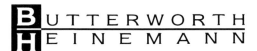

Preface

This is a text which attempts to bridge the gap between the pocket book vade-mecum and the 5 kg tome.

What follows is inevitably didactic for reasons of space. A practical approach, without being exhaustive, has been my aim. Sections begin with normal findings and basic physiology. A symptom based problem-solving approach follows, and is supplemented by a discussion of individual disorders. Where relevant, recent advances and controversy concerning the management of problems are included. A selection of references, hopefully not too idiosyncratic, complement the text.

Within these pages I hope to help those taking on further paediatric responsibilities in hospital and community, and who may be studying for postgraduate examinations.

The child is referred to usually as he, as he is generally more vulnerable, but no sexism is intended.

Without peer review this work would have been riddled with inaccuracies and more than one school-boy howler! I am pleased to record my thanks to the following, in the hope that this small public acknowledgement of their help is at least partial recompense: Mike Burch, Joseph Caser, Jonathon Cripps, Jane Deal, Penny Fallon, Sally Flew, Sue Holder, Peter Husband, Simon Nadel, Tony Oakhill, G C Rastogi, David Stewart, Sam Walters, Hamish Watson, Alan and Nicola Wilson.

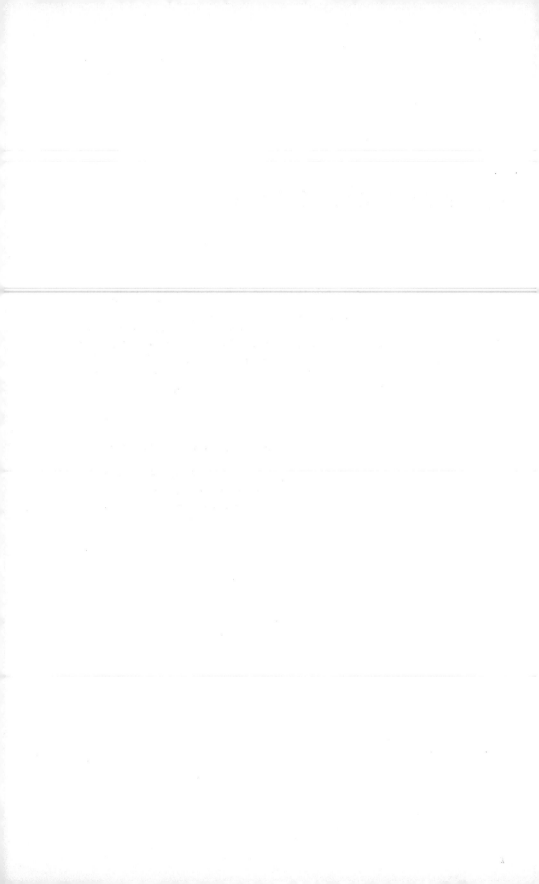

Acknowledgements

Grateful thanks to Betty Bass and Dr Abraham of the Central Middlesex Hospital for providing the EEG illustrations.

Permission to use illustrations was granted by: Blackwell Scientific Publications, of Tanner's puberty ratings (Figs 8.1–8.3); Clement Clarke International Ltd, of the respiratory function chart (Fig. 12.5); Lady Limerick, of compiled infant mortality rates (Fig. 1, p. 3); Royal College of Physicians, of sexual abuse diagrams (Figs 3.3–3.5).

Abbreviations

Abbreviations have been kept to a minimum, and the following will be found in the text:

AD Autosomal dominant inheritance
AR Autosomal recessive inheritance
CT Computerized tomography
EEG Electroencephalograph
ESR Erythrocyte sedimentation rate
FBC Full blood count
LP Lumbar puncture
MRI Magnetic resonance imaging
US Ultrasound
WBC White blood count
XL Sex linked inheritance

Introduction

CHILDREN, HEALTH AND THE ROLE OF THE MEDICAL SERVICES

The role of paediatricians continues to expand, and encompasses the health of children both within the community and hospital, as the artificial barriers to a comprehensive childrens' service are brought down.

To put hospital practice into context, parents care for 80% of all childhood illness without recourse to professionals, and only 3% are referred on by the primary care team.

CHILDREN'S RIGHTS

The statement of children's rights, adapted from the United Nations declaration, emphasizes how education, legislation and economic factors are the larger forces controlling the health and well-being of the world's children:

1. Equal rights regardless of sex, race, or religion.
2. Special protection to be enabled to develop fully. The right to education, play and recreation.
3. Adequate food, housing and medical care.
4. Special care if handicapped.
5. Protection against neglect, cruelty and exploitation.

To this end, the specific contribution that medical services as a whole can make are the WHO and UNICEF goals of:

1. Growth monitoring. Regular weighing to detect infant malnutrition.
2. Rehydration. (Oral rehydration therapy (ORT) has saved millions of lives.) Clean water supply for all by the year 2000.
3. Breast feeding.
4. Expanded vaccination programme
5. Family planning to improve survival.
6. Maternal nutrition and education level improved.

AUDIT OF CARE

Crude measures, such as annual mortality rates, have served well in comparing success over time, nationally and internationally (Figure 1). As rates decline, new challenges emerge, such as combating cot deaths and the sudden infant death syndrome.

The annual death toll in the UK for the 0–16 year age group

Total: 10 500 children aged 0–16 years.
4000 in the newborn period.
5000 suddenly from accidents, cot deaths, and infections.
1500 die from degenerative diseases or severe handicap (800), malignancy (400), and organ failure (300).

Audit of care in the 1990s

Audit is now an obligatory component to contracts made between NHS hospitals whether of trust status or directly managed by a Health Region. It needs to be confidential, credible, practical, regular and relevant. It is the systematic critical analysis of medical care and has four components.

1. Resources: the facilities (hospital, beds, laboratories, etc.) and personnel (doctors, nurses, therapists, management, etc.) available, and the patients.
2. Process: the assessment, treatment and management of patients. Quality assurance is the application of acceptable standards to the process (ranging from waiting times, availability of notes, delay in communicating with family practitioners, to review of the recording of history taking, examination, appropriateness of investigations and their interpretation, correctness of diagnosis and treatment. It includes parental and children's perceptions of the services, e.g. courtesy, value of the consultation, ward facilities, staff).
3. Outcome: measured traditionally by death rates, more recently by quality of life of outcome of the process, e.g. leukaemia survival in specialist centres versus district hospitals, and reduction in intelligence follows cranial irradiation when compared with chemotherapy.
4. Change: the result of appraisal, change in the process (e.g. by teaching or in management protocols) may be indicated. To complete the audit cycle, this then becomes the subject of subsequent audit.

Practical audit

Guidelines for case review of neonatal, in-patient, out-patient, and community notes, as well as the running of audit meetings are available from the British Paediatric Association (1991). Topic or criteria audit measures the effectiveness of services, e.g. detection of abnormalities such as undescended testes, congenital dislocation of the hip, or sensory deficits (see Monitoring child health surveillance, in the Community section), and the management of conditions like febrile convulsions and asthma.

Further reading

BPA Working Group (1990) Paediatric Audit. British Paediatric Association.

Joint Working Group (1991) Guidelines for the Management of Convulsions with Fever. *British Medical Journal*, **303**, 634–636

Oberklaid F, Barnett P, Jarman F, Sewell J (1991) Quality Assurance in the Emergency Room. *Archives of Disease in Childhood* **66**, 1093–1098

Ross Russell R I, Helms P J (1990) Audit–Where do we go from here? *Archives of Disease in Childhood* **65**, 1107–1108

THE CARE OF CHILDREN IN HOSPITAL

Society's expectations of the nature and delivery of services are changing. The National Association for the Welfare of Children in Hospital (NAWCH) charter is the standard against which we must measure our performance, as perceived by the children and their parents.

1. Admission is a last resort, when care cannot be equally well provided at home or on a day basis.
2. Parents should be able to stay with their child provided it is in his/her best interests.
3. The child and parents have a right to be informed and involved in decisions appropriate to age and understanding.
4. The right to protection from undue physical and emotional distress, and respect for privacy during admission.
5. Care among others of similar age and maturity, in their own clothes, by appropriately trained staff in an environment suitably orientated and equipped, with opportunity for play and recreation and with facilities to continue their education.

THE CONSULTATION: A GENERAL GUIDE

1. Welcome

A warm welcome and smile helps put children at their ease.

Toddlers often initially have eye avoidance. A toy to play with, on the accompanying adult's lap, will give them time to adjust; forcing your attentions can be counterproductive.

2. History taking: an outline

Direct questions appropriate to age and maturity, for example about their age, how they came to the clinic, TV programmes, pop music and football, what they like most, and least, at school.

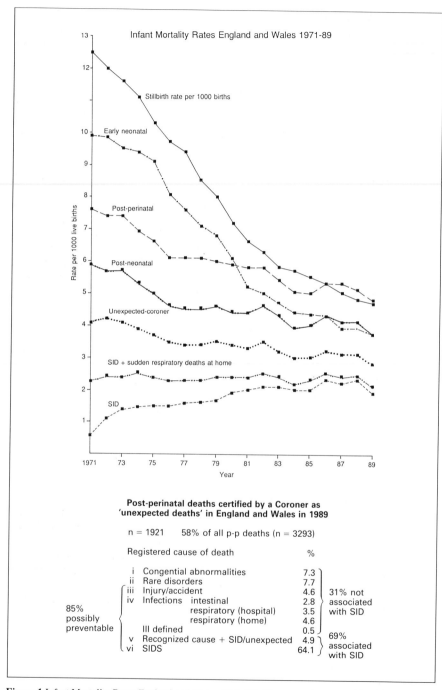

Figure 1 Infant Mortality Rates England and Wales 1971–89. 'Unexpected - coroner' in 1989 comprised 70% sudden infant death, 30% with underlying cause. (Compiled by S R Limerick from unpublished OPCS data analysed by A Gardiner).

i Enquiry as to the main complaint 'why have you come?' may be addressed to the child first, unless from the referral letter it is likely to be embarrassing, e.g. for enuresis. The real reason for the consultation may not be the stated-one, so asking the parents 'what are you worried about most?' may be more revealing. Ignore their concerns at your peril!

   Record dates or days before consultation, not days of the week. Medication, names, doses, duration and effects need to be noted. School non-attendance is an indicator of illness, family anxiety and behavioural issues.

ii Pregnancy and birth history. Maternal health: previous pregnancies and outcome, infection, rubella status, handling cat litter, drugs, alcohol, smoking, medication, bleeding, blood pressure. Quickening, US timing and result.

   Birth: gestation, onset spontaneous/induced, duration, presentation, complications, delivery. Birth order and weight.

   Newborn: Apgar score is often known. Resuscitation, cyanosis, breathing difficulties, congenital abnormalities may have delayed the infant joining the mother. Abnormal sleeping or feeding, convulsions, jaundice, and time of passage of meconium often relevant to problems presenting in infancy.

iii Growth and development. Feeding: breast and its duration, or bottle, time of introduction of solids, a dietary history of milk intake and content of meals for the last 24 hours, where and how meals are taken, frequency and description of bowel motions.

   Weights +/- height and head circumference from the parent held record are invaluable.

   Developmental milestones: detail is related to relevance, but should always be ascertained.

   Behavioural problems: sleep, feeding, temper, whether happy, recent alteration may indicate emotional upset/abuse.

   Habits such as pica. Later drugs, smoking, alcohol, solvent abuse in relation to abnormal behaviour.

iv Past medical history. Illness, accidents, hospital attendance, operations, immunizations, allergies.

   Foreign travel or visitors from abroad, especially Africa or Asia, is often relevant.

v Systems review.

vi Family history. A properly constructed genetic chart of parents and siblings, deaths, terminations and miscarriages. Consanguinity must be noted. Grandparents and other relatives may need to be included.

   Enquire as to inherited disease: atopy, epilepsy, mental retardation, diabetes, system disease relevant to the history, e.g. urinary tract infection and reflux. Increasingly, sexually transmitted disease is relevant.

vii Social history. Accommodation, parental employment, stable partner or single parent may be a crucial factor.

3. Physical examination

Note general appearance, height, weight, and if relevant, head circumference. (Details of systems examination are included in each section.)

i Confidence building activities include asking to look at the child's hands, and if preschool play 'Round and round the garden'. The latter evaluates the degree of supination, tests sensation and allows palpation of the axillae for lymphadenopathy! 'This little piggy' similarly permits initial handling of the lower limbs.

ii In puberty and adolescence the rule is to respect the privacy of the individual, i.e. treat like Royalty. Examination may at times be as piecemeal and with as much subterfuge as for a fractious toddler.

iii Unpleasant procedures are best left to last by which time you will have been sized up. Time taken will encourage cooperation for the next step. A spatula can be replaced by a teaspoon handle. Voluntary mouth opening is preferable, as the alternative is to restrain the child sitting on an adult's lap. An apprehensive girl may prefer to have her *mother* touch the genitals to demonstrate the introitus.

Encouraging the child to play with the instrument, e.g. an auriscope, and jointly to hold the handle as the speculum is introduced into the external canal allows the child to feel in control. Similarly, a perineal swab can be taken by the child, after an initial dummy run with a buccal swab, the examining person guiding her hand for both.

COUNSELLING PARENTS AND CHILDREN WHO HAVE SEVERE, ACUTE OR CHRONIC DISORDERS

Breaking bad news

This situation arises across the whole spectrum of paediatric practice, and for that reason sits as comfortably in the introduction as anywhere.

Typical situations: birth of a baby with Down's syndrome, spina bifida, diagnosis of mental handicap, blindness, a fatal illness, cancer.

1. When to tell: as soon as the diagnosis is reasonably secure, but not necessarily precise. For example, Down's syndrome is clinically evident, but chromosome culture not yet available, or acute lymphoblastic leukaemia from a bone marrow examination but no chromosome or cell-type information.
2. Delay leads to significant parent dissatisfaction.
3. Parents should be informed together, in a quiet room, with a nurse and a junior doctor present to know what facts have been relayed.
4. Sketch in the overall picture, avoid giving too many facts.
5. Give time to allow discussion, including the normal needs of the child for loving care, family life and routine.
6. Guilt is common. Reassurance is essential.
7. Arrange follow up to continue discussion. Provide information and literature as they want it. Consider parent support group, and introduction to other suitable families similarly affected. Consult the Contact a Family directory of specific conditions and rare syndromes in children with their family support networks.

Parental reactions, which may not progress beyond the initial stage:

1. Initial disbelief, shock or anger.

2. Adjustment, often with depression.
3. Resolution, acceptance.

Common responses include searching for second opinions (refusal to accept diagnosis), rejection or its apparent opposite, overprotectiveness. Crusading zeal may mask anger or depression. Child abuse is more likely.

Family pressures: main burden of care is on mother; increased incidence of marital breakdown and sibling difficulties in vulnerable families can be ameliorated by support and advice. Strengthening family bonds, empathy, and siblings entering caring professions, are positive outcomes.

Cultural patterns: isolation and prejudice are especially common among some ethnic minorities.

Conveying the diagnosis of cystic fibrosis and diabetes mellitus may elicit similar bereavement reactions on the part of the parents, depending on their previous experience and conceptions.

Illness, death and bereavement – the child's perspective

Responses by children to being told about illness with long term or severe implications:

1. Anger: directed at parents, family, professionals.
2. Mourning: loss of previous abilities/imposition of restrictions by the treatment.
3. Guilt: causality – imagined wrong doing or own bad thoughts responsible. These may be experienced by siblings, who may also need help.

Telling children

Honesty is necessary, but not brutality.

Work with the parents: their emotional reactions will greatly influence the child.

Knowledge of the implications of the disease for that individual child, its effects on function and self-image, to be able to give relevant explanations.

Acceptance of illness

This takes time, and various coping mechanisms are used by the child: intellectualizing about the illness; ritualization of behaviour. Denial may be constructive, allowing the child to carry on, or be obstructive, preventing cooperation with treatment, and is especially prevelant in adolescence.

The professionals must 'roll with the punches', and not be rejecting but supportive in the emotional upheavals.

Concept of death, with relevance to child's own mortality and bereavement

Under 3 years have no understanding. Over half of 5 year olds and nearly all 8 year olds understand death to be irrevocable, with cessation of all bodily functions, and that it happens to all.

Studies of children with cancer suggest stages in understanding, through observation of others' and their own experience as the illness progresses: 1. I am very sick; 2. I have an illness that can kill people; 3. I have an illness that can kill children; 4. I may not get better; 5. I am dying.

Asking the child what he thinks is wrong allows discussion about issues from which the parents may want to shield him, or themselves.

In the case of bereavement, a simple explanation of the cause of death may remove guilt or confusion. The finality of death may be eased by talk of Heaven, but not so as to cause frustration at being unable to go there! Depression, regression, and behaviour disturbance is common, and if prolonged is termed adjustment disorder, which benefits from psychiatric intervention.

Further reading

National Association of Health Authorities (1988) The Care of Dying Children and their Families
Delight E, Goodall J (1990) Love and loss. Conversations with parents of babies with spina bifida managed without surgery 1971–1981. *Developmental Medicine and Child Neurology*, Supplement 61

Chapter 1

Genetics

A congenital malformation is an anatomical or structural abnormality present at birth. Fifty per cent of deaths and 40% of hospital admissions under 15 years old are due to congenital malformations and genetic disease.

In the UK 20000 births of a total of 700000 have a major malformation, chromosomal or genetic disorder, i.e. 3% (65% are sporadic, 35% inherited). This doubles to 6% by the end of the first year as more are detected (Table 1).

Table 1.1 Incidence of congenital and genetically inherited disorders per 1000 births

Congenital malformations	sporadic	20
	inherited	2
Mendelian	single gene	8
Chromosomal	sporadic	2
	inherited	0.6

INHERITED DISORDERS

Despite their individual rarity (there are over 4000 Mendelian inherited disorders) the risk of passing on an inherited disease is present in 3% of parenting couples, for example 20000 of the UK population are at risk of developing Huntington's chorea (Table 1.2).

DYSMORPHOLOGY

Malformations resulting from abnormal intrauterine development.

Definitions

Malformation

A primary structural defect arising during development of an organ or tissue.

i Single defect, e.g. cleft palate, congenital heart disease. If it occurs in isolation is usually multifactorial, with a low risk of recurrence.

ii Multiple malformation syndrome, e.g. Down's syndrome; mental handicap is often associated. Recurrence risk is related to aetiology: single gene, chromosomal, congenital infection, or environmental.

Table 1.2 Incidence and carrier rate of some inherited diseases

	Per 10,000 births	*Carriers as % of population*
Dominant		
(1 in 2 offspring affected)		
Adult polycystic disease	0.8	The carrier rate is the same as the
Huntington's chorea	0.7	incidence of the disease, i.e. most
Neurofibromatosis	0.3	have an affected parent and the mutation rate is very low or absent.
Recessive		
(1 in 4 offspring affected)		
General: Cystic fibrosis	5	4
Phenylketonuria	2	1
Ethnic groups:		
Mediterranean ⎫		
⎬ Thalassaemia	from 3 to 70	3 to 17
Asians ⎭		
Blacks Sickle cell	from 1 to 200	2 to 25
Ashkenazi Jews Tay-Sachs	3	4
X Linked		
(1 in 2 males affected,		
1 in 2 females are carriers)		
Fragile X mental retardation	7	About twice as many carriers as
Duchenne muscular dystrophy	1	there are affected, mainly among
Haemophilia	0.5	the female relatives

Disruption

Extrinsic force/influence on initially normal development. Examples:

i Amniotic bands → amputations, facial clefts.

ii Infection, e.g. chickenpox → vascular occlusion → bowel atresia. Recurrence is unlikely.

Deformation

Abnormal form, shape or position due to mechanical forces.

i Maternal: uterine cavity malformed, reduced space from fibroids, multiple gestation, oligohydramnios → talipes, lung hypoplasia, Potter's facies.

ii Fetal: diminished movement → arthrogryposis.

Dysplasia

Abnormal organization of cells into tissues and its morphological result, e.g. achondroplasia, osteogenesis imperfecta.

Sequence

Initial abnormality due to a malformation, deformation or disruption results in secondary effects, e.g. Robin sequence of posterior placed tongue → cleft palate, micrognathia; Potter's syndrome of renal agenesis→ reduced liquor → pulmonary hypoplasia, deformation of face, limbs.

Associations

The occurrence together of certain malformations more often than expected by chance, without a known underlying cause. Often eponymous, e.g. Goldenhar association or called by the acronym of the abnormalities found, e.g. CHARGE = coloboma, heart defects, atresia of choani, growth and mental retardation, genital abnormalities, ear abnormalities. See also VATER/VACTERL.

CRITICAL PHASES OF INTRAUTERINE DEVELOPMENT

Weeks 1+2 Preimplantation: maximum vulnerability but effects limited in the surviving embryo because of the totipotency of embryonic cells which die or regenerate a damaged part completely.

Weeks 3–9 Embryonic or Organogenesis period: 3 germ layers by third week, folding of embryo longitudinally and transversely in 4th week. *Organs are most susceptible to teratogenic damage at their first appearance*, e.g. Thalidomide (effects seen at 21–34 days fetal age), fetal alcohol, rubella (Table 1.3).

Weeks 10–40 Fetal period: growth and maturation phase, although differentiation is not complete and organs are still susceptible to teratogenesis (e.g. rubella leading to deafness and intrauterine growth retardation, stilboestrol causing virilization, etc), while damage alone becomes more evident, e.g. cytomegalovirus.

Table 1.3 Known teratogens (10% of all birth defects)

Drugs	Thalidomide and diethylstilboestrol (historical), antimetabolites
	Alcohol, anticonvulsants, warfarin, vitamin A, inhalation anaesthetics
Metabolic conditions	Diabetes mellitus: neural tube defects, sacral agenesis
	Maternal phenylketonuria: microcephaly, mental retardation, congenital heart defects
Environmental	Mercury: Cerebral palsy
Infections	Cytomegalovirus, syphilis, rubella, toxoplasmosis, varicella

NB: overall fetal loss is 50–75%, the majority in the first trimester, the main reason being chromosomal abnormalities which are found in 50% of all conceptions.

CONGENITAL INFECTIONS (ALSO SEE NEONATAL PROBLEMS, INFECTIONS)

Affect 3% of all pregnancies, but the incidence of long term teratogenic abnormality and organ damage is very much lower.

Factors include:

   i Timing, e.g. rubella early in gestation → organ malformation in 30%, negligible after 16 weeks.

  ii Placental resistance to transfer, e.g. Cytomegalovirus (CMV) affects up to 5% of pregnancies but only 0.5% fetuses infected.

Incidence

1. *T*oxoplasma: 1 in 1000 births.
2. *O*thers: e.g. syphilis, varicella; HIV: 200 annually and increasing.
3. *R*ubella: despite a vaccination programme 1 in 6000 pregnancies still infected in the late 1980s.
4. *C*MV: 1 in 5000 births, although 10 times as many fetuses infected.
5. *H*erpes simplex acquired at birth causing encephalitis in 1/20,000.

The traditional acronym TORCH is considered too restrictive, not just a question of attribution, but also has active treatment implications.

Example: syphilis and disseminated Herpes simplex are indistinguishable from traditional TORCH in the acute phase. However, delay in treatment may damage/ kill. A specific IgM and *Treponema pallidum* inhibition test is required, and treatment initiated 'blind' with acyclovir if the latter is negative, to cover Herpes.

Clinical manifestations of toxoplasmosis, CMV, rubella

1. All share: growth retardation, microcephaly, mental retardation, acute encephalitis and hepatitis.
2. Infection specific

   i Deafness in CMV (progressive in some, i.e. absent at first) and rubella.

  ii Cataracts in CMV and rubella (also glaucoma in latter), choroidoretinitis in rubella, toxoplasmosis.

 iii Cerebral calcification in CMV, toxoplasmosis.

 iv Heart defects in rubella: stenotic branched pulmonary arteries, patent ductus arteriosus.

Identification of morphological syndromes/genetic disease

(after Dr Robin Winter)

A syndrome is a recognizable pattern of abnormality, or malformation of function, or structure, due to a single cause.

1. Find a good 'handle' to diagnosis, i.e. a prominent relatively uncommon feature, e.g. good = webbed neck in Turner's syndrome, poor = cleft lip +/− palate found in 150 associated conditions.
2. Constellation of features which are recognized as a whole (Gestalt), e.g. face of Down's, William's, fetal alcohol syndrome.
3. More evident with age, e.g. mucopolysaccharidoses, degenerations.

4. Siblings and family have associated characteristics. Examples:

   i Deafness occurs in osteogenesis imperfecta, Pendred's syndrome, and hereditary nephritis.

   ii Skin pigmentation/nodules and/or only Lisch nodules in the eyes of relatives with neurofibromatosis.

5. Three or more minor malformations (e.g. polydactyly, hypertelorism, ear pits/tags): 90% of infants will have one or more associated major malformations, or cerebral palsy. One in five of these have multiple malformations.

Assessment of the dysmorphic individual

Half of dysmorphic children have an identifiable disorder.

1. Family history of fetal loss, physical and mental abnormality.

   i Ethnic group and consanguinity are important determinants of genetic disease, e.g. the Pakistani custom of cousin marriage doubles the normal risk of serious disease and malformation. With incest it rises to 1 in 2.

   ii A pedigree of 3 or 4 generations should be drawn up.

2. Pregnancy:
   - Drugs, alcohol and medication timing and duration of exposure.
   - Growth, e.g. oligohydramnios.
   - Diminished fetal movement is a clue to neuromuscular disorders.
   - Abnormal uterus, e.g. fibroids, septate uterus causing deformation.
3. Examination: List abnormal features, development, and neurology.
4. Investigations commonly indicated: skeletal survey, chromosomes, ultrasound scan of heart, kidneys and head. (CT of head may be preferred especially if the fontanelle is closed or small.) Biochemical tests are for the most likely inborn error or metabolic condition (e.g. hypercalcaemia in William's syndrome), especially if already present in a parent or sibling; usually blood and urine for amino acids, urine for glucose, reducing substances, ketones.

PRACTICAL GENETIC COUNSELLING

The what, why, prognosis and parenting questions that must be addressed:

1. What it is and why it occurred. The communication of the diagnosis.
2. Prognosis: implications for the individual and the family; the risks of recurrence.

   Counselling is non-directive. It seeks to help the couple make the right choice for themselves. Marital separation or artificial insemination are rarely seen as alternatives, so prenatal diagnosis is useful if applicable.

Imparting information and counselling parents

Essential points in any informed discussion:

   i Randomness of nature, unless clearly familial or inheritable. 1 in 40 children are born with a major defect, most of unknown cause.

   ii Describe the origin of the defect if known, e.g. failure of neural tube closure at 28 days in spina bifida, extra chromosome at the time of formation of an individual in trisomy 21.

   iii Incidence and likely recurrence.

Some specific situations, drawing attention to the implications for the child and family

Discussion must have a balance of fact with compassion and ease the feelings of guilt and recrimination parents are likely to have.

1. Major malformation, no therapy available or benefit likely, e.g. trisomy 13 or 18.

   i Often a high incidence of spontaneous loss during pregnancy.

   ii Experience has shown that no intervention appears to improve function.

   iii Letting nature take its course with no medical intervention is the most humane approach.

2. Chronic handicap present or the potential for disability is there:

   i Origin, examples: phenylketonuria has genetic and metabolic consequences, trisomy 21 needs chromosome investigations.

   ii Features. Describe and demonstrate those present or anticipated, e.g. Marfan's syndrome: arachnodactyly, lens dislocation, later dissection of the aorta.

   iii Implications for life, schooling, work, social/marriage.

   iv Therapy may be possible, e.g. secondary preventive surgery of early aortic dissection, growth hormone (GH) replacement if GH deficient, medication and physiotherapy in cystic fibrosis.

   v Prognosis with treatment.

   vi Acknowledge acceptance of the needs of that individual, not a blanket approach.

   vii Parent support groups and syndrome societies have valuable supporting roles. Found in the Contact a Family Register.

3. Single, usually corrigible abnormality, e.g. congenital dislocation of the hip, talipes, cleft lip and palate, congenital heart disease (CHD).

   i This is a normal child, the defect is not necessarily handicapping. Stress normality in terms of development, function, activities, and social relationships.

   ii Treatment plan involves discussing the type of intervention, if any, its timing and likely and realistic expectations of outcome.
Examples

    a. The majority achieve acceptable speech after cleft lip and palate surgery, some need further surgery (pharyngoplasty) and most need speech therapy.

    b. Complex CHD may be curative or palliative, with a possible need for later procedures/transplant.

   iii Emphasis is on localization of the problem in the context of the life of the whole child, i.e. avoiding 'medicalizing' him/her.

Counselling for single gene disease, autosomal and sex linked conditions

1. Risks of recurrence

The complications, and variation in severity of the condition need to be shared with the parents and family. Thalassaemia major is an example of how advances in education, screening and obstetric intervention can change parental expectations. Affected Greek Cypriot families previously voluntarily limited family size to an average of two children. Now population screening → prepregnancy counselling and selective termination → family size expands to the cultural norm of three or four children. This is not yet happening with affected Asian families.

2. Spontaneous mutations

Eighty per cent of achondroplastics have normal parents, 50% of Duchenne dystrophics have no family history, i.e. a new mutation in that individual or the mother. Investigations may be morphological or DNA linkage/oligonucleotide studies (see below).

3. Dominant with variable penetrance

'Skipped generations' from grandparent to grandchild, the parent apparently unaffected, e.g. von Recklinghausen, tuberous sclerosis, Alagille syndrome: triangular face, deep set eyes, broad nose root, congenital heart and biliary tree defects. Such patterns of inheritance may be due to genomic imprinting: see below.

4. XL, usually recessive

i.e. male affected, female normal unless she has a single X as in Turner's XO. Females are protected by the presence of two X chromosomes, only one of which need be active in each cell (Lyon's hypothesis).

Rare XL dominant conditions occur in which the female carrier may be symptomatic, e.g. nephrogenic diabetes insipidus, vitamin D resistant rickets.

Counselling for chromosomal disease

i Non-disjunction

Failure in the ovum or sperm of normal division into 23 single chromosomes, two of a pair being present. Usually sporadic in most autosomal and all sex chromosome abnormalities.

ii Mosaic

Some children/parents are mosaic (mixed normal and abnormal chromosomes in different tissues) for the condition, and pass on the condition. Look for a 'forme fruste' in one of the parents.

iii Translocations

Combinations of chromosomes stuck together to a greater or lesser extent. Translocations are often sporadic, but always require parents' chromosomes to be examined.

iv Genomic imprinting

Abnormal development may occur if chromosomal material from either parent is missing, e.g. deletion on chromosome 15 (15q 11-13) in mother = Angelman syndrome, and the same deletion in father = Prader-Willi syndrome. This occurs through:

   a. Deletion on the long arm of chromosome 15 of the parent.
   b. Uniparental disomy (two chromosome 15 from the same parent).

Counselling in multifactorial Disease

1. Genetically inherited susceptibility is present in 30% of the population, brought out spontaneously or by the environment, e.g. cleft lip and palate incidence is 1 in 1000 births. Empirical risk of recurrence after one affected child is 1 in 25, after two children or one + affected parent the risk increases to 1 in 10.
2. The risk may be reduced, as in spina bifida by periconceptional folic acid supplementation.
3. Where a sex ratio exists, if the index case is the less common sex then the recurrence risk for siblings may be higher:

	sex ratio	M index	F index
e.g. Pyloric stenosis	M:F = 5:1	1 in 25	1 in 10

Environmental Hazards

Advice on drugs in pregnancy, e.g. steroids, anticonvulsants (but weigh up risk of exacerbation of asthma or epilepsy if reduced). Abstinence/reduction in alcohol consumption. Immunization against rubella if no antibodies are present.

High and Low risk in genetic counselling

More than 1 in 10 = high risk, e.g. autosomal dominant (1 in 2), or recessive (1 in 4) or 1 in 2 males for sex linked conditions.
   Less than 1 in 10 = low risk, e.g. insulin dependent diabetes.
   Risk can change from low to high in multifactorial diseases as in cleft lip and palate and spina bifida if more than one family member is affected.

PRENATAL DIAGNOSIS

Aims

Informed choice; reassure appropriately; termination of severely affected fetus; planning optimal treatment of the affected fetus, e.g. exomphalos.

Ethics

Informed consent is essential, with the knowledge that abortion may be an option. Antenatal diagnosis can be offered even if anti-abortion, either to reassure or allow preparation for the handicapped child.

Methods

1. *Identify risk groups by*

i Maternal age (Down's).
ii Blood screening ethnic groups (e.g. Asians, Blacks for haemoglobinopathies).
iii Affected family member (e.g. Huntington's, α-1 antitrypsin deficiency, cystic fibrosis, Duchenne, inborn errors, spina bifida).
iv Maternal screening blood test (Rhesus antibodies, α fetoprotein raised in spina bifida, low in Down's syndrome [+ oestriol + HCG = triple test]).

2. *Definitive investigations*

i Obstetric ultrasound detects congenital malformations at 18–20 weeks : commonly head, heart, spine, kidneys.
ii Chorionic villus sample (CVS) first trimester at 10–12 weeks.
iii Amniocentesis in second trimester at 16-18 weeks: liquor for

  • alphafetoprotein raised in spina bifida.
  • bilirubin spectrometry in rhesus disease.
  • biochemistry in inborn errors where an enzyme test is unavailable/unreliable, e.g. some forms of adrenogenital syndrome.
    Risk of fetal loss from CVS is about 1–2%, amniocentesis 0.5–1.0%, both slightly higher than background spontaneous abortion rates at that stage in pregnancy. An increase in limb defects may occur in early CVS. False positives/negatives result from contamination by maternal blood or placental chromosomal mosaicism.

iv Fetoscopy for haemoglobinopathies and coagulation disorders (blood), for skin disorders, e.g. ichthyosis, epidermolysis bullosa (skin). Risk of fetal loss 5%.

3. *CVS and amniotic fetal cells for:*

i Chromosome identification and fetal sexing for X-linked disorders.
ii Enzymes for known enzyme deficiency.

iii   Gene identification

  a. Oligonucleotide DNA probes specific for the gene locus, e.g. in sickle cell and cystic fibrosis both the affected homozygote and carriers are accurately identified, i.e. 0% or 100%. Others include: thalassaemias α and β, HbS, some haemophilias.

  b. Cutting up DNA with enzyme scissors (restriction endonucleases) produce restriction fragment length polymorphisms (RFLPs) allows identification of:

   • a unique 'fingerprint' for that individual.
   • gene mapping – sites very close to the gene causing the disease, e.g. Huntington's chorea, α–1 antitrypsin, Duchenne muscular dystrophy. Only useful if the family is informative i.e. has an identifiable DNA pattern, and it needs at least one other member to be affected for comparison. As random cross linkage occurs 1 in 30 times by chance, the prediction is a 97% or 3% likelihood of having the gene, not 100% or 0%.

  c. The polymerase chain reaction enables a lot of DNA to be made available from just a few cells, e.g. amniotic fluid, buccal cells obtained by mouth rinse, to do a or b.

  d. Rubella virus by RNA specific DNA probe.

CVS preliminary results are available in 1–3 days, accurate result 7–10 days, amniotic cells 1–3 days for DNA studies but 2–3 weeks for chromosomes.

Further reading

Leader (1991) Imprinting makes an Impression *Lancet ii*, 413–414.
Royal College of Physicians (1989) Prenatal diagnosis and genetic screening, community and service implications. *Journal of the Royal College of Physicians of London*, **23**, 215-219.

SOME SELECTED CHROMOSOMAL ABNORMALITIES

Down's syndrome

Incidence

1 in 600 births, commonest chromosomal abnormality and single commonest cause of mental retardation.

Aetiology

1. 47 chromosomes: non-disjunction, occurs in 97% of cases, rising with maternal age to an incidence of >2% at 40 years. Recurrence risk 1%.
2. 46 chromosomes: translocation found in 2%, usually inherited from a carrier parent with balanced material from 46 chromosomes on 45 chromosomes. Recurrence risk for 14/21 type is 15% if maternal, 1% if paternal, for either parent with 21/21 it is 100%.
3. Chromosome mosaicism in 1%, may not be present in all tissues.

Clinical appearance

Characteristic facies and features are a combination which may occur in isolation in normal individuals but not so many altogether. Short stature, hypotonia, short hands, single palmar crease, sandle toe, typical facies.

Problems specific to Down's syndrome (also see Mental Handicap)

1. Mental handicap. Majority have IQ<50, a small number are at the lower end of the normal range and may be independent. Stimulation programmes, e.g. Portage scheme, provide welcome support but are sadly limited in improving outcome. Presenile dementia with Alzheimer-like brain appearance is of interest as both conditions are linked to chromosome 21 disorders.
2. Ethical problem of surgery for gut abnormalities and cardiac abnormalities. The needs of the child, and inability to predict future accomplishments, weigh in favour of intervention. Full discussion with the parents usually determines the correct approach.

    i Congenital heart abnormalities, mainly ostium primum, in 40%. Many are inoperable, with early pulmonary hypertensive changes and intractable heart failure.
    ii Duodenal atresia 10%, Hirschprung's disease 3%. Early identification of Down's syndrome allows informed discussion with the parents and surgeon.

3. Hypothyroidism of the autoimmune variety later in childhood.
4. Care problems:
    Infancy – hypotonia, poor feeding, chronic nasal discharge and respiratory infection due to defective WBC function.
    Childhood – persistent middle ear fluid. Behaviour problems develop. Training routines in feeding, dressing, washing, toileting help.
    Adolescence – atlantoaxial instability in 10%. Advise to report symptoms of neck pain, torticollis or limb weakness if taking part in sporting activities. A screening neck X-ray is indicated only in those engaging in trampolining, diving, or contact sports, according to the Chief Medical Officer of the DSS, and Mencap. Others recommend annual screening from 5 years old.
5. Parental rejection is independent of the timing of revelation of diagnosis. Guilt is often prominent, and may lead to refusal for permission to operate. Adoptive parents appear free of these stigmatized feelings.

Prognosis

Survival to 5 years in 90%. Death in infancy is from congenital heart disease, Hirschprung's disease and infection. Adult life expectancy: 50% reach 60 years old, compared with almost 90% of the general population. Residential care is ultimately likely for the majority as their parents become infirm through age.

Further reading

Leader (1987) Atlantoaxial Instability in Down's syndrome. *British Medical Journal*, **294**, 988–989.
Elliott S, Morton R E, Whitelaw R A J (1988) Atlantoaxial instability and abnormalities of the odontoid in Down's syndrome. *Archives of Disease in Childhood*, **63**, 1484–1489.

Trisomy 18

Incidence

1 in 3000 births. Sporadic in 90%, only 10% due to a parental translocation.

Clinical

Small for dates, microcephaly with prominent occiput, micrognathia, overlapping of index and little finger on middle and ring fingers, rocker bottom feet, dislocated hips. Short sternum. Spastic. Malformations of brain, heart. Apnoea is common, and often the immediate cause of death.

Prognosis

Mental retardation severe, 90% dead by 1 year.

Trisomy 13

Incidence

1 in 5000 births. Nondisjunction is usual, with <1% recurrence risk, but 5% have a parental translocation with a 10% risk of recurrence.

Clinical

Microcephaly, microphthalmia/colobomata, cleft lip +/− palate, polydactyly, exomphalos; brain, heart and external genitalia malformations.

Prognosis

Mental retardation severe, 90% dead by 1 year.

SEX CHROMOSOME ABNORMALITIES

X0, Turner's syndrome

Incidence

1 in 2500 girls, majority are 45 XO, others have an altered X chromosome structure or are mosaic 45X/46XX, rarely 45X/46XY. Finding normal 46XX chromosomes in the blood indicates mosaicism, and a need to look at the chromosome content of other tissues, or the individual has Noonan's syndrome.

Clinical

1. Morphology: puffy hands and feet at birth, lasts days to weeks; webbed neck (due to cystic hygroma of the neck in early fetal life); shield-shaped chest, increased carrying angle at elbow, pigmented naevi, short fourth metacarpal.
2. Growth in height is normal for 4 years, and falls away as the ovaries involute. Without treatment average adult height is 142 cm.
3. Malformations: 95% have ovarian dysgenesis, 50% are deaf (secretory otitis media), 40% renal (horseshoe), 20% heart (coarctation, aortic stenosis, bicuspid aortic valve).
4. Intelligence is low average, only 10% are mentally handicapped. Learning difficulties with maths and geography are common.

Treatment

1. Surgical treatment for cardiac lesions, grommets for ears, plastic surgery for neck webbing.
2. Height. Growth hormone from mid-childhood improves height prognosis. Some add oxandrelone. Early introduction of oestrogens is counterproductive.
3. Gradual introduction of tiny doses of ethinyloestradiol in early adolescence over 2–3 years building up to a cyclical oestrogen–progestogen regimen, develops secondary sexual characteristics and reduces osteoporosis.
4. If a Y chromosome is present remove the gonads as 50% are neoplastic by adult life.
5. Counsel the parents and later the girl on infertilty, but emphasize the potential for normal sexual relationships.

Further reading

Brook C G D (1986) Turner syndrome. *Archives of Disease in Childhood,* **61**, 305–309.

XXY, Klinefelter's syndrome

Incidence

1 in 1000 boys, and 1–2 per 10,000 are 46XY/47XXY mosaic.

Clinical

Long limbs, tall for the family, feminine shape to the body and body hair. Gynaecomastia in 30%.

Reduced verbal skills, normal performance IQ.

100% infertile, increased cryptorchidism, small penis, delayed puberty. Reduced libido.

Increased emotional immaturity, loneliness, and unemployment. Testosterone therapy is useful.

XYY

Incidence

1 in 1000 boys.

Clinical

Tall, more antisocial personalities than average as a group. Finding it on antenatal investigation is not, however, an indication for termination.

CHROMOSOMAL DELETIONS

Angelman's syndrome

Long arm chromosome 15 interstitial deletion (see genomic imprinting).

Clinical

Global developmental delay, ataxia, paroxysmal laughter (happy puppet), seizures, microcephaly.

Prognosis

Severe mental retardation, rarely learn to speak.

Cri du chat

Short arm chromosome 5 (5p-). Usually sporadic, occasionally due to a parental translocation with an associated high risk of recurrence.

Incidence

1 in 50 000

Clinical

Mewing cry as infants, in many.
Malformation of the brain, eyes (cataracts, optic atrophy), heart.

Prognosis

Mental retardation is severe. Survival to adult life is possible.

Retinoblastoma

Incidence

1 in 20 000

Deletion on the long arm of chromosome 13 in the tumour (sporadic) or all cells (familial). The gene locus is identifiable by RFLP, and 90% of families are informative.

1. Forty per cent are familial, bilateral, with early onset, i.e. by 18 months. Mental handicap is common.
2. Later onset in the sporadic form, average 2.5 years old, tumour is unilateral, intelligence normal.

The 'two hit' theory of causation:

Familial: −Inheritance of one retinoblastoma gene, it requires a relatively minor genetic/environmental insult to change one other gene (one hit).

Sporadic: −More insults needed to alter two genes (two hits).

Clinicopathology

Small round cells, multiple sites, grow forward into the vitreous or subretinal layers, causing retinal detachment. Both produce a *white pupillary reflex*, (exclude cataract, coloboma, retinopathy of prematurity, *Toxocara canis*, Coates disease), loss of vision and squint. May spread into the brain, → raised intracranial pressure.

Treatment

Irradiation to small tumours, otherwise enucleation. Unilateral disease usually requires the latter.

Prognosis

1. Early diagnosis, i.e. familial with previously affected individual: cure in 100%, avoiding eye removal.
   RFLPs identify infants at risk, otherwise screen all sibs 3-monthly for 2 years, then progressively less frequently to 10 years.
2. Normal presentation: survival 85−100%

Aniridia, retardation, high risk of wilms' tumour/gonadoblastoma (ARW syndrome)

Interstitial deletion on the short arm of chromosome 11

Clinical

Mental retardation, boys often have ambiguous genitalia.

Prognosis

Regular abdominal US for early diagnosis of malignancy determines survival.

Prader-Willi syndrome

Interstitial deletion on the long arm of chromosome 15 in 50%.

Clinical

1. Characteristic face, long silky hair, gracile limbs, small hands and feet, hypo-plastic genitalia (easier to diagnose in boys!).
2. Severe hypotonia from birth and feeding difficulties.
3. From 2–3 years appetite is pathological (temper tantrums +++), with gross obesity.
   - Mental retardation is mild to moderate.
   - Short stature, hypogonadotrophic hypogonadism.
   - Diabetes mellitus responsive to oral hypoglycaemic agents.

Treatment

Strict calorie control when appetite increases. Behaviour modification programme and locked cupboards help. Fenfluramine may have a short-term role. Administering growth hormone can be justified in some cases with short stature, mild retardation.

Fragile X syndrome

Incidence

Up to 1 in 1000 males; 30% of female carriers are also mentally slow. The gene locus has been identified by DNA studies. The 'fragile site', detected using folate deficient culture medium, at the end of the X chromosome is only a marker.

Clinical

1. Prepubertal lack of discriminating features: Larger head and taller than average, some ligamentous laxity.
2. From puberty onwards: large jaw, ears, prominent forehead, large testes.
   Mental retardation is moderate, some show autistic features.

Investigation

Worth doing chromosomes, requesting that fragile sites be looked for, in a retarded male or female of normal appearance and head size, even with a negative family history.
   Antenatal diagnosis by CVS and DNA probe is now possible in some centres.

Table 1.4 Some single gene diseases diagnosable by DNA probes. (By identifying the gene product, i.e the protein produced, it is a first step in understanding the biochemical basis, and hence potential reversal of its effects.)

Disease	Chromosome number
Autosomal dominant	
Adult polycystic disease	16
Huntingdon's disease	4
Myotonic dystrophy	19
Neurofibromatosis type 1 (Von Recklinghausen)	17
Neurofibromatosis type 2 (bilateral acoustic neuromas)	22
Osteogenesis imperfecta	7/17
Polyposis coli	5
Retinoblastoma	13
Autosomal recessive	
21 hydroxylase deficiency	6
Alpha-1-antitrypsin deficiency	14
β-thalassaemia	11
Cystic fibrosis	7
Gaucher's disease	1
Sickle cell anaemia	11
Tay-Sach disease	15
Wilson's disease	13
Sex linked recessive (X chromosome)	
Duchenne/Becker muscular dystrophy	
Fragile X syndrome	
Haemophilia A and B	
Hunter's syndrome	
Lesch-Nyhan syndrome	

SOME SELECTED SYNDROMES

Noonan's syndrome

AD with variable penetrance, i.e. other family members and generations may show minor features without the full blown syndrome.

Clinical

Turner-like physically. Congenital heart disease and mental retardation are common. Affects both sexes equally.

William's syndrome

Sporadic occurrence. A subgroup may have increased sensitivity to vitamin D.

Clinical

'Elfin' face (coarse lips, upturned nose), failure to thrive, hypertension, supravalvular stenosis, mental retardation.

Investigation

Hypercalcaemia found in 50% in the first 1–2 years. X-ray the orbits and metaphyses to detect increased calcification.

Treatment and prognosis

Lower serum calcium with low calcium containing milks. Omit vitamin D. Steroids occasionally help for their calciuric effect. Prevents renal damage, improves weight gain. Unfortunately the mental retardation is not altered.

Fetal alcohol syndrome (FAS)

Incidence

> 1 in 1000 births, up to 1% in Northern France. Severity is proportional to intake. Risk is 30–50% for a chronic alcoholic mother.

Clinical

Florid FAS after 8–10 or more units of alcohol per day. As little as 10 units a week in the first trimester will reduce birthweight. (1 unit = 1/2 pint of beer, a glass of sherry or wine, a measure of spirits).

1. Growth impaired, both pre- and postnatally.
2. Microcephalic. Mental retardation is mild to moderate. Clumsy, with tremor. Often hyperactive.
3. Face: short palpebral fissures and nose, and thin top lip. Hypertelorism.
4. Malformations: ventriculoseptal and atrioseptal defects, renal defects.

Prognosis

Stillbirths and malformation rate doubled even in moderate drinkers.

Russell-Silver syndrome

Sporadic, may be part of a spectrum of small for dates infants.

Clinical

1. Face is triangular with small chin, frontal bossing.
2. Growth: prenatal and postnatal impairment. Feeding difficulties are prominent. Fasting hypoglycaemia in infancy. Adult height 150 cm.
3. Asymmetry of body, limb size and length, variable in frequency.

Treatment

Response to growth hormone shows accelerated closure of epiphyses, thus preventing any long term gain.

SOME SELECTED NON-RANDOM ASSOCIATIONS: USUALLY SPORADIC

Goldenhar Association

Incidence

1 in 3000

Embryology

First and second branchial arch developmental defect due to insufficient migration of neural crest cells into the first and second branchial arches during the fourth week of fetal life.

Clinical

Facial asymmetry due to maxillary/mandibular hypoplasia; eye epibulbar dermoids; preauricular skin tags, external ear deformities with conductive hearing loss. Occasional mental retardation.
    Vertebral anomalies.

VATER/VACTERL

Mesoderm insult at 4–7 weeks gestation. Two or more of the following:

*V*ertebral defects, *a*nal atresia, *t*racheo*e*sophageal fistula, *r*adial aplasia and *r*enal abnormality. *C*ardiac and *l*imb abnormalities expand this to VACTERL.

Further reading

Green E D, Waterston R H (1991) The human genome project. Prospects and implications for clinical medicine. *Journal of the American Medical Association*, **266**, 1966–1975
Harper P (1988) *Practical Genetic Counselling*. Third edition London:Wright.

Standard references for illustrations of syndromes and their origins

Goodman R M, Gorlin R J (1983) *The Malformed Infant and Child*. New York:Oxford University Press.
Moore K L (1988) *The Developing Human. Clinically Oriented Embryology*, fourth ed. Philadelphia: Saunders.
Smith D W (1981) *Recognizable Patterns of Human Deformation*. Philadelphia:Saunders
Smith D W (1989) *Recognizable Patterns of Human Malformation*, fourth ed. Philadelphia:Saunders.

Chapter 2

Neonatology

Ninety to 95% of liveborn babies are healthy. Five to 10% are ill and/or low birth-weight and need special care. One per cent need intensive care.

DEFINITIONS

1. Growth and size for gestation

Three categories:

  i   Appropriate for gestational age (AGA).
  ii Small for gestational age (SGA) or small/light for dates. Variously defined as <10th centile or 2 standard deviations below the mean. Contains both normal small infants and growth retarded infants.
  iii Large for gestational age (LGA) or large for dates.

2. Low birthweight (LBW) babies

LBW = 2500 g or less at birth. Comprises both AGA and SGA infants; 7% of all births.
  Subdivided further into

  a. Very low birth weight (VLBW) = 1500 g or less, 1% of all births.
  b. Extremely low birth weight (ELBW) = 1000 g or less, 0.3% of all births.
  c. Previable = <500g or 22 weeks' gestation or less.

STILLBIRTH AND INFANT MORTALITY

Weight, maturity and survival

Weight is the single most important variable influencing survival. This is applied in birthweight specific perinatal mortality (Table 2.3). For example, the 7% of births under 2.5 kg comprise 65% of perinatal deaths, and the 1% less than 1.5 kg contribute 40%.

Mortality statistics, perinatal and infant

Table 2.1 Definitions and mortality rates for England and Wales, 1989

i   *Rate per thousand live and stillbirths*
  a   Stillbirth: born dead after 28 completed weeks of gestation 4.6
  b   Perinatal death: stillbirths and death in the first week of life (early NND) 8.2
ii   *Rate per thousand livebirths*
  a   Neonatal death (NND) and neonatal mortality rate (NMR) = within 28 days of delivery of a
      liveborn infant at any gestation 4.8
      Early NND = death in first 6 days of life 3.7
      Late NND = 7–27 completed days of life 1.1
  b   Infant mortality rate (IMR): Deaths under one year (includes NND) 8.4
  c   Post neonatal mortality rate (PNMR): Deaths in the first year after the neonatal period, i.e.
      PNMR=IMR–NMR 3.6

An increasing number of deaths are postponed from the early to the late NND period due to intensive care

Table 2.2 Trends in infant mortality, 1975-89 for England and Wales (rate per thousand)

Year	Stillbirth	Neonatal MR	Post NMR	Infant MR
1975	10.3	10.6	4.8	15.5
1980	7.3	7.6	4.3	11.9
1985	5.5	5.3	3.9	9.2
1989	4.7	4.8	3.6	8.4

Table 2.3 Birthweight specific perinatal
mortality rates for England and Wales 1987

<1500 g	322
1500–1999	87
2000–2499	22
2500–2999	6.5
3000–3499	2.6
>3500	2.1

Over the period 1983 to 1987 survival among those <1500 g improved by 30%, and
by 50% in those 500–999 g birthweight, despite an increase in proportion and absolute numbers.

Weight and gestation are each independently important in survival, particularly
in extreme prematurity (Table 2.4). (Example taken from McIntosh N (1988) Clinical issues. *The British Medical Bulletin*, **44**, 1119–1132.)

Table 2.4 Relation of weight, gestation and survival

Weight (g)	Gestation (weeks)	Survival (%)
<750	<26	13
750–1000	<26	47
<750	26 or more	33
750–1000	26 or more	65

Deferred deaths

Intensive care defers death in addition to preventing deaths from congenital abnormality, prematurity and its complications, and asphyxia. They account for most late neonatal deaths, and 30% of post neonatal deaths.

Causes of stillbirth and neonatal mortality, as rates per 1000 (England and Wales 1987).

In the UK approximately 0.5% of babies are stillborn and 0.5% liveborn die in the first month.

1 Stillbirth

   i Birth asphyxia 1.7 (intrapartum 0.8, maternal abruption 0.6, hypertension 0.3)
  ii Congenital malformation 0.4
 iii Unexplained 1.4

2 Livebirths

Over 50% of deaths occur in VLBW infants under 1.5 kg.

   i Congenital malformations 1.6
  ii Prematurity (90% <1.5 kg) 1.4
 iii Respiratory disorders (50% have respiratory distress syndrome) 1.2
 iv Asphyxia 0.3
  v Infection 0.3

Table 2.5 Relative contribution to PMR by gestation

	Preterm	*Term*	*Post-term*
Germinal layer haemorrhage (GLH)*	++++	-	-
Respiratory	+++ RDS*	+	meconium aspiration
Congenital malformations	++	+++	+
Asphyxia	++	+	+++
Sepsis	+	+	+

RDS = respiratory distress syndrome. Mortality of ventilated infants with RDS reduced from 80% in 1965 to 17% in 1983.
*GLH *plus* RDS is the final common pathway in most very sick prematures.

3 Multiple births

50% are 2.5kg at birth, compared with 6% of singletons. Relative risk compared with a singleton pregnancy: of stillbirth x 4, death in the first year x 5.

SIMPLIFIED CLASSIFICATION OF PERINATAL DEATHS, AND ITS APPLICATION TO PERINATAL ADULT

A logical subdivision of the major pathological findings at autopsy, linked to the clinical situation, enables interpretation of perinatal mortality data. (After Wiglesworth JS (1980) Monitoring perinatal mortality. A pathophysiological approach. *Lancet*, **ii**, 684–686.)

1. Normally formed macerated stillborn infants, i.e. intrauterine asphyxia, growth retardation.
2. Congenital malformations (stillborn or neonatal death).
3. Conditions associated with immaturity (neonatal death).
4. Asphyxial conditions developing in labour, e.g. acute asphyxia, trauma, infection (fresh stillbirth or neonatal death).
5. Other specific conditions (e.g. bacterial infection, fatal inborn errors.)

Audit using the classification

Enables identification of preventable versus inevitable losses, and an audit of effectiveness of obstetric intervention and neonatal care.

Further division by birthweight highlights possible inadequacies, e.g. excess of (i) >2500 g asphyxial deaths may be due to lack of monitoring equipment or expertise (ii) <2000 g deaths from immaturity due to lack of special/intensive care provision.

Factors to take into account in interpreting neonatal mortality statistics nationally and internationally.

1. Registration.

In the UK, a stillbirth less than 28 weeks may be classified as an abortion, and thus not registered, but a live birth must be registered, regardless of gestation. Figures may be distorted by local attitudes of the medical staff to labelling such infants. In future, delivery after 22 weeks may be used for international comparisons.

2. General factors

   i Maternal age (best between 20–29 years)
   ii Parity (best second or third baby)
  iii Social class (class I NMR is 60% of class V, despite 40 years of a health service equally available to all).
  iv Legitimacy. Among the illegitimate the NMR is higher by 20%.
   v Region. NMR is lowest in East Anglia, highest in Yorkshire.

These factors combined increase the risk substantially, e.g. a para 3 in Yorkshire has a PMR 50% higher than for each factor alone.

3. Genetic, cultural and environmental factors

   i Relatively high PMR and congenital malformation rate among the Pakistani community (2–3 times national average) in the UK may be related in part to first cousin marriage.

  ii Low birthweight rates are related to many factors. In some developing countries they comprise up to 50% of all births.

 iii Low PMR in Scandinavia is due in part to a lower incidence of malformations, especially neural tube defects (NTD), and low birthweight. In Sweden for example, the incidence of <2.5 kg infants was 4.2% in 1987, versus 7.9% in England and Wales.

  iv Environmental factors operate, e.g. rate of NTD is high in Ireland, but, in the same genetic population, lower in Americans of Irish descent in the USA (folate levels in the diet?).

4. Antenatal screening

For chromosomal, metabolic and structural defects resulting in the abortion of affected fetuses alters the PMR.

5. Comparisons

When making 'like with like' comparisons of the impact of neonatal care on PMR and neonatal mortality between units, it is permissible to exclude lethal malformations, and to stratify by birthweight.

POSTNEONATAL MORBIDITY AND MORTALITY

1. A relatively slow fall in PNMR compared with rates at other ages is due to:

   i Increased survival of VLBW infants, succumbing beyond the neonatal period. Examples:

    a. Due to bronchopulmonary dysplasia (BPD).

    b. Sudden infant death syndrome (SIDS) is inversely related to birth weight. Per 1000 births: term = 2, preterm = 9, VLBW = 10, VLBW and ventilated = 15

  ii Congenital malformations, especially cardiac, due to palliation prolonging survival beyond the neonatal period (Table 2.6).

    Additional factors: maternal age, parity, social class, place of birth, infant's place of birth, birthweight and legitimacy, as in NMR. Seasonal variation is important, with SIDS more common in the winter.

Prevention

Improved care in cold weather (avoid overheating? see SIDS), breast feeding, reduce parental smoking; increased vigilance during illness, for example using the Baby Check system to identify serious illness.

Table 2.6 Causes of post-neonatal mortality (rate per 1000)

Sudden infant death syndrome 1.4
Congenital anomalies 0.8
Conditions originating in the perinatal period (e.g. BPD, hydrocephalus, infection) 0.2
Accidental death 0.2

2. Morbidity
   i Increased hospitalization among the VLBW for wheeze and respiratory infection.
   ii Among ELBW (<1000 g) multiple handicaps are often suffered:

   Cerebral palsy 15%.
   Mental handicap, hydrocephalus, epilepsy 13%.
   Sensorineural deafness 4%.
   Visual defect 10%, blind 3%.
   Bronchopulmonary dysplasia 10–20%.
   School learning difficulties, hyperactivity 20 - 30%.

   iii Of all VLBW (<1500 g) 5–10% are disabled, but they represent only 3% of all moderately and severely handicapped whose aetiology is 75% congenital, 5% birth asphyxia, 2% other perinatal causes, 17% unidentified

COST–BENEFIT OF NEONATAL CARE

Measuring outcomes by morbidity and mortality are indicators of the effectiveness of the services and the resources allocated. The perinatal mortality rate (PMR) has shown a continuous reduction, despite a 30% increase in the numbers of <1.5 kg very low birthweight (VLBW) infants since 1980. Delivery in a hospital with level III (highest grade) intensive care significantly improves survival and quality of outcome in those less than 28 weeks gestation.

Cost

1. Survival of VLBW handicapped infants who would otherwise have died, a potentially intolerable burden to their family.
2. Chronic disorders requiring prolonged/multiple hospital admissions, and community support.
3. Financial drain on resources. Inverse relationship between birth weight of survivor and cost of treatment.

Controversy: an example of how to halt this trend, by the introduction of artificial surfactant treatment, reducing complications and duration of intensive care reduces costs.

Benefit

1. Lowered risks for the majority due to improvement in care.
2. Despite requiring expensive resources (technology, medical, nursing, laboratory services) as neonates, the return to society in productive years of life gained is high.

Table 2.7 Common obstetric problems, and intervention strategies important to paediatrics

Situation (gestation in weeks)	Management
Premature labour 26–34 weeks	1. Tocolytic: ritodrine (not given if hypertensive or bleeding). 2. Corticosteroids accelerate lung maturation: give for 48 h, repeated weekly to 33 weeks (omitted if infection present)
Premature rupture of membranes less than 34 weeks	1. Buy time with tocolytics, as prematurity is more serious than potential infection. Give antibiotics and deliver if an offensive vaginal discharge or maternal pyrexia develops. 2. After 34 weeks expedite delivery
Preterm breech less than 32 weeks	Caesarian section minimizes asphyxia and trauma, with no increase in respiratory distress syndrome
Intrauterine growth retardation from 28 weeks	Caesarian section, as above, if evidence of progressive growth failure +/- fetal distress
Prolonged pregnancy beyond 42 weeks	Consider induction to avoid dangers of stillbirth, dystocia, postmaturity, meconium aspiration

Further reading

Cole T J, Gilbert R E, Fleming P J, Morley C J *et al* (1991) Baby check and the Avon infant mortality study. *Archives of Disease in Childhood*, **66**,1077–1078.
Macfarlane A (1988) The ups and downs of infant mortality. *British Medical Journal*, **296**, 230–231.

CHANGES AT BIRTH

Physiological changes, needs at birth, and complicating pathological processes

1. Temperature control

Aim

To maintain normal body temperature at least energy cost. Neutral thermal environment is the temperature surrounding the baby that achieves this goal. Higher or lower temperatures result in more energy expenditure. The smaller and less mature, the greater the heat provided needs to be.

Result of impaired control

1. Hypothermia: increases morbidity and mortality. Effects include reduced surfactant production → hypoxaemia → grunting. Increasing acidosis, consumption of oxygen and calories → hypoglycaemia, eventually to sclerema and even death.

    During resuscitation a wet newborn's temperature can fall 0.25°C per minute unless dried, swaddled, and placed in a warm environment.
2. Overheating: hyperosmolality, weight loss, more jaundiced, recurrent apnoea/cot death.

Cold stress response

Is dependent on:

1. Ability to adopt flexed position reducing surface heat loss.
2. Subcutaneous fat insulation.
3. Thermogenesis from brown fat laid down towards term.

All are reduced in the preterm, low birthweight infant.

Heat conservation

1. In the sick/premature losses occur from:

    i   Radiant heat: loss reduced by plastic tunnel/shield sealed at one end, bubble foam sheet.
    ii Convection: loss by convective air incubators, radiant warmers.
    iii Conduction: reduced by insulated or heated mattresses.
    iv Evaporative loss through the premature's skin. Applying oil can reduce this.
        Servocontrolled incubators may mask fluctuations in temperature due to sepsis or cerebral abnormality.

2. Term infants: effective heat conservation with appropriate number of layers of clothing and blankets in a draught-proof cot.

2. Oxygenation and gas exchange

i Fetal:

Brain and myocardium preferentially receive the most oxygenated blood. Gas exchange is dependent on:

a. An intact placenta.
b. Carriage of sufficient oxygen by high haemoglobin mass (16 - 20 g/dl).
c. The ability of fetal haemoglobin to be 95% saturated at half the tension needed by adult haemoglobin (6 kPa versus 12 kPa).
d. The Bohr effect of raising pH by exchange of CO_2 across the placenta increases transfer of oxygen from mother's circulation into the fetus.

ii Respiration and the first breaths

Stimulus to breathing: hypoxia, rise in P_aCO_2, fall in blood pH, and cooling of the facial trigeminal area are each potent stimulants of respiration.

Initiation: inspiratory effort generates negative pressures of 10–30 cm, sometimes up to 30–60 cm H_2O. Functional residual capacity (FRC) is achieved within 30 minutes.

Lung fluid in the fetus equals FRC (25–30 ml/kg). Some fluid is expressed by the chest squeeze during vaginal delivery. The majority is absorbed equally via lymphatics and across pulmonary capillary membranes in the first 24–48 h.

3. Circulatory changes at birth

The fetal circulation

i   Placenta holds the same amount of blood as is in the fetus.
ii Oxygenated blood returns to the fetus via the umbilical vein.
iii Half passes directly to the inferior vena cava via the ductus venosus, the other half passes through the liver first.
iv In the right atrium the septum secundum diverts a third of the flow into the left atrium, ensuring the coronaries and the brain of the highest possible P_aO_2.
v   The oxygenated two-thirds from the inferior vena cava is joined by desaturated blood draining from the superior vena cava into the right heart. This is ejected into the pulmonary artery, but most of that is diverted down the patent ductus arteriosus into the descending aorta. Only 10% of the cardiac output reaches the lungs.

From fetal to adult circulation

i   The baby breathes: this increases pulmonary blood flow fivefold. Aeration of lungs causes P_aO_2 to rise, P_aCO_2 to fall, and pulmonary vascular resistance (PVR) to fall, rapidly at first, tailing off over 4 or more weeks. Pulmonary BP drops from 100% to 10% of systemic.
ii Clamping the cord: results in a fall in inferior vena cava flow, rise in systemic vascular resistance.
iii Separation of right and left heart by closure of foramen ovale. Mechanism is due to a rise in left atrial pressure as a consequence of:

increased return of (oxygenated) blood from the lung.
reduced pressure from inferior vena cava as the umbilical vein is occluded.

iv Rise in P_aO_2: **Ductus arteriosus closure**. The ductus is 5–10 mm in diameter, with a thick intima with spirals of smooth muscle. The muscle contracts and the lumen occludes in 10–15 h. The intima is obliterated by fibrous tissue in 2–4 weeks but can be re-opened within this period by hypoxia or fluid overload, i.e. patent ductus arteriosus (PDA).

Physiology

a. Prostaglandin (PG) E_1 relaxes the smooth muscle to maintain patency.
b. PGF_{2a} and oxygen encourage closure.
Sensitivity to oxygen increases with gestation.

Pharmacological manipulation of the ductus arteriosus

a. To facilitate closure of the ductus in prematures, (up to 50% <1500 g have PDA, mainly related to hypoxia during RDS). Induced by the prostaglandin inhibitor indomethacin.
b. To prevent closure. Where closure may result in severe hypoxaemia and death. Prostaglandin E i.v./orally permits the ductus to shunt between right and left heart when required, e.g. transposition of the great vessels, pulmonary or aortic atresia/severe stenosis, coarctation of the aorta.

v Ventricular wall thickness
Equal at birth, the adult ratio is achieved by 6 months. Thickness is proportional to the work done.

Circulatory pathophysiology of hypoxia

Hypoxia induces a return to the fetal circulation. A vicious cycle may operate, with several entry points, applicable in asphyxia, respiratory distress syndrome, meconium aspiration, and congenital heart disease.

i Hypoxia, hypercapnia or acidosis individually or jointly result in severe pulmonary vasoconstriction, inducing pulmonary hypertension and fetal pattern of flow across the foramen ovale (right to left).
When a large communication exists between right (R) and left (L) heart the PVR falls more slowly than usual. (Cardiac failure from L to R shunts therefore usually occurs after the neonatal period).
ii Ductus arteriosus reopens due to hypoxia, shunting blood away from the lungs.
iii Surfactant production is impaired, causing alveolar collapse, further hypoxaemia and acidosis and reinforcing the cycle.

4. Energy requirements

These comprise minimal expenditure plus needs for growth (the infant gains 10–25 g per day). Additional requirements exist in the small for dates or any infant stressed through illness, hyperpyrexia, cardiac failure etc (Table 2.8).

Table 2.8 To calculate needs in kcal/kg/day (1 kcal = 4.2 J)

1. Minimum expenditure	60 kcal (covers BMR, specific dynamic action of food, activity, stool losses)
2. Needs for growth = 4 kcal/g wt gained Therefore:	40 kcal for 10g/kg/day
3. Total requirements in health	100–120 kcal/kg/day
4. In the small for dates/stressed infant(higher BMR, extra needs for catch-up growth)	120–140 kcal/kg/day

Need for glucose is 4–6 mg/kg/min. Greater than 8 mg/kg/min is pathological.

Energy stored in the term infant as liver glycogen is sufficient for 6–10 h basal activity. Lipolysis from adequate fat stores, present in the appropriately grown more mature (Table 2.9), or provision of calories is an essential early requirement.

Newborn infants are capable of using ketone bodies as energy substrate for the brain, i.e. they have a major glucose-sparing effect.

Table 2.9 Body composition changes with gestation

Gestation (weeks)	Weight (g)	Water (%)	Fat (%)	Protein(%)	Energy (kcal)
24	700	90	0.1	9.0	300
28	1100	85	3.0	9.5	500
34	2200	80	7.5	11.0	2500
40	3300	75	11.0	12.0	5000

5. Blood volume and blood pressure (BP)

Blood volume 90 ml/kg at birth, reduces to 80/kg in first days.
BP:

i Fetal mean 30–40 mmHg	One week after birth
ii Prematures 30–50 mmHg	60–80 mmHg
iii Term 50–70 mmHg	independent of gestation

6. Excretion

i Urine

Newborns have a low glomerular filtration rate, proportional to gestational age and postnatal age, e.g. in ml/min/m^2, 5 ml at 28 weeks, 12 ml at 40 weeks, increasing to 25 ml from birth to 2 weeks old.

Production less than 0.5 ml/kg/h gives rise to dehydration or renal failure.

Sodium less conserved in the VLBW and needs supplementation.

Concentrating ability less than half that of the adult kidney, and less able to acidify urine, i.e. more vulnerable to destabilizing by metabolic acidosis.

ii Meconium

Consists mainly of bile pigment. Passed within 24 h in 95% of infants. Delay may be due to organic obstruction, prematurity, opiates, Hirschsprung's disease, cystic fibrosis or meconium plug, and always needs careful assessment.

iii Skin

Weight loss in the first few days is largely due to water loss by evaporation, increased 2-fold by radiant heater. Method of warming must be taken into account when assessing daily fluid requirements.

EXAMINING THE NEWBORN 'TOP TO TOE'

Aim

1. To detect congenital abnormalities.
2. Assess the transition to effective normal respiration, the effects of delivery and gestation (after gestational age assessment) on the infant.
3. Identify the presence of disease or infection.

General observations

Is growth appropriate for gestation? If SFD: congenital infection, malformation, chromosome defect? If LFD: infant of diabetic mother, Beckwith syndrome?

Scrutinize the face and body for asymmetry, midline abnormalities, and characteristic facies, e.g. Down's, Apert's, syndromes.

Colour

1. Pallor in asphyxia, anaemia, shock, infection.
2. Cyanosis: central, traumatic or peripheral.
3. Jaundice: >100 μmol/l is clinically identifiable.
4. Red: polycythaemia, may become cyanosed on crying.

Head and neck

1. Scalp/skull

   i Mis-shapen

      a. Caput (from birth, boggy, crossing suture lines) or
      b. Cephalhaematoma (after 24 h, limited by sutures).
      c. Moulding or craniostenosis. If persistent, and an X-ray confirms premature fusion of suture(s) early referral to a neurosurgeon is indicated.

   ii Anterior fontanelle:

      a. Bulging. Cerebral oedema, raised CSF pressure, crying.
      b. Overriding sutures from compression, dehydration, or failure of brain growth.

   iii Measure head circumference 1 cm above the nasal bridge, from the third day to allow for effects of moulding to disappear.

2. Choanal atresia

   i Bilateral. Inability to adapt to mouth breathing may result in sudden death or respiratory distress with cyanosis relieved by crying, from birth. Patency checked by occluding each nostril with mouth closed, or passing a nasogastric tube with a radiopaque line. If hold-up occurs insert an oral airway and then X-ray.

ii Unilateral. Later onset of symptoms with a persistent unilateral purulent discharge.

3. Eyes

For discharge, size (two-thirds adult at term, appears larger in buphthalmos), colobomas, and lens opacity. Sclera usually bluish. Ophthalmoscopy for cataracts: +3 lens at 10 cm. Sitting baby up encourages eyes to open.

4. Mouth

Common normal variations: epithelial cells (Epstein's pearls) on the palate or gum margins; 'tongue tie' = short frenulum, which does *not* require a surgical 'snip'. Bluish retention cysts (ranulae) on the floor of the mouth and mucocele of the salivary duct resolve spontaneously.

i   Clefts of the lip/palate. May be lip/alveolar notch only, cleft palate associated with lip pits (Van der Woude syndrome AD) or micrognathia (Robin sequence).
    Bifid uvula +/- submucous cleft may be missed unless torch and spatula are used.
ii Micrognathia, with posteriorly placed tongue → cleft palate = Robin sequence: feeding and airway difficulties.
iii Macroglossia: local haemangioma, or syndrome, e.g. Beckwith's syndrome (macrosomia, exomphalos, hypoglycaemia) and Pompe's disease. Large tongue from hypothyroidism or mucopolysaccharidosis appears later.
iv Neonatal teeth: remove, as invariably they loosen, may interfere with feeding and be aspirated.
v   Excessive salivation: oesophageal atresia. Nurse and transport head up, using a double lumen tube to aspirate the proximal pouch.

5. Ears

Check shape, size, position, and presence of the external canal.
Low set = top of helix below a horizontal line drawn from the outer canthus of the eye; seen in renal abnormalities, Potter's syndrome.
'Simple' in Down's syndrome.
Preauricular sinuses and skin tags are common. Occasionally associated with first branchial arch malformations.

6. Neck

i   Midline: thyroid swelling, sinuses or thyroglossal cyst.
ii Anterior triangle: sinus/cyst near anterior border of sternomastoid is a branchial cleft malformation.
iii Sternomastoid 'tumour' in that muscle's lower third after the first week.

iv Cystic hygroma transilluminates. Early surgery indicated if increasing in size and involving airway. Non malignant; total excision is the aim, but not at the expense of vital structures.

v Webbing in Turner's syndrome. Short, with reduced mobility, in Klippel-Feil syndrome (fused cervical vertebrae).

vi Feel for fractures of the clavicles; if the arm is weak a nerve injury may also be present.

Upper limbs

For symmetry of length, normal shape and number of digits. Accessory digits: often symmetrical, familial, and common in Africans. Consider Ellis van Crefeld syndrome or trisomy 13. Tie off if a narrow pedicle, otherwise refer to the plastic surgeon.

Chest

i Respiratory effort (including flaring, neck extension, sternal recession, abdominal see-saw motion), rate, and symmetry of chest movement.

Asymmetry is an emergency until proven otherwise: pneumothorax, lung collapse or compression by diaphragmatic hernia or lobar emphysema.

In diaphragmatic hernia, delay transfer to a surgical unit until stable, and electively ventilate; mortality has consequently been reduced from 50% at 6 h to 7% at 24 h. Such cases are still prone to persistent pulmonary hypertension postoperatively, when tolazoline, prostacyclin, and in the last resort ECMO (extra corporeal membrane oxygenation) are effective.

Auscultation: bronchial breath sounds are normal. Fine crackles (crepitations) after the first few hours are not.

ii Cardiovascular system: pulses, (using the right radial as reference to detect coarctation of the aorta), rate, volume.

Heart: apex beat is usually in the 4th intercostal space in the midclavicular line. Murmurs in the first 24 h need to be reviewed, but are rarely abnormal. Persistence of a loud murmur should be investigated.

Severe heart disease may be present without a murmur.

Abdomen

1. Observation

i Peristaltic waves may be normal in thin prematures, otherwise it is a sign of obstruction.

Scaphoid abdomen = diaphragmatic hernia.

ii Hernial orifices best examined while crying.

  iii Umbilicus: 2 vessels found in 1% of newborn. Only investigate low birth-weight, or malformed, infants for abnormality of kidneys.

  iv Exomphalos, gastroschisis: place the baby in a sterile plastic bag, or cover the intestines and membranes with cling film or place them in a surgical glove. This protects, reduces water loss, and avoids hypothermia induced by applying wet saline swabs. Urgent surgical referral.

  v Distension due to organomegaly/ascites/obstruction or flatus.

2. Palpation

Masses are usually renal: 80% due to hydronephrosis or multicystic kidney. The remaining 20%: posterior urethral valves, polycystic kidney, renal vein thrombosis, pelvic kidney, adrenal haemorrhage, hydrocolpos, and solid tumours (neuroblastoma is commonest), ovary, teratoma, kidney, liver.

  i Kidneys are palpated by flexing the legs and gently squeezing between the fingers, at the back, and thumb locating the kidney from in front.

  ii Liver is normally 2–3 cm below the right costal margin. If lower consider cardiac failure, hydrops etc, or pressure from above, e.g. tension pneumothorax, subcapsular haematoma, or haemangioma.

  iii Spleen is tipable in up to 30% of normal infants. Enlarged by infection, rhesus isoimmunization, and hepatic causes.

3. Auscultation

For bowel sounds: ileus is common in infants sick from any cause, but always consider necrotizing enterocolitis, meconium ileus, intestinal duplication, volvulus, Hirschprung's disease.

Anus

Position, patency and tone ('winking' on stroking). Passage of meconium occurs within 24 h in 95% of infants. Delay is considered in gastroenterological problems.

Genitals

Ambiguity, chordee, hypospadius. Hydroceles are common, but failure to resolve by a year is an indication for surgical referral.

Lower limbs

Length, shape, postural/fixed talipes, hips (for examination see Orthopaedics).

    Talipes: failure to correct on tickling, or to overcorrect by passive movement is an indication for early orthopaedic referral. Similarly for metatarsus varus, which usually corrects spontaneously.

Back

Mongolian blue spot is normal in dark-skinned races, and up to 10% of Caucasians.

1. Spinal deformity, spina bifida/overlying marker, e.g. hairy patch, lipoma. Sacral dimple is usually blind ended.
2. Sacrococcygeal teratoma, a mass immediately posterior to the anus: 4% are malignant at birth, becoming 25% by 2 years, i.e. early surgical referral is indicated.

Neurology examination

Factors affecting observations include alertness, timing after the feed, intercurrent illness, and medication. Often carried out as the general examination progresses.

Behaviours to watch

Lethargy, hypotonia: due to prematurity, drugs, asphyxia, sepsis, shock, intracranial bleed, RDS, post-ictal, inborn errors, or a neurological condition, e.g. Prader-Willi syndrome.

Irritability, hypertonia: hunger, asphyxia, drug withdrawal, kernicterus.

Abnormal movements, apnoea: caused by asphyxia/birth injury, sepsis, hypoglycaemia, hypocalcaemia. (Seizures often also involve abnormal eye movements, with sucking activity).

Look for asymmetry due to (often transient) hemiplegia after asphyxia/birth injury.

Cranial nerve examination

Not a routine, but as clinically indicated.

II Sight: turns to diffuse light, or fixing on a red ball held 10 cm away.
III, IV, VI Occular muscles: ptosis, pupillary constriction to light (III), doll's eye reflex (III, VI).

Persistent squint is always abnormal.
V Facial sensation: rooting reflex, cardinal points, blink to puff of air.
VII Facial movement: grimace/cry, affected side fails to move and eyelid to close fully.
VIII Hearing: quiets to voice/rattle, startle to clap.
X Gag reflex.
XI Head turns in direction of travel on examiner rotating on his own axis, baby held horizontal.
XII Tongue: stripping action on examiner's finger introduced into the mouth.

Tone and power in term infant as indicators of hypotonia and weakness

(See Behaviours to watch.)

Pull to sit = palmar grasp, with active flexion of arms and neck. Marked head lag is abnormal.

Sitting, chin rises from chest. Failure to do so or snapping backwards is abnomal.

Prone, supported under abdomen, the head and neck in line horizontally, hips and knees gently flexed. Infant 'draped over hand' posture is abnormal.

Primitive reflexes as aids to diagnosis

Moro: absence in hypoxia or depressed consciousness, asymmetric in hemiplegia, absent response in arm(s) in brachial plexus lesions.

Asymmetric tonic neck reflex: obligatory response is abnormal at any age, and due to cerebral injury or raised intracranial pressure.

Commoner focal weaknesses due to nerve injury

1. Facial (labour/forceps compression): differentiate from absence of the depressor muscle of the angle of the mouth associated with congenital heart disease.
2. 'Waiter's tip' posture: Erb's C5, 6 +/- C4. Associated with cyanosis, and laboured respirations in phrenic nerve involvement, diaphragmatic paralysis confirmed on fluoroscopy.
3. 'Claw hand': Klumpke's C7, 8, T1 +/- Horner's syndrome, which is associated with subsequent failure of iris pigmentation.

Prognosis: most Erb's resolve within days to weeks, a few within 3 months. Longer implies neurotmesis/axonotmesis, needing neuroplasty or muscle tendon transfers later. Klumpke's is less common and more likely to persist.

Gestational age assessment and its accuracy

1. Antenatal

   i Maternal dates, from last menstrual period: accurate in the 60% with regular cycles and certain dates.

  ii Bimanual palpation and quickening from 16 weeks for multiparous, 17 weeks for nulliparous: to within 2 weeks.

 iii US crown rump length between 7 and 14 weeks, biparietal diameter 14–24 weeks: to within one week.

2. Postnatal

Affected by depression or excitation of the infant's brain, and the effects of intrauterine growth retardation causing flaking, wrinkled skin, reduced ear cartilage and breast tissue, loss of subcutaneous fat, and poor growth of the external genitalia.

   i Physical characteristics of skin, ear lobe and breast size (Parkin J M, Hey E N, Clowes J S (1976) Rapid assessment of gestational age at birth. *Archives of Disease in Childhood*, **51**, 259–263.)

  ii Combination of neurological and physical state as a score (Dubowitz L, Dubowitz V, Goldberg C (1970) Clinical assessment of gestational age in the newborn infant. *Journal of Paediatrics*, **77**, 1-10). This is the most widely used system. Accurate to within 14 days in 95% when used between days 1–7 of life in babies >1.5 kg. Overestimation by 2 weeks is common below this weight (Sanders *et al.* (1991) Gestational age assessment in preterm neonates weighing less than 1500 grams, *Pediatrics*, **88**, 542-545).

Twins

Incidence

1 in 80: the monozygous (MZ) rate is constant world wide, 1 in 200, due to the splitting of a single egg in the first 14 days. Dizygous (DZ) is variable, familial, and expressed only in mother, the result of multiple ovulation, and commoner in Africans.

Placentation

1. Single vs separate placenta? As 30% of MZ have separate placentae, and DZ may have a fused dichorionic placenta, this is not a reliable guide.
2. Monochorionic placenta: only found in MZ. In practice it is often difficult to determine the absence of chorion between the two amniotic sacks after delivery.

Zygosity

Determined by
   i placentation
  ii sex, facial features, hair colour
 iii blood groups, up to 15 required for 95% confidence
 iv DNA fingerprinting or HLA typing in transplantation/genetic disease investigation.

Problems

1. Mortality increased, × 9 MZ, × 3 DZ.
2. Prematurity and respiratory distress syndrome, especially second twin. Infection commoner in first twin, presumed due to ruptured membranes.
3. Common in MZ twins:

   i At birth: malformations (also increased concordance, e.g. for cleft lip and congenital heart disease), low birthweight, large disparity in birth weight, feto-fetal transfusion via artery to vein anastomosis (recipient polycythaemic, hypertensive, heavier).

   ii Later illness: high concordance (50% or more) for epilepsy, diabetes, asthma, acute lymphatic leukaemia under 5 years. (DZ twins' risks are as for any other sibling.)

4. Infectious fevers 90% concordance for twins, MZ and DZ.
5. Parental factors. Death of a twin induces the same intensity of grief reaction as for a singleton. Increased risk of stress related child abuse.

ASPHYXIA

1. Intrauterine hypoxia is manifest by abnormal fetal heart patterns, fresh meconium, and reduced fetal movements. It may be acute, chronic (small for dates/growth failure), or acute on chronic. Blood gases show hypoxaemia, low pH with metabolic acidosis, and at times, hypercapnia.
2. Intrapartum asphyxia may be:

   i   Acute.
   ii Acute on chronic due to placental insufficiency.
   iii Prolonged, during labour, due to oxytocin infusion or cord compression.

Incidence

1–2% of newborns require active resuscitation.

Causes of asphyxia

Maternal, fetal or placental.
   Majority (70%) are due to prematurity or asphyxia (acute, acute on chronic, and chronic).

1. Maternal factors: sedation, hypertension (pregnancy induced, chronic), eclampsia, acute hypotension (bleed, epidural), maternal disease or diabetes, age <19, >35 years.
2. Fetal: obstruction (malpresentation, cephalopelvic disproportion), multiple birth, premature, postmature, growth retarded, hydrops.
3. Placental: abruption, placenta praevia, cord prolapse, bleed into mother or other twin.

Evaluation

Descriptive assessment is the most valuable, but the Apgar score has the merit of universality and is a guide to the need for and response to resuscitation (Table 2.10).

Taken at 1 and 5 minutes. If the score is <5, repeat at 5 minute intervals until greater than 5, or 30 minutes has elapsed.

Table 2.10 Apgar score

Item	0 points	1 point	2 points
Appearance	White	Blue	Pink
Pulse	Absent	<100/min	>100/min
Grimace on suction	No response	Grimace	Cough/sneeze
Activity	None	Spontaneous flexion	Active
Respiratory effort	None	Irregular gasps	Regular, crying

Resuscitation

Planned (i.e. standing by in the delivery room), if possible. Indications for being called to attend before delivery has occurred:

1. Fresh meconium seen.
2. High risk of asphyxiated delivery.
3. Acute blood loss suspected.

1. Meconium aspiration

Efforts are directed at prevention, although aspiration prior to delivery occurs in some cases.

i Suck out nose and oropharynx as the head is delivered.
ii Some advise to clamp the chest as it is delivered, to help prevent aspiration, though this may already have taken place in utero. Take the infant to the resuscitair.
iii Direct laryngoscopy now if not already performed on the bed as the head was delivered. If meconium is below the cords, intubate with the largest endotracheal (ET) tube possible, aspirate directly via the tube or largest catheter possible.
iv Reintubate if the tube becomes blocked by meconium, and continue to aspirate until clear. Have several ET tubes ready.
v If condition deteriorates, e.g. heart rate falls below 60/minute, start IPPV with 100% oxygen. Aspirate the stomach to prevent inhalation of swallowed meconium.

2. Asphyxia

Initial action according to score at 1 minute:

If respirations are shallow, irregular or absent: dry the skin, place under a radiant heater, apply suction to the mouth and nose.

Then proceed:

Apgar score (+ frequency)	Action
0 (0.1%)	Intubate, ventilate, cardiac massage, drugs. First mechanical inspiration held for 3–5s to improve lung inflation. 30–40 respirations/min at pressures up to 30 cm H_2O. (Occasionally higher pressures are needed in large infants. Higher respiratory rates may be useful in severe asphyxia, resulting in a more rapid fall in CO_2 and consequent rise in pH.)
1 (0.2%)	Intubate, ventilate, massage if heart beat <60/min.
2–3 (0.5%)	Oropharyngeal suction and ventilation by bag and mask with effective seal on baby's face.
4–6 (5%)	Oxygen by funnel, tactile stimulation.

Heart rate, respiratory effort and colour are the best indicators of the need for resuscitation. Tone and reflex irritability are a function of gestation.

Maintain temperature during and after resuscitation. Resuscitate under radiant heater, then dry off, wrap in towel (silver swaddler may be ineffective if hypothermic).

Drugs for resuscitation

   i Arrest: via umbilical venous catheter give 10% glucose 10 ml/kg, 10% calcium gluconate 1 ml/kg. Repeat after 4 minutes and give adrenaline 0.5 ml of 1/1000 i.v./via endotracheal tube. Intracardiac drugs are rarely justified.

  ii Sodium bicarbonate (3 ml/kg for failure to establish spontaneous respiration by 5 minutes) administration is contentious. Experimental evidence shows it worsens intracellular acidosis, and efforts should be directed at improving cardiac output.

 iii Glucose if hypoglycaemic, tested for early in resuscitation. Glucose is not given 'blind', unless in an arrest, as hyperglycaemia is associated with a worsening of acidosis, a hyperosmolar state leading to germinal layer haemorrhage and possible death.

 iv Hypovolaemia/pallor an indication for plasma or O negative blood 10–30 ml/kg.

  v Naloxone 0.1mg/kg i.v./i.m. (recommended dose has been increased) to counter maternal analgesia. Contraindicated in maternal drug addiction.

 vi Vitamin K is given in all cases, if unable to take orally i.m.

3. *Acute blood loss, shock*

Signs: persistent pallor, tachycardia, poor pulse volume, (low mean blood pressure <40 mmHg) despite adequate ventilation.

Insert umbilical venous catheter, take blood for Hb, PCV, group, cross match, pH and blood gases.

i   Transfuse 15 ml/kg of the freshest immediately available O rhesus negative blood if clinically imperative or if the haematocrit is <40%. Do a partial exchange if <25%.
ii 20 ml over 3 mins, the rest as clinically indicated.
iii Further plasma expander as required.

(Resuscitation advice adapted from Royal College of Obstetricians and Gynaecologists (1990) *Resuscitation of the Newborn* Part 1 and 2).

Persistent failure to establish respiration

Consider:

1. Central.

i   Maternal analgesia or sedation.
ii Asphyxia, birth injury.
iii Prematurity.

2. Respiratory

i   Laryngeal: spasm from suction catheter.
ii Lung: pneumothorax, meconium aspiration.
iii Congenital: hypoplastic lung in Potter's syndrome, displaced/hypoplastic lung in diaphragmatic hernia.

3. Circulatory failure due to acute blood loss: revealed/concealed into mother, fetal tissues, or twin.
4. Hypoglycaemia and acidosis.

Duration of resuscitation and prognosis

Continue for 30 minutes before abandoning the attempt, as 80% of survivors are normal (Table 2.11).

Table 2.11 Prognosis (US Collaborative Perinatal Project)

Apgar score	Age in minutes	Handicapped (%)	Mortality (%)
0–3	1	2	18
	5	5	44
	>10	20	80
4–6	1	<1	4

Prognosis is independent of gestational age.

Effects of asphyxia

1. Hypotension   → Myocardial damage, cardiac failure.
   - → Renal failure, reduced urinary flow.
   - → Hepatic damage, hyperammonaemia.
   - → Consumption coagulopathy.
2. Hypoxia and reduced cerebral blood flow → watershed infarcts, germinal layer haemorrhages = hypoxic-ischaemic encephalopathy (HIE). Reduction in brain high energy phosphates and accumulation of lactate occurs.

Hypoxic-ischaemic encephalopathy (Table 2.12)

Pathophysiology

   i Watershed zone infarction = ischaemia. Typically found following hypotension. Cerebral blood flow (CBF) is normally held constant by autoregulation in term infants. A fall in CBF → infarction at the 'watershed' or boundary zones between the major arteries in cortex and periventricular white matter. Result: cortex and subcortex necrosis → cysts and periventricular leucomalacia (PVL).
  ii Germinal matrix haemorrhage (GMH) → intraventricular haemorrhage (IVH). In prematures especially, the germinal matrix's periventricular capillary bed is poorly supported by glia, is unable to autoregulate the blood flow and therefore 'pressure passive'. Haemorrhage follows sudden fluctuations in blood pressure, hypoxia, rise in CO_2, or fall in pH.

   The bleed may distend the ventricle which impairs the venous return of the adjacent parenchyma. Venous infarction (VI) may follow and become cystic in 2–4 weeks. Bleeds are graded according to extent and severity, and correlate with prognosis. Grade I = subependymal haemorrhage. Grade II = IVH alone. Grade III = IVH + ventricular dilatation. Grade IV = III + parenchymal haemorrhage.

   Whether a lesion is ischaemic or haemorrhagic is difficult to distinguish on US. (Also see prematurity and GMH).

Table 2.12 Hypoxic-ischaemic encephalopathy

Mechanism	Distribution	Cerebral lesion
1. Focal arterial or venous occlusion	Stroke, dense hemiplegia, unilateral or bilateral	Parasagittal cortex and subcortial white matter
2. Ischaemia→PVL GMH + VI	Lower limbs mainly (diplegia)	Periventricular white matter (US grade III and IV)

Clinical progression

Manifestations may be none to severe (Table 2.13).
1. First 12 h: initial lethargy, or unresponsiveness, floppy, normal pupil and eye movement reflexes. Seizures* in 50%. Breathing irregular, high pitched cry.

2. 'Hyperalertness' by 12–24 h. Jittery ++. May have a hemiplegia due to focal ischaemic lesion in term infants, or diplegia in prematures. Frequent seizures, apnoeas.
3. 48–72 h may see a return of coma and loss of spontaneous movement. Absent brainstem reflexes are likely to be associated with a bulging fontanelle due to cerebral necrosis = poor prognosis.

*Seizures in term infants tend to be multifocal myoclonic, often 'subtle' with unusual eye movements, spontaneous suckling, +/- apnoea, rarely clonic. Tonic seizures are more common in prematures.

Table 2.13 HIE graded by severity and distribution

Grade of HIE	Clinical pattern	Seizures	Cerebral oedema
Mild	Jittery, irritable	-	-
Moderate	Lethargy, floppy, primitive reflexes +++	+ 'subtle'	Variable
Severe	Coma, brainstem dysfunction	+++	Present

Investigations

1. Disturbances of blood glucose and calcium, and liver enzymes, are common.
2. US changes aid diagnosis and prognosis. Small ventricles may be normal or due to cerebral oedema, increased echogenicity infarcted areas. The development of periventricular cysts >3 mm predicts cerebral palsy.

Procedure available in selected centres:

1. Electrophysiology: abnormal sensory evoked potentials and EEG changes of the 'burst supression' type have a poor prognosis.
2. Monitoring intracranial pressure can identify abnormal peaks.
3. Near infrared spectrophotometry. Changes in energy levels reflect the severity of hypoxia or circulatory impairment. The test has powerful predictive ability.

Management

1. Support of homeostasis: temperature, BP, urine, glucose, calcium. Dopamine infusion at a renal dose (2 μg/kg/min), +/- dobutamine to support BP.
2. Combat brain swelling: restrict fluid, mannitol; controlled ventilation may be necessary.
3. Control seizures. Prophylactic phenobarbitone does not alter the prognosis for brain damage. Discontinue after a week unless persistent neurological signs +/- EEG abnormalities.

Prognosis

Persistent unresponsiveness for a week has a poor outlook.
 Death 10–20%, mental handicap, cerebral palsy, epilepsy in 50% of survivors.
 Seizures with HIE have 30–50% mortality, >50% have severe handicap.

LOW BIRTHWEIGHT

Incidence

In UK 7% are low birthweight (LBW), of which 60% are appropriately grown for gestational age (AGA). Of the LBW, 80% are 1.5–2.5 kg, 20% are <1.5 kg.

In developing countries 10–30% of all births are LBW. The majority are small for gestational age (SGA).

Increase in incidence in the UK was noted in the 1980s and attributed to:

1. Including fetuses previously classified as previable.
2. More born to <20 and >40 year old mothers.
3. The poor, i.e. changes in the socioeconomic climate.

The ratio AGA:SGA varies with the country's nutritional and economic status.

Causes of premature LBW infants

1. Unknown in 50%, but linked with socioeconomic disadvantage.
2. Incompetent cervix.
3. Elective prematurity for eclampsia, pregnancy induced hypertension. Diabetes and rhesus disease are now less likely to be managed by early delivery.
4. Antepartum haemorrhage: abruption, placenta praevia.
5. Premature rupture of membranes.
6. Infection: e.g. maternal urinary tract infection, history of pelvic inflammatory disease, possibly ureaplasma urealyticum and chorioamnionitis.
7. Teenage mother: reduced antenatal care, increased pregnancy induced hypertension.

Prevention

1. Improving socioeconomic wellbeing as in Japan and Sweden where LBW rate has fallen to 4%.
2. Identifying high risk pregnancies.
3. Intervention by bed rest, cerclage, and tocolytics may be beneficial in selected cases.

Table 2.14 Problems of the premature

Early, i.e. within the first 3 days	Later
1 Immaturity: hypoxia, apnoea	1 Sepsis, necrotizing enterocolitis
2 Periventricular bleeds	2 Jaundice
3 Respiratory distress syndrome	3 Bronchopulmonary dysplasia
4 Homeostasis: hypoglycaemia, hypocalcaemia, hypothermia, salt and water balance	4 Osteopenia of prematurity
	5 Anaemias: iatrogenic, dilutional, nutritional, folic acid and vitamin E
5 Persistent ductus arteriosus	6 Retinopathy of prematurity
6 Sepsis	7 Cerebral palsy, mental handicap
7 Functional ileus/nutrition	8 Parental attachment and support
8 Jaundice (anticipatory treatment)	9 Growth impairment and educational difficulties

Outcome for premature infants, AGA and SGA

1. Morbidity and mortality (Table 2.15)

Table 2.15 Morbidity and mortality by birthweight and intrauterine growth, (including change in incidence over 25 years)

Birthweight	Change in mortality 1960–1985	Handicapped 1985	Healthy 1960–1985
AGA* <1000 g	92–50%	10–15%[x]	2–35%
<1500 g	72–30% Term × 200*	10%	7–60%
1501–2500 g	Term × 40*		
SGA	same as AGA§	× 6 AGA§	

* Compared with term infants of normal birth weight.
§After removing those SFD with congenital malformations, congenital infections and chromosomal abnormalities.
x Often multiply handicapped: see postnatal morbidity.
*Reference: McCormack M C (1989) Long-term follow-up of infants discharged from neonatal intensive care units, *Journal of the American Medical Association*, **261**, 1767–1772

2. Assessing neurodevelopmental progress

Allowing for prematurity requires age correction: 40 weeks – infant's gestational age in weeks. Subtract this from the infant's chronological age.
Achievements at school correlate with:

   i Correction for prematurity in the first year, and uncorrected age after a year.
  ii Slowing of head growth at 6 months of age, an ominous sign. Educational difficulties and special educational needs greater.

3. Growth

In the VLBW, growth continues to catch up over 2–3 years, but remains unsatisfactory in 15%.
    Poor growth in bronchopulmonary dysplasia, malabsorption after necrotizing enterocolitis, and large periventricular bleeds.

4. Head growth

The circumference accelerates by 6 weeks of age, even to the 90–97th centile due to the flattening effect of gravity. Continued crossing of centiles should prompt cranial US for hydrocephalus (up), or cerebral atrophy (down).

5. Hearing loss

Incidence 10-fold greater than normal after hypoxia, in the VLBW, and those needing intensive care.

6. Retinopathy of prematurity

Incidence is inversely proportional to birth weight and gestation, and 7–10% in ELBW.

7. Complications

Of respiratory distress syndrome see below.

Small for gestational age infants

Definition

See above.

Causes of SGA infants

Fetal growth retardation, timing and aetiology

First trimester

Congenital malformation, chromosomal abnormality, congenital infection.

Third trimester

1. Maternal malnutrition (severe, prolonged).
2. Alcohol and street drugs proportional to intake.
3. Toxaemia, established hypertension.
4. Smoking in up to 40% of SFD.
5. Multiple pregnancy.
6. Maternal disease, e.g. congenital heart, sickle cell, uterine malformation.

Factors not directly related to disease: race, altitude, female sex, maternal height and weight, birth order, interpregnancy interval, socioeconomic group.

Antenatal detection of growth retardation

1. Clinical

    i   Serial fundal–symphysis height.
    ii   Kick chart (value uncertain in preventing intrauterine death).

2. Biochemical.

Raised α-fetoprotein in the first half of the pregnancy.

3. Fetal US

    i   Small head in the second trimester or slowing of growth from 30 weeks.

ii Reduced abdomen:head circumference ratio in the third trimester in placental insufficiency.

iii Malformation.

4. Placental US

Doppler wave form abnormalities.

Prevention

1. Treat maternal disease, dependency, malnutrition.
2. Low dose aspirin–500g heavier than control.
3. Bed rest is of unproven value, but often recommended.

Appropriate assessment when intrauterine growth retardation is detected

1. US to identify if the fetus is abnormal, and repeat measurements to establish the trend.
2. Monitor for fetal heart rate (FHR) abnormalities, and low fetal biophysical profile (amniotic fluid volume, fetal tone, movement, breathing and variability of FHR).
3. Doppler: absent end diastolic wave pattern is predictive of hypoxia.
4. Invasive tests to consider: chorionic villous biopsy (CVB) for karyotype, viral studies, amniotic fluid for AFP; cordocentesis for blood gases is of doubtful value and is hazardous.

Indications to expedite delivery of IUGR fetus

1. Failure to grow in utero. Abdominal delivery may prevent fatal hypoxia of vaginal delivery.
2. Abnormal FHR or biophysical profile prior to or during labour.
3. pH <7.20 in labour.

Problems of the SGA

1. Hypoxia. Intrauterine/intrapartum hypoxia may cause death/brain injury.
2. Hypothermia. Large surface area for weight.
3. Hypoglycaemia. Reduced/absent glycogen stores.
4. Meconium aspiration during fetal distress.
5. Polycythaemia.
6. Pulmonary haemorrhage, now rare, occurs in asphyxiated infants with congestive cardiac failure.
7. Abnormal neurology:

    i Seizures: hypoxia, hypoglycaemia, hypocalcaemia.
    ii Jitteriness: increased hunger drive, drug withdrawal.
    iii Apathy: poor feeding in some.

Predicting outcome in the SGA

1. Growth 'channel' below the 10th centile is found in 30–50%, and comprises two groups:

    i   With small head circumference before 34 weeks' gestation.
    ii Normal growth velocity in small normal infants, regardless of gestation.

2. 'Catch up' growth in light for dates occurs within the first year.
3. Neurological outcome is dependent on:

    i   Underlying cause of being SGA, e.g. chromosomal, malformation, congenital infection.
    ii Complications suffered, e.g. hypoxia, hypoglycaemia.
    iii Small head before 26 weeks gestation has a 6-fold likelihood of abnormal neurodevelopmental progress at a year.

4. SGA is associated with increased heart disease, strokes and mortality in adult life.

CLINICAL MANAGEMENT OF EARLY PROBLEMS WITH ONSET IN THE FIRST 3 DAYS OF LIFE

1. Immaturity: hypoxia, apnoea

i Hypoxia

See asphyxia.

ii Apnoea

Definition

Pathological if >20 seconds, with bradycardia, cyanosis, hypertension followed by hypotension.

Incidence

Recurrent apnoea is 1% overall. Frequency inversely related to prematurity, 75% <30 weeks, 7% at 35 weeks.

Pathophysiology

a. Central (50%) have an open airway. Possible mechanisms:

    Chemoreceptor failure $\rightarrow$ diminished responsiveness to hypercarbia or hypoxia, e.g. prematurity.
    Laryngeal reflex to reflux or aspiration of milk or water.
    Raised environmental temperature.

b. Obstructive (10%): closed airway, e.g. Robin anomaly, neck posture, reflux, hypopharyngeal tissues 'collapse'. Chest wall seen to be moving, but not inflating.
c. Mixed (40%): central → obstructive.

Causes

a. Infant is otherwise well.

   i Immaturity: in the first week, VLBW, and <32 weeks gestation.
   ii After a feed in:
     VLBW prematures (distended abdomen, airway obstruction by feeding tube)
     Term infants (aspiration, especially with cows' milk).
   iii Clinically sick infant.

Worsening RDS, asphyxia, intracranial bleed, infection, metabolic disorder. See below for causes and investigation.

Management

a. Single apnoea: Observation alone if a single, brief apnoea.

   i Aspirate/stimulate/resuscitate.
   ii Only use oxygen if bradycardic; in recurrent apnoea hyperoxia could result, contributing to retinopathy of prematurity.
     Continuous oxygen if P_aO_2 is low. Monitoring respirations, ECG, and oxygen tension/saturation is mandatory if supplemental oxygen is given.
   iii Check temperature (abnormal in infection; in prems hyperthermia may induce apnoea), and for hypoglycaemia and anaemia. Take appropriate steps.

b. Recurrent apnoea of prematurity (diagnosed by exclusion).

   i Respiratory stimulant: xanthine, e.g. oral caffeine (easier to give, fewer side effects than theophylline) 10 mg/kg loading dose, 2.5 mg/kg once daily; theophylline oral/i.v. loading dose 6 mg/kg, maintenance 2–8 mg/kg/24 h in 3 divided doses. Blood xanthine levels of 5–20 mg/l for caffeine, 5–15 mg/l for theophylline, are to be aimed for.
   ii Continuous positive airway pressure (CPAP) of 8–12 cm via a nasal prong + theophylline.
   iii Endotracheal intubation if CPAP is inadequate. As the lungs are relatively normal use 25% oxygen and set the ventilator accordingly: 3–5 cm H_2O peak end expiratory pressure (PEEP), peak inspiratory pressure 10–15 cm H_2O, rate 5/min as sighs.
   iv Ventilate as required if apnoea persists. Inspiratory time should be short, 0.3–0.6 s. Ratio inspiration:expiration 1:3.

Increasing oxygen requirements and pressure may herald bronchopulmonary dysplasia.

2. Germinal matrix haemorrhage and periventricular bleeds

See hypoxic-ischaemic encephalopathy

Incidence

40%, inversely related to gestation, increased with RDS. The majority occur within the first 48 h. Unusual after 34 weeks' gestation. Pneumothorax with hypotension, secondary to RDS, greatly increases the risk and severity of the bleed.

Pathophysiology

Germinal matrix haemorrhage is characteristic, mainly at the head of the caudate nucleus, from its poorly supported capillary network.

Clinical

Often silent, may present as apnoea, bradycardia or fits, loss of eye movements, abnormal tone. Sudden collapse with a drop in Hb, BP, and bulging fontanelle has a poor prognosis.

Metabolic effects: hyperglycaemia, hyponatraemia, persistent metabolic acidosis.

US changes

Damaged white matter detected on US as cystic spaces or ventricular dilatation from atrophy or hydrocephalus from blockage of CSF pathways.

Grading: I = blood in germinal matrix only, II = blood fills lateral ventricle, III = II + distended ventricle, IV = parenchyma involved.

Prognosis

1. Immediate: large haemorrhages 50% mortality, hydrocephalus common in survivors. Medium size bleeds have a 10% mortality.
2. Long term: see Table 2.16.

Table 2.16 Predicting cerebal palsy and mental handicap after changes in US of the neonatal brain

US appearance	Outcome	Normal (%)
1 Normal US or isolated periventricular haemorrhages without parenchymal involvement	Excellent	95
2 Echodensity or 'flare' which resolves	Good	85–90
3 Cavitations in periventricular white matter persisting 2 weeks or more.	Poor	25 or less

Further reading

Anthony MY, Levene MI (1993) Neonatal cerebral ultrasound. In *Recent Advances in Paediatrics*, pp. 85–102 (David TJ, ed). Churchill Livingstone, Edinburgh.

3. Respiratory difficulties

Normal rate 30–40 breaths/minute, but >60/min requires investigation.

Causes of respiratory distress, apnoea, cyanosis

a. Septicaemia
b. Raised temperature (incubator temperature set too high)
c. Respiratory disease:

Acquired
    i Hyaline membrane disease
    ii Transient tachypnoea of the newborn (TTN)
    iii Aspiration:
    meconium, stomach contents
    iv Pneumothorax
    v Pneumonia
    vi Pulmonary haemorrhage

Congenital
    i Upper airway: hypoplastic jaw + cleft palate (Robin sequence), choanal atresia, oesophageal atresia
    ii Lower airways: pneumonia, lung hypoplasia, cysts, lobar emphysema, diaphragmatic hernia

d. Circulatory
    i Cardiac failure
    ii Congenital heart disease
    iii Persistent pulmonary hypertension

e. Neurological
    i Asphyxia, birth injury, IVH, immaturity, drugs
    ii Seizures
    iii Neuromuscular weakness, e.g. myasthenia gravis, myotonia congenita

Differential diagnosis of common causes

1. By history
    i Perinatal difficulties, with asphyxia and meconium aspiration.
    ii Prolonged rupture of membranes, offensive liquor, or maternal pyrexia in congenital pneumonia.
    iii Intubation at birth precedes pneumothorax, but it also occurs spontaneously or with RDS.
    iv Caesarean section: transient tachypnoea.

2. By clinical examination:
    i Obstructed breathing due to Robin anomaly, eased in prone.
    ii Pink on crying, cyanosed when attempting nose breathing = choanal atresia.

iii Persistent mucusiness and 'blowing bubbles' in oesophageal atresia +/- tracheosophageal fistula.
iv Asymmetric chest movement, hyperinflated one side: pneumothorax, lobar emphysema.
v Concave abdomen, grossly shifted mediastinum: diaphragmatic hernia.
vi Periods of hyperventilation, apnoea, subtle fits, signs of raised intracranial pressure: drug withdrawal, seizures, intracranial bleed.
vii Frothy pink tracheal fluid in pulmonary haemorrhage.

3. By time of onset

i Within 4–6 h of birth:

  a. Premature: hyaline membrane disease.
  b. Term: meconium aspiration.
  c. Any gestation: pneumothorax, asphyxia, transient tachypnoea of the newborn, anemia.
  d. Transposition of the great arteries: failure to become pink.

ii After 4 h:

  a. Pneumonia.
  b. Congenital heart or lung malformation.
  c. Metabolic acidosis: sepsis or inborn error.

Investigations

1. A Hb for anaemia. WBC total $<6 \times 10^9/l$ or neutrophil count $<2 \times 10^9/l$ or presence of band forms suggest infection.
2. Chest X- ray identifies lung disorders, although the 'diagnostic' cardiac outline may be present in only 50% with structural cardiac defects.
3. Blood gases identify type of decompensation.
4. Swabs from ear, throat, umbilicus for culture, gastric aspirate. Gram stain aids rapid identification. Blood culture. Maternal high vaginal swab in suspected congenital pneumonia.
5. Oxygen wash out helps distinguish respiratory from cardiac disease, ECG and cardiac US a cardiac malformation from persistent fetal circulation.
6. Metabolic screen for inborn errors.
7. Head US, EEG if seizures suspected or confirmed.

Respiratory distress syndrome

Definition

Respiratory distress syndrome (RDS) or hyaline membrane disease (HMD) is due to surfactant deficiency. Surfactant is produced by type II alveolar cells, stored in lamellar bodies, and composed mainly of lecithin (L) and sphyngomyelin (S).

Incidence

1% of all births, 25% of deaths. Up to 70% of VLBW infants are affected under 32 weeks' gestation. Frequency and severity decreases with maturity. Rare at term. Factors:

1. A ratio of L:S of <1.5 has a 70% incidence, 1.5–2.0 a 40% incidence, >2:1 RDS unlikley.
2. Increased incidence in: male infants, prematurity, perinatal asphyxia, maternal diabetes, caesarean section without labour, second twin, after a previous infant had RDS.
3. Reduced incidence: stressful pregnancy (pregnancy induced hypertension, hypertension, infection), maternal drug addiction, intrauterine growth retardation, giving corticosteroids.

Pathogenesis

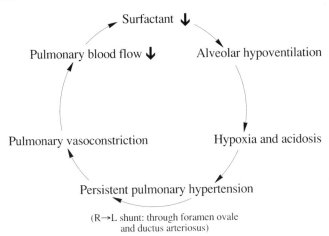

(R→L shunt: through foramen ovale and ductus arteriosus)

Histology: Alveolar disruption, eosinophylic hyaline membrane (HM) formation in RDS (HM also found in pneumonia and cardiac failure).

Prevention

1. Prevent prematurity.
2. Accelerate surfactant production.

  i Dexamethasone for 1–7 days reduces RDS incidence by 70%, independent of gestation, race and sex. Fewer deaths, less intracranial haemorrhage and necrotizing enterocolitis.
  ii Thyroid releasing hormone in addition to steroids may further reduce RDS by 50%.

3. Below 28 weeks consider Caesarean section.

  i Incidence of RDS is not increased at this gestation.

ii Premature breech delivered by section has reduced RDS and germinal matrix haemorrhage (GMH).

Clinical

Onset within 4 h of birth, of breathlessness, tachypnoea, expiratory grunting (back pressure keeping alveoli open) and sternal recession (cartilage comprises most of the anterior chest wall).

Reduced air entry, tachycardia, floppy; oedema, ileus and delay in passing meconium.

Pneumonia, metabolic disturbance, and pneumothorax, all present in a similar way.

Progress

Cyanosis and apnoea have serious prognostic significance.

Peak of illness at 2–3 days, improving as surfactant production increases. Its course lasts 5–10 days, and may be protracted in the VLBW requiring ventilatory assistance.

Chest X-ray has a ground glass appearance, with an air bronchogram not only behind the heart, a common and normal finding. A 'white out,' i.e. solid lungs on early X-ray, indicates severe RDS is likely.

Management of RDS

1. At delivery:

   i   Minimize hypoxia and heat loss. Place in a neutral thermal environment as soon as practicable.
   ii Elective intubation below 30 weeks' gestation if the Apgar score is less than 5 at 1 minute.
   iii Artificial surfactant given prophylactically, or, more logically, as 'rescue' therapy during IPPV reduces mortality from 30% to 20%, the severity and duration of RDS, pneumothoraces by half, from 37% to 16%, and possibly the incidence of bronchopulmonary dysplasia and intracerebral bleeds.

2. Oxygenation: maintain P_aO_2 at 8–12 kPa (60–100 mmHg). Continuous monitoring of blood oxygen tension or saturation, and intermittent blood gas analysis is required (see retinopathy of prematurity).
3. Maintain pH >7.20

   i   Plasma expansion 10–20 ml/kg is the first line treatment if the mean BP is below 30 mmHg, as the infant may be underperfused.
   ii Sodium bicarbonate, always if base deficit is >10 mmol/l, and depending on clinical state between 5–10 mmol/l, aiming for half correction of base deficit.

4. Antibiotic, especially to cover for Group B streptococcus: penicillin + gentamicin (or ceftazidime if anti-pseudomonal cover is desired).
5. Fluids, electrolytes, nutrition. Nil by mouth, as ileus common.

i Fluid balance limited preferably to 60 ml/kg in the first day, a maximum 80 ml/kg in the first 3 days to avoid opening the ductus arteriosus by fluid overload.

ii Glucose 10–15%, for 1–2 days; add sodium, calcium, and aminoacids to minimize catabolism.

Once on the ventilator the positive chest pressure prevents aspiration, so it is safe to feed via a nasogastric tube if the bowel is functioning. Must stop 12 hours prior to extubation and for 6–12 h after.

Others prefer the nasojejunal position, to minimize aspiration, but this increases the risk of necrotizing enterocolitis.

6. Haemoglobin. Maintain >12 g/dl by transfusion during the acute phase.

7. Mechanical ventilation

Indications
a. Electively in the ELBW <1000g
b. Clinical failure to establish effective ventilation; onset of apnoeas; irregular, exhausted respiration.
c. Blood gases poor: in 60% oxygen P_aO_2 < 8kPa (60mmHg) P_aCO_2 > 8 kPa (60mmHg)

Principles
1. Normal lungs require low pressures (12–14 cm H_2O) to inflate, inspiration 0.2 s, expiration 0.4 s (I:E ratio of 1:2) based on the time required for the lung to inflate to 60% of its maximum at that level of airway resistance and lung compliance. Examples: apnoea of prematurity, post surgical.
2. Low compliance as in RDS, requires relatively more inspiratory to expiratory time to inflate the lungs, and high inspiratory pressures with positive end expiratory pressure (PEEP) to keep the alveoli open. Each of these manoeuvres raises the mean airway pressure (MAP) which is optimally around 12–14 cm H_2O in RDS. If CO_2 accumulates, increase the minute volume by raising the respiratory rate or tidal volume, or lowering the PEEP.
3. High resistance as in meconium aspiration requires prolonged expiration time, no PEEP, and slow rates.

Initial ventilator settings
1. Respiratory rate of 30–40/minute is usual, with inspiratory time 0.2–0.6 s.
   In the VLBW 60–140/min may be more 'physiological' and baby synchronizes better with the ventilator to give improved oxygenation and pH, lower incidence of pneumothorax.
2. i Peak pressure initially 25 mm Hg
   ii Ratio inspiration:expiration 1:1
   iii Gas flow 5 - 10 l/min.

3. Continuous distending pressure of 4–6 cmH_2O keeps alveoli open.
4. Failure to synchronize with the ventilator may be an indication for transiently raising inspiratory pressure +/- plasma infusion. If fighting continues or high pressures of 30–40 cm H_2O continue to be needed for exceptionally stiff lungs, change sedation from oral to i.v., or paralyse with pancuronium 0.03–0.04 mg/

kg. The risk of pneumothorax by breathing against the ventilator is thereby reduced.

Sedation   An endotracheal tube in situ is very uncomfortable, resulting in impaired homeostasis. Infuse morphine 0.05 mg/kg/h. Chloral via the nasogastric tube helps keep the dose down.

Subsequent alteration to ventilator settings   In order of adjustment, while improving ventilation, to minimize atelectasis, bronchopulmonary dysplasia and pneumothorax:

1. Oxygen increased to no more than 95%.
2. Alter I:E ratio–prolonging inspiration raises P_aO_2, i.e. I:E ratio of 1:1 (1:2 used for ventilating healthy lungs).
3. Respiratory rate – raise to reduce CO_2 retention. Sometimes better to accept raised P_aCO_2 than to go on to increase peak inflation pressure.
4. Lastly, raise inflation pressure, in 5 cmH$_2$O steps.
   Once improving, reduce peak pressure, oxygen and rate in that order to minimize barotrauma, pneumothorax, and bronchopulmonary dysplasia.

Trouble shooting rapid onset of hypoxia or cyanosis: steps 1, 2, 3.

1. No chest wall movement – hand ventilate with 100% O_2, bag and mask.

   i Improvement indicates ventilator leak or stiff lungs needing higher pressures.
   ii Poor/no response: tube partially or totally blocked, or infant extubated.

2. Chest wall moving = ventilator working.

   i Check whether

      a. Tube in right main bronchus.
      b. Adequate oxygen concentration, rate, or inflation pressure.

   ii Fighting, i.e. non-synchronized:

      a. Increase oxygen concentration to 95%.
      b. Increase respiratory rate in steps of 10/min or double to 60–90/min.
      c. Raise inflation pressure in steps of 5 cm H$_2$O up to 40/5.

   Opiate i.v. or pancuronium is indicated early if fighting continues.
3. Failure to improve: look for pneumothorax (usually rapidly identified by transillumination using a cold light source), sepsis, bleed, hypotension, hypoglycaemia, metabolic acidosis, necrotizing enterocolitis, patent ductus arteriosus.
4. Additional manoeuvres:

   i   Tolazoline or prostacyclin vasodilator for failure to improve (persistent pulmonary hypertension/persistent fetal circulation).
   ii High frequency jet ventilation.
   iii Trial of extracorporeal membrane oxygenation (ECMO) in the most severe cases of RDS or persistent fetal circulation, is currently being evaluated.

5. Weaning
Duration of ventilator dependency (support + weaning) 3–10 days over 28 weeks, for earlier gestation 2–4 weeks is common.

As RDS resolves:

   i Reduce peak pressure in steps of 2–4 cm H_2O to 20/4.
   ii Oxygen steps of 5–10% down to 40–50%.
   iii Rate to 25–30/min., in that order. Monitor blood gases after each adjustment.

Once achieved, start intermittent mandatory ventilation 5–10/min. Limit inspiration time to 0.5 s to reduce duration of weaning. IMV is often unnecessary in rapidly improving larger infants.

If gases are satisfactory for a few hours in 30–40% O_2, allow spontaneous respiration with PEEP of 3–4 cm. Reduce to 2 cm for 8–12 h before extubation.

Add theophylline if weaning is slow. This regulates respiration, improves diaphragmatic function and reduces pulmonary artery pressure.

Failure to wean   Causes include patent ductus arteriosus, (re)infection and secretions, recurrent apnoea, and bronchopulmonary dysplasia.

High frequency jet ventilation has a place in the management of bronchopulmonary dysplasia.

Prognosis   Mortality 12% overall, 20% of ventilated infants.

Incidence of complications among <1500 g

1. Respiratory, acute phase:

   i Pneumothorax in up to 35% of ventilated infants has a mortality of 70% in ELBW.
   ii Pulmonary interstitial emphysema: 20% – mortality high if bilateral.

2. Respiratory longer term:

   i Laryngeal stenosis: in up to 7% of ELBW, 2% overall. Use Coles tube for resuscitation only, change to unshouldered tube for more prolonged IPPV, to prevent injury.
   ii Bronchopulmonary dysplasia or Wilson Mikity syndrome in 15%. Respiratory symptoms and infection, and hospital readmission rate all increased. Persistent abnormalities of lung function.

3. Intraventricular haemorrhages 35%.
4. Neurological handicap 10–20%.

Further reading

Cooke R W I (1990) Developments in the management of respiratory distress syndrome. In *Recent Advances in Paediatrics* vol. 9, ed T J David. Edinburgh:Churchill Livingstone

Crowley P, Chalmers I, Keirse M J N C (1990) The effects of corticosteroid administration before preterm delivery: an overview of the evidence from controlled trials. *British Journal of Obstetrics and Gynaecology*, **97**, 11-25

Hennes H M, Lee M B, Rimon A A, Shapiro D L (1991) Surfactant replacement therapy in respiratory distress syndrome. *American Journal of Diseases of Children*, **145**, 102–104

4. Patent ductus arteriosus (PDA)

Rare in term infants, common (20–30%) in the VLBW with RDS.

Pathophysiology

Onset of signs at 3–4 days old.

1. Due to failure of ductus arteriosus to close and of the normal fall in pulmonary vascular resistance.
2. Reopening of the ductus due to acidosis and hypoxia.
3. Increased circulatory volume keeps ductus open due to excess fluid intake.

Chest X-ray shows cardiomegaly, congested lung fields + changes of RDS.

Limiting fluid intake to 60–80 ml/kg/day in the first 3 days reduces the incidence of PDA.

Management

i   Restrict fluid , diuretics, increase PEEP if on IPPV.
ii Failure to respond after 1–2 days and <34 weeks and <10 days old: restrict fluid + oral indomethacin 0.2 mg/kg 12 hourly × 3 or 0.1 mg/kg/daily for 6 days. Complications: impaired renal function → fluid retention, gut haemorrhage.
iii 'Stuck on ventilator'. Inability to wean is an indication for surgical ligation on the intensive care nursery.
iv The less severe PDAs can be left as they tend to close spontaneously around the expected date of delivery; failure to do so is an indication for surgery.

5. Functional ileus, subnutrition

Problems arising: hypoglycaemia, hypocalcaemia, salt and water balance. See relevent sections.

6. Jaundice

Early phototherapy indicated in the acidotic, hypoglycaemic premature, all risk factors for kernicterus. See below.

OTHER RESPIRATORY PROBLEMS

1. Transient tachypnoea of the newborn (TTN)

Definition

Tachypnoea due to retained lung fluid, commoner after caesarean section, asphyxia, and in infants of diabetic mothers.

Clinical

Onset often predictable from the perinatal history. Commonly a term infant with signs of respiratory distress. Chest X-ray shows prominent vascular markings and interlobular fissures, with well inflated lungs. Resolution over 2–3 days.

Relatively mild course is usual, requiring up to 40% oxygen, rarely needing ventilation. May only be diagnosable in retrospect.

Management

1. Oxygen.
2. Antibiotic until pneumonia/sepsis excluded by culture and rapid progress.
3. Withold feeds until the respiratory rate falls below 60/min. Maintenance hydration and glucose i.v.

   Prognosis excellent.

2. Pneumothorax, other air leaks

Spontaneous in 1% of term infants, the majority are asymptomatic. Rising incidence with RDS (5%), PEEP (10%), and ventilated (20%) prematures, and up to 40% with the meconium aspiration syndrome.

Pathophysiology

Rupturing alveolus allows air into the pleural space by either of two routes:

1. Overdistended from air trapping, bursts into the subpleural space, e.g. meconium aspiration.
2. Air tracks towards the hilum along the bronchovascular bundle, especially in prematures being ventilated, and results in pulmonary interstitial emphysema (PIE) in 20%. In half of these it reaches the hilum and a pneumothorax, pneumomediastinum or rarely a pneumopericardium develops.

Tension pneumothorax: acute lung collapse $\rightarrow$ shunting $\rightarrow$ rise in CO_2 and increased likelihood of germinal matrix haemorrhage.

Management

Fibreoptic cold light transillumination, confirmed by chest X-ray if time and baby's condition permit. Insert chest drain at anterior axillary line, fourth intercostal space, and attach to an underwater seal. Small pneumothoraces and PIE are better left.

3. Bronchopulmonary dysplasia

Definition

The need for supplemental oxygen after 28 days of age, with characteristic hyperinflated and cystic lungs on X-ray.

Pulmonary interstitial emphysema is a forerunner. Similar X-ray changes are found at an earlier stage in RDS, pneumonia, and cardiac failure.

Incidence

Inversely related to gestation and birthweight. Affects up to 50% of those less than 1 kg, increasing to 70% if ventilated for more than 2 weeks. Rare over 2 kg. Annually, up to 1000 cases are likely in the UK, 7000 in USA.

Pathophysiology

Histology: squamous metaplasia, fibrosis and thickening of pulmonary arterioles seen.

Biochemistry: proteolytic enzymes released by inflammatory cells contribute to the damage, further worsened by the consequent release of toxic free radicals.

Clinical correlates:

1. Injury to the premature lung by barotrauma.
2. High inspired oxygen concentration.
3. Associated factors: intubation, secretions and infection, e.g. ureaplasma urealyticum (?). Exacerbated by a soft chest wall due to metabolic bone disease of prematurity.

Compensatory growth of the lung postnatally alleviates much of the damage done.

Management

1. Prevention: superoxide dismutase, vitamins E and A, bovine surfactant, early use of PEEP or continuous negative extrathoracic pressure (CNEP) may each be beneficial. Trials are in progress.

   Reduce peak pressures and oxygen as soon as possible during mechanical ventilation.
2. Medication:
   Steroids in the absence of infection.

   i   ELBW requiring continued ventilatory support, over 2 weeks old.
   ii In established BPD, prednisolone 0.5 mg/kg/day reducing over 3 weeks.

   Bronchodilators ipratropium or salbutamol by nebulizer are helpful if wheezy.
   Diuretics improve lung compliance.

   Antibiotics for bacterial and chlamydial infection; antifungals; ribavirin for respiratory syncitial virus (RSV) given promptly may halt progression to respiratory failure, to which these infants are prone.
3. Oxygen. Maintain normal blood oxygen saturation of 95–98% via a catheter, placed in the nasopharynx, or taped below the nares, to prevent pulmonary vascular resistance rising. Home care, expert visiting nurse support, and providing an oxygen concentrator through the family practitioner reduces separation, hospitalization, infections, and costs.
4. Pertussis immunization from 2 months is essential.

Prognosis

Before discharge from hospital the mortality rate is 15%.

Readmission to hospital with respiratory infection 60%, death 10% (12 × controls) from infection (especially RSV) and cot death.

Further reading

Northway W H (1990) Bronchopulmonary dysplasia: then and now. *Archives of Disease in Childhood*, **65**, 1076–1081

4. Wilson Mikity syndrome

The gradual onset of respiratory distress, hypoxia and apnoea in prematures a few days old, with no preceding severe respiratory disease. Cystic spaces seen on X-ray.

Treatment as for BPD. Resolution over weeks or months. Prone to recurrent chest infections for the first 2–3 years.

5. Meconium aspiration syndrome

Incidence

Although 10% of births have meconium stained liquor, if golden it is old, and requires no active measures.

Active intervention in the 0.2–2% passing fresh meconium improves morbidity and mortality.

Common in the postmature growth retarded. Prematures rarely pass meconium, except in Listeria infection.

Prevention

The presence of thick green meconium mandates sucking out the mouth and nose when the head is on the perineum. Clear the larynx under direct vision immediately, intubate and applying suction to the endotracheal tube, or aspirate using the largest possible catheter.

Failure to do so allows the meconium to be inhaled, causing ballvalve hyperinflation → pneumothorax, atelectasis → shunting of blood, hypoxia, and persistent pulmonary hypertension.

Clinical

Meconium stained skin, marked respiratory distress, hyperinflated chest. Pneumothorax occurs in 10–20%.

Chest X-ray

Coarse mottled densities with patches of hyperinflation in both lung fields.

Management

1. Oxygen, i.v. fluids, ventilate using short inspiratory times. High peak pressures often required, increasing the danger of pneumothorax. To minimize this risk, sedate +/- paralysis. Artificial surfactant may have a role. Extracorporeal membrane oxygenation is under trial.
2. Tolazoline, or prostacyclin (prostaglandin I_2) for persistent fetal circulation.
   Controversial: magnesium sulphate i.v. may improve survival (Abu-Osba Y K, *et al* (1991) Treatment of severe persistent pulmonary hypertension of the newborn with magnesium sulphate. *Archives of Disease in Childhood*, **647**, 31–35).
3. Infection is rarely a problem but antibiotics are usually given (as it has been shown experimentally that *E. coli* flourish).

Prognosis

Death is usually due to persistent fetal circulation, when mortality is 20–40%.

6. Pulmonary haemorrhage

Definition

Production of frothy pink pulmonary fluid with low haematocrit, in an acutely ill infant; mainly due to acute cardiac failure, associated with hypoxia from asphyxia, RDS, or pneumonia, hypothermia, and bleeding disorders. Now rare, except in <750 g given Exosurf.

Management

Correct coagulation, transfer if necessary, ventilate, give broad spectrum antibiotics.

INFECTION

Incidence

One to 3/1000 neonates develop severe tissue infection, septicaemia, meningitis, pneumonia, etc. Premature infants have a 10–fold risk due to immature defences, more invasive management and longer time in hospital.

Minor infections are common, 1–5%, e.g. sticky eye from chlamydia, *E. coli*, staphylococcal pustules, paronychia. Prompt treatment prevents progression/dissemination.

Historical perspective

1940s Predominant organism was the group A streptococcus until the penicillin era.
1950s Staphylococci until penicillinase resistant antibiotics were developed.
1960s Gram–negative organisms flourished.

1970s The group B beta-haemolytic streptococcus (GBS) became the most important pathogen. Up to 25% of pregnant women carry GBS in their vaginal flora and a half of their infants are colonized, but only 1% of these develop disease (they lack the specific antibody). Annual incidence of severe GBS disease in the UK is 0.3 per 1000 live births.

1980s *Staphylococcus epidermidis* recognized as a common septicaemic organism in the VLBW.

Prevention of spread within the nursery

1. Hand washing: simple soap on lying in wards, chlorhexidine, iodine compounds or alcohol splash when caring for sick infants. Masks are dangerous if repeatedly touched, as often happens.
2. Avoid overcrowding, encourage rooming in and breast feeding.
3. In special care nurseries: adequate staffing levels, incubators to isolate potentially infected infants. Minimum of invasive procedures. Consider hyperimmune IgG prophylaxis in the VLBW if infection in the nursery is common.
4. Containing an outbreak.

    i Handwashing reinforced.
    ii Cohorting. To prevent spread, the cohort of infected babies is nursed in one room, and subsequent admissions in another room. Nursing staff are allocated to one or other group, but not both. Gowning up is a reinforcing 'barrier' advocated by some.

Education of the public

Primary prevention

    i   Avoidance of possible Listeria containing foods.
    ii Safer sex if the male partner has HIV or genital herpes.
    iii Gloves for handling cat litter, food waste, and gardening prevents toxoplasmosis.
    iv Vaccination: against GBS, hepatitis B.

Controversy: should CMV negative women work in day care infant facilities as 30% of infected infants continue to excrete CMV for 3–5 years? No evidence that such a policy would be effective.

Secondary prevention

The work of sexually transmitted disease clinics, antenatal testing for syphilis, contact tracing.

Risk factors

1. Sepsis risk factors:

    i   Preterm.
    ii Prolonged rupture of membranes.
    iii Maternal fever, offensive liquor.

2. Difficult delivery and birth asphyxia.

Organisms implicated and manner of spread to infect the infant

1. Transplacentally: toxoplasmosis, rubella, cytomegalovirus, parvovirus, Listeria, syphilis, Echovirus, Coxsackie virus, chickenpox, rarely TB, malaria.
2. Via maternal genital tract: GBS, gonococcus, herpes simplex virus.
3. Environmentally via hands, indwelling catheters, endotracheal tubes etc.

In Europe and USA, GBS is the most significant bacterium involved in early septicaemic and pneumonic infections (and meningitis at 2–14 days), but after 48 h Gram negative organisms predominate (*E. coli, Pseudomonas aeruginosa, Klebsiella pneumoniae*) and *Staphylococcus aureus, Staph. epidermidis*, occasionally *Haemophilus influenzae, Strep. pneumoniae*.

Other organisms to consider: viruses (herpes, nosocomial RSV and rotavirus), fungi (i.v. lines), chlamydia (maternal), pneumocystis (prematures), mycoplasma, ureaplasma (?).

Presentation

1. Meconium stained liquor in premature delivery (such staining is unusual), consider *Listeria monocytogenes*.
2. Clinical signs of infection are non-specific: respiratory distress, apnoea, cyanosis, vomiting, diarrhoea, abdominal distension, irritability, lethargy, hyper- or hypothermia.
3. Site: Pneumonia in 60%, septicaemia 30%, meningitis and soft tissue infection 10%.

Some characteristics of the organisms

1. GBS and *L. monocytogenes* present similarly:

   i   Early onset: mortality 20–50%. Stillbirth or sepsis in *L. monocytogenes* from transplacental spread. First day pneumonia, septicaemia, meningitis in GBS type II and III, acquired during delivery.
   ii Late onset: previously healthy term infant, age >7 days to 3 months, as meningitis (*L. monocytogenes* type IVB, GBS type III). Mortality 10%.

Suitable antibiotics: penicillin or ampicillin/amoxycillin together with gentamicin act synergistically against both organisms.

2. *Staphylococcus epidermidis*.

Entry via invasive procedures in the LBW, e.g. long lines, especially if lipids infused. Low grade septicaemic presentation common, also with pleural effusions, abscesses, meningitis (usually via a ventricular shunt), necrotizing enterocolitis, or endocarditis.

Mortality low (5%).

Vancomycin for 7–10 days is usually sufficient.

Differential diagnosis

1. Of apnoea, shock, acidaemia:

    i <6 h from birth: sepsis.
    ii After 24–48 hours, with hypoglycaemia: inborn errors, midgut volvulus.
    iii Elevated blood pH in urea cycle defects.

2. Cyanosis with tachypnoea: differentiate by microbiology, chest X-ray, ECG, and if uncertain, cardiac echo.

    i Congenital heart disease +/- persistent pulmonary hypertension (PPH).
    ii PPH secondary to sepsis, hypoxia, aspiration.

Table 2.17 Early and late infection characteristics

	Early (<48h old)	*Late (>48h old)*
Incidence	2/1000	8/1000
Source	Maternal	Environmental>maternal
Bacteria	GBS, *E. Coli, Listeria,* Occasionally *Strep. pneumoniae,* H. influenzae	*Staph. aureus, Staph. epidermis,* Gram negative (*E. coli, Klebsiella, Pseudomonas, Proteus*), *Serratia*
Candida		Sick prem, on TPN, antibiotics long line, systemic in 2% of infants <1.5 kg
Viruses	Rubella, CMV, toxo, Coxsackie	HSV, Enterovirus, RSV
Gestation	Premature>>term	Preterm>term, 15% of <1.5 kg
Presentation	RDS like, shock, PPH	1. Deteriorating on IPPV 2. Change in behaviour
Investigations	FBC, blood glucose, IgM, CXR, septic screen*	As for early infection. Routine surveillance cultures are unhelpful.
Management	Support BP, antibiotics, policy ventilate	As for early infection. Particular care with antibiotic to avoid resistant organisms emerging
Mortality	40–50%	5–25%, mainly premature

Investigations
* Cultures of blood, CSF, urine, throat and external auditory meatus swab, stain gastric aspirate for rapid identification. Counterimmune electrophoresis for bacterial products in urine, CSF, for GBS, E. coli K$_1$ antigen. C-reactive protein if rapidly available is useful to monitor progress.
    In early onset always obtain a maternal high vaginal swab.

Appropriateness and interpretation of investigations

1. WBC and differential:
    i WBC <5 × 10^9/l
    ii Neutrophil count: ratio of immature (band forms) to total (I/T) >0.2
       Factors to consider in interpretation:

        a. High WBC and I/T ratio after asphyxia, maternal toxaemia.
        b. WBC and neutrophil count rise during the first 12 h after birth then fall. A change in count opposite to that expected may be significant.

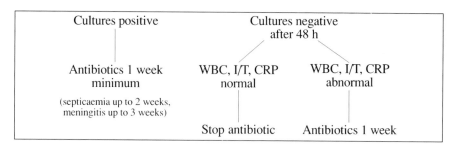

Figure 2.1 Algorithm for antibiotic treatment using culture and acute phase reactants.

2. Acute phase reactants: C-reactive protein (CRP): latex CRP positive or >20 mg/l. Erythrocyte sedimentation rate >20 mm in the first hour. Interleukin-6 is under evaluation.
3. Radiology and US for specific changes in chest, or detection of underlying renal anomaly, collection of pus etc.
4. Suspected viral infection: specific IgM for congenital infection, IgG antibody titres, urine for CMV, rubella; swabs, stool and CSF for enterovirus.

Prevention of infection and the use of prophylactic antibiotics

1. Premature birth accounts for 4–5% of all births, and routine antibiotic prophylaxis is not indicated. Direct efforts at preventing prematurity.
2. Prolonged and premature rupture of membranes. Defined as longer than 24 hours, the incidence is 3%.

   i Term infant: swabs, blood culture and observe. Temperature or clinical deterioration are indications for broad spectrum antibiotic administration.
   ii Preterm infant: immediate broad spectrum antibiotic cover after swabs and blood culture have been obtained. If cultures are negative after 48 h, and baby is well, stop treatment.

3. Meconium aspiration: increased risk of *E. coli* infection experimentally, so antibiotics are often given.
4. GBS isolated from mother's vagina: penicillin prophylaxis

   i In term infants of limited benefit in preventing early onset, none in preventing late onset infection.
   ii To mothers in premature labour, if the membranes have ruptured for more than 12 h it is effective.

5. Renal tract reflux/obstruction suspected from antenatal US: trimethoprim 2 mg/ kg daily until resolution/intervention recommended by many.
6. Prophylaxis is contentious in the following situations:

   • In umbilical cord care (delays normal separation).
   • Endotracheal intubation and IPPV without sepsis as a cause.
   • Antifungals to prevent candida superinfection during antibiotic administration in the very low birthweight.
   • Acyclovir in babies of mothers with recurrent genital herpes.

7. Staff and maternal infections.
   i Open pustules: staff must stay away until they have resolved, mothers should cover the lesion; both are swabbed and treated.
   ii Herpetic lip and finger lesions: topical 35% idoxuridine for 3 days, returning to work after 24 h of treatment and wearing a mask.

Management

The limited repertoire of the sick neonate's responses to different disease processes dictates that treatment must:

1. Cover many disparate conditions while searching for a diagnosis (which may not be conclusive!).
2. Be instituted early to minimize or prevent a downward spiral.

General principles

1. Evaluation to determine:
   i 'At risk' of infection: term infants before treatment, and preterm infants in the first 48 h after taking samples and commencing treatment.
   ii In the presence of clinical signs: culture the blood, CSF, urine. Evaluate WBC, immature:total granulocytes (I/T) ratio, C-reactive protein (CRP). Start antibiotics (Figure 2.1).
   Antibiotic policy: broad spectrum, according to local sensitivity patterns, initiated before the results of microbiology, acute phase reactants or biochemistry for inborn errors, are available.

   a. Early infection: penicillin and aminoglycoside (usually gentamicin) act synergistically in GBS and listeriosis.
   b. Late infection: ceftazidime (effective against *Staph. epidermidis* and *Pseudomonas*) + ampicillin/penicillin, or penicillin + gentamicin as for early infection + vancomycin for *S. epidermidis*.
   As initial signs of sepsis and necrotizing enterocolitis are similar it may be prudent to add metronidazole cover.
   IgG (Sandoglobulin) i.v. 'rescue' has a place in the sick VLBW.
   Antifungal drugs: amphotericin B and 5-flucytosine, in combination, for systemic fungal infection, which occurs in up to 2% of VLBW (<1500 g), treat for 10 days. Fluconazole may be an alternative.

2. Monitor carefully for temperature instability.
   Beware, using servo control of the infant warming system masks it.
3. Biochemical monitoring: hypoglycaemia, acidaemia, hyponatraemia common.
4. Blood pressure support, by volume expanders, inotropes. Watch urine output for renal failure.
5. Check Hb as haemolysis due to infection and iatrogenic falls in Hb are common.
6. Oxygen, IPPV for cyanosis/hypoxia, apnoea, hypercapnoea, gross abdominal distension due to air or fluid.

7. Feeding is often stopped as ileus is common in sick infants. Rapid improvement following the giving of fluids i.v. may be due to an amino acid inborn error ameliorated by stopping milk feeds (protein load).

Specific infections

1. Pneumonia

Commonly bacterial. After the first few weeks also consider:

    i Fungal (repeated antibiotics in VLBW).
    ii Chlamydial (previous conjunctivitis).
    iii Viral, e.g. cytomegalovirus (blood transfusion) → persistent pneumonitis and recurrent episodes of wheeze.

Differential diagnosis

Aspiration, asphyxia, cyanotic congenital heart disease, metabolic, RDS, TTN.
    GBS septicaemia/pneumonia, with early shock and acidosis, is indistinguishable from RDS.

Management

As for RDS, especially antibiotics: penicillin (ensure in high dose) + gentamicin or ceftazidime.

Prognosis

Mortality 10–50%, may be related to the rapidity with which antibiotics are started.

2. Ophthalmia neonatorum

Definition

Any mucopurulent conjunctivitis in the first 3 weeks of life.

Incidence, epidemiology and prophylaxis

Affects 5–10% of all newborns.
    Organisms include staphylococci, haemophilus, chlamydia and *Neisseria* gonococcus. Prophylaxis against the latter, worldwide (*except* UK, and some others) is with silver nitrate 1% solution.

    i *Neisseria gonorrhoeae*: UK incidence 20–40 cases annually. Golden yellow discharge onset within 24 h of birth, may be delayed to up to 4 weeks.
    ii *Chlamydia trachomatis*: onset a week after birth, inclusion body conjunctivitis in over half of colonized infants, up to a quarter develop pneumonia. No long-term visual abnormalities. Diagnosis by culture (gold standard), fluorescent monoclonal antibody or enzyme immunoassay (60–70% pick-up).

Management, according to rapidity of onset and recurrence

i Acute onset = gonococcal until proven otherwise, penicillin irrigation to the eyes, hourly, until discharge abates. Confirmation of intracellular Gram negative diplococci: from the stain differentiation of *N. meningitidis* from *N. gonorrhoeae* is essential to avoid an explosive gaff! Antibiotic of choice is still penicillin, or cefotaxime if resistant. Isolate infant and mother.

ii More gradual onset: neomycin drops (effective against bacteria, not chlamydia) for 48 h. No improvement is an indication for investigation for chlamydia and change to tetracycline drops. If confirmed add oral erythromycin for 2 weeks to prevent pneumonia. The parents should also be treated to prevent recurrence.

iii Recurrent conjunctivitis = blocked tear duct, receives saline drops 6 hourly, or chloramphenicol drops bilaterally if a profuse discharge or eyelids swell. The duct usually opens by 3 months old, but may be probed at a year if still blocked.

3. Meningitis

See Infectious diseases.

Table 2.18 Drugs: Antibiotic dosages in the newborn

	single dose/kg	*frequency/24 h*
Amoxicillin, Ampicillin	30 mg	2 × if < 7 days old, 3–4 thereafter
	in meningitis 50 mg	
Ceftazidime, or cefotaxime	25 mg, increased to 50 mg	2 × if < 7 days old, after the first week
Cefuroxime	in meningitis	increased to 3 ×
Carbenicillin	100 mg	<2 kg 2–3 ×, >2 kg 3–4 ×
Flucloxacillin	30 mg	<2 kg 2 × in week 1, to 4 × in week 2, >2 kg 4 ×
Gentamicin <7 days old	2.5 mg	<28 weeks once, 29–35 weeks 18 hourly, >36 weeks 12 hourly.
>7 days old	2.5 mg	>1 kg 2 ×, <1 kg every 18 h
renal failure	1.5–2.5 mg/kg	Interval determined by drug level after 1st dose. Blood levels normally after 3rd dose: trough prior to dose <2 µg/ml, peak at 1 hour post dose 5–10 µg/l.
Metronidazole	75 mg	3 ×
Netilmicin	similar to gentamicin in dosage and blood levels.	
Penicillin 1<2 kg	25000u	
2 kg with GBS	50000u	}2 × if <7 days old
2 >2 kg	25000u	}3 × if >7 days old
2 kg with GBS	50000u	}3 × if <7 days old
Piperacillin	100 mg	}4 × if >7 days old
Trimethoprim prophylaxis	2 mg	2 ×
therapeutic	4 mg	1 ×
Vancomycin	15 mg	2 ×
		2 × if <7 days old, others 3 ×

4. Pyogenic arthritis

See Orthopaedic problems. Uncommon, may be multifocal. Presentation as systemic illness usual in preterm infants.

5. Urinary tract infection

See Renal problems.

6. Otitis media

Especially common in ventilated infants, and cleft palate.

Further reading

de Louvois J, Harvey D (1990) *Infection in the Newborn.* Chichester:Wiley
Williamson J B, Galasko C S B, Robinson M J (1990) Outcome after acute osteomyelitis in preterm infants. *Archives of Disease in Childhood,* **65,** 1060–1062

Congenital infection

An increasing recognition of the wide variety of organisms and presentations has led to a call for the abolition of the restrictive acronym of TORCH (Table 2.19).

Table 2.19 Some characteristics of the 'classical' TORCH infections

Organism	Annual UK incidence	Transmission	Stage in gestation	Percent infected	Damage to fetus
Toxoplasma	2/1000	Cats faeces, undercooked meat	0–3/12	25	Severe in 75%
			6–9/12	65	Mild/subclinical
Rubella	Falling, was 1/1000	Children. Rarely, a reinfection	1–3/12	50	Severe MD, CHD etc
			3–5/12	10	Deaf, retinitis.
CMV	3/1000	Primary	0–9/12	40	Severe 5%
		Secondary (sero+ve mother).	0–9/12	1	Asymptomatic 100%
Herpes 1 and 2	1/40 000	1. Primary genital infection	Intrapartum	40	Moderate/severe
		2. Recurrent, rarely occurs	Intrapartum	?	Moderate/severe
Syphilis	4/year	Primary or secondary stages	0–9/12		Stillbirth, premature, hydrops, death; may be asymptomatic

Note: generally the stage of gestation influences the severity of the damage suffered, and recurrent viral transmission of rubella is rare but no less severe when it occurs.

1. 'Classical' TORCH = Toxoplasma, Other (e.g. syphilis), Rubella, Cytomegalovirus (CMV), Herpes simplex (HSV).

i Features common to all.

(Findings vary between individuals).
- Low birthweight
- Prematurity
- Haematological: anaemia, purpura

- Hepatitis picture: jaundice, hepatosplenomegaly
- CNS: seizures, encephalitis, microcephaly, mental handicap
- Failure to thrive

ii Selective findings

- Eyes:
  a. Cataracts, microphthalmia: rubella>>toxoplasmosis, rare in HSV, never in CMV.
  b. Retinopathy
  - pepper and salt = rubella.
  - punched out chorioretinitis = CMV, toxoplasmosis (maybe unilateral and progressive), HSV.
  c. Glaucoma: rubella.
  d. Keratitis: HSV.
- Deafness: rubella, CMV both > toxoplasmosis, syphilis.
- Cerebral calcification: in toxoplasmosis widespread, CMV periventricular, less common and obvious in others.
- Hydrocephalus: toxoplasmosis, HSV.
- Patent ductus arteriosus, pulmonary branch stenosis: rubella.
- Osteochondritis in syphilis, rubella.
- Pneumonia, myocarditis: CMV, rubella, syphilis.
- Skin rashes: vesicles in HSV, condylomata in syphilis, mulberry 'muffins' in rubella.

Investigation

1. Antenatal indications:
  i Maternal illness, e.g. rubella-like rash (includes parvovirus B19), discharge and pelvic pain (sexually transmitted disease).
  ii At risk of HIV and hepatitis B (HBV) through life style or partner(s), and HBV by race (Far East, Africans).
  iii All pregnancies are screened for syphilis and rubella status, but the latter is no indicator of recent infection, and rubella IgM is needed for confirmation.
  Controversy : Screening for CMV and toxoplasmosis have been recommended for the UK.

  a. In CMV infection only 5% of fetuses are severely damaged, so termination on viral studies alone would destroy disproportionally many more healthy fetuses.
  b. Toxoplasmosis: in France termination or antiprotozoal treatment is offered in proven infection initially detected on screening; in the UK it would be uneconomic as confirmed cases are less common (only 14 in 1990), and many more mothers are initially non-immune, requiring repeated investigation.

2. To avoid over-investigation for congenital infection
As similar signs and symptoms are present in a wide range of other diseases, for example in the SGA, consider:

- First whether due to maternal disease/smoking/drug abuse.

- Secondly a congenital malformation may be due to a chromosome abnormality.
- Finally look for congenital infection, especially if cataracts or skull calcification are present.

Samples helpful in the detection of congenital infection
1. Antenatal maternal blood, fetal blood, amniotic fluid:

    i Maternal blood for specific IgM for CMV, toxoplasma, rubella, parvovirus, in addition to the usual tests for syphilis, HIV, HBV.
    ii Cordocentesis for fetal specific IgM, for parvovirus IgM in non-immune fetal hydrops, or presence of the viral genome DNA/RNA (in rubella).
    iii Amniotic fluid for viral culture.

2. Postpartum blood samples from infant and mother, for specific IgM. Paired samples, at delivery and an interval of 3–6 months, to exclude passive transfer of maternal antibodies if an initially positive result is obtained. Infection is not excluded by a negative result!
3. Viral culture of urine or throat swab for rubella, CMV, herpes; CSF culture for herpes.

Management of antenatally acquired infection
1. Counselling of risk, effects, outcome possibilities.
2. Termination. Considerations in early pregnancy:

    i Indicated in toxoplasmosis or rubella.
    ii CMV not justified as risk of damage is low.
    iii HIV: see Infectious diseases for discussion.

3. If pregnancy is too advanced or termination unacceptable: fetal sampling for IgM, viral studies etc.
   If infection is confirmed as toxoplasmosis, give spiramycin alternating with pyrimethamine + sulphadiazine in 3 weekly courses throughout pregnancy. After birth, continue treatment for the first year of life.
4. Syphilis: penicillin i.m. during pregnancy. LP at birth for WBCs. If more than 25 WBCs/mm^3, or previously untreated, give penicillin i.v. for 10 days.

Vertically acquired at delivery:

1. Herpes simplex

Table 2.20 Clinical presentation and prognosis of herpes simplex infection in the neonate

Age (days)	Clinical presentation (% of total)		Deaths (%)	Damaged (%)
9–11	Disseminated	50	80	20
	Treated with acyclovir →		20	50
10	Localized mucocutaneous	20		
	(some go on to CNS involvement)			
15–17	CNS involvement*	30	15	60

* Type 2 infection has worse outcome than type 1 (mentally handicapped 80% vs. 20%).

Prevention of neonatal herpetic infection
1. Primary infection: caesarian section with ruptured membranes <4 h is effective. Otherwise start acyclovir prophylactically.
2. Recurrent genital herpes has only a small risk, so it is permissible to observe closely for the first 2 weeks of life and start acyclovir only if symptoms develop.
3. Mothers with active HSV: isolate during the hospital stay. If labial, wear a face mask when feeding or handling their infant and apply acyclovir to the lesion. If genital, careful handwashing emphasized.

Controversial: exclude care staff with active herpes lesions? Absolutely if a herpetic whitlow. Education in the prevention of primary genital herpes during pregnancy?

Management: Acyclovir 10 mg/kg 8-hourly for 14–21 days. Recurrence of infection in 1 - 2%, despite a full course, may lead to encephalitis.

2. *Cytomegalovirus*   A third of seropositive mothers shed the virus in their breast milk. Although over a half of their infants become infected they are asymptomatic, i.e. actively immunized!

3. *Hepatitis B*   See below and Infectious diseases.

2. Other important presentations and viruses to consider

i Symptoms within the neonatal period

- Coxsackie B: meningoencephalitis, carditis with shock, hepatitis.
- Parvovirus B19: transplacental passage is common (30%), miscarriage or stillborn hydrops probably rare.
- Polio: paralytic illness onset < 5 days, mortality 50%.
- Echovirus 11: responsible for some neonatal unit outbreaks. Jaundice with fulminant hepatitic failure, onset in first week.
- Varicella (VHZ)

  a. First trimester infection: skin scarring, muscle atrophy, mental retardation in 5%.
  b. Late pregnancy: clinical maternal chickenpox within 7 days of delivery (before or after) carries high risk of severe infection. Give infant anti–varicella-zoster IgG (VZIG) 250 mg, and acyclovir only if symptomatic.

ii No symptoms until after the neonatal period

  a. Hepatitis B: usually 'silent' becoming chronic, very occasionally fulminant hepatitis in infancy.
     Prevention: vaccination and specific IgG within 24 hours of birth, revaccination at 1 and 6 months.
  b. Human immunodeficiency virus (HIV): 25% become symptomatic, from 2–3 months onwards.

Further reading

Public Health Laboratory Service (1990) *TORCH Screening Reassessed.* 61, Colindale Avenue, London NW9 5DF

Whitley R, Arvin A, Prober C, Corey L (1991) Predictors of morbidity and mortality in neonates with herpes simplex infection. *New England Journal of Medicine*, **324**, 450–454

NEWBORN SEIZURES

Seizures are generally symptomatic in the newborn. In term infants perinatal hypoxia accounts for half, infection, hypoglycaemia and hypocalcaemia 12% each. The remainder are caused by congenital malformations, drug withdrawal, other metabolic disturbances, and idiopathic around the fifth day. Rarely, they may be familial.

Incidence

Clinically evident in 1% of all infants, 3% of admissions for intensive care.

Continuous EEG monitoring detects seizure activity in 25% of neonates with congenital malformations, hypoxia, sepsis, metabolic disturbance, or germinal layer haemorrhages, though less than half are overt.

History

1. Check maternal history for drugs, seizures in utero, and family for consanguinity, other neonates affected, e.g. inborn errors, recurrent fetal loss, or tuberous sclerosis.
2. Details of the labour and delivery for prematurity, difficulty, prolonged rupture, maternal pyrexia or vaginal discharge, water intoxication from syntocinon infusion.

Cause by time of onset

Day 1:   birth asphyxia and birth injury; hypoglycaemia; subarachnoid haemorrhage; congenital infection.
Day 2:   intracerebral bleed, hypoxia; hypoglycaemia.
Day 3:   hypocalcaemia (see later section); inborn errors (as milk intake builds up and placental dialysis effect ends).
Days 4–7:   hypogalcaemia, meningitis, drug withdrawl, fifth day fits (i.e. of unknow causation).

Clinical

Well organized symmetrical tonic–clonic seizures are rare.
Term infants commonly show:

• Focal or multifocal clonic seizures.

- 'Subtle' signs including facial jerks, sucking movements, abnormal eye movements, eyelid fluttering. These may be brainstem release phenomena from the inhibitory control of the forebrain.
- Abnormal tone in the trunk and limbs.
- Respiratory abnormalities: apnoea or rapid respiratory bursts.
- Tonic seizures in birth asphyxia, which carry a poor prognosis.

Prematures: tonic fits, apnoea commonly associated with them.

Organization of the brain accounts for the manifestations. The premature behaves at a brainstem level; the term infant has relatively mature temporal lobe function.

Differentiate from jitteriness, which is:

- Rhythmic, with equal amplitude and rate in both flexion and contraction.
- Stimulus sensitive, eased by relaxing the limb into the position of comfort.
- Has no facial involvement.

Clonic convulsive movements have a rapid and slow phase, and continue to push the examining hand away.

Investigation

The routine biochemistry and microbiology for a sick newborn, including CSF. US for malformations and germinal layer haemorrhages. EEGs are difficult to interpret, especially in prematures, but may be predictive.

Management

1. Hypoglycaemic seizure: glucose bolus 0.5 g/kg, followed by 10% glucose infusion to maintain blood glucose above 2.5 mmol/l.
2. Hypocalcaemic seizures temporarily respond to i.v. 10% calcium gluconate. Best is 0.1 ml/kg of 50% magnesium sulphate im.
3. Status epilepticus: diazepam 0.5 mg/kg i.v. If unresponsive paraldehyde 0.1 mg/kg i.m. or rectally 50:50 with arachis oil.
4. Frequent seizures:
    i Phenobarbitone 20 mg/kg loading dose, followed by 5 mg/kg/24 h.
    ii Clonazepam 0.25 mg/kg loading dose, followed by an infusion of 0.1 mg/kg/day.
    iii Phenytoin 15–20 mg/kg i.v. may give superior control with less respiratory and neurological depression, but interfere with cerebellar development.
5. Pyridoxine 100 mg i.v. is worthy of trial if no other cause is found. Confirm by administering concurrently with EEG to demonstrate ablation of epileptiform pattern.
6. Treat the underlying cause.

Duration of anticonvulsive therapy

1. If neurological intact and seizure free: discontinue within the neonatal period.
2. Persistent neurological signs but seizure free: EEG helpful at 3–6 months to decide whether to continue.

3. Cerebral malformations: continue as 80% chance of recurrence.

Prognosis

The cause determines prognosis. If none is found 60% are normal. Early onset and prolonged seizures have a poorer outcome.

Birth asphyxia, severe intracerebral bleeds and meningitis 30–50% mortality, >50% have severe handicap.

Drug withdrawal, hypoglycaemia and hypocalcaemia, and the rare pyridoxine dependency, each has a good prognosis if identified and treated rapidly.

Further reading

Leader (1989) Neonatal seizures. *Lancet*, ii, 135–137

Maternal narcotic addiction

Drugs: heroin, methadone (maintenance treatment while 'coming off' heroin), alcohol, phenobarbitone, benzodiazepines, codeine etc.

Pregnancy is 'at risk' because

1. Poor antenatal care compliance is common.
2. Complications increased: toxaemia, premature rupture of membranes, sexually transmitted disease, breech, cord prolapse, stillbirth.
3. Fetal complications: more likely to be premature or small for dates with opiates. Alcohol and phenobarbitone are both associated with an increased risk of congenital abnormalities.

Clinical signs

Onset within 2 days, occasionally up to 4–6 weeks.

Likelihood of symptoms is dependent on the amount and duration of drug taking, e.g. heroin – half affected, increasing to three quarters if taken >1 year, and more severe if the last dose <1 day before delivery.

Less respiratory distress syndrome and jaundice due to enzyme induction.

Presentation

1. CNS: 'hyper' (activity, reflexes, tone, cry, yawn, tremor), seizures (10–20% of methadone babes), myoclonic jerks, disturbed feeding and sleep behaviours.
2. Respiratory: tachypnoea, aspiration syndromes, apnoea.
3. Autonomic (with opiates): temperature, diarrhoea, vomiting, tachycardia, sneezing, 'snuffles', tears, colour changes.

Management

Naloxone may cause acute withdrawal and is contraindicated for respiratory depression at delivery.

1. Supportive: swaddle, frequent feeds, i.v. fluids if vomiting.
2. Medication:

    i Opiates: morphine or paregoric (preferred in USA).
    ii Sedation: phenobarbitone or chlorpromazine (UK).

   Weaning off within 5–15 days, exceptionally up to 6 weeks.
3. Social: starts before delivery. Encourage cooperation with social services.
   Consider a child protection plan and arrange a meeting of hospital and community support (staff of the drug dependency unit, social worker, health visitor, general practitioner etc.) when the pregnancy is notified, and before discharge.
   Increased risk of family break up, death of parent, child abuse.
4. Follow up: supervision of weaning off drugs, looking for failure to thrive and possible developmental delay. Risk of sudden unexplained death is increased.

Further reading

Williams M J H (1990) Infants of drug dependent mothers. In *Recent Advances in Paediatrics* vol. 9, ed T J David Edinburgh:Churchill Livingstone, pp109–122

JAUNDICE

Clinical jaundice = serum bilirubin >100 μmol/l (6 mg/dl).

Incidence

1.Unconjugated

    i   Physiological, seen in 50% of term infants, 85% of prematures.
    ii Breast milk jaundice in 2.5% of healthy term infants.
    iii By contrast, severe rhesus isoimmunization now occurs only 1 in 6000 pregnancies. ABO is now a relatively more common cause, but is rarely severe.

2. Conjugated in infancy

Abnormal if >20–40 μmol/l (1–2 mg/100 ml).

    i   Early neonatal: congenital infection, galactosaemia or inspissated bile from severe haemolytic disease.
    ii Late neonatal and first few months: neonatal hepatitis syndrome, 1 in 3000, biliary atresia 1 in 10000. Rarer still is α-antitrypsin deficiency, for although the incidence is 1 in 5000 only 10% develop liver disease.

Pathophysiology

Abnormality in the production, isomerization and excretion of bilirubin.

1. Breakdown of haem in the reticuloendothelial system

    i   75% comes from old red blood cells (RBCs).

ii 25% comes from bone marrow haem not incorporated into RBCs plus haem proteins broken down to unconjugated bilirubin by haem oxygenase (HO) and cytochrome haem.

The enzyme HO can be inhibited by tin protoporphyrin (TPP), and the haem then excreted in bile. TPP works in ABO incompatibility in term infants, and may have a prophylactic role in sick prematures.

1g Hb = 600 µmol (35 mg) unconjugated bilirubin. In the healthy newborn 0.5 g Hb is broken down each day.

More RBCs are broken down if polycythaemic (small for dates, infants of diabetic mothers, delayed cord clamping) or extensive bruising is present.

2. Bilirubin toxicity

Unconjugated bilirubin is fat soluble and when transported in serum, bound to albumin, it is safe. When the albumin binding capacity is exceeded, the free fraction (not albumin bound) of unconjugated bilirubin may cross the blood–brain barrier to cause kernicterus. The basal ganglia become bilirubin stained. The infant is initially hypotonic and lethargic, develops opisthotonus and fits. Death ensues in 50% of those affected. Survivors suffer dyskinetic cerebral palsy, sunset eyes sign, mental handicap and high frequency deafness.

Phototherapy works by light energy isomerizing unconjugated bilirubin to a more water soluble product, which passes through the liver rapidly.

Symptomatic levels associated with kernicterus:

i   Term: 425–510 µmol/l (25–30 mg/dl).
ii Rhesus: 340–425 µmol/l (20–25 mg/dl).
iii Preterm 'low-bilirubin kernicterus' may be asymptomatic, and found only at necropsy, at levels as low as 170 µmol/l (10 mg/dl). It is probably related to injury to the blood–brain barrier, allowing albumin to cross and stain the basal ganglia and cerebral cortex.

Controversy: developmental impairment and bilirubin levels below those causing kernicterus. Persistent abnormalities in behaviour and electrophysiological function have not been consistently found.

Thus, the precise level of bilirubin at which brain damage occurs is unknown, but risk factors include:

i   Less than 2 weeks old.
ii Increasing prematurity.
iii Bilirubin displacement from albumin by acidosis, asphyxia, infection, low albumin, hypoglycaemia, hypothermia, drugs, (e.g. i.v. diazepam, sulphonamides).
iv Excessive haemolysis in ABO/Rhesus incompatibility, glucose 6–phosphate dehydrogenase deficiency, septicaemia, congenital spherocytosis.

3. Intrahepatic abnormalities in biliary metabolism

Cytoplasmic ligands complex with unconjugated bilirubin, enabling the enzyme glucuronyl transferase to conjugate it with glucuronic acid to water soluble, conjugated bilirubin.

   i Unconjugated hyperbilirubinaemia is due to:

      a. Immaturity of enzyme in prematures and many term infants, and in hypothyroidism.

      b. Hypoglycaemia and hypoxia both decrease the efficiency of the enzyme glucuronyl transferase (GT).

      c. GT is inhibited in breast milk jaundice, possibly by 3-α 20-β pregnanediol?

      d. Absent or reduced GT enzyme activity in Crigler-Najjar syndrome (AR) type I and II respectively, probably also in Gilbert syndrome which affects 6% of the adult population and becomes manifest when fasting or stressed.

   ii Both unconjugated and conjugated hyperbilirubinaemia in:

      a. Metabolic disease causing liver damage: α-1-antitrypsin deficiency, cystic fibrosis, galactosaemia, fructosaemia.

      b. Urinary tract infection (mechanism unknown).

   iii Conjugated hyperbilirubinaemia
   Failure of cellular excretion: with normal liver function tests, in Dubin-Johnson and Rotor syndrome (both AR).

4. Biliary obstruction through inflammation or structural abnormality

Bilirubin glucuronide is converted to stercobilin or broken down by bacteria in the gut to free bilirubin and reabsobed via the enterohepatic circulation.

   In obstruction, the liver function tests and bilirubin are abnormal, as in 3 ii. Only further tests can distinguish between them all.

   i Reduced conjugation and excretion. The commonest causes of persistent conjugated hyperbilirubinaemia are both probably caused by reovirus 3 infection.

      a. Neonatal hepatitis syndrome. Differentiate from cytomegalovirus, herpes, coxsackie B, syphilis and toxoplasmosis by serology.

      b. Biliary atresia.[131I] Rose Bengal and [99mTc] Disida scan to differentiate from neonatal hepatitis (see below).

   ii Obstruction: choledochal cyst.

   iii Parenteral nutrition (due to periportal inflammation?).

   iv Inspissated bile from severe haemolysis, e.g. rhesus incompatibility.

5. Delayed passage of meconium

Allows greater reabsorption of bilirubin via the enterohepatic circulation, e.g. prematurity, prolonged bowel transit time in obstruction, and in pyloric stenosis.

Indications for investigation (Table 2.21)

1. Clinical jaundice:

    i   Early onset <24 h old.
    ii Sick infant of any age.
    iii Persistent, i.e. for >1 week at term, >2 weeks if premature.

2. Biochemical jaundice

    i   Rising >85 µmol/l (5 mg/dl) per day in serum, or 17 µmol/l per hour in a sick or premature infant.
    ii Conjugated serum bilirubin >25 µmol/l (1.5 mg/dl) or bilirubinuria on 'Combistix' testing.
          Conjugated hyperbilirubinaemia >40 µmol/l (2 mg/dl) is always pathological.
    iii Total serum bilirubin >300 µmol/l (18 mg/dl) in a term infant aged 3–5 days, and in a premature infant at 200 to 250 µmol/l (12–15 mg/dl), taking gestational age into account.

Clinical approach

1. Family history of an affected parent (spherocytosis) or sibling: e.g. ABO, Rhesus; breast milk jaundice has a 25% recurrence; glucose-6-phosphate deficiency (XL) in a brother; possibly Gilbert syndrome (AD).
2. Pregnancy complications:

    i   Infections: toxoplasmosis, rubella, cytomegalovirus, syphilis.
    ii Gestational or established diabetes.
    iii Hypertension causing a small for dates baby.

3. Labour resulting in operative delivery, extensive bruising. Oxytocin may be a factor.
4. Examination:

    i   General: bruising, cephalhaematoma, pallor or polycythaemia; infection especially umbilical; distended abdomen or delayed passage of meconium; hepatosplenomegaly.
    ii Behaviour: often lethargic, poor feeding.
          Rarely, rigidity, cerebral cry, apnoeas, opisthotonus and fits = kernicterus.
    iii Look for syndromic features:

        a. intrauterine infection, e.g. microcephaly, cataracts, purpura, hepatosplenomegaly.
        b. Down's syndrome.
        c. Alagille syndrome (chromosome 20 partial deletion) = bile duct hypoplasia, pointed chin, vertebral, heart and eye anomalies.

    iv Excreta:

        a. urine: clear/yellow if unconjugated; dark from bilirubinuria in conjugated obstructive jaundice (if presence is confirmed by urine dipstick it must be investigated).

b. acholic stools are proportional to the degree of biliary atresia/obstruction, and develop after a few weeks.

Table 2.21 Day of onset of jaundice and appropriate investigation

Age	Cause	Investigation
Day 1–2	1 Rhesus, ABO 2 Congenital infection 3 Spherocytosis	Haemoglobin, PCV, reticulocyte count, blood film, mother and baby's blood group direct Coombs' test, septic screen. Extended TORCH screen if conjugated hyperbilirubinaemia found. If indicated do parents' film, osmotic fragility
Day 2–5	1 Physiological 2 Infection 3 Extravisated 4 G-6-P-D 5 Spherocytosis	As above, excluding reticulocyte count unless pallor is present. Septic screen, excluding lumbar puncture unless specifically indicated. G-6-P-D blood test. Do pyruvate kinase level if haemolytic and all other tests are negative.
Day 6–10	1 Infection 2 Breast milk jaundice 3 Hypothyroid 4 Galactosaemia	Septic screen, thyroid function, liver enzymes to exclude hepatitis, urinary reducing substances (Clinitest) for galactosaemia. NB Galactosaemia and infection may be present together; Clinitest is not reliable, so if likely, do galactose-1-phosphate uridyl transferase level
Day 11+	1 Neonatal hepatitis 2 Biliary atresia 3 Choledochal cyst 4 Urinary tract infection 5 Alpha-1-anti trypsin 6 Tyrosinaemia 7 Fructosaemia	If bilirubin is mainly conjugated: TORCH screen. Blood for liver function, alpha-1-antitrypsin phenotype, galactosaemia. Urine: Clinitest, urine culture. Sweat test. US of abdomen for choledocal cyst and biliary tree appearance. To differentiate 1 from 2: (i) [^{131}I]Rose Bengal and [^{99m}Tc] Disida scan: <10% of dose excreted in urine = obstruction. (ii) Liver biopsy: the histological pattern has an 80% concordance with findings at laparotomy of hepatitis or obstruction. 6 requires blood and urine amino acid chromatogram and sugars. DNA probe for 7, as the loading test is dangerous.

Management

1. Adequate fluid and caloric intake to prevent worsening jaundice.
2. Unconjugated hyperbilirubinaemia
   Bilirubin 'action' charts combine gestation, weight and age in days to determine when phototherapy or exchange is indicated.

   i Phototherapy. Blue light (450 nm) is most effective, usually mixed with white.

Indications:

    a. Immediately after birth if rhesus isoimmunized.
    b. Bilirubin rising rapidly, or premature.
    c. Very low birthweight and sick, serum bilirubin >100 μmol/l (6 mg/dl).
    d. Healthy term infants: wait until 50–100 μmol/l (3–6 mg/dl) below the exchange level, i.e. at 350 μmol/l.

       Rebound rise on stopping phototherapy is common.

       Extra water is given to replace increased losses via stool (very loose, frequent, green and frothy), and the skin (vasodilation and increased blood flow).

  ii *Exchange transfusion* for urgent reduction, especially rhesus isoimmunization.

Indications:

    a. Haemolysis: rising serum bilirubin level at >17 μmol/l (1 mg/dl) per hour or cord blood bilirubin >100 μmol/l (6 mg/dl).
    b. Well infant: two crude guides applicable after 30 weeks
       Gestational age + 0, e.g.36 weeks = 360 μmol/l (21 mg/dl).
       By weight: <1 kg = 170 μmol/l (10 mg/dl), 1.5 kg = 250 μmol/l (15 mg/dl), 2.5 kg = 300 μmol/l (17 mg/dl).

Safe exchange level is reduced by (i) acidosis (ii) hypoglycaemia (iii) Septicaemia, by 50 μmol/l for each factor.

       Use rhesus negative blood ABO compatible with mother's blood, CMV negative, less than 5 days old, warmed carefully to 37°C. Twice blood volume exchange (180 ml/kg) replaces 90% of fetal cells.

       Often combined with phototherapy before and after exchange.

       Late anaemia. Persistent haemolysis for 6–8 weeks can lead to severe anaemia, usually when phototherapy prevents an exchange.

       Complications of exchange include:

  i Vascular: air/blood clot emboli, thrombosis leading eventually to portal hypertension, or necrotizing enterocolitis.
  ii Cardiac failure, arrhythmias.
  iii Metabolic: hypoglycaemia, hypocalcaemia, hyperkalaemia, acidosis.
  iv Infection: bacterial, viral, e.g. CMV (prevent by ensuring blood is screened).

3. Conjugated hyperbilirubinaemia due to obstruction

  i Laparotomy/Kasai drainage operation for biliary atresia. Majority have no external biliary tree to connect to the bowel, so a portoenterostomy is made. Ascending infection is common postoperatively.

    Prognosis: Death within a year without surgery. 80% become jaundice free if operated on by 60 days. They have a 90% 5 year survival. Success rapidly diminishes if operation is delayed. Liver transplant for treatment failures: 60% + survival a year later.

  ii Infants with neonatal hepatitis syndrome do badly after laparotomy, so supportive histology and excretion tests are essential preoperatively.

    Prognosis is otherwise moderately good: 7% mortality, 90% recovering normal liver function by a year. A few develop cirrhosis with ascites, some have learning disorders.

iii α-1 antitrypsin deficiency: no specific treatment, but as long as cholestasis persists, give Pregestimil, daily oral vitamins A 5000 IU, D up to 10000 IU, E 100 mg, K 5mg.

Prognosis: 25% each are normal, have a biochemical liver abnormality, cirrhosis in childhood, or are dead from cirrhosis by adult life. Transplant is curative. Antenatal diagnosis of the abnormal PiZZ phenotype allows selective termination.

BLOOD GROUP INCOMPATIBILITY AND HAEMOLYSIS IN THE FETUS

Pathophysiology of Rhesus isoimmunization

Rhesus(Rh) blood group antigens comprise three pairs, Ce, Dd, Ee; D is the most important as it is the most potent. To be Rh positive, as 87% of Caucasians are, is a dominant character. About 50% are heterozygote. If father is heterozygote (Dd) and mother Rh negative (dd) there is a 1:2 risk of isoimmunization.

Transplacental feto-maternal bleeding, which occurs during most normal pregnancies, (and may induce mild Rh disease even in a first pregnancy in 5%), but particularly at delivery, is the main cause of isoimmunization (Table 2.22)

Fetal rhesus D positive cells cross to the maternal circulation and provoke an IgG antibody response if she is rhesus negative, unless fetal cells are quickly removed from the maternal circulation due to ABO incompatibility.

In the next Rh incompatible pregnancy a small bleed (as little as <1 ml!) can cause a large IgG response. These antibodies cross the placental barrier and attach to fetal red cells (the basis of the direct Coombs' test) which are then destroyed by the fetus' own reticuloendothelial system (Table 2.23). Erythropoeisis in the liver increases. Reticulocytosis, anaemia, and ascites with hypoalbuminaemia develop.

Pathophysiology of ABO incompatibility

Usually the mother is group O with naturally occuring IgG A and B haemolysins, reacting with blood group A or B fetal red cells.

Table 2.22 Blood group , frequency and timing of affected pregnancies

Group	Frequency of affected pregnancy	Time of first manifestation
Rhesus	5% of ABO compatible = 1 in 80 of all pregnancies	After sensitization, previous pregnancy termination, blood transfusion
ABO	1 in 20 of all pregnancies, but most are very mild and clinically insignificant	First pregnancy, baby group A or B

Table 2.23 Blood group, Coombs' test and severity

Blood group antigens	Coombs' test	Severity of haemolysis
Rhesus D, as C*D*e or c*D*E, is the commonest	Direct +++	Mild 50%, moderate/severe 30% stillbirth/hydrops 20%
ABO	Direct + or Indirect +/++	Mild/moderate Hydrops does not occur
Duffy, Kell	Indirect +	Mild usually, but rarely hydrops does occur

Management of pregnancy

1. Maternal anti D antibody levels (>1 µg/ml), or titres, at booking, and 28, 32, 36 weeks' gestation. Regular antibody estimation is needed, once it is detected, to identify a rise indicating a worsening of the haemolytic process.
2. Amniocentesis for rising antibody or previously severely affected infants from 24 to 26 weeks.
3. Liley chart to assess the optical density of the liquor at 450 nm, the bilirubin band, compared with normal liquor. Action accordingly: intrauterine transfusion, deliver prematurely or at term.

At delivery

1. Immediate exchange if hydropic or Hb <8 g/dl.
2. Early exchange, by 6 h, if cord bilirubin >85 µmol/l (5 mg/dl) and/or Hb <11g/dl, or bilirubin is rising at >17 µmol/l (1 mg/dl) per hour.

Severely affected/hydropic infant's special problems.

1. Hypoglycaemia secondary to pancreatic hypertrophy.
2. Hypoalbuminaemia may need correction pre-exchange, to reduce free unconjugated bilirubin and so the risk of kernicterus. Disseminated intravascular coagulation is common, and needs blood product support.
3. Cardiac failure helped by diuretics but monitor for hypovolaemia.
4. Respiratory failure due to respiratory distress syndrome, anaemia, ascites, cardiac failure.

Causes of hydrops

Unknown in 50%, others include:

1. Anaemia: Rhesus, fetal alpha thalassaemia, bleed into mother or twin.
2. Parvovirus B19 infection.
3. Cardiac failure: cardiac arrhythmias and congenital malformations, placental venous thromboses and angiomata.
4. Hypoproteinaemia: congenital infection or nephrotic syndrome.
5. Chromosomal: Turner's syndrome, trisomy 13, 18.

Prognosis: Death in 65% or more, despite intensive resuscitation.

Prevention of rhesus isoimmunization

Anti-D globulin (100 µg) is given to all Rh negative women for

1. Fetal loss: spontaneous or therapeutic termination.
2. Manoeuvres: amniocentesis, external cephalic version.
3. Antepartum haemorrhage.

Further reading

Newman T B, Maisels M J (1990) Does hyperbilirubinaemia damage the brain of healthy full-term infants? *Clinics in Perinatology*, **17**, 331–358

Hussein M, Howard E R, Mieli-Vergani G, Mowat A P (1991) Jaundice at 14 days of age: exclude biliary atresia. *Archives of Disease in Childhood*, **66**, 1177–1179

CARDIAC PROBLEMS

(Individual conditions discussed in cardiology).
Antecedent factors include family history, infection (rubella), drugs and alcohol in pregnancy, maternal diabetes.

Commonest cardiac causes of severe distress in the first week of life

1. Hypoplastic left heart syndrome.
2. Transposition of the great arteries.
3. Coarctation of the aorta syndrome.
4. Multiple major cardiac defects.
   Other congenital anomalies are frequently present, examples:

1. Chromosomal: trisomy 21 (ventriculoseptal defect, atrioventricular canal), Turner's syndrome (coarctation of the aorta, aortic stenosis).
2. Characteristic facies: Smith-Lemli-Opitz (VSD, PDA), de Lange syndrome (VSD, Fallot's tetralogy).
3. Limb abnormalities: Ellis-van Crefeld (ASD, single atrium), TAR = thrombocytopenia-absent radius (ASD, Fallot's tetralogy).

Presentations are of three main types: cyanosis, heart failure, shock

1. Cyanosis

Cardiac causes

Transposition of the great arteries, atresia or severe stenosis of pulmonary or tricuspid valve, total anomalous pulmonary venous connection (TAPVC) with obstructed venous return.

Differential diagnosis

1. Central cyanosis abolished by breathing 90% oxygen for 10 minutes (basis of hyperoxia test) is indicative of pulmonary disease, confirmed on X-ray (Table 2.24).

    Persistent pulmonary hypertension (persistent fetal circulation) cannot be distinguished from CHD clinically, or necessarily by the hyperoxia test. Perinatal asphyxia, meconium aspiration etc, with normal heart on ECG and chest X-ray support the diagnosis, echocardiogram confirms; see Cardiological problems.
2. Otherwise well baby: examples

    i Traumatic cyanosis due to cord compression around the neck.
    ii Polycythaemia with >5 g/dl desaturated Hb.
    iii Pigmented lips in dark skinned babies–the tongue is pink.

3. Airway obstruction: examples

    i Robin sequence: micrognathia and cleft palate.
    ii Choanal atresia: inability to pass nasal catheter.

4. Shocked due to sepsis, metabolic acidosis from inborn error, or asphyxial birth causing myocardial ischaemia.
5. Asphyxia/injury/bleed affecting the brain, manifest through seizure, cyanosis, hypoglycaemia, hypothermia, autonomic disturbance.

Table 2.24 Identification of likely lesion in cyanotic CHD from the chest X-ray and ECG

Chest X-ray

1. Decreased pulmonary vascularity	*2. Normal/increased pulmonary vascularity +*
i ECG: right ventricular hypertrophy	*normal heart shadow + normal ECG*
a. Pulmonary stenosis + VSD	Transposition of great arteries (TGA)
b. Fallot's tetralogy	
ii ECG: left ventricular hypertrophy	*3. Increased pulmonary vascularity*
a. Pulmonary atresia with intact septum	i ECG right ventricular hypertrophy
b. Tricuspid atresia	Total anomalous pulmonary venous
iii ECG: right atrial hypertrophy	connection
Ebstein's anomaly	ii ECG normal/LVH
	a. TGA + ventriculoseptal defect
	b. Truncus arteriosus
	iii ECG normal/RVH
	Hypoplastic left heart syndrome

Management

1. Prostaglandin E_1 infusion while definitive investigations continue. Oral prostaglandin will maintain ductus arteriosus patency while awaiting palliative shunt, e.g. for pulmonary or tricuspid atresia.
2. Correct metabolic acidosis.
3. May require IPPV and tolazoline or intrapulmonary artery prostaglandin I_2 for persistent pulmonary hypertension, as a disease entity, or complicating underlying CHD.
4. Balloon atrial septostomy to improve mixing in transposition of the great arteries (TGA).

5. Operation:
   Urgent for total anomalous pulmonary venous connection.
   Definitive atrial "switch" operation in TGA may be done as a primary procedure, or a Mustard's operation later.
   Fallot's repair in late infancy.

2. Heart failure

Causes

   i Obstruction to left heart outflow, e.g. hypoplastic left heart, coarctation of the aorta syndrome, severe aortic stenosis.

  ii Multiple major heart defects: truncus arteriosus, arteriovenous canal, single ventricle, TAPVC and others.

 iii Hyperdynamic, through shunt, as pulmonary resistance falls: large ventricular septal defect and patent ductus arteriosus (PDA). Other than prematures in the first week with PDA associated with fluid overload and RDS, the onset of failure is usually after the neonatal period.

Symptoms and signs

- Excessive weight gain >30 g (1 oz) per day despite poor feeding.
- Tiring during feeds is characteristic.
- Tachycardia >180/min.
- Respiratory rate >60/min.
- Barking cough, sweating, wheeze and fine crackles with left ventricular failure.
- Liver enlargement, +/- sacral oedema, in right heart failure.

Differentiate from other causes

1. Pulmonary disease: RDS, meconium aspiration, pneumonia, transient tachypnoea of the newborn.
2. Sepsis, metabolic acidosis, asphyxial brain injury.
3. Hydrops due to anaemia (rhesus, α-thalassaemia), hypoproteinaemia (infection, nephrotic syndrome) or severe cardiac tachy/brady arrhythmias.
4. Cardiac: arrhythmias, myocarditis. Always auscultate the head for a bruit, suggestive of an arteriovenous malformation.

Investigations

1. ECG and chest X-ray characteristics of CHD sought (Table 2.25). Look for evidence of an arrhythmia, or potential for it, e.g. delta wave; ST-T wave changes are seen and creatine phosphokinase requested if myocardial damage is suspected, usually due to asphyxia or coxsackie B infection.
2. Sepsis: acute phase reactants, WBC total and a ratio of >0.2 immature:total neutrophils, help determine the need for antibiotics after a septic screen is done. However, remember sepsis may also precipitate previously asymptomatic CHD.
3. Metabolic: severe metabolic acidosis is a feature of CHD, sepsis and inborn errors. Monitor for hypoglycaemia, a common association in these stressful con-

Lesion	Cyanosis	Heart failure	Heart shape	Pulmonary vascularity	Electrocardiogram
Pulmonary atresia with VSD	Severe	None		Reduced	RAD RVH
Pulmonary atresia with intact septum	Severe	Occurs when RV very small	Hollow pulmonary arc; uptilted apex	Reduced	Normal axis LVH or decreased right ventricular activity for age
Tricuspid atresia	Severe	None	RA +	Reduced	LAD LVH RAH
Tricuspid atresia with high pulmonary flow	Slight or moderate	Frequently	Square heart. RA + Pulmonary arc hollow	Increased	LAD LVH RAH
Severe pulmonary stenosis with ASD	Slight initially, gradually increasing	Rare in first month	RA + Pulmonary arc +	Reduced	RAH + + RVH
Ebstein's disease	Moderate	Rare in first month	Large RA	Reduced	RAH Right bundle branch block
Transposition with intact septum	Rapidly becomes severe	Second to fourth week	Large RA. Narrow pedicle Egg-shaped heart	Normal or increased	RVH

Condition	Cyanosis	Heart failure	Heart shape	Pulmonary vascularity	ECG
Total anomalous PVC with obstruction	Rapidly becomes severe	Liver enlarged if drainage below diaphragm	Normal size	Pulmonary venous congestion	RAH RVH
Hypoplasia of left heart	Slight at first, increasing by third day	First few days of life and is severe	General enlargement	Increased + pulmonary venous congestion	RVH RAD
Coarctation of aorta	Slight	In first week; left heart failure frequent	General enlargement	Increased + pulmonary venous congestion	RVH RAD
Truncus	Slight or moderate	In first few weeks	Pulmonary arteries high up or not seen	Increased	RVH but may be LVH or combination of RV + LV
Atrioventricular canal	None	In first few weeks	RA + PA + RV + LV +	Increased	LAD, rsR pattern in $V_3R + V_1$. Usually combined ventricular hypertrophy
Normal heart with enlarged thymus	None	None	Broad pedicle	Normal	Normal

ditions. Introduction of protein, or unusual smell, are helpful pointers to metabolic investigations.

4. Asphyxia: head US may show 'bright' echoes, consistent with oedema after asphyxia. History, low Apgar score and blood pressure are pointers.
5. Anaemia/hydrops: Hb, antibody levels, bilirubin, Hb electrophoresis.

Table 2.25 Identification of likely lesion in acyanotic CHD from chest X-ray and ECG

Chest X-ray

1. Normal pulmonary vascularity + normal heart
i ECG: normal/RVH
  Pulmonary valve stenosis
ii ECG: normal/LVH
  a Ventriculoseptal defect
  b Patent ductus arteriosus
  c Non-critical aortic stenosis
	2. Normal pulmonary vascularity + enlarged heart
	i ECG: normal/arrhythmia
	  a Paroxysmal tachycardia
	  b Heart block
	ii ECG: LVH
	  a Arteriovenous malformation
	  b Critical aortic stenosis

3 Increased pulmonary vascularity + enlarged heart
+ ECG: shows left axis deviation
Atrioventricular canal
	iii ECG: RVH
	  a Hypoplastic left heart syndrome
	  b Coarctation of the aorta syndrome
	iv ECG: RVH or LVH
	  a Atrioventricular valve incompetence
	  b Myocarditis
	  c Endocardial fibroelastosis

General management

(See Cardiology for detailed assessment and management of the individual conditions).

1. Congestive cardiac failure

   i Oxygen: beware of clinical worsening, due to closure of the ductus arteriosus, if either systemic or pulmonary circulation is ductus dependent.
   ii Maintain blood pressure.

     a. Packed cells if low Hb, albumin if hypovolaemic.
     b. Pressor agents dobutamine, dopamine increase systemic vascular resistance, reducing the right to left shunt.

  iii Frusemide in high flow states due to VSD, ASD, to reduce pulmonary and systemic venous congestion.
  iv Captopril or hydralazine cause vasodilatation and so reduce left ventricular after-load in VSD, PDA, and dilated congestive cardiomyopathies.
   v Digoxin in asphyxia or cardiomyopathy to improve efficiency. Contraindicated where heart is working maximally against obstruction, e.g. pulmonary stenosis, Fallot's tetralogy.
  vi Correct acidosis, glucose, calcium and other electrolyte abnormalities.
 vii Fluid restriction to 100–120 ml/kg/day is a short term measure only, otherwise inadequate calorie intake occurs.
     Drug dosages: see Cardiological problems.

2. Infection, often a precipitant, may require an antibiotic. Ribavirin has a role in respiratory syncitial virus infections complicated by heart failure due to underlying CHD.
3. Ventilatory support for respiratory failure.
4. Management of individual lesions: see Patent ductus in Neonatal problems, others in Cardiology problems.

3. Shock

Clinical

Ill, greyish pallor, poor peripheral circulation, pulses weak, low BP. Laboured breathing, air hunger, floppy. May be a consequence of deteriorating heart failure, or arise de novo.

Differential diagnosis

Cardiac	Non-cardiac
Hypoplastic left heart	Sepsis
Coarctation of the aorta syndrome	Hypovolaemia due to fluid or blood loss
Heart failure (see above)	Asphyxia
Pericardal effusion	Inborn error
Pneumopericardium	

Investigations and differentiation of causes

1. History, ECG and chest X-ray for hypoplastic left heart and coarctation of the aorta are similar (both may be present). Lower BP in legs than arms identifies coarctation. Echocardiogram is essential; it will also determine other causes of heart failure, and the presence of a pericardial effusion.
2. Low haematocrit due to blood loss (allowing time for haemodilution), history of poor intake or excessive loss, elevated urea and creatinine, each point to hypovolaemia.
3. Other causes: sepsis, asphyxia, inborn errors, see above.

Asymptomatic murmurs indicative of underlying CHD

Murmurs shortly after birth are often related to duct closure.

1. An ejection systolic murmur radiating from left sternal edge to the pulmonary area may signify obstruction due to severe pulmonary stenosis or Fallot's tetralogy.
2. Short duration/pansystolic murmur. These, due to high flow systolic murmurs of VSD, PDA, appear later in the neonatal period as the pulmonary vascular resistance falls.
3. Palpate for wide pulse pressure of PDA, obtain upper and lower limb BP for coarctation of the aorta.

Management

Persistence beyond 48 h of a murmur grade 3/6 or more, especially if associated with a thrill, calls for investigation.

1. Inform parents of possible heart condition warranting ECG and chest X-ray.
2. Alert them to symptoms of heart disease, especially with feeding, to avoid delay in seeking medical help.
3. Echocardiography, and early cardiological referral (urgent if coarctation) if ECG or chest X-ray abnormal or symptoms appear.
4. Provided signs are unequivocally due to a simple, asymptomatic lesion, e.g. small VSD, pulmonary stenosis or a PDA, then non-cardiological follow-up may continue. Persistence beyond a year needs cardiological referral.

Innocent/functional murmur

Intensity grade 1–2/6, usually over lower left of precordium, vibratory and low pitched. Reassure parents. If it fails to disappear after a few days, observe, review until satisfied as to its benign nature.

HAEMATOLOGICAL PROBLEMS

Normal Hb, reticulocyte and white blood cell (WBC) indices:

	At birth	*Age at lowest values*
1 Hb (g/dl)		
Term	17 +/– 3	9–11 at 6–8 weeks
Prematures	15 +/– 2	7–8 at 4–6 weeks in VLBW
2 Reticulocytes (%)	3–7	1% or less by day 7
3 WBC ($\times 10^9$/l)	9–36	Neutrophils 60% in the first week, thereafter lymphocytes predominate until mid-childhood

Anaemia at birth

1. Revealed: placenta praevia, cord rupture.
2. Concealed:

Acute

   i   Feto-maternal bleed (a few millilitres is common, and up to 20% of circulating blood volume in 1% of newborn).

   ii Feto-placental: lost from baby → placenta if baby held above uterus before clamping, or cord is tightly wound round the neck, preventing venous return to the fetus.

Chronic

   i   Feto-fetal in monozygotic twins is common and recognized by >5 g/dl difference between them.

ii Haemolytic disease, e.g. rhesus.

iii Feto-maternal.

3. Infant: internal into presenting part, e.g. breech → buttocks, or vertex →subaponeurotic. Also trauma → organ rupture, e.g. intracranial, liver, adrenal.

Clinical

Acute salient features: *pallor*, air hunger, shock or hypotensive, tachycardia.

In chronic loss, may have adapted to a degree, +/– hepatosplenomegaly due to extramedullary erythropoiesis. Hydrops due to heart failure is a bad prognostic sign.

Management

1. Oxygen, and IPPV if necessary.
2. Arterial line, blood for Hb, haematocrit, group and Coombs' test, bilirubin, cross-match. Do coagulation tests if oozing at puncture sites.
3. Transfuse 20 ml/kg over half an hour of albumin or if very severe, O negative blood. Continue until the BP is stable.
4. Save placenta and cord for careful inspection, do a Kleihauer test on maternal blood film (maternal cells 'ghost', while fetal cells remain intact in acid medium). Check Hb: it takes 3–6 hours to haemodilute after a fresh bleed, but in a sick infant do not delay treatment to confirm this.

Progressive anaemia in the newborn period

1. Iatrogenic: keep a record of blood volumes taken.
2. Unexplained sudden fall = acute bleed, causes include:

   i Vascular, e.g. intracerebral, arteriovenous malformation.

   ii Coagulation disorder: haemorrhagic disease of the newborn, consumption coagulopathy.

3. Progressive fall >1.5 g/dl per week: haemolysis or occult bleeding.
4. Dilutional and nutritional anaemias appear towards the end of the neonatal period (Table 2.26).

Management

Maintain Hb of sick infants >13–14 g/dl by transfusion.

Identify site of acute bleed clinically or by US of the head and trunk. Blood tests as for acute anaemia, treating as results dictate.

Late onset anaemia.

Table 2.26 Time of onset and likely aetiology of late onset anaemia

4–6 weeks: Early dilutional anaemia of prematurity
6–8 weeks: Physiological anaemia (nadir of RBC production)
6–10 weeks: Vitamin E deficient haemolytic anaemia
8–12 weeks: Folic acid, copper deficiency } in ELBW/VLBW
9–12 months: Iron deficiency (especially premature infants)

Pathophysiology of late anaemias of infancy

1. Physiological anaemia

   i Fetal RBC survival shorter than adult RBCs.
  ii Lower haemoglobin mass needed to carry the oxygen requirements ex utero as saturation is higher.
 iii Erythropoietin levels fall and moderate tissue hypoxaemia has to develop before juxtaglomerular cells produce it.

2. Anaemia of prematurity

   i Rapid somatic growth with same haemoglobin mass, so a dilution occurs.
  ii Iatrogenic.

3. Nutritional anaemias

   i Iron: present mainly in circulating haemoglobin, stored as initially high Hb falls, enough until weaning, i.e. 6–9 months. The low Hb mass in the premature (or after blood loss) is rapidly exhausted. Classically the exclusively milkfed premature presents at 9–18 months with irritability, failure to thrive, pallor, tachycardia, systolic murmur and splenomegaly.
  ii Folic acid: megaloblastic anaemia is possible as infants' requirements are many times adults'.
 iii Vitamin E: normocytic, raised reticulocyte and platelet count. May have periorbital, labial or scrotal oedema.
 iv Copper: iron deficiency indices with neutropenia in a premature infant given total parenteral nutrition. Low serum copper or caeruloplasmin diagnostic. X-ray changes are unlikely to be confused with child abuse, see Community problems.

4. Rhesus isoimmunized infants

Those not exchanged at birth continue to haemolyse. Check for anaemia every 1–2 weeks for the first 8 weeks of life. Transfuse if symptomatic.

Management

1. Supplements for all VLBW infants: iron 2–4 mg/kg/day, folic acid 5 mg, vitamin E 50 mg daily from the fourth week of life.
2. Blood transfusion at 1–3 months old for anaemia of prematurity. Indications: tachycardia, tachypnoea, episodes of apnoea or bradycardia, lethargy, poor weight gain, (usually present at 7–8 g/dl). If reticulocytes >5%, delay, to avoid transfusion and further suppression of the bone marrow. Give semi packed cells, 20 ml/kg or calculate needs from the formula:

    Volume required = (Hb desired - Hb actual) × wt in kg × 4

    CMV negative blood should be used, otherwise up to 20% of recipients become infected.
3. Synthetic erythropoietin for anaemia of prematurity, as well as in renal failure, shows promise.

Bleeding

1. Haematemesis and melaena

Haematemesis

1 Coffee grounds:
   i Gastritis
   ii Swallowed maternal blood
   iii Local trauma: nasogastric tube
   iv Stress ulcer
   v Drugs: indomethacin, tolazoline
2 Profuse:
   i Bleeding disorders–DIC, NEC, haemorrhagic disease of the newborn
   ii Severe acid ulceration, Meckel's diverticulum

Melaena

1 Profuse:
   i Disseminated intravascular coagulation (DIC)
   ii Necrotizing enterocolitis (NEC)
   iii Haemorrhagic disease of the newborn
   iv Swallowed maternal blood

2 Streaking: local trauma

3 With mucous: infection

Likely site by clinical state and amount of blood present

1. Well, usually streaks or coffee grounds.

    i First day, swallowed maternal blood likely (occasionally profuse).
    ii Otherwise: gastritis, local trauma, haemorrhagic disease of the newborn likely.

2. Sick, usually profuse: necrotizing enterocolitis, disseminated intravascular coagulation (DIC), severe acid ulceration.
3. Bleeding from other sites: DIC, haemorrhagic disease of the newborn.

Management

1. Initial assessment.

    i   Has vitamin K been given? If a sick premature have indomethacin or tolazoline been given (both increase bleeding tendency)?
    ii Investigate Hb, platelets, coagulation status unless simply swallowed maternal blood, mild gastritis/oesophagitis or local trauma.

2. Observation only.

    i   Maternal blood: infant <7 days old. Differentiate swallowed blood by Apt's test: mix 5 parts water with 1 part infant's vomit/stool. Centrifuge, then add 1ml 1% sodium hydroxide to 4 ml supernatant. Pink = HbF, yellow-brown = maternal HbA.
    ii Gastritis: a few 'coffee grounds' in vomit in a well infant, said to be due to swallowed debris during delivery and eased by gentle stomach irrigation.
    iii Trauma: upper GI tract from feeding tubes and airways; or perianal, e.g. hard stool, thermometer (stop rectal temperature taking). Usually transient.

3. May require active resuscitation if active bleeding or hypotension present.

    i   Acid ulceration: usually well with oesophagitis; blood loss may be significant in stress ulcer, acid secreting mucosa in bowel duplication or Meckel's diverticulum, resulting in shock. Barium studies, ^{99m}Tc scan for acid secreting tissue. H_2 blocker, e.g. cimetidine, reduces acid secretion.
    ii Abdominal distension: necrotizing enterocolitis or volvulus; plain X-ray is usually diagnostic.
    iii Bleeding disorder: see 2 below.

2. Bleeding disorders

Bruising, purpura, oozing from puncture sites. Due to low platelets, lack of, or consumption of, coagulation factors, or capillary abnormality.

Normal values

1. Platelet count: as for older ages, abnormal <150 × 10^9/l.
2. Tests of coagulation: in prematures the partial thromboplastin time (PTT) is up to twice the adult norm; the range for prothrombin time, fibrinogen and fibrin degradation products is similar to term and older infants.
3. Coagulation factor levels are 25% of adult values.

History

1. Family and pregnancy history for:

    i   Inherited bleeding tendency, e.g. haemophilia, hereditary protein C deficiency.
    ii Maternal drugs depress vitamin K dependent factors: anticonvulsants, coumarin anticoagulants. Heparin does not pass the placental barrier.
    iii Maternal immune thrombocytopenia (ITP): by passive transfer of IgG. The level of IgG antibodies and platelets are prognostic factors. Maternal systemic lupus erythematosus presents similarly.

iv Maternal platelet alloantibody (like Rhesus), usually against platelet antigen 1. Can occur in the firstborn. Management is corticosteroids to mother in the last 2 weeks before elective delivery, check fetal platelets and deliver by caesarian section if <50 × 10⁹/l.
v Maternal infection: congenital CMV, rubella, toxoplasmosis.

2. Delivery: traumatic, asphyxiated, premature, prolonged rupture of membranes.

Clinical approach

1. Well or sick?

Well
i Inherited deficiency: haemophilia, protein C deficiency
ii Maternal thrombocytopenia or alloantibody
iii Haemorrhagic disease: breast fed, maternal anticonvulsants
iv Vascular malformation bleed, and severe liver disease
v Bone marrow infiltration/abnormality

Sick
i Consumption coagulopathy; cold, hypoxia, acidosis, sepsis
ii Vascular injury; ventricular bleed
iii Mechanical platelet injury (in NEC, renal vein thrombosis, Kasabach-Merritt giant haemangioma)
iv Total parental nutrition

Investigations and management

1. Blood gases showing acidosis, hypoxia, RDS, shock, infection (neutropenia): treat trigger factors aggressively.
2. Falling Hb and haematocrit (repeat to detect haemodilution). Transfuse.
3. Abnormal coagulation test:

    i Prolonged PT if vitamin K dependent. Give vitamin K_1.
    ii Prolonged PTT, low fibrinogen and raised FDPs if factors are being consumed. Replace using cryoprecipitate, and give vitamin K_1.

4. Platelets: give concentrate if <30 × 10⁹/l and bleeding. To halt consumption treat the trigger.

    i If due to maternal ITP give prednisolone 2 mg/kg, or i.v. Sandoglobulin. Thrombocytopenia may persist for up to 3 months.
    ii In maternal alloimmune type fetal thrombocytopenia and <40 × 10⁹/l transfuse with mother's platelets if symptomatic, as hers will not have the antigen.

5. Splenomegaly: congenital infection screen, and bone marrow aspiration, if pancytopenia or abnormal cells in the peripheral blood, looking for aplasia or leukaemia.
6. Identify sites of bleeding, e.g. cranial US for intracerebral bleeds, barium contrast X-ray or technetium scan for ulcers and duplications in gastrointestinal bleeding.

Prevention

1. Vitamin K_1 for classical haemorrhagic disease (HD) of the newborn. (Incidence, without prophylaxis, is up to 0.5%. Onset within the first 7 days in a well infant, of bruising, bleeding from the gastrointestinal tract, umbilicus, and into cephal-haematomata.)

   i   To all babies, whether or not breast fed, 500 μg orally at birth.
   ii Mothers on anticonvulsants in late preganacy and labour, 100 μg i.m. at birth.
       Late onset HD is rarer, 50% die or brain damaged, ideopathic or due to liver disease or malabsorption. Prevent by giving oral vitamin K, 500 μg day 7–10 and week 4–6.

2. The benefit of giving 'prophylactic' plasma or ethamsylate in high risk neonates is unproven.

   Controversy: are i.m. vitamin K and childhood leukaemia causally linked?

3. Haemolytic conditions

See also Jaundice.
Broadly divide into immune and non-immune haemolysis.

Immune: blood group incompatibility	*Non-immune; infection, RBC abnormality*
Rhesus	1 Infection: congenital and acquired
ABO	2 Enzyme: G6PD deficiency, pyruvate kinase
Duffy, Kell, Kidd etc.	3 Shape: hereditary spherocytosis
	4 Hb: alpha thalassaemia
	5 Rare: Vitamin E, pyknocytosis

   Investigations: Hb, film, reticulocytes, platelets, blood group, Coombs' direct and indirect, TORCH, enzyme levels especially if an Asian boy; Hb electrophoresis if hydropic.

Differential diagnosis

Spherocytes are seen in infection and ABO incompatibility as well as hereditary spherocytosis, though absence of a family history should not deflect one as 25% are sporadic.

GASTROINTESTINAL PROBLEMS

Physiology of the neonatal digestive system.

1. The stomach's hydrochloric acid secretion is high in the first 24 h of life, then reduced for the first few months of life before it gradually increases throughout childhood. Stomach emptying occurs within 1–2 h.
2. Enzyme activity:

i Lactase is lower in prematures, which may cause intolerance. Activity wanes in black children, so much so that intolerance of milk may follow. Stool carbohydrate content up to 0.5%, on Clinitest, is normal in infancy.
ii Lipases and fat digestion. Lingual lipase from von Ebner's gland in the base of the tongue actively digests fats to form triglycerides in the stomach. Breast milk lipases need to be activated by bile salts. Pancreatic enzyme secretion is low (10% of adult activity), as is the bile acid pool, especially in prematures. This reduced activity results in 'physiological steatorrhoea'.

3. Gut transit time is 18–24 h in the neonate. Stool colour: scrambled egg in breast fed; formula milk stools are pale yellow to grey-green, depending on the type of fats the manufacturers use.

Gastrointestinal symptoms

Antenatal indicators of potential complications

1. A history of maternal hydramnios alerts to swallowing disorders due to neuromuscular weakness and high intestinal obstruction, including oesophageal atresia and duodenal atresia. Suspect if >10 ml/kg of stomach contents are aspirated after delivery. Hydramnios is present in 25% with bowel obstruction.
2. Maternal drug dependence may present with vomiting and diarrhoea.
3. US identifies dilated stomach due to duodenal atresia. Check for Down's syndrome
4. Family history: cystic fibrosis (meconium ileus), pyloric stenosis, Hirschprung's disease, inborn errors presenting with vomiting, e.g. congenital adrenal hyperplasia.

Vomiting

Within the first 3 days of life

1 Feeding problem
2 Gastric irritation, swallowed blood
3 Obstruction: duodenal atresia, stricture, web, annular pancreas, Ladd's bands, mid-gut volvulus, meconium ileus/plug, Hirschsprung's, anal atresia
4 Ileus: premature, respiratory distress, low K⁺
5 Infection: sepsis, pneumonia
6 Neurogenic: asphyxia, birth injury, intracerebal bleed

End of first week onwards

1 Hiatus hernia
2 Infection
3 Necrotizing enterocolitis
4 Metabolic disorders: inborn errors, e.g. congenital adrenal hyperplasia; renal failure
5 Obstruction: pyloric stenosis volvulus, ileal stenosis, small left colon, Hirschsprung's disease, anal atresia
6 Cows' milk protein intolerance

Nature of vomit or aspirate, and management

1. Bile stained

First thought must be obstruction or ileus, although 50% turn out to have no detectable cause. May be confused with swallowed meconium stained liquor.

Pass nasogastric tube to decompress the stomach. Establish parenteral route for feeding, colloid support, antibiotics, and coagulation factors as required, and deal with the primary cause.

    i   Obstruction. Incidence 1 in 1000. Usually well initially. Enquire if mother had polyhydramnios. Dehydration and jaundice result from vomiting.

       Meconium may be passed in high obstructions but no changing stool is seen.

       Pointers to lesions and associations:

       a. Small intestinal atresia, midgut volvulus. Erect abdominal X-ray: 'double bubble' in duodenal atresia, or fluid levels. Barium may show site of obstruction, e.g. Ladd's band, or abnormally sited duodenum if malrotated.

       b. Large bowel, e.g. Hirschsprung's disease: no gas in rectum on X-ray, barium diagnostic.

       c. Anal stenosis/atresia: associated with genitourinary abnormalities, and the VATER association.

    ii Ileus: usually unwell at presentation: necrotizing enterocolitis and meconium ileus each have characteristic x-ray changes. Ileus also seen in sepsis, and prematures with RDS.

2. Blood stained

(See haematemesis) Swallowed maternal blood, nasogastric tube, stress ulceration, drugs, haemorrhagic disease of the newborn, severe necrotizing enterocolitis, disseminated intravascular coagulation.

3. Undigested feed

Due to delayed emptying (see list above) or overfeeding.

    i   If aspirate is <30% of the previous feed and infant is well, replace it in the stomach, which may only require longer between feeds to empty, or smaller volumes more frequently.

    ii   If large aspirates persist, review, consider reduction in oral feed or resting the gut. Abdominal X-ray is helpful.

    iii If septic, stop feeds, obtain cultures, start antibiotics.

    iv   Consider inborn errors, as their presentation often appears 'septic'. Stop feeds. See inborn errors.

    v   With diarrhoea. Initially consider gastroenteritis or maternal medication. Persistent diarrhoea is unusual, and associated with intolerance of lactose (stool >1% sugar) or cows' milk protein, or rarely, congenital chloridorrhoea (AR, an enzyme defect, causing metabolic alkalosis, with low serum Cl^- and K^+).

Haematemesis and malaena

See above.

Acute abdominal distension

Causes

    i   Air swallowing is a common feeding difficulty, which needs attention to technique or teat hole size.

'H' type oesophageal fistula is rare, detected by passing a nasogastric tube. Insert the open end under water while slowly withdrawing it, when bubbling during expiration or crying confirms its presence.
ii Intestinal due to obstruction and ileus.
iii Congestive cardiac failure. Hepatomegaly and ascites are associated with obvious symptoms and signs.
iv Tension pneumothorax pushing liver and abdominal contents down.

Delay in passing meconium

Normal passage of meconium in term infants: 95% within 24 h, 99% by 48 h.

Causes in first 48 hours

Condition	Assessment, diagnostic features
1 Prematurity	Delay is especially common if sick
2 Maternal opiate analgesia or dependence	Lethargy/withdrawal symptoms
3 Obstruction:	
i structural: anal atresia, stenosis, vesicorectal malformations	Distended abdomen. Inverted X-ray to demonstrate obstructed rectum
ii Meconium plug, meconium ileus	X-ray: 'bubbly' large bowel contents
iii Hirschsprung's disease	Rectal exam may seem therapeutic. Be warned!

Subsequent failure to pass stool

Cause	Associated findings
1 Breast feeding	Thriving, gaining weight, normal stool
2 Underfeeding	Poor weight gain, green pellet-like stool
3 Constipation	Excessive straining, hard stool, anal fissuring
4 Ileus: sepsis, low K^+, necrotizing enterocolitis	Ill, distended abdomen. Fluid levels on X-ray
5 Surgical obstruction: intestinal stricture, web, volvulus, intussusception	Initially well, barium examination diagnostic
6 Hypothyroidism	Difficulty feeding, prolonged jaundice

Embryology and the development of some gut disorders (Figure 2.3)

1. Oesophageal atresia: the caudal part of the foregut is divided by a septum into trachea and oesophagus by 7 weeks' fetal age. Deviation of the septum posteriorly prevents this. A fistula between the two is common.
2. Duodenal stenosis or atresia: the lumen is filled with epithelial cells at 5 weeks due to their proliferation, and obstruction results from failure of vacuolization and recanalization by the eighth week of fetal development.

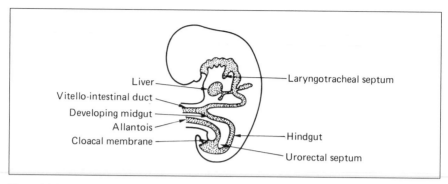

Figure 2.3 Fetal gut development

3. Intestinal stenosis or atresia: a similar mechanism to duodenal lesions in some cases, but the majority are vascular in origin, due to infarction as the intestines return to the abdomen at 10 weeks. Malrotations may cause vascular compromise later in gestation.
4. Malrotation: failure of the intestines to rotate anticlockwise through 270° as the midgut returns to the abdomen results in malfixation. The width of the mesenteric fixation may be narrow, allowing the guts to swing on a pedestal, and the bands to pass across the duodenum to cause obstruction.
5. Omphalocele is a failure of the midgut to return to the abdomen.
6. Anorectal anomalies result from failure of growth or deviation of the urorectal septum. This grows downwards towards the cloacal membrane, between the allantois and the hindgut. Arrested growth above the membrane results in high malformations, with fistula between bowel and bladder or vagina. Low anomalies result in ectopic anus or anal atresia which may have a fistula into the urethra in boys or vulva of girls. A covered anus occurs if the anal membrane fails to break down at 8 weeks.
7. Hirschsprung's disease is due to failure of migration of autonomic ganglion cells in the wall of the gut to reach the descending colon/anorectal junction at 5–7 weeks.

SURGICAL PROBLEMS PRESENTING IN THE NEWBORN

Facial clefts

Cleft lip and palate (CL&P)

Incidence

1 in 1000, malformation occurs at 6–8 weeks' fetal age.
Aetiology
Multifactorial: include familial, male predominance, maternal anticonvulsants during organogenesis, trisomies 13 and 18.

Risk of recurrence is 5%, greater if bilateral, and other family members affected.

Cleft palate

Incidence

1 in 2500, fewer familial cases than CL & P, except Stickler syndrome (AD with myopia, deafness, micrognathia, and Marfanoid appearance). Steroids have been implicated. Risk of recurrence is 2%.

Pierre Robin sequence of micrognathia and cleft palate is due to pressure of the tongue preventing lateral palatal shelves from joining in the midline at 7 weeks' fetal age. The tongue falls back into the airway unless nursed on the side or in prone. The retrognathia improves spontaneously over the first year of life.

Management of facial clefts

A team approach is essential, medical (plastic surgeon, orthodontist, ENT surgeon, paediatrician), speech therapist, feeding advisor, parent support group.

1. Consider cause, chromosomes, genetic opinion and counselling.
2. Photographs of affected babies pre- and postoperative are shown to parents immediately after birth to instil reality and confidence.
3. Flanged teats help establish feeding.
4. Surgical timetable.

    i   Cleft lip–first few days of life preferred by some plastic surgeons, others wait until 3 months old.
    ii Cleft palate is closed at 8–12 months, i.e. early, to encourage normal speech. Secretory otitis due to eustachian tube dysfunction occurs in all, so grommets are often inserted at closure.
    iii Tidy ups, and pharyngoplasty for nasal escape in late childhood.
    iv In adolescence, midface hypoplasia due to the early surgery for CL&P is evident and may require maxillofacial surgery combined with orthodontics.

5. Speech therapy.

Anterior abdominal wall defects

Exomphalos	*Gastroschisis*
Incidence: 1 in 3000	1 in 5000
Site: Umbilical. Transparent sac containing intestine +/- liver depending on size of defect	To right of umbilicus, loops of bowel matted together. No covering
Other malformations: Common. Look for Beckwith syndrome, trisomies 13, 18	Unusual.

Management

Place baby's trunk in a sterile polythene bag to minimize heat and fluid losses. If primary closure is impossible, a silastic sac is sewn over and used to return the abdominal contents over 1–2 weeks. Some huge omphaloceles are slowly epithelialized by applying mercurochrome, avoiding surgery, and needing prolonged parenteral nutritional support.

Bladder extrophy

Incidence 1 in 10000 M>F.

Failure of mesenchymal cells to migrate into the area in the fourth fetal week prevents development of the anterior abdominal wall and anterior bladder.

Findings: epispadius, usually undescended testes, widely separated pubic bones, anteriorly sited anus. Upper renal tract is initially normal.

Early closure is indicated.

Chest problems

Diaphragmatic hernia (DH)

Incidence

1 in 2000

Pathophysiology

Foramen of Bochdalek remains open, especially on left side, allowing herniation of abdominal organs into the chest.

Compression causes hypoplastic lung in utero, and expansion of intestines with air after birth further embarrasses cardiorespiratory function → hypoxia and severe metabolic acidosis.

Persistent pulmonary hypertension is a major potential cause of death.

Eventration: membrane-like diaphragm, allows abdominal contents to bulge into the chest, with the same clinical features as DH.

Clinical

1. Respiratory distress. Reduced chest movement and air entry on the affected side. The heart is displaced, usually to the right.
2. Scaphoid abdomen.

Post-neonatal presentation: failure to thrive, abdominal pain and vomiting, dyspnoea during feeding.

Diagnosis

Chest X-ray shows multiple 'cysts', simulating staphylococcal pneumonia.

Management

1 Deflate, with free drainage of the gut via a nasogastric tube.
2 i   Secure the airway by endotracheal intubation.
  ii Prevent hypoxia secondary to lung compression by the liver and progressively air-filled intestines, by sedating, paralysing and mechanical ventilation. Tolazoline, prostacyclin and finally extracorporeal membrane oxygenation (ECMO) for severe persistent pulmonary hypertension (PPH).

3 Surgery after satisfactory stabilization.

Prognosis

Dependent on:

1. Severity of lung hypoplasia (respiratory distress aged <12 h has a bad prognosis) and 'malignant' nature of PPH in some infants.
2. Bohn's predictive index of P_aCO_2 >40 + mean airway pressure × respiratory rate if >1000 = 100% mortality has been dramatically reduced to 40% by applying ECMO.
3. Delay in diagnosis.

Oesophageal atresia/Tracheo-oesophageal fistula (TOF)

A proximal blind pouch and distal tracheo-oesophageal fistula is the common association (80%). For embryology, see this section's introduction.

Incidence

1 in 3000.

Clinical presentations

1. 'Mucousy', excessive bubbliness from birth or a cyanotic episode before or during the first feed.
2. Abdominal sign: if a fistula is present and large, distension may result; if no fistula, the abdomen is scaphoid.
   Associated malformations in 50%, often syndromic, e.g. VATER, VACTERL.
3. Recurrent choking during feeds and/or chest infections. Always consider 'H type' TOF (5%).

Management

Nursed head-up in prone prevents regurgitation of acid stomach juice into the trachea via a fistula, if present.

Suction applied to a double lumen Replogle tube in the oesophageal pouch, prevents aspiration (Figure 2.4). Nil by mouth.

Surgical repair depends on oesophageal length: primary repair end to end, or staged repair of feeding gastrostomy and defunctioning cervical oesophagostomy, followed by colon transplant. Sham oral feeding must continue during this period to avoid subsequent feeding problems.

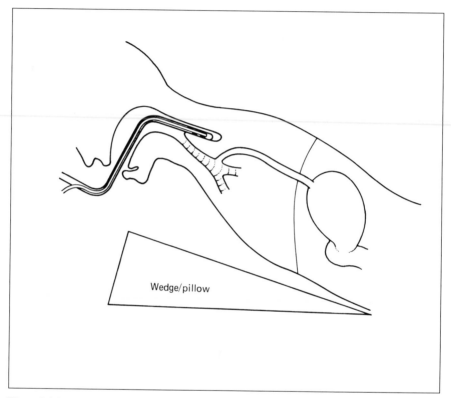

Figure 2.4 Oesophageal atresia with tracheosophageal fistula, drained in the head up position, Replogle tube in place

Prognosis

The mortality of 20% is mainly dependent on the associated anomalies.

Intra-abdominal problems

Small intestine and duodenal stenosis or atresia

Incidence

Approximately 1 in 5000 for each.

Site, lesion and associations

Ileum: atresia, lumenal diaphragm or stenosis. Multiple atresias in 5–10%. Cystic fibrosis is associated.

Duodenum: also consider compression by an annular pancreas or Ladd's bands with malrotation. Half are associated with other abnormalities, e.g. Down's syndrome, malrotation, congenital heart disease.

Clinical

1. Antenatal: hydramnios in pregnancy.
2. Vomiting: bile stained in 75%, or clear if above the ampulla of Vater.
3. Little or no meconium passed.

Investigation

Plain X-ray shows dilated proximal gut, e.g. 'double bubble' and absent or reduced gas beyond the obstruction. Fluid levels are common. Calcification, as in meconium peritonitis, is indicative of antenatal perforation.

Barium enema distinguishes small from large bowel atresia, meconium ileus and Hirschsprung's disease.

Surgery to bypass obstruction or relieve compression. Complications and mortality, up to 20–30%, are usually due to associated malformations.

Malrotation

The mesentery is short, the attachment often obstructing the duodenum, and allows the bowel to twist round its root –>volvulus (Figure 2.5).

Associated with exomphalos, diaphragmatic hernia, duodenal atresia, meconium ileus.

Clinical

1. Bile-stained vomiting, which may be intermittent as the bowel twists and untwists.
2. Volvulus is found in 50%, with blood in stool from venous obstruction, and shock. Infarction, then gangrene, may result.

Investigation

Plain X-ray: double bubble of duodenal obstruction and airless abdomen from absorbed air in volvulus.

Barium meal: the jejunum is to the right of spine, the caecum placed abnormally high. Barium enema shows the abnormal caecal position.

Differential diagnosis

In the first month of life: other causes of acute obstruction. Later: repeated gastro-enteritis, recurrent abdominal pain with vomiting, 'cyclical vomiting'.

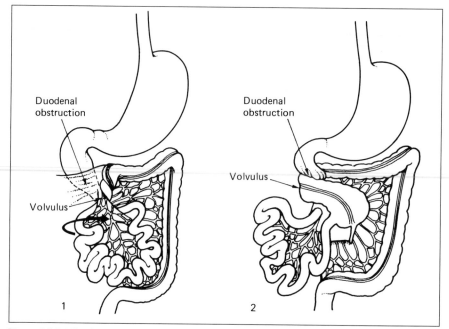

Figure 2.5 1. Mixed rotation and volvulus
2. Midgut volvulus

Treatment

Laparotomy, undo volvulus, tack down the mesentery while broadening its pedicle.

Meckel's diverticulum and duplications (Figure 2.6)

Site

Meckel's diverticulum: on the free border of ileum, not far from the ileocaecal valve, a remnant of the vitello-intestinal duct. Present in 1% of people but symptomatic in only 1 in 3000.

Duplications: mesenteric side of the bowel anywhere along the gastrointestinal tract; encysted or communicating with the bowel.

Pathophysiology

May contain acid secreting gastric mucosa, resulting in pain and or obstruction due to pressure on the adjacent bowel, or painless haemorrhage, or perforation.

Investigation

Barium examination and technitium-^{99m} for ectopic gastric mucosa. US scan may reveal cystic duplication. X-ray of vertebrae for hemivertebrae or split vertebrae, which are commoner in duplications.

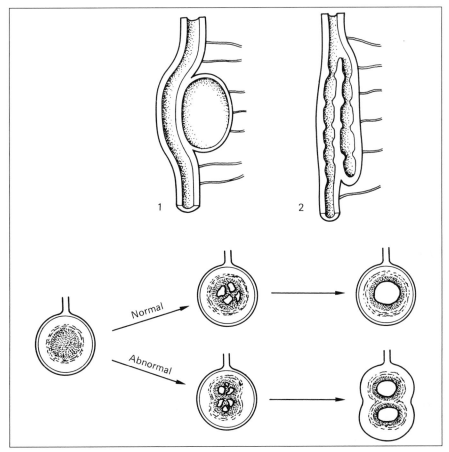

Figure 2.6 Duplications　1. Cystic
2. Double lumen, blind ended loop.

Treatment

Surgical removal if causing symptoms.

Meconium ileus

Cause

Thick viscid meconium, due to cystic fibrosis, 10% presenting in this way. Colon contains pale meconium pellets.

In one half of meconium ileus one of the following complications arise: → intra-uterine perforation → meconium peritonitis, calcification, volvulus of the dilated ileum → strangulated bowel→ atresia.

Clinical

Abdominal distension, bilious vomiting, palpable loops of bowel mainly in the right iliac fossa. Meconium plug on rectal examination.

X-ray: fluid levels, gas bubbles in the meconium, faecal masses in the colon. Abdominal calcification may be present.

Barium enema: descending colon is narrowed. Matted, dilated small intestinal mass.

Management

Decompression by gastrograffin enema or defunctioning ileostomy and resection of any atretic bowel. Perform sweat test.

Prognosis for the chest in cystic fibrosis is no worse as a result of meconium ileus.

Meconium peritonitis

Causes

Meconium ileus in 50%, bowel atresia, Hirschsprung's disease, or intrauterine volvulus.

Pathophysiology

Bowel perforation, followed by leakage of meconium into peritoneum. If it occurs in utero it may show as intra-abdominal calcification on X-ray.

Meconium plug

Lower bowel obstruction due to inspissated meconium 10–12 cm long, often relieved by rectal examination or barium enema. Always test for Hirschsprung's disease and cystic fibrosis.

Hirschsprung's disease

Incidence

1 in 5000, short segment M:F = 4:1, long segment M = F. Risk is 3% among siblings, and in Down's syndrome.

Pathophysiology

Absence of myenteric and submucosal plexus in the colon causes it to be continuously in tonic contraction. Obstruction results.

Involvement

75% rectosigmoid, 5% whole colon.

Presentation

90% in infancy, but often after the neonatal period.

1. Delay in passing meconium >24 h (also occurs in 5% of normal infants).
2. Intermittent bouts of poor feeding, bilious vomiting, abdominal distension, relieved by passage of offensive stool and flatus.
3. Failure to thrive
4. Enterocolitis is commoner in the neonatal period and may result in perforation. Severe fluid loss and shock result. May occur even after successful surgery.
5. Rectal examination (PR): tight grip on the finger by the bowel, no 'give' into the rectal chamber, and faeces not palpable. Gush of faeces after withdrawal is 'gratifying' but a false reassurance.

Investigation

Plain X-ray should be taken before a rectal examination: dilated loops of bowel and fluid levels.

Barium enema: delay for 12–24 h after rectal examination as the latter deflates the obstructed bowel by passive stretching of the aganglionic segment, and removes the characteristic 'ice cream cone' shape, at the transitional zone, in short segment disease.

Rectal manometry: a positive test result is failure of relaxation of internal sphincter after inflating a balloon in the rectum.

Suction rectal biopsy and staining for acetyl-cholinesterase is diagnostic: absent ganglion cells, large nerve trunks.

Treatment

1. Colostomy first, in infants, to avert the danger of enterocolitis.
2. Anorectal pull-through, at about a year, preserves sensation and sphincter function.

Prognosis

Enterocolitis may be fatal if recognition is delayed. Mortality <5%. Incontinence/ constipation is equally common after any one of the preferred operations. A short-gut syndrome may result, in very long segment or total colon Hirschsprung's.

Anorectal anomalies: imperforate anus

Incidence

1 in 4000.

Associations

Other malformations are found in 50% (always look for VACTERL association–see Genetic problems). Prematurity is common.

Level of lesion and sex, related to severity

Boys: high lesions are more common than in girls.

1. High = ends above levator ani, communicates via fistula with bladder/urethra in 80% of boys. Require colostomy initially. Problems with sensation and continence after pull-through are common in childhood, but persistence usually results in reasonable continence.
2. Low = ends below levator ani, may be only a 'covered anus', 90% of boys have a fistula to the perineum, discharging meconium or mucus. After surgery, dilation by finger/dilators is often needed in early infancy.

Girls usually have low lesions. High lesions open into the vagina and bladder fistulae are therefore uncommon.

If no fistulous discharge, and anus is imperforate, do an 'invertogram', a lateral X-ray of the baby in the upside down position, after 12 h of age. Air above a line between pubes and sacroccygeal junction = high lesion in which a cystogram may also show a fistula.

Acquired potential surgical problem

Neonatal necrotizing enterocolitis (NEC)

Definition

Damage to the bowel wall from many causes, including infection, manifest as abdominal distension, blood passed rectally, and intraluminal air. Onset in the first 1–3 weeks commonly.

Incidence

Up to 10% of babies <1.5 kg at birth, rare in term infants. Overall, 3/1000.

Aetiology

Outbreaks occur within neonatal units, suggesting infection of damaged/ischaemic bowel. Factors: hypoxia, hypovolaemia, fluid overload, umbilical catheterization and exchange transfusion, patent ductus arteriosus, hyperosmolar feeds, and nasojejunal feeding of high solute milk formula. Prevention is by avoiding or minimizing these factors.

The precise cause is unknown. Breast milk is protective.

Clinical

1. Vomiting, especially if bilious, indicating ileus/obstruction.

2. Abdominal distension, progressing to ileus. Ascites. Oedema of abdominal wall with bluish skin discoloration in advancing disease.
3. Blood in faeces, from streaks to shedding of mucosa.
4. Non-specific: hypotonia, lethargy or apnoea. Associated with pallor, hypotension, hypothermia, jaundice.

Diagnosis

Based on clinical findings plus X-ray: initially a distended loop of small bowel or caecum, then intraluminal air (pneumatosis intestinalis) whose appearance is as a 'railway line' double gut wall shadow, progressing to perforation showing usually as free air above the liver, or gas in portal venous system.

Thrombocytopenia and disseminated intravascular coagulation are common in sicker infants.

Hirschsprung's disease to be excluded in previously well, term infants.

Management

1. Treat shock, anaemia, coagulation disorders, electrolyte and acid–base disturbances. Mechanical ventilation for apnoea or severe acidosis, and respiration embarrassed by the abdominal distension.
2. Stop oral feeds. Remove umbilical catheter and nasojejunal tube, if present, replacing it with a nasogastric tube for drainage and regular aspiration.
   Start parenteral nutrition, continue for 7–10 days.
3. Antibiotics (e.g. penicillin + gentamicin) and metronidazole.
4. Daily X-ray. Laparotomy for resection of non-viable bowel if deterioration continues. Perforation alone is not an indication, as more survive with conservative treatment, if it works within 2–3 days, than if taken to surgery.
5. After symptoms have subsided for about a week, milk may be introduced, usually as Pregestimil as post NEC malabsorption can be a problem.

Complications

Strictures and subsequent subacute obstruction 2–6 weeks later; malabsorption; second attacks can occur.

Prognosis

Worse in girls, <1.5 kg birth weight, onset in the first few days, with coagulation disorders, low platelet count, positive blood culture. Mortality 10%, and 25% after perforation.

OXYGEN TOXICITY RELATED DISORDERS

In addition to bronchopulmonary dysplasia and the Wilson-Mikity syndrome already discussed.

Retinopathy of prematurity (ROP)

Definition

Damage to the developing retina by relative or absolute hyperoxia.

Pathophysiology

Hyperoxia (absolute, or relative to the in utero exposure) → retinal vessel vasocon-striction → tissue ischaemia → proliferation of blood vessels in response.

Associated factors: hyperoxia, adult haemoglobin. Vitamin E deficiency is now discounted.

Incidence

Forty per cent of VLBW show changes. Most are minor and regress, but 7–10% of survivors weighing under 1000 g at birth have significant visual impairment.

Findings

On the equator of the eye globe, a demarcation line (stage 1), then a ridge form (stage 2). Fibrovascular proliferation follows (stage 3). Progresses to bleeds, and retinal detachment either partial (stage 4) or total (stage 5).

Management

Examination for ROP starts at 4–8 weeks old.
Cryotherapy may prevent progression to blindness.

METABOLIC PROBLEMS

Hypoglycaemia

Definition

Blood glucose <2.6 mmol/l (46 mg/dl) after 3 days old.

Evidence accumulating that brain dysfunction occurs at <2.6 mmol/l (46 mg/dl) *at any age or gestation*. A redefinition of hypoglycaemia is implied, and previous standards (<1.7 mmol/l (30 mg/dl) in term infants and <1.1 mmol/l (20 mg/dl) in preterm/small for dates) no longer apply.

Incidence

All births 0.4%. Infants of diabetic mothers 50%, (10–20% symptomatic), gestational diabetes 20% (25% symptomatic), low birth weight infants 6% (80% symptomatic).

Causes of neonatal hypoglycaemia

1. Transient neonatal

  i Ketotic: decreased production
    Small for dates, premature, cold stress, trauma, cerebral hypoxia or malformation, sepsis. Starvation via fluid restriction, e.g. acute renal failure, hypoxic-ischaemic encephalopathy. Maternal labetalol.
  ii Non-ketotic: hyperinsulinism.
    Infant of diabetic mother, severe rhesus isoimmunization, Beckwith-Wiedemann syndrome (exomphalos, macroglossia, gigantism (EMG) syndrome).

2. Persistent neonatal and early infancy

  i Decreased production (ketotic).

    a. Enzyme defect: direct effect in glycogen storage diseases, and indirect as in maple syrup urine disease, galactosaemia, fructose intolerance.
    b. Hormone deficiency: growth hormone, glucocorticoids.

  ii Hyperinsulinism (non-ketotic): islet cell hyperplasia alone or with Beckwith-Wiedemann syndrome, discrete adenoma, and nesidioblastosis (increase in islet cell tissue throughout the pancreas, occasionally familial AR).

Clinical

Macrosomia: hyperinsulinism. Check the core temperature, which may be low.
  Jaundice favours galactosaemia, sepsis.
  Hepatomegaly: alone in glycogen storage, with spleen in rhesus isoimmunization.
  Non-specific: jitteriness, convulsions, apnoea, lethargy, hypotonia.

Investigation

1. Blood glucose during the hypoglycaemic episode.
2. If persistent and recurrent hypoglycaemia despite treatment:

  i Ketones in blood or urine.
  ii Blood for insulin level (hyperinsulinism), cortisol (hypoadrenalism), growth hormone (hypopituitarism), and lactate (elevated in von Gierke's glycogen storage disease).

3. Severe persistent metabolic acidosis: consider inborn errors, blood and urine for organic acid and amino acid screen.
    Hyperinsulinism is likely when:

  i Non-ketotic hypoglycaemia present.
  ii Insulin level is inappropriately high for the blood glucose level.
  iii Glucose infusion >8 mg/kg/min is required to maintain normoglycaemia.
  iv Glycaemic response to glucagon when hypoglycaemic.
  v Low branched chain amino acid levels in blood when hypoglycaemic.

Management

1. Milk feed is better than a glucose feed, 3 ml/kg followed by hourly feeds for 12h.
2. Coma/seizure: 1 ml/kg 25% glucose i.v. over 4 min, then oral feed or 10% glucose infusion, 60–90 ml/kg/day slowly tailed off to avoid rebound if hyperinsulinaemic. If glucose remains low give 15–20% dextrose infusion, then hydrocortisone 2.5 mg/kg 12-hourly if still <2.6 mmol/l.
3. In hyperinsulinism: diazoxide orally regularly (up to 25 mg/kg/day) adding chlorthiazide, which potentiates it, or try somatostatin infusion short term. Glucagon (0.1 mg/kg) for rescue.
   Surgery for resistant nesidioblastosis (95% of pancreas removed), and islet cell adenoma.

Prognosis

The underlying condition determines prognosis. Delay in diagnosis and glucose stabilization in nesidioblastosis, and possibly Beckwith-Wiedemann syndrome, is associated with a high likelihood of mental handicap.

Clinical syndromes

Infant of a diabetic mother (IDM)

Diabetic pregnancies 0.5%. Problems are not so frequent in gestational diabetes, which complicates 2% (more in Asians) of all pregnancies.

Problems

1. Macrosomia: obstructed labour, asphyxia, traumatic delivery resulting in brachial plexus injury. Excessive fetal size reduced by improved management of diabetes during pregnancy. Prolonged, severe maternal diabetes may result in small for dates infants.
2. Hypoglycaemia

   i Transient in first 6 h, avoided by maintaining stable maternal blood glucose 4–7 mmol/l during labour.
   Asphyxia during delivery: may require glucose during resuscitation. Always establish dextrose infusion via a peripheral vein to avoid rebound hypoglycaemia.
   ii Lasting 12–48 h.
   Stress related hypocalcaemia common, resolves spontaneously, may contribute to the fine tremulousness that characterizes the IDM in the first 2–3 days.

3. Respiratory distress.

   i RDS: Surfactant qualitatively different, despite normal lecithin:sphyngomyelin ratio.
   ii Retained lung fluid after caesarian section for macrosomia.

4. Polycythaemia: stiff lungs, renal vein thrombosis, physiological jaundice common in IDM.
5. Congenital malformations 2–3 times normal incidence.

   i Congenital heart disease (ventricular septal defect, coarctation, transposition of the great vessels), transient obstructive hypertrophic cardiomyopathy– avoid inotropes.
   ii Sacral agenesis.
   iii Left microcolon.

Prognosis

Perinatal mortality 2–3 times infants of similar gestation. Tenfold risk of diabetes in childhood.

Further reading

Lucas A, Morley R, Cole T J (1988) Adverse neurodevelopmental outcome of moderate neonatal hypoglycaemia. *British Medical Journal*, **297**, 1304–1308
Aynsley-Green A, Polak J M, Gough M H, Keeling J, Ashcroft S H, Turner R C, Baum D (1981) Nesidioblastosis of the pancreas: definition of the syndrome and the management of the severe neonatal hyperinsulinaemic hypoglycaemia. *Archives of Diseases in Childhood* , **56**, 496–508

Inborn errors of metabolism

Features of individual defects of carbohydrate, amino acids and organic acids, and urea cycle are discused in Metabolic problems.
   Individually rare, features in common include:

1. Family history of consanguinity, neonatal death.
2. Onset of symptoms after introduction of milk feeds, ameliorated by their withdrawal.
3. Clinical syndromes mimicking other conditions:

   i 'Septic' in many organic acidaemias, urea cycle defects and aminoacidopathies.
   ii Others 'hepatitis' like in galactosaemia etc.
   iii Vomiting in congenital adrenal hyperplasia, and galactosaemia, in which condition infection may coexist, i.e. check septic (especially if jaundiced) infants for reducing sugars in urine.
   iv Neurological: lethargy, hypotonia, progressing to apnoea, seizures, and coma. Onset may be rapid (<3 days old) in organic acid and urea cycle defects.

4. Biochemistry

   i Hypoglycaemia is a common presentation in many inborn errors.
   ii Base deficit, hyponatraemia, hyperkalaemia, raised urea after the first 3–5 days suggests congenital adrenal hyperplasia.

iii Base deficit >15 mmol/l + ketosis may be an amino aciduria (+ characteristic smell? e.g. phenylketonuria, maple syrup).
iv   Metabolic alkalosis + hyperammonaemia = urea cycle defect.
v   Persistent obstructive jaundice in galactosaemia.

Investigations

Platelets and WBC (often low in organic acidaemia). Plasma electrolytes and urea. Blood and urine for aminoacids, organic acids; blood gases, plasma ammonia, galactose-1-phosphate uridyl transferase in erythrocytes. Plasma 17-hydroxyprogesterone for 21-hydroxylase deficiency.

Management

1. Resuscitate, IPPV, correct metabolic acidosis, hypoglycaemia, electrolyte and fluid disturbance. The onset may be related to the introduction of milk feeds, so blood and urine should be taken as the feeds are stopped. See Metabolic problems for details of investigation.
2. Stop milk feeds until certain that protein and lactose (containing glucose and galactose) are not harmful.
3. Peritoneal dialysis removes toxic organic acids and urea metabolites.
4. Dietary/drug management of individual conditions.

Hyperglycaemia

Definition

>9 mmol/l.

Causes

1. Preterm infant on i.v. dextrose 10% or parenteral nutrition.
2. Stress-induced: septicaemia, intracranial bleed, asphyxia.

Management

Identify cause, and treat. Reduce glucose infusion rate if appropriate, correct any dehydration or electrolyte imbalance that may have resulted.

Hypocalcaemia

Definition

Serum calcium <1.8 mmol/l.

Physiology

Normally present as half ionized, half protein bound. It is the ionized fraction that determines whether the infant is symptomatic. Acidosis increases ionization, and hypoproteinaemia the ionized fraction, so symptoms are less likely in these states.

Transient neonatal hypoparathyroidism

1. Early: first 1–3 days. Usually asymptomatic, and spontaneously improves.

    i Prematurity.
    ii Stress: asphyxia, birth injury, sepsis, infant of diabetic mother, surgical conditions.

2. Late: 4+ days old, with excessive jitteriness, occasionally multifocal convulsions:

    i   Maternal hyperparathyroidism due to lack of vitamin D, more prevalent in Asians, suppresses parathormone secretion in the fetus.
    ii The neonatal kidney does not excrete phosphate readily. In the presence of maternally induced hypoparathyroidism, the high phosphate load in unmodified cow's milk leads to elevated serum phosphate, suppression of calcium.
    iii Hypomagnesaemia: associated with (i) and (ii) and seizures which may not improve until serum magnesium rises.

Drug doses

1. Treatment with calcium gluconate

    i   Asymptomatic: leave unless premature, sick and prolonged QT on ECG. Give calcium gluconate 10% as 5–8 ml/kg/day.
    ii Jitteriness: oral supplements 200–500 mg/kg/day.
    iii Seizures: 10% i.v. 2 ml/kg slowly over 20 minutes. If repeated consider i.v. infusion, check magnesium.

2. If Mg^{2+}<0.8 mmol/l give magnesium sulphate 50% 0.5 ml/kg 12 hourly × 2.
3. Vitamin D as 1-alpha calcidol in hypoparathyroid states and maternal hyperparathyroidism.

Persistent hypoparathyroidism

Rare in newborn: DiGeorge's syndrome, pseudohypoparathyroidism.

Osteopenia or metabolic bone disease of the premature (MBDP)

Osteopenia = reduced bone density on X-ray. Also seen are cupping and splaying of epiphyses, and fractures if severe, i.e. combination of rickets, osteomalacia and osteoporosis.

Pathophysiology

Eighty per cent of calcium and phosphorus accretion of the fetal skeleton normally occurs in the third trimester.

Maternal calcidiol (25 hydroxycholecalciferol) crosses the placenta and is converted by the fetal kidney to calcitriol (1:25 dihydroxycholecalciferol).

1. MBDP results from the increased need for phosphate and calcium in the VLBW group.
2. At risk

    i   Breast fed/standard formula/total parenteral nutrition low in calcium and phosphorus,
    ii Respiratory distress with fluid restriction, and if frusemide administered.

    Exacerbated by prematures' reduced absorption of calcium and phosphate from the intestine, and reabsorption from the renal tubule.
3. Vitamin D levels and metabolism normal.

Investigations

1. Serum
    Raised alkaline phosphatase (>5 × adult).
    Phosphate low for newborn (at upper limit of the adult range).
    Calcium normal or raised, calcidiol and calcitriol normal.
2. X-ray changes seen from 6 weeks old:
    Grade 0 = normal bone, I = rariefaction only, II = metaphyseal changes– fraying and cupping, and subperiosteal new bone formation, III = I + II + fractures.

Treatment

If phosphate <1.6 mmol/l give additional phosphate at each feed as the neutral salt.

Prevention

Of limited efficacy:

1. Fortify human milk with phosphorus as disodium phosphate 0.5–1 mmol/100ml or use preterm formula, until infant weighs 2 kg.
2. Vitamin D, 1000 iu/day for the first 3 months.

Prognosis

Good, a self-limiting condition with little morbidity. Alkaline phosphatase >5 × adult maximum in first month is associated with reduced growth in length in first 18 months, and may impair full growth potential.

Further reading

Bishop N (1989) Bone disease in preterm infants. *Archives of Disease in Childhood*, **64**, 1403–1409
Gertner J M (1990) Disorders of calcium and phosphorous homeostasis. *Pediatric Clinics of North America*, **37**, 1441–1465

ENDOCRINE DISORDERS

Thyroid

1. Hypothyroidism

Incidence

1 in 5000

Clinical

Neonatal presentation classically as prolonged jaundice and feeding difficulties. Rarely as a palpable goitre or respiratory obstruction due to retrosternal goitre in synthesizing enzyme defect (dyshormogenesis).

Investigation

Guthrie card for screening TSH level; >20 IU/l indicates need for repeat testing. Unusual to go onto radioisotope studies or US unless goitrous. Most glands are ectopic sublingual, some absent, others involuting or large due to dyshormogenesis.

Replacement

Start with 25 µg/day of thyroxine (or 8–10 µg/kg). Check T4 at 2 weeks, 6 weeks, 3 months, then 3 monthly until 2 years old. Maintenance dose is based on 100 µg/m², aiming to keep the T4 in the upper part of the normal range.

Review diagnosis at one year to identify those with transient hypothyroidism due to maternal blocking antibodies (5–10%). Method: replace T4 with T3 20 µg for 1 month, then stop it for 2 weeks before taking blood for TSH, T4 +/- isotope scan. Restart T4 and advise when results are to hand.

2. Thyrotoxicosis secondary to maternal hyperthyroidism

Although hyperthyroidism occurs 1–2 per 1000 pregnancies, neonatal Graves' disease, due to transplacental immune–mediated IgG thyroid stimulating antibodies (TSAbs), is rare. May present in utero as persistent fetal tachycardia, or from birth, occasionally in the second week, with tachycardia, jitteriness, proptosis, with voracious appetite, sweating, loose stools. Reduced mental potential may occur from premature fusion of skull bones.

Treatment

1. In utero: for persistent fetal tachycardia, even if mother has had surgical removal for Graves' disease. Continue infant's antithyroid drug, with thyroxine replacement, after delivery.
2. Newborn: iodide inhibits release, antithyroid drugs synthesis, of thyroid hormone. If the sympathetic system is acutely overactive, give propranolol.

Drug doses

Iodide (Lugol's solution) one drop 3 times a day
Propylthiouracil 5 mg/kg/day (4 divided doses)
Propranalol 1–2 mg/kg/day (4 divided doses)

Half life of TSAbs 3 months, so continue for several weeks and withdraw slowly.

GENITOURINARY PROBLEMS

Antenatal US has led to an increased awareness of the frequency of underlying abnormalities and the need for prevention of progressive renal damage in selected cases. Many resolve with conservative management, hence the label of 'transitional uropathy' for the findings in this period.

Incidence

Up to 8 per 1000 fetuses = 0.65% at birth, now the commonest organ system affected by anomalies.

Selected congenital renal abnormalities often detected antenatally by US

Findings

1. Persistent dilatation of all or part of the urinary tract: pelviureteric obstruction 70%, vesicoureteric obstruction 15%, vesicoureteric reflux 12%, posterior urethral valves 3%.
2. Cystic changes or reduced renal parenchyma.
   Bilateral in 30%.

   Incompatible with life in 12%, due to lung hypoplasia as a part of Potter's syndrome–common associations are oligohydramnios, small for dates, limb contractures, Potter's facies–low set ears, epicanthus, squashed face. Amniotic surface covered by clumps of epithelial cells described as 'amnion nodosum'.

Causes

Bilateral agenesis/dysplasia, obstruction to urethra especially in boys, and polycystic kidneys.

Management

Most lethal malformations are seen by 20 weeks' gestation, and the less serious by 28 weeks. Conservative management is indicated antenatally. Postnatal aim is to preserve renal function, prevent urinary infection and subsequent scarring.

Antenatal US dilated, possibly obstructive uropathy

1. Confirmatory US within 7 days of birth. Action:

   i Normal: reassure.
      The GFR is low in the first 2–3 days, so dilatation may be absent. Delay the US or repeat later.
   ii Bilateral dilatation (30%) due to bladder neck obstruction (usually posterior urethral valve) or bilateral pelviureteric junction (PUJ) obstruction requires imaging urgently (Figure 2.7).

      a. A micturating cystourethrogram will identify the cause.
      b. A ^{99m}Tc diethylene triamine pentacetic acid (DTPA) scan is useful to show poor excretion in PUJ obstruction and the possible need for nephrostomies.

   iii Unilateral dilatation (70%). Start trimethoprim prophylaxis, to prevent infection and renal scarring, continuing it for the first year.

      a. At a month repeat the US.
         If dilatation is confirmed do a DTPA scan to determine if due to:
         large, poorly functioning pelvis, or obstruction at PUJ or ureteric orifice. Many improve spontaneously in the first year, so surgery should be reserved for severe impairment or deteriorating function due to obstruction when GFR <10–20 ml/min/1.73m^2.
         Failure to demostrate dilatation: stop prophylaxis, reassure.
      b. At 3 months an MCU may reveal associated vesico-ureteric reflux. Continue prophylaxis and follow up with US and DTPA until reflux resolves.

Prognosis

In PUJ obstruction in the first year 80% improve on prophylaxis alone. The 20% who deteriorate are among the initially more severely affected, but as early prediction by imaging is not accurate careful follow up is essential.

Controversy

1. Fetal/neonatal US may fail to identify 50% of those later found to have reflux nephropathy.
2. To preserve/improve function, pyeloplasty in the first year in the moderately obstructed kidneys is advocated. However, the natural history of the condition is insufficiently known and requires a randomized study.

Further reading

Thomas D F M, Gordon A C (1989) Management of prenatally diagnosed uropathies. *Archives of Disease in Childhood*, **64**, 58–63

Homsy W L, Saad F, Laberge I, Williot P, Pison C (1990) Transitional hydronephrosis of the newborn and infant. *Journal of the American Urological Association*, ii, **144**, 579–583

Ransley P G, Dhillon H K, Gordon I, Duffy P G *et al* (1990) The postnatal management of hydronephrosis diagnosed by prenatal ultrasound. *Journal of Urology*, ii, **144**, 584–587

Scott J E S, Lee R E J, Hunter E W, Coulthard M G, Matthews J N S (1991) Ultrasound screening of newborn urinary tract, *Lancet, ii*, 1571–1573

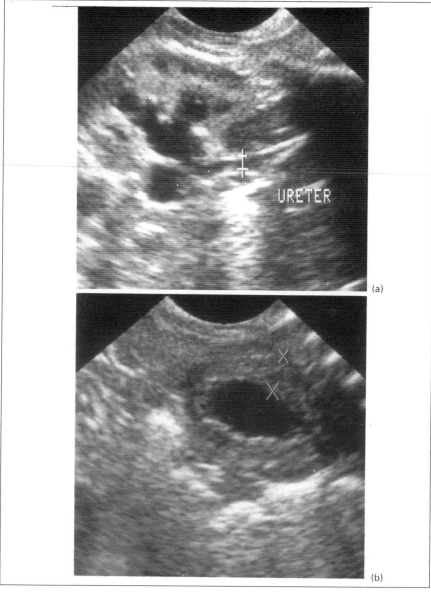

(a)

(b)

Figure 2.7 On US the right kidney (a) has a grossly dilated pelvicaliceal system with clubbing of the calyces, and the dilated ureter (marked) is also seen. The left kidney (not shown) is similarly affected. (b) The bladder wall is markedly thickened, shown x - x. Posterior urethral valve confirmed at operation.

Anuria from birth

Urine is often passed at birth, but may be unobserved. Failure to pass any within 24 h requires assessment, when the infant will fall into one of the following groups:

1. Well, normal on examination.
2. Dysmorphic:

   i Respiratory distress from lung hypoplasia: Potter's sequence, secondary to renal aplasia, severe neonatal polycystic disease (AR, family history?) or bilateral obstruction of the urinary tract.
   ii Prune belly with atonic collecting system.

3. Large kidneys and/or bladder on examination, due to obstruction of urinary tract.
4. Sick, asphyxiated, shocked: see below.

Immediate management

1. Observe, if well, and wait for urination.
2. Pass a catheter. Release of a large volume requires a micturating cystogram (posterior urethral valves, atonic bladder). US for kidney substance, size of collecting system and bladder.

   Further management see Renal problems.

Anuria/oliguria

Definition

A urine output of <0.5 ml/kg/h. Biochemical indication of abnormal renal function:

1. Term: rising plasma potassium >7mmol/l, urea >10 mmol/l, increasing by >1 mmol/l/24 hours.
2. In the infant <1.5 kg these values are not unusual, due to fluid restriction, i.e. prerenal 'failure', so guides to renal failure are:

   i Plasma creatinine above the upper limit for gestation and post-natal age, increasing by >50 μmol/l/24 h.
   ii Urinary sodium >40 mmol/l.
   iii Urine:plasma osmolality ratio <1.1

   If pre-renal failure is likely, a loading test of 15 ml/kg of normal saline over 1 h followed by 2 mg/kg frusemide will show whether urine can be formed. Care is needed to avoid aggravating hypovolaemia if already fluid restricted.

Causes of newborn renal failure

1. Pre-renal, leading to acute tubular necrosis/cortical necrosis in some.

   i Asphyxia at birth, and in severe respiratory illness.
   ii Hypotension: hypovolaemia due to blood loss, sepsis, coarctation of the aorta.

2. Renal:

   i Congenital: agenesis/dysplasia, rarely nephrotic syndrome.
   ii Urinary tract infection.

iii Renal vein thrombosis.

3. Obstructive: bilateral pelvi-ureteric obstruction, posterior urethral valve, urethral stricture.

Management

As for older infants.

Haematuria

Must be distinguished from vaginal bleeding and, in boys especially, urate crystals on the nappy.

Causes

1. Profuse:

    i Bleeding in sick infants with disseminated intravascular coagulation, or well with haemorrhagic disease of the newborn.
    ii Renal vein thrombosis.

2. Mild to moderate

    i Urinary tract infection.
    ii Bladder neck obstruction, hydronephrosis.

3. Usually microscopic

    i Suprapubic aspiration.
    ii Emboli from umbilical arterial catheter.

Investigations are usually self-evident from associated features.

Ambiguous genitalia

1. The primary aim of assessment is to establish the sex of rearing by identifying the cause, using the flow chart, shown in Figure 2.8.
2. US of the internal organs if the chromosomes are XX or XX/XY and abnormality is not due to congenital adrenal hyperplasia or maternal androgens.
3. The adequacy of the phallus for function and appearance are the final arbiters. If surgery to external genitals is needed it should be completed by 2 years old (leave fashioning the vagina until puberty) to minimize psychological trauma.
    Remove dysplastic intra-abdominal testes as the risk of malignant change is increased.

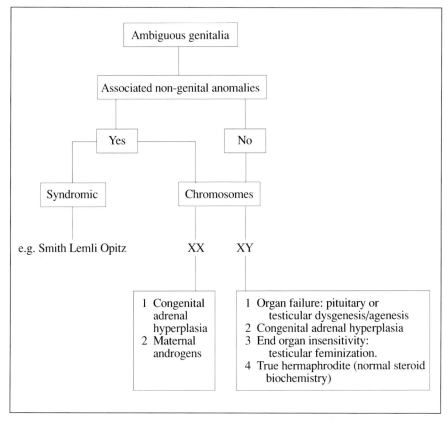

Figure 2.8

Recommended reading

Gomella T L (1988) *Neonatology: Basic Management, On-call Problems, Diseases, Drugs*. London: Prentice-Hall.

Harvey D, Cooke R W I, Levitt G A (1989) *The Baby Under 1000 g*. London:Wright

Roberton N R C (1986) *A Manual of Neonatal Intensive Care. 2nd edn.* London:Edward Arnold

Whitelaw A, Cooke R W I (1988) The very immature infant—less than 28 weeks' gestation. *British Medical Bulletin*, **44**, no 4. (particularly McIntosh N, on clinical issues).

Yu V Y H (1986) *Respiratory Disorders in the Newborn*. Edinburgh:Churchill Livingstone

Standard texts

Levene M I, Tudehope D, Thearle J (1987) *Essentials of Neonatal Medicine*. Oxford:Blackwell

Roberton N R C (1991) *Textbook of Neonatology* 2nd edn. Edinburgh:Churchill Livingstone

Chapter 3

Community Paediatrics

Care of children in the UK is based on the Family Doctor service and the increasingly integrated Community and District Hospital services. The aim is total care, by breaking down the barriers between care-giving groups.

Community paediatricians monitor general community health levels, and immunizations. They target the identification of individual children with health needs or in danger of less than optimal health and development, promote injury prevention, and health education.

The recommendation of a National Personal Child Health Record held by the parents reflects professionals' belated recognition of parental primacy in child care and making use of community-based services.

CHILD HEALTH SURVEILLANCE (CHS)

Definition

The prevention of disease, the early detection of problems affecting growth and development and the positive promotion of health. It includes the following activities.

1. Primary prevention: immunization.
2. Secondary prevention. The early detection of disease in the presymptomatic phase, e.g. phenylketonuria (PKU), hypothyroidism, congenital dislocation of the hip (CDH).
3. Tertiary prevention. Minimizing secondary effects, e.g. speech, language and behaviour disorders in sensorineural deafness, and postural deformities in cerebral palsy.
4. Health promotion, e.g. accident prevention in the home, on the roads; the dangers of passive smoking; good nutrition.

Primary prevention

In the developing world immunization annually prevents 750000 deaths from measles, 320000 pertussis, and polio and tetanus 200000 each.

World Health Organisation target for the year 2000 is for all children to be immunized; in 1990 70% were covered, a rise from 5% in 1974.

Cost to immunize such a child with six vaccines is $10 (BCG, diphtheria-tetanus-polio (DPT), polio, measles) under the WHO Expanded Program on Immunization.

A measure of the efficacy of vaccines: benefit to cost ratio

Benefit = prevention of morbidity and mortality, cost = complications of vaccination.

Ratios for a developed country, e.g. USA, is measles 12:1, rubella 8:1, pertussis 11:1.

Herd immunity and vaccination targets

Minimum targets for polio, measles, mumps, pertussis is 90% by second birthday. Only 100% is acceptable for rubella if all cases of embryopathy are to be prevented.

A new accelerated vaccination schedule was introduced in May 1990, in an effort to improve uptake of diphtheria, tetanus, polio and pertussis. England and Wales achieved 90% for diphtheria, tetanus and polio, and rubella, in 1991, and 85% for pertussis.

Introduced in 1988, measles/measles-mumps-rubella (MMR) vaccination uptake was already 89% by 1991, from Health Authority vaccination returns to COVER (Cover of vaccination evaluated rapidly), a reporting scheme organized by the Communicable Disease Centre, Colindale, in 1987, and has been successful in interrupting the triennial mumps epidemic.

Reasons for low immunization uptake

1. Inaccurate or misleading advice from doctors, nurses.
2. Parental refusal: perceived low risk of serious complications, allegations of vaccine damage in the media.
3. Organizational: low priority for money and staff.

Scale of disease prior to introduction of MMR into the UK in 1988

Measles: 1.5 million deaths in the developing world. Even in UK there were 95 000 cases in 1988, compared with USA 5000 (but by 1991 the UK had fewer than 10 000 while the USA experienced an unprecedented upsurge to 30 000!).

Complications: 1 in 15 affected. In UK 1.4% hospitalized.

Deaths 20 annually. Most vulnerable: leukaemics in remission, or other underlying abnormality (see priority groups below). Ten died from subacute sclerosing panencephalitis.

Mumps: the commonest cause of hospital admission for meningoencephalitis in UK at 1200 annually for <15 years old, an estimated 20 cases of nerve deafness, and 5–10 deaths.

Rubella: laboratory confirmed congenital infections 164 in 1987.

Priority groups for vaccination

Asthma, cystic fibrosis, bronchopulmonary dysplasia, congenital heart disease, Down's syndrome, small for dates, prematures, HIV antibody positive.

Table 3.1 Vaccination schedule

Vaccine	Age
DTP Hib, OPV × 3 doses	2, 3 and 4 months
MMR**	12–18 months
DT and polio preschool booster	4–5 years
Rubella and BCG	10–14 years
Tetanus and polio	15–18 years

OPV: oral polio virus vaccine
Hib: Haemophilus influenza type b
**Primary vaccine failure in 2–5% with measles vaccination has led to the introduction of a booster dose in USA.

Administration

1. BCG: intradermal, otherwise ineffective, into deltoid insertion, (or lateral aspect of upper thigh in girls). Interval of 3 weeks between BCG and giving a live vaccine. Never give to immunosuppressed and HIV positive individuals.
2. In each arm if giving more than one live vaccine at the same time, or separate by 3 weeks.
3. Anaphylaxis is a rare but important danger. Always have appropriate drugs and equipment available.

Special situations

1. Prevention of vertical transmission of hepatitis B from mothers: see also Hepatic problems

   i Carriers or recently infected.
   At risk:
   ii Chinese>Asian>Black. All but Caucasians should be screened.
   iii Drug addicts, prostitutes, partners of bisexual men, occupational exposure.
   Administration: hepatitis B vaccine and immunoglobulin within 48 h of birth. Repeat vaccination at 1 and 6 months.

2. Neonatal BCG in UK in inner cities with high proportion of Asians.
3. Measles vaccination at 6 months in countries with high incidence of morbidity and mortality in infancy, e.g. Africa.
4. Pneumococcal vaccine for sickle cell disease, nephrotic syndrome, post splenectomy in children over 2 years old. Plans to vaccinate all from 1993.

Specific concerns

1. Pertussis

Vaccine-related encephalopathy. Adverse media comment resulted in a fall in acceptance rate from 80% to 30% in the 1970s. The prospective National Childhood Encephalopathy Study found an attributable risk of 1 in 300000 vaccinations.

When cases of Reye's syndrome and proven viral infections are excluded, no statistical correlation with damage or death exists.

Efficacy of vaccine: 20% after 1st, 60% after 2nd and 80% after 3rd dose protected, and severity of cyanosis and convulsions reduced in those infected.

Only absolute contraindications are

  i Severe local indurated swelling of most of upper arm circumference or lateral thigh following a previous injection.
  ii General reaction with temperature >39.4°C within 48 h, persistent screaming >2 h, unresponsiveness, anaphylaxis, or convulsions within 72 h.

Problem histories for assessment of risk/benefit:

  i   Cerebral damage documented in the neonatal period.
  ii Personal history of convulsions.
  iii First degree relative with idiopathic epilepsy.

Nicoll and Rudd (1989) state: 'Although chances of reactions may be higher in immunizing these children, they should still be protected as benefits outweigh the risks'.

Antipyretic treatment for (i) and (ii) is indicated—paracetamol for 36 h after vaccination, 10 mg/kg/dose, up to 4 doses in 24 h.

2. Measles-mumps-rubella (MMR)

A personal/family history of convulsions is not a contraindication, so long as parents are aware of the febrile response 5–10 days later, and the need for antipyretic treatment at that time.

Incidence of febrile convulsions is five times less frequent than in natural measles, plus a 10–fold reduction in subacute sclerosing panencephalitis. Meningoencephalitis after MMR is rare, (1:200000), down from 1 in 400 in wild mumps. Parotitis may occur in the third week for 24 h. Neural deafness after vaccination is very rare.

General contraindications

1. Acute febrile illness: delay vaccination for one week.
2. Anaphylaxis following egg (still relevant regarding influenza, but measles and MMR vaccine components now grown in chick fibroblast) or specific antibiotic (traces of neomycin and kanamycin in mumps and MMR vaccine).
3. Immunodeficient or immunosupressed, e.g. prednisolone 2 mg/kg/day for >1 week, or on antimetabolites: live vaccines are prohibited. Exception is MMR in HIV, and acute leukaemia in remission for >6 months.

   Give immunoglobulin i.m. after exposure to measles, chickenpox. Parents must be aware of the need for treatment after contact. Measles vaccination is essential for siblings and close contacts. Inactivated polio vaccine only, not live oral polio vaccine (OPV).
4. No live vaccines to pregnant women except after exposure to polio or yellow fever where the need for protection outweighs the risk to a fetus.

False contraindications to be ignored

1. Family/personal history of atopy (asthma, hay fever, eczema).
2. Receiving antibiotics, inhaled or topical steroids.
3. Infant breast feeding, jaundiced after birth, below a specified weight.
4. Mother pregnant.
5. Previous history of measles, pertussis, or rubella infection.
6. Prematurity: do not delay, as early immunization protects against pertussis, i.e. start at 2 months old.
7. Stable neurological condition, e.g. cerebral palsy, Down's syndrome.
8. Over the age required by the vaccination schedule.

New immunizations

1. *Haemophilus influenzae* type B (Hib) vaccine. In the UK the annual estimated incidence of systemic infection (septicaemia, epiglotitis, septic arthritis, pneumonia) prior to Hib introduction 380 cases, meningitis 250, with 20 deaths.

2. Under development

Varicella, respiratory syncitial virus, rotavirus vaccine.

Further reading

Bellanti J A (ed) (1990) Pediatric vaccinations: update 1990. *Pediatric Clinics of North America*, **37**, no 3
Committee on Infectious Diseases (1991) The relationship between pertussis vaccine and brain damage: Reassessment. *Pediatrics*, **88**, 397–400
Department of Health (1990) *Immunisation against Infectious Disease* (1990). London:HMSO
Dyer C (1988) Judge 'not satisfied' that whooping cough vaccine causes permanent brain damage. *British Medical Journal*, **296**, 1189–1190
Nicoll A, Rudd P (1989) *Manual on Infections and Immunizations in Children.* Oxford:Oxford University Press
Nicoll A, Elliman D, Begg N T (1989) Immunisation: causes of failure and strategies and tactics for success. *British Medical Journal*, **299**, 808–812

Secondary and tertiary prevention: surveillance and screening

Changing concepts about universal screening at regular intervals

1. The majority of severe handicaps are identified at birth or follow up of small babies, or parental concern.
2. Be selective. Use parental participation, check lists, appropriate 'opportunistic' counselling and enquiry at vaccination visits, and at times of sensory testing.
3. Only use items with proven benefit and cost-effectiveness.
   Early detection is beneficial to parents and therefore management of the child's handicap.
   Non-attenders, travellers, the homeless and the potentially abused need greater attention to avoid being overlooked.

Required knowledge and skills to operate a core screening programme

1. Development: able to assess normal, atypical and abnormal. These skills are used in surveillance.
2. Sensory testing: vision and hearing.
3. Detection of physical abnormality: e.g. congenital dislocation of the hip (CDH) and congenital heart disease (CHD).
4. Understanding parental behaviour: normal and abnormal. See Breaking bad news, Child abuse, Behavioural problems.
5. Knowledge of the types of interventions available in child development, relationships between local child health services and other agencies, the roles and skills of colleagues. See District handicap team, and special educational needs.

The Child Health Computing System

Organized on an NHS Regional basis, it is a record initiated at birth for every child. It provides the information for calls for vaccination and surveillance, and the result. May also cover school health programmes.

Körner data

Agreed 'core' information on individuals and community services (immunization, health surveillance) is collected for assessment of work done, and cost effectiveness. Computer compatible, ideal for number crunching, e.g. for child health surveillance, the minimum data set agreed is:

1. Age and sex of the child.
2. Location of surveillance (home, surgery, clinic, school).
3. Result of surveillance (no action/continued observation/referred).

SCREENING AND ASSESSMENT

Screening for suspected abnormality using tests such as the Denver Developmental Screeening Test or the Woodside Test for health visitors have strict pass/fail criteria which do not evaluate performance. Many normal children may be referred, while a hemiplegic child or even one with Down's syndrome may pass. *Screening* is a rapid means of identifying children who are well but may have a disability. *Assessment* determines whether they have and its type, severity, and cause.

Universal screening for developmental abnormalities is no longer recommended in the UK following the reviews of Hall (1989) and Butler (1989):

1. Lack of precision in identification of normal or abnomal.
2. Unpredictability of childhood development.
3. Lack of proof of efficacy of much of intervention strategies.

Surveillance is still required for those families identified as reluctant to use services, with poor rearing skills, or paralysed through anxiety.

Recommended screening procedures in all children

(Abstracted from Hall D M B (1991) *Health for All Children. A Programme for Child Health Surveillance.* 2nd edn. Oxford: Oxford University Press. (Chapter 17, the Report of the second joint working party on Child Health Surveillance, is essential reading).

Replaces universal developmental screening with a *selective* approach using procedures of proven efficacy. More frequent or more complete evaluation is done as indicated by family history, parental or professional concern.

'The aims of a child health surveillance (CHS) program, in collaboration with parents and carers, are:

1. All children have the opportunity to realize their full potential in terms of good health, well-being and development.
2. Remediable disorders are identified and acted upon as early as possible.'

An integral part of CHS is health promotion, at appropriate ages. Accident prevention, passive smoking, identification of children in need (disabled, deprived, abused etc), and good nutrition are topics listed.

Selective hearing tests between 1–5 years

Routinely and periodically in Down's syndrome and cleft palate. All with language delay, dysarthria, or repeated secretory otitis media, and behaviour difficulties should have an audiological assessment.

Vision

Squint and amblyopia: treat early as >4 years by occlusion is of limited effectiveness.

Discontinued vision tests: 0–3 years the graded balls test, matching toys, hundreds and thousands. At 3+ years the Sheridan Gardiner STYCAR 5 and 7 letters test, and Snellen chart are also considered inaccurate screening tests.

Personnel required

Family doctor where physical examination is required, otherwise Health Visitors or Practice Nurses with special training in hearing and vision testing, and the taking of heights.

Monitoring child health surveillance

To ascertain whether the scheme outlined above is working, and reaching all children. Each health district is to monitor efficiency and effectiveness.

Table 3.2 Timetable of child health surveillance

Age	Parental guidance and screening procedures
Week 1	1 Review: Family history, pregnancy, birth factors. Parental concerns elicited.
	2 Complete physical examination: include weight, head circumference. Examine: eyes for red reflex, look for congenital abnormalities, auscultate for congenital heart disease (CHD).
	3 High risk of hearing deficit is an indication for referral for auditory response cradle, or brainstem evoked response hearing test (gold standard).
	4 Testicular descent
	6% are undescended at birth. Fully descended testes do not ascend later.
	5 Congenital dislocation of the hips (CDH)
	Check at birth and at 10 days. 10% of CDH present later, i.e. they must be tested regularly until the infant is walking.
	6 Blood screening tests
	i Phenylketonuria by Guthrie card.
	ii Hypothyroidism by T4 or TSH.
	Half the children who become hypothyroid present after infancy so there is a continuous need for clinical awareness aided by the regular measurement of height as well as weight.
	iii Screening in some Health Regions for haemoglobinopathies, and cystic fibrosis by trypsin levels.
	7 Health education
	Feeding and nutrition, baby care, sleep position, sibling management, crying and sleep problems, transport in cars, passive smoking, accident prevention (scalds from baths, bottles, fires), immunization, reasons for blood screening tests.
6 weeks	1 Check the history, ask about vision and hearing, and parental concerns, ascertain whether in a hearing loss high risk group and refer if necessary.
	2 Parent check list for advice on detecting hearing loss is given. See figure 3.1.
	3 Weight. Plot on parent held chart.
	4 Physical examination including for CDH and CHD.
	5 Health education: immunization, nutrition, dangers of fires, falls, overheating, scalds; signs of illness and appropriate action.
6–9 months	1 Discuss parental concerns about health and development.
	2 Ask about vision and hearing.
	3 Weight. Plot on parent held chart, and height if indicated.
	4 Hearing using distraction testing.
	Discontinue screening cover test for squint altogether, as poorly performed by non-specialists. Action: refer to orthoptist if a squint is reported.
	5 CDH Look for the classical signs. (Cerebal palsy is a special risk group.) Surgery is required from now on, and the results become poorer.
	6 Testes. Treatment before 18–24 months may improve fertility so all high scrotal and suprascrotal testes should be referred to a paediatric/interested surgeon.
	7 Health education: accident prevention anticipating mobility consider safety gates, fire, plug and cooker guards; choking, sunburn. Dental prophylaxis, nutrition. Car transport, passive smoking dangers reinforced. Developmental needs.

Table 3.2 Timetable of child health surveillance (*continued*)

Age	Parental guidance and screening procedures
	Assessments from this age onwards may be done by Health Visitors or trained Practice Nurses, and not Doctors, excepting auscultation of the heart and examination for testicular descent.
18–24 months	1 Parental concerns at this age are especially about behaviour, vision, and hearing. If doubt over either of the latter two arrange detailed specialist testing, do not do test yourself as responses are difficult to interpret at this age. 2 Check walking, and that gait and hips are normal. 3 Confirm he is saying some words, and understands when spoken to. 4 Weight, and height provided it is accurate. Refer if –3 standard deviations or decreasing velocity. 5 Anaemia is common at this age, taken as <11 g/dl. Target the deprived urban and ethnic minorities. 6 Health education: accident prevention of falls from heights including windows, drowning, suffocation, poisoning, road safety. Nutrition. Behaviour problems, avoidance and management. Developmental needs, socialization, e.g. playgroup. 7 Notify children who may have special educational needs under the Education Act 1981, or the Children Act 1989 in whom health or development is likely to be impaired without special provision by the Local Authority.
36–48 months	'Pre-school examination' 1. Physical exam, especially squint, hearing. Height. Testicular descent. CHD. Listen especially to the second sound: single in pulmonary stenosis, fixed splitting in atrioseptal defect. 2. Development and behavioural issues. 3. Immunizations: ensure completed. 4. Health education: accident prevention of fires, drowning; road safety. Dental hygiene, nutrition.
5 years	School entry exam by School Health Service. May be abandoned if preschool checks are effective. 1 Check vaccination status, in discussion with parents anticipate potential learning difficulties. 2 Height: as above. 3 Refractive errors and amblyopia by vision screening: Snellen chart preferred. 4 Hearing screening: sweep audiometry.
8 years	Screening for refractive errors.
11 years	Screening for refractive errors, colour vision.
10+ years	Adolescent scoliosis in 3 in 1000 girls. Screening now discontinued as low specificity (66% were treated unnecessarily).

Routine sensory testing: see Developmental assessment for details.

Table 3.3 Monitoring child health surveillance

Efficiency of surveillance	Effectiveness of surveillance
Is response rate adequate?	Is population covered by geography and service provision?
Non-responders/lost to follow up pursued	Expected numbers of disorders detected and followed up?

Sensitivity and specificity, yield and predictive power of screening adequate?

The target population is the annual cohort of children, to minimize the effect of highly mobile families being missed.
Management's responsibility is to match/redistribute clinics and personnel to achieve optimal service.

Figure 3.1 Parent check list for hearing

When your health visitor sees you, please tell her the answers to the following questions:	Here are some things you can look out for yourself at home:
1 Is there any deafness in your family?	1 Shortly after birth your baby should be startled by a sudden loud noise. He should blink or open his eyes widely to such sounds.
2 Did you have any illness during this pregnancy?	2 By 1 month your baby should still if you make a sudden prolonged sound.
3 Was your baby in a special care unit after birth?	3 By 3 months he should quieten or smile when you speak even when he cannot see you.
4 Has your baby had any illness since birth?	4 By 6 months your baby should turn immediately towards your voice across the room or to very quiet noises made on each side.
5 Does your baby get frequent colds or ear infection?	5 By 9 months your baby should listen attentively to familiar everyday sounds, e.g. key in the door, rattle of cutlery, and turn towards very quiet sounds made out of sight. He should show pleasure in babbling loudly and tunefully.
6 Are you worried about baby's hearing?	6 By 1 year your baby should respond to his/her name and other words such as 'bye bye' and 'no'.

Adapted from advice to parents from the Hounslow and Spelthorne Health District

Sensitivity is the ability of a test to identify correctly children with a disorder, specificity identifies those without the disorder.

Yield is the ratio of population screened to those detected; a measure of cost effectiveness.

Predictive power is used to assess whether the levels of specificity and sensitivity are high enough to be useful in population screening.

Examples where monitoring may identify deficiencies:

1. Age at diagnosis of sensorineural deafness.
2. Prevalence of amblyopia at school entry.
3. Age at operation for CDH, or undescended testes.
4. Children with special needs notified to the Education Authority, their number and the number of multi-disciplinary assessments.

Special needs register

Contains details of children with disease, disability and handicap. It is used for surveillance, planning and allocation of resources.

Role of community paediatricians

Increasingly taking on the role of coordinating all health services for the total paediatric population of a district.

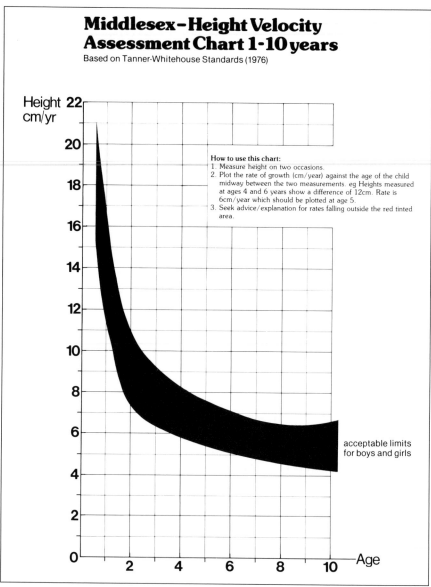

Figure 3.2 Middlesex Height Velocity Assessment Chart 1–10 years. Measure on two occasions, plot the rate of growth in cm/yr against the age midway between the two measurements. (Reproduced from Archives of Disease in Childhood (1983) p. 840, by kind permission of the Copyright holders Castlemead Publications, ref 65.)

1. Child health

   i Prevention through monitoring and improving vaccination uptake by feedback to primary care teams, promoting health education, parent counselling.

  ii Health screening.

iii Audiology services.
iv Clinical role in Child Development Centres, the diagnosis and continuing care of children with chronic disabilities.
v Maintain registers of children with special needs.

2. School health service: assessment for Special Educational Needs under the Education Act 1981. Continued assessment of these children in nurseries, ordinary and special schools. Screening for sensory defects. Advice to local education authority, teachers, careers officers.
3. Adoption and fostering adviser to local social services.
4. Child abuse: clinical role and as advisers in emotional problems, liason with Social Services departments.
5. Planning and developing services.
6. Developing outcome measurements. Examples: age at diagnosis of deafness, dislocated hip, cerebral palsy, severe growth hormone deficiency; % of children's squints not identified before starting school, or orchidopexy after 6 years of age.

School Health Services

These may vary from one health authority to another. The team comprises a doctor (vocationally trained general practitioner or community doctor) and school nurse for every school. The nurse screens for vision, hearing, height (schedule above), and is most accessible to pupils and teachers.

Doctor's duties

1. If a preschool medical has not been done, auscultation for murmurs, and testicular descent checked.
2. Identification of physical or neurodevelopmental problems from medical records, parental information and teachers' observations, and subsequent clinical examination.
3. Immunization records checked and maximum uptake promoted.
4. Health education promotion. To facilitate by discussion with teachers, making material available.
5. Define policies, with the Head Teacher: e.g. the giving of medicines in school (not normally a teacher's responsibility), pupils' absences for medical reasons, emergency situations.
6. Support and advice concerning the 2% of children with Statements of special educational needs under the Education Act, and the 18% of children with less severe special needs: asthma, behaviour problems, epilepsy, diabetes.

HEALTH PROMOTION

Definition

The process of enabling people to increase control over and improve their health. Involves reducing inequalities in health, encouraging public participation, working together with local organizations.

People make their own decisions in their own time.

Follow-up of media campaigns by health visitors improves uptake of measures, e.g. injury prevention, immunizations.

Parental participation in health education

Opportunities: at birth, development checks, and acute episodes. A useful promoting aid is the recently introduced parent-held record.

1. Immunization, to encourage uptake, dispel myths.
2. Accident prevention.
3. Awareness and avoidance of sexual abuse.
4. Normal developmental problems: sleep disturbance, negativism and their management, variations in development and warning signs of delay or impairment.
5. Common ailments: diarrhoea, fever, wheeze.
6. Feeding: encouraging breast feeding, change to door step milk at 12 months, vitamin supplementation in prematures and Asians.
7. Dental care, fluoride toothpaste, regular checks.

Adolescence and health education

Age appropriate messages:

1. Secondary school discussion of attitudes to drugs, alcohol, smoking, sexual relationships, contraceptives, AIDS, child care, breast feeding.
2. Self-referral ('drop in') clinics. Adolescents seeking advice on growth and development, sexual problems, emotional difficulties including drug abuse.

Deprivation

The following are identified as increased among the deprived: infant mortality, low birthweight, teenage pregnancy, single parent family, poor use of health services including antenatal clinics and immunization, child abuse, ill health.

- Behaviour and coping is learned. A cycle of deprivation continues from generation to generation.
- Inner city children are twice as likely to be emotionally disturbed and educationally retarded as their rural and suburban peers. School absence, attendance at special school for moderate learning difficulties, and misbehaviour are all more common.

Intervention strategies

School health education on contraception, smoking, alcohol, child development. Disappointing results to date.

Personal contact by Health Visitor to encourage antenatal visits and vaccination uptake.

Early stimulation 'Head start' programmes pioneered in the USA have had disappointing results in the long term.

Behaviour modification. Necessary by 7 years to prevent antisocial behaviour in adolescence, i.e. needs early recognition and referral to child guidance.

Ethnic minorities

Disadvantaged economically, higher unemployment. Language and culture separates them from the host community.

Conflicts arise between home and school attitudes to behaviour, and among Asians the relative freedom of their Caucasian peers.

Racial discrimination and harassment at school age reflected in behaviour disturbances.

Child rearing practices lacking stimulation and self worth result in under achieving at school and work, as among some West Indians.

Tuberculosis from foreign visitors; TB, malaria and intestinal infections acquired during visits abroad.

Medical problems more common in some ethnic communities

Asian

1. Increased perinatal mortality and congenital malformations. See Neonatal problems. Related to poorer weight gain in pregnancy, vegetarian diet, and consanguinity. About half of Pakistani marriages in the UK are between first cousins (3% extra risk) and uncles with nieces (5–10% extra risk of malformation).
2. Infection: congenital rubella as Asian brides coming to the UK are usually unvaccinated; hepatitis B (3–10% are carriers); open TB.
3. Nutritional deficiencies:

   i   Rickets both in infancy and adolescence.
   ii Iron deficiency anaemia.
   iii Lead poisoning from cosmetics ('surma') or sikor clay used for indigestion.

4. Others: β-thalassaemia, and glucose-6-phosphate dehydrogenase (G6PD) deficiency are not uncommon. α-Thalassaemia is common but usually of the mild variety (see Haematological problems).

   Nephrotic syndrome and congenital hypothyroidism are more common than among other UK children, though diabetes is less common.

African and Afro-Caribbean

1. Perinatal mortality rate is only slightly higher, related to economic factors, while congenital malformations are lower than average, except for polydactyly. Dizygotic twins are more common.
2. Haemoglobinopathies: sickle cell disease, SC disease and S-thalassaemia, G6PD deficiency.
3. Nutritional deficiencies in Rastafarian children.

Mediterranean

Haemoglobinopathies: β-thalassaemia, G6PD deficiency.

Jewish

Inborn errors: degenerative, e.g. Tay-Sach's, Niemann-Pick and adult Gaucher's disease.

Far Eastern: Chinese and Vietnamese

1. Hepatitis B high risk group.
2. Haemoglobinopathies: α-thalassaemia (Hb Barts) and β-thalassaemia, G6PD deficiency.

Further reading

Black J (1989) *Child Health in a Multicultural Society.* London:British Medical Journal

Atypical families

Single parent families

Almost 30% of children are registered at birth in mother's maiden name only, but many are the product of stable relationships. Total 1 million, with 1.6 million children. Problems of homelessness, inadequate housing, and deprivation are prominent.

Divorce and reconstituted families

A third of UK marriages are dissolved.

Effects on the child: preschool children may regress in behaviour, and under 8 years often feel guilty and responsible for the break–up. Long-term problems requiring help may emerge in 20%.

Remarriage is common, resulting in step-relationships with attendant behaviour problems. Repeated divorce/separation is increasing, exposing children to multiple stressful adjustments.

Adoption

Incidence of abuse and behavioural difficulties slightly higher than the majority of the population, as many are reconstituted families. Even if much wanted by a childless couple there is no guarantee of parenting success.

Adverse environmental influences

Inner city overcrowding, the housing shortage

The incidence of death and disease is higher in slums and high rise flats; maternal isolation and depression increase above the fourth floor. Overcrowding and lack of sanitation increase disease. Reduced facilities increase antisocial behaviour.

Further reading

Polnay L (1985) *Community Paediatrics*. Edinburgh: Churchill Livingstone

ACCIDENTS AND INJURY PREVENTION

Accidents are the commonest cause of death after the neonatal period. Identified as an area where there is clear scope for improvement.

Death rate for England and Wales (E & W) is 700 annually, 55% involving vehicles.

Table 3.4 Fatalities to children under 15 in England and Wales

Type of accident	Deaths	%
Road		
Pedestrians	260	31
Vehicle occupant	96	11
Cyclists	73	9
Home		
Burns, fires	119	14
Suffocation	34	4
Home and elsewhere		
Drownings	63	7
Falls	40	5
Choking on food	50	6

Others, individual cases: electrocution 15, falling object 14, poisoning 13.

(Figures for England and Wales 1989, Department of Trade and Industry).

Morbidity of accidents to children

1. Short term: Accident and Emergency department

    i Attendances 2 million annually:
       40% cuts and bruises.
       25% sprains and fractures.
       20% head injuries.
       3% each foreign body in orifice, eye injuries.
       2% each burns and scalds, poisonings, inhalations and ingestions, bites and stings.
    ii 120 000 admitted.

2. Long term: permanent injury, loss of function, and hence skills to society and possible drain on community resources. Numbers unknown.

Vulnerability and age

Infancy

Falls from changing table. Reaching and placing objects in the mouth. Premature mobility in baby walkers leads to falls, injuries against radiators, into fires.

Toddler

Exploratory behaviour, no sense of danger. Guard drugs, cookers, electrical appliances, open fires, windows, gates etc.

Preschool

Trainable to avoid these dangers, but lack reasoning to perceive them.

School age

Early years characterized by increasing risk taking on bikes and skateboards in the street and park.

In adolescence peer pressure and desire to conform to the group increase the risks of alcohol, substance abuse and sexual activities. Self-poisoning may result from depression or acting out behaviour.

Accident prone children are more likely in emotionally deprived and disorganized families, and to have attention deficit and impulsive behaviour.

General guidelines on prevention

Anticipatory guidance begins from the newborn period.

1. Safe transport in cars (safety seats available from some hospitals).
2. Safe bedding, nursery furniture.
3. Safe toys, and playgrounds with padded areas.
4. Child-resistant containers for medication, household caustics.
5. Hazards in the home minimized:

- Safety glass in doors, bannisters on stairs, secure latches for windows, swimming pools fenced, gates to the road.
- Equipment: flex tidy for electrical kettle, guards for fires, cookers; covers to electical plugs; paraffin stoves properly used.
- Smoke detectors, fire blanket in kitchen, matches hidden, cigarettes put out.

6. Lead-free surma (an Asian eye cosmetic) and petrol.

Traffic accidents

Annual incidence

Deaths: 400 (100 car occupants, 250 pedestrians, 50–100 cyclists). Seriously injured: 9000. Boys especially at risk on bikes, M:F = 9:1.

Prevention

1. In the car. Mandatory use of baby seats, seat belts in front and back seats became law in 1989. Must be properly anchored, and fit (booster may be required), otherwise child may balloon under, catching the jaw.
2. Pedestrians. Road safety training, reflective clothing at night.
3. Helmet (approved design) for cycling, and cycling proficiency courses.

Drowning

Deaths annually: 40, near drowning 80.
   Site: unsupervised bath at home, garden ponds, private swimming pools, occasionally lakes and rivers, and the sea.
   Possible associated factors to question: seizures, head injury, drugs. Commonest in the preschool child, then adolescent boys.

Mechanisms

Sudden immersion in very cold water results in the diving reflex found only in young children—apnoea, shunting of blood to head and heart. Eventually gasping leads to inhalation, finally hypoxia and cardiorespiratory arrest.
   As little as 1–3 ml/kg water may actually enter the lungs.
   Fresh water drowning is exacerbated by hyperkalaemia and cardiac arrhythmias; salt water death is slower, by asphyxia.
   Action: vigorous resuscitation is almost always warranted. If cold/icy water, resuscitation should continue for at least an hour, even if initially pupils are fixed and dilated, and until the core temperature >33°C. Management of near drowning is respiratory support, warming, alkali, and countering cerebral oedema.

Prognosis

Cold water is better than warm, as hypothermia protects. Half of 'lifeless' children survive after fresh water, 70% after salt water immersion. Recovery may take 4–6 months; 30% mild handicap, 5% severe.

Scalds and burns

Annual incidence

Deaths 100, admitted to hospital 3000.

Flame burns and inhalation

1. Most fires are caused by cigarette smoking, followed by faulty heating equipment or electrical wiring. Non-flammable night clothes and fire guards have greatly reduced flame injuries.
2. Thermal injury has occurred if the nasal hairs are sooty or singed.

3. Respiratory failure results from airway obstruction, bronchoconstriction, asphyxia, and the effects of the gases.

   i Carbon monoxide (CO) poisoning is the commonest cause of death in the home from incomplete combustion in gas appliances or an accidental fire. CO has 200 × Hb affinity of oxygen. Half-life of COHb = 2–5 h.

     a. Acute poisoning → coma, convulsions, death at COHb >50%. Appearance is often pale, but venous blood looks arterial. Ischaemic changes and extrasystoles on ECG.
       Treatment is 100% oxygen, or hyperbaric oxygen (located at designated hospitals and Royal Navy diving schools).
     b. Chronic exposure to low concentrations → headache (COHb 20–30%), 'flu'-like, or symptoms like food poisoning (COHb 30–50%).

   ii Cyanides common in house fires from combustion of foam and synthetic fabrics. Acute poisoning → sudden death.

Prevention

Avoid smoking in bed. Smoke alarms. Keep matches, candles out of reach.

Scalds

Hot water or oil from cup, kettle or cooking pot in the kitchen/dining area account for the majority. Bathroom scalds occur in preschool children.
    Beware of deliberate immersion.

Prevention

Cooker guards, keeping pot handles to the back/ or side. Coiled kettle flexes. Hot drinks or smoking avoided while a child is held. Check bath temperature, supervise running in the water. Water heater temperature set at 54°C (usually 60–70°C in the UK) will not scald.

Contact burns

Coming in contact with hot surfaces, e.g. cigarettes, hot plate, toaster, iron, radiant heater.
    Distribution over buttocks, hands and feet is more likely in deliberate injury.
    Irregular burn from accidental brush against hot object, e.g. cigarette, must be distinguished from the clear cut edges of a burn of abuse.

Electrical burns

Mouthing of a live connector or poorly insulated cable producing lip/mouth burns, insertion of fingers/metal implements into sockets cause hand burns. Both may result in electrocution.

Swallowed foreign bodies

1. Preschool children swallow stones, coins, ring pulls of drink cans, mercury cells. Ulceration, perforation, and stricture can occur. Oesophageal hold up requires urgent endoscopy.
2. Sharp and long objects are the most likely to cause perforation. Abdominal pain and tenderness, with failure of an object to progress radiologically in 24 h, are indications for surgery.

Inhaled foreign bodies

See Respiratory problems.

POISONING

Annual incidence

Deaths 15–20
Hospitalized 14000
Attend A & E departments 40000

Factors

Age 1–3 years, boys > girls, summer:winter ratio is 2:1

Types

Medications 80% of fatalities, 55% of total, household products the remainder.
   Plants and seeds rarely cause serious problems.
   In contrast, kerosene is the single most important ingestant in developing countries.

Ingestants

General principles

1. Emergency support for respiratory depression/shock.
2. History of ingestant, dose, time, onset of symptoms and progression, first aid measures at home.
   Other likely situations:

   i   Sudden inexplicable illness in a 1–5 year old, visiting a grandparent who is taking medication, or in an adolescent under stress/truanting.
   ii Family illness, e.g. diarrhoea (lomotil) or celebration (alcohol).
   iii Consider Munchausen by proxy.
   iv Older child 'drunk' or in coma from substance abuse.

3. Examination for specific clinical signs.
4. Stomach emptying if within 2 h of ingestion (up to 24 h for salicylates), *except when there is suspicion of ingesting hydrocarbons, corrosives, or lipoid substances.*

>   i Ipecacuanha syrup BP if conscious.
>
>   - At 6–18 months 10 ml, up to 12 years 15 ml, >12 years 30 ml.
>   - Then a drink of 200 ml water/juice, and encourage emesis by moving about.
>   - Repeat if no emesis in 15–30 minutes. Investigations are planned according to the likely cause and course of illness.
>
>   ii Gastric lavage with water/antidote if unconscious, with cuffed endotracheal tube if the gag reflex is absent. Monitor blood glucose and gases, BP, and input/output closely.

5. Activated charcoal
   1 g of activated charcoal has a surface area of $1000 m^2$ for absorbtion.
   Mechanisms: immediate contact (absorption) in the gut, interruption of the enterohepatic circulation of drugs secreted in bile (e.g. tricyclics), and gut dialysis against the intestines' rich capillary network.
   Action: within 2 h of ingestion, give 50 g activated charcoal. Useful in mild to moderate aspirin poisoning and especially effective against tricyclics (but not heavily ionized substances like strong acids or alkalis, iron, heavy metals, lithium, or cyanides). Administered with magnesium sulphate as a cathartic to reduce further absorption. Repeated doses in theophylline, tricyclic, and anticonvulsant poisoning further remove the drug.
6. Contact the regional poison information centre if the ingestant is known.
7. Arrange urine and blood screening if illness suggests poisoning, especially if abuse is likely.
8. Psychiatric referral if deliberate self poisoning.

Majority ingest little, and can go home from the A & E department provided no late complications are expected, and:

>   i Enough time has passed since ingestion.
>   ii Asymptomatic.
> iii The parents are reliable.
>   iv The primary team can be informed.

Hydrocarbons

Kerosene (paraffin), is the commonest ingestant and killer in developing countries.
   Danger of aspiration pneumonitis, so emesis best avoided.
   Toxic hydrocarbons, e.g. carbon tetrachloride, cause coma, pneumonitis, liver and kidney damage.

Household substances

Bleach (mildly corrosive), ammonia, dishwasher powders. Drain cleaners are highly corrosive, containing sodium hydroxide or sulphuric acid.

Management

Copious water to wash skin and milk to drink. Monitor for respiratory obstruction. Check pharynx for burns , may need early diagnostic oesophagoscopy (this procedure may cause perforation if delayed), antibiotics, and gastrostomy if confirmed. The use of steroids is controversial.

White spirit (turpentine substitute): the main danger is aspiration pneumonitis.

Medications/Iatrogenic poisoning

1. Benzodiazepines are the most frequently taken, but are rarely serious.
2. Tricyclics, antidepressants and opiates have replaced salicylate, iron and barbiturates as the most important causes of morbidity and mortality.
3. Digoxin is the leading cause of iatrogenic deaths.
4. Contraceptive pill. Although relatively common, it is not a management problem.

Prevention

1. Prescribing all medications in small amounts, in child-proof bottles or blister packs, unless otherwise requested, has resulted in a reduction in aspirin and paracetamol ingestion admissions from 9000 to 2000 annually in the UK.
2. Household substances should be sold with child-proof screw lids, in powder or dilute form, in original containers, with appropriate warning labels.
3. Such substances to be stored in cupboards with locks or child resistant catches.
4. Tricyclics should not be prescribed to children who are, or have siblings, under 5 years.

Aspirin

Less common now in under 12 year olds, partly due to recommendations regarding Reye's syndrome. Rarely iatrogenic now as rheumatic fever is uncommon.

Delayed absorption is common, especially if enteric coated tablets ingested. An early blood salicylate level at 2–3 hours (normally peak time) can therefore mislead.

Clinical

Anxious, sweating, tachycardia, tinnitus, vomiting → delerious, convulsions, coma. Fever, tetany early on, progressing to hypotension, pulmonary and cerebral oedema, renal failure and death.

Investigations

Salicylate serum levels at 6 h:
    Mild: <2.9 mmol/l
    Lethal: >8.8 mmol/l
Initial respiratory alkalosis gives way to metabolic acidosis; hypoglycaemia and hypoprothrombinaemia may occur. Coma occurs late.

Treatment

1. Emesis or gastric lavage up to 24 h after ingestion. Instil 1% sodium bicarbonate, leave activated charcoal.
2. Encourage excretion of salicylate:

   i Oral fluids, alkalinize urine with i.v. bicarbonate, consider diuretic.
   ii Dialysis or exchange transfusion in severe cases.

Digoxin

Specific antidote Digibind ligand.

Iron

Phases

1. Within 1 h–vomiting, bloody diarrhoea, then shock and steady deterioration to acidosis, may progress to coma and death.
2. Silent period with apparent stabilization for 10–15 h.
3. Relapse into coma, convulsions due to liver failure, brain swelling.
4. Long term: stenotic scarring of antrum/pylorus causing obstruction weeks later.

Investigation

Urgent serum iron, >1.25 µg/l = significant poisoning. Abdominal X-ray may show radiopaque tablets.

Management

1. By mouth: emesis, and pass nasogastric tube to wash out stomach with solution of 1% sodium bicarbonate and desferrioxamine 2 g/l. Post wash out instil 5 g desferrioxamine.
2. Parenteral: desferrioxamine i.m. 0.5 g immediately, and in severe poisoning infuse i.v. until urine changes from red to normal colour.
   Avoid overvigorous treatment of mild poisoning. Anaphylaxis with i.v. desferrioxamine, and in the longer term, iron deficiency, may result.

Lead

Antidote is now DMSA. See lead encephalopathy.

Opiates, including diphenoxylate

Naloxone 400 µg i.v. and i.m., repeat every 3 minutes up to 2.5 mg total.

Organophosphorus insecticides e.g. malathion.

Oxygen, enough atropine to atropinize, plus pralidoxime mesylate (a cholinesterase reactivator).

Paracetamol (acetaminophen)

Stage 1: minor nausea, vomiting, sweating in first 24 h. Stage 2: feel better in next 24 h. Stage 3: at 2–4 days = liver failure. Stage 4: resolution by 7 days.

Acetylcysteine (AC) must be given within 16 h of ingestion to be effective, though unlike adolescents and adults, liver failure is rare in children under 6 years, as they conjugate more of the drug, and metabolize less via cytochrome p450 which when swamped produces a hepatotoxic intermediate metabolite.

Action line for treatment is at peak plasma concentrations, at 4 h, >1.2mmol/l (180mg/l) and 0.2 mmol/l (30 mg/l) at 15 hours, the same as adults. AC orally: 140 mg/kg then 70 mg/kg 4-hourly for 17 doses.

Phenothiazines or metoclopramide causing dystonic reactions

Procyclidine hydrochloride 2.5 mg <1 year, 5 mg thereafter.

Tricyclics

Coma, seizures, myocardial depression with shock, tachyarrhythmias with characteristic ECG of broad QRS complexes, heart block.

Avoid antiarrhythmics, as correcting acidosis may suffice. Pacing occasionally required.

Diazepam for seizures.

Further reading

British Medical Association and The Pharmaceutical Society of Great Britain. *British National Formulary* London:Pharmaceutical Press

Reviews by various authors, compiled in the following journals:

Childhood Injuries in the United States (1990) *American Journal of Diseases of Children*, **144**, 625-727

Injuries and Injury Prevention (1985) *Pediatric Clinics of North America*, **33**, 1

Pediatric Toxicology (1986) *Pediatric Clinics of North America*, **33**:2 and **33**:3

CHILD CARE PROVISIONS

Adoption

Definition

The taking up of parental rights and duties under the 1975 Children's Act, usually by the husband adopting the child on marrying the mother.

Most are through the Social Service department of the local authority, with statutory supervision by a Medical Advisor.

Placement for adoption

Earliest is 6 weeks old, final adoption order 3 months later. Mainly comprise children with special needs (80% of total). The dearth of healthy Caucasian infants for adoption has resulted in older infants and children with handicaps, black or mixed race, being placed with Caucasian families.

Transcultural adoption (Black babies with Caucasian families) is deprecated by the British Association of Fostering and Adoption Agencies as preventing optimal development of racial identity.

Adoption Contact Register: with maternal permission, the name and address of the natural parent/relative can be revealed to the child after the age of 18 years old. Alternatively the individual may ask for the information from their birth record.

CARE

The Children Act 1989 principles:

1. The child's welfare is paramount. A court order is only made where not to do so would be harmful, and after considering that particular child's circumstances, wishes and needs.
2. Parental responsibility and involvement maintained, including the right to representation in court proceedings affecting their child.
3. Identification of children in need of local authority services through disability, being in care, on child protection registers, or with educational problems; to provide services and ensure those who would benefit know of them, and to promote care within the family.
4. Child care and protection legislation revised in the following areas:

Looked after by local authority (LA)

Accomodation provided where parents are absent/ill or child lost/abandoned. Child can be removed at any time by the parent without 28 days notice as required under previous 'Voluntary care' legislation. If the child is abandoned, LA may seek Care Order if in the child's best interests.

Child minder

Looks after children < 8 years old for reward. Registration with the local authority is required by law.

Foster care

For more than 28 days by someone not a relative.

Police protection

Without a court order this lasts up to 72 h, during which an Emergency Protection Order may be asked for. It applies when a constable believes a child may be harmed by removal from a hospital, or by staying at home. Inquiries into possible abuse must follow immediately.

Emergency Protection Order (EPO)

Replaces the Place of Safety Order.

Any person (in practice working through the Local Authority) can apply to a Magistrate in the Family Proceedings Court for an EPO to detain a child for up to 8 days (renewable for a further 7 days once only) when care proceedings are likely or the child is about to leave the country.

Parents must be notified, and have access unless the court specifies otherwise. They can challenge the EPO in court, or ask for it to be stopped after 72 h if they were not in court when it was given.

The child's home should be the safe place. In suitable cases, removal of the alleged abuser is preferred to removing the child to a hospital or residential home.

Medical or psychiatric or other assessments can be ordered by the court. Application for a Care Order or Supervision Order may follow.

Child Assessment Order

A child at risk of harm, and previous medical or psychiatric appointments have been refused or not attended. Not for emergencies. Time for completion 7 days.

Care and Supervision Orders

The family proceedings court requires the demonstration of significant harm (ill-treatment, impairment of health or development), present or future, attributable to parenting or lack of parental control.

A guardian ad litem is appointed by the court to represent the interests of the child.

An interim Care or Supervision Order may be given for 8 weeks, with a single extension of up to 4 weeks, to allow assessments and social investigations to be completed.

Care Order

The local authority has care and control, even though the child may still be at home. Can be removed to a children's home or foster parents if cooperation is lacking.

A child guilty of a criminal offence is no longer subject to a Care Order, but a Supervision Order can still be made.

Supervision Order

The supervisor (social worker/probation officer) is to befriend, advise, and assist the child and his family. A 'responsible person' is named by the Court (usually the parent). He/she must inform the supervisor of the current address and allow contact. If this or entry is refused a search warrant can be obtained.

Education, training, or 'intermediate' care can be required; medical and/or psychiatric treatment may be a part of the Order. Lasts 1–3 years.

Ward of Court

The High Court takes over responsibility, as a last resort and if the above framework fails. Acts 'in the best interests of the child' and becomes the child's guardian.

Both Care Order and Ward of Court orders remain in force to 18 years unless changed by the Courts.

Education Supervision Order

For children not attending school and of compulsory school age. Lasts 1 year, can be extended to 3, annually. Replaces the need for a full Care Order.

Family Assistance Order

To give expert advice for up to 6 months, usually during difficulties in separation or divorce.

Further reading

Department of Health (1989) *An Introduction to the Children Act.* London:HMSO
Miles M (1991) Implications of the children act for paediatricians. *Archives of Disease in Childhood,* **66,** 457–458

CHILD ABUSE

Definition

Unacceptable treatment of a child by an adult.

Epidemiology of abuse: emotional, neglect, physical, sexual

Prevalence

Four per cent of children under 13 years.

Incidence

Increased from 0.6 to 3.5 per 1000 from 1977 to 1988 in England and Wales. Reflects better public and professional awareness rather than true increase in incidence.

Distribution of reasons for placing on Child Protection Register: grave concern 40%, physical abuse 30%, sexual abuse 15%, neglect 15%.

Mortality

One in 10000 children annually (estimate).

Table 3.5 Characteristics of those involved in abuse

Child	Abuser	Relationships
First born	Young	Unstable with cohabitee
Often scapegoated	Known to Social Services	Isolated socially or geographically
Preschool>school age	Parent (of child) or cohabitee	
	Abused by others*	
	Personality disordered	

*Increases the risk of abusing by a factor of 20

Definitions of types of abuse

Emotional abuse

Persistent or severe emotional ill-treatment causing severe adverse effects on behaviour, development or health; includes coldness, hostility, rejection or constant denigration, seriously distorted emotional demands or extreme inconsistency.

Neglect

Failure to provide adequate food, shelter, clothing, physical protection or medical care.

Failure to thrive may result from emotional abuse or neglect (see deprivational failure to thrive).

Emotional deprivation and neglect are the most difficult to prove to be due to criminal intent.

Physical abuse

Injury inflicted or knowingly not prevented by the person caring or responsible for the child. It includes:

- Explanation for injuries improbable.
- Deliberate poisoning.
- Fabricating illness (Munchausen by proxy).
- Drowning and smothering attempts.
- Leaving unattended or inadequately supervised.

Sexual abuse

The involvement of dependent, developmentally immature children and young persons in sexual activities they do not truly comprehend, to which they are unable to give informed consent, or that violate the social taboos of family roles.

Liasion between agencies on the report of a case of suspected child abuse

Based on the Butler-Sloss recommendations following an inquiry into child abuse in Cleveland, in the North-East of England, in 1987.

Local policies and procedures are agreed by the Area Child Protection Committee, on which health, police, child protection agencies (NSPCC in the United Kingdom) and the social services are represented.

Child Protection teams have been established in many parts of the UK. Police officers and social workers interview and investigate cases together.

Guidelines ensure rapid exchange of information between the agencies so that appropriate advice can be given quickly.

Action taken by the team includes an interview with the child, if mature enough, before medical involvement, to establish the nature and extent of the abuse. This prevents unnecessary examination.

Failure of the parent to cooperate can be overcome by an EPO. *A duty of care to the child over-rides all other professional considerations of confidentiality.*

Medicine, the law and abuse. The Doctor's role

1. To be aware of medical and forensic findings on examination.
2. A duty to ensure the proper recording of findings and collecting of evidence, especially in sexual abuse.
3. To write reports to social work departments, provide statements to the police.
4. Attend court to give evidence and/or express an expert opinion.

Note taking

As any injuries may be the subject of extensive social work, and/or criminal investigation, pay careful attention to:

1. *Timing* (chronology) of events in the history.
2. *Date and time* of first interview and examination, and subsequent meetings with the parents/guardians.
3. *Draw* the injuries, with measurements of the size of the lesions.
4. *Negative* findings are also important, e.g. no bruising, normal genitalia, intact anus, etc.
5. *Immediately* make the entry in the clinical notes, dated and signed, not sometime later. Always have a witness with you (nurse, social worker, doctor) when interviewing. The name should be recorded in the notes.

TYPES OF ABUSE

Physical abuse/non- accidental Injury (NAI)

Definition
The result of acts or omissions by parent, cohabitee or guardian.

Incidence

One in 2000 children annually, of which 2% are killed, 30% seriously injured.

History

1. Tell-tale signs

- Inadequate explanation for injuries.
- Inconsistencies in story and timing of events when repeated to different people.
- Delay in coming forward.
- Repeated injuries with visits to different hospitals.

2. Attitudes

- Aggressiveness towards professionals and denial are common.
- Parents may collude or accuse each other.
- Child may shield and deny parental involvement.

3. Family history

Of brittle bones, premature deafness in osteogenesis imperfecta, bleeding or bruising must be enquired after.

4. Developmental history

Retardation? cause? behavioural problems, how are they handled?

Examination

Demeanor

Silent watchfulness or drugged appearance? May be wary of, name or indicate, the perpetrator.

Injuries

Carefully measure all injuries and draw them. The ages of bruises, burns and cuts to be estimated
1. Bruising is the commonest injury.

    i Immobile infants are unlikely to suffer these accidentally.

    ii A uniform colouring of the bruises indicates they occurred at the same time. Bruises of different hues signify more than one incident.

    iii Predominant colour: red = 1 day, blue = 1–3 days, greeny-yellow = 5–10 days, yellow >8 days.

    iv Sites, distribution of characteristic injuries, and mechanism:

- Face, especially the cheeks: linear or finger tip marks.
- Bilateral black eyes = direct blow to the nose, and fractured.
- Black eye/purpura in the orbit: blow from fist.
- Pinna: purpura over and behind pinna, +/- bleeding from the meatus: a blow from the open hand.
- Trunk and limbs: grip marks, finger tip marks from shaking, or swinging.

- Buttocks, trunk, limbs: 'rings' from teeth bite marks, or linear bruises from ligatures or belt marks.

2. Burns and scalds
   Perfect circular burn–cigarette burns most likely on exposed areas. Often deep if deliberate.
   Stocking scald/ linear burn–immersed/held against his will.
3. Fractures/separation of epiphyses (haematoma often overlying)

   i Long bone: Mid shaft–direct blow; spiral–twisting; epiphyseal shearing–swinging the body by the limb.
   ii Ribs: shaking/squeezing, direct blows.
   iii Skull: suspect NAI if multiple, depressed, not parietal, wide and growing.

4. Soft tissue injury
   Subarachnoid and subdural haemorrhage: drowsy, fits, decerebration. Retinal haemorrhage is common. Mechanism: direct trauma, and shaking the trunk vigorously backwards and forwards.
   Torn frenulum: a blow, or forced bottle feeding.
   Ruptured internal organs: direct blows, may present as an acute abdomen.

Investigations

1. Growth: height and weight centiles.
2. Photographs.
3. Platelets, coagulation; calcium, phosphate, copper if premature/parenterally fed.
4. Skeletal survey, including lateral of ribs. Repeat 7 days later if uncertain, by which time callus will show.

Suspicious fractures on X-ray

Skull: multiple/complex, depressed, wide, growing, especially of occipital bone or more than one bone.
Long bones: metaphyseal, or in different stages of repair. Spiral fractures without adequate explanation.
Scapulae, outer end of clavicle, and ribs: these suggest direct injury.

Differential diagnosis

Very premature: metabolic bone disease shows rickets and osteopenia; serum alkaline phosphatase high.
Brittle bones: wormian skull bones, abnormal long bone X-ray structure.
Scurvy, vitamin A intoxication, infantile cortical hyperostosis: characteristic X-ray findings.
Copper deficiency: osteopenia, neutropenia, hypochromic anaemia.

Diagnosis

- Injuries suggestive of physical abuse.

- Explanation inconsistent with injuries.
- Injuries of different ages.

Misdiagnoses

Impetigo, Mongolian blue spot, normal periosteal new bone formation (laid down in layers, symmetrically), bone disorders, congenital insensitivity to pain, bleeding disorders.

Management

Protection of the child is paramount. Child protection team must be notified, preferably before examination.

1. Admit to hospital/other, with parental cooperation or under Emergency Protection Order.
2. Evaluate other children in the home, admit if at risk.
3. Case conference arranged.
   Temporary fostering, during social/psychiatric work to evaluate risk of re-uniting, may become long term if return to the family is unworkable.

Outcome

Returned to family 60%; death 2%; severe injury 30%; re-injury 10-30%; growth failure 30%
Handicap resulting: cerebral palsy, epilepsy, mental handicap.

Further reading

Carty H (1988) Brittle or battered. *Archives of Disease in Childhood*, **63**, 350–352
Newton R W (1989) Intracranial haemorrhage and non-accidental injury. *Archives of Disease in Childhood*, **64**, 188-190
Taitz L (1991) Child abuse: some myths and shibboleths. *Hospital Update*, **17**, 400-408 A pithy account, and an attack on the 'expert witnesses' in NAI.

Deprivational failure to thrive and short stature

Definition

Short proportionate stature, with low growth velocity, but catch-up growth occurs when away from the family.
Found at any age in childhood.
Endocrine investigation shows reversible growth hormone deficiency.

Symptoms

1. Abnormal feeding behaviour: pica, stealing food, eats alone or separate from the family. Gorging outside the home.
2. Diurnal enuresis, faecal smearing or encopresis.

3. Delayed mental development, delayed puberty.
4. Immaturity in appearance and behaviour. Unhappy, anti-social.

Useful signs

Blue and cold extremities, frozen watchfulness or over-affectionate to strangers.

Investigations

1. Exclude organic causes by clinical examination, delayed bone age. See Growth problems.
2. Parental attitudes explored. Often critical, dismissive. As sexual abuse occurs in association, may need a social work enquiry.

Treatment

Change in parenting attitudes may not be possible. For the child's long–term physical growth, emotional and mental development, removal from the home may be necessary.

Munchausen by proxy (Meadow's syndrome)

Definition

The victim is of preschool age. Symptoms or signs are deliberately fabricated or induced, usually by mother.

Lying by mother about medical, social and family background is common. Associated with unexplained deaths of previous siblings.

False clinical signs

- Seizures, apnoea (the latter may be induced by suffocation).
- Recurrent bleeding from mouth, anus, bladder is common. The blood is smeared on, usually from finger prick/menses.
- Intermittent coma due to smothering, hypnotics, anticonvulsants, insulin, salt.
- Rashes from scratching and applying caustics to cause blisters.
- Restrictive diets for 'allergies', 'hyperactivity' resulting in malnutrition.
- Temperature: thermometer warmed, charts altered, in hospital by the parent.

Observation

Symptoms absent during continuous observation. Rarely, smothering has been witnessed during video surveillance.

Occasionally a physical condition may be present, but the features are grossly and persistently exaggerated.

Investigation

1. Verify history. May be reported to be witnessed by others who cannot corroborate.
2. Suspect if occurrence of symptom in hospital is only in mother's presence and her exclusion results in their disappearance.
3. Check body fluids: is the blood in urine/faeces/haemoptysis etc the child's blood group? Unexpected drugs, insulin, abnormal biochemistry?

Diagnosis

1. Inability to find a diagnosis or symptoms only manifest when mother is present.
2. Mother usually has some medical background, e.g. nurse or medical family, but no overt psychopathology.
3. Previous death or severely ill sibling with undiagnosed condition.

Treatment

1. Confrontation.
2. Child protection team notified. If danger of removal arrange for Emergency Protection Order. Case conference and plan for return home under supervision, or other provision if too hazardous, and offering psychological help.

Further reading

Meadow R (1984) Factitious illness—the hinterland of child abuse. *Recent Advances in Paediatrics No.7* London:Churchill Livingstone

Child sexual abuse (CSA)

Definition

The exploitation of a child for the sexual gratification of an adult.

Prevalence

Estimated to be 10–20% of under 16 year olds.
Three levels of severity:

1. Non-physical event, 60%, the majority occurring only once, (e.g. indecent exposure, shown or photographed in pornographic poses).
2. Physical acts in 30%: mainly fondling, kissing, biting, by adult, touching private parts by adult or the child.
3. Penetration in 5–10%: oral, vaginal, anal; includes rape, intracrural (= between upper thighs) intercourse or buggery.

Incidence

One per 1000 annually, from 0.17 in 1979; likely to be a rise in notification, not the true rate.

Ratio of girls:boys = 2:1, peak age 3–5 years old, though boys may be under reported.

Perpetrators

Three-quarters are relatives, usually male: father, step-father or cohabitee, and teen-age brother or uncle; grandfathers and mothers are less commonly implicated.

Unrelated men (often in authority, e.g. teachers, activity leaders, or trusted family friend), and baby sitters comprise the rest.

Prognosis as an adult after abuse in childhood: increased depression, anxiety dis-orders, drug and alcohol abuse by a factor of 2–12-fold.

The family

Marital disharmony is common; drugs and alcoholism; occasionally prostitution, previous CSA in another child. Mothers may be colluding and could be the last per-son to turn to.

Rarely a personality disordered or psychotic parent.

Presentation

1. Disclosure by the child to a trusted adult (always to be believed, until completed enquiries can confirm or refute the possibility).
2. Partial disclosure

    i By word– 'about another little girl I know' meaning herself.
    ii Or action – showing inappropriate knowledge of sexual caress or act of inter-course.

3. Information or allegation by parent, relative, others.
4. While investigating other forms of abuse.
5. Physical or behavioural complaints in which abuse is one of the possible causes.

A. Physical conditions

    i   Vulvovaginitis, vaginal discharge.
    ii Vaginal bleeding, especially in the premenstrual child – always check puber-tal stage.
    iii Recurrent lower abdominal pain or dysuria with sterile urine cultures.
    iv Faecal soiling, constipation, rectal bleeding, anal soreness.
    v   Non–accidental injury (15% of NAI cases).
    vi Pregnancy under 16 years old and identity of father unknown.

B. Behavioral problems which should arouse suspicion, especially if previously 'normal'.

    i Inappropriate sexuality in dress or attitudes to adults, preoccupation with sexual fantasies (may also occur in schizophrenia).
    ii Unexplained changes in behaviour.

iii Truanting or school failure, running away from home.
iv Suicide attempt.

Initial response

1. Suspicion of CSA should trigger discussion with an experienced paediatric colleague or social services.
2. The differential diagnosis is discussed, and action agreed.
3. Once agreed, the parent(s) or guardian(s) are informed of the need for investigation of suspected CSA, in a non–confrontational way even when they are suspected abusers.

A full interview is then planned, in as suitable a place as possible, not a police station (unless it has a rape suite and the child has recently suffered this assault and evidence could be lost) or room in the A & E department.

A single interview, conducted jointly by a social worker and police officer with expertise with child interviews, is desirable, in the presence of an adult not implicated and whom the child may trust (parent, teacher or social worker known to the child).

Asking questions as to fact, about the keeping of 'secrets', or detecting a wish to protect the abuser out of love or fear, and the use of anatomically correct dolls, require gentleness and patience.

A video recording may be made to relieve the child of repeated questioning, is part of the case records, must be preserved, and kept safe, and may be used in evidence in court in the UK.

Examination

1. Refusal. The child has this right (under the Children Act), provided the doctor is of the opinion the child understands the consequences.
2. Examination must be limited to one: a cursory one may already have taken place in establishing a need for investigation. To avoid further emotional trauma by repeated examination ('professional abuse') a joint examination by police surgeon and paediatrician may be called for, especially when forensic specimens (for semen, blood, fibres etc) are likely to be taken. The doctor's sex is less important than their manner. Proceed as follows:

   i Recent abuse <72 h before. All clothing must be kept, placed in plastic bags. No teeth cleaning or bathing until examined.
   ii A paediatric history of health, development, behaviour.
   iii Height, weight, general examination, 'head to toe' direction, meanwhile engaging the child and observing her responses.
   Look for burns, bruising, teeth marks. Significant sites are neck, breasts, below the waist, thighs, genitalia; grip marks on upper arms, the knees.
   Age the bruises by their colour.
   Draw a diagram of the lesions.

3. Genital examination.

    i Girls 'frog-legged', lying supine with hips flexed, soles touching, and blanket draped from waist to knees. The prone knee-chest position is only recommended when needing a better view of the posterior margin of the hymen.

   ii Draw and describe injuries such as bruising, erythema from rubbing, tears. Holding the labia apart by gentle lateral pressure at their lower end allows the vaginal orifice to be assessed.

- The maximum normal vaginal opening up to 4 years is 4 mm, and 10 mm before puberty. More than 15 mm is suggestive of abuse if signs of trauma are present. Congenital absence of the hymen in otherwise normal girls is unknown.
- The hymen and posterior fourchette may be torn or scarred; hymenal 'bumps', and notching at 12 o'clock, without tear or scar, is normal. An auriscope head or hand held lens (× 2–4 magnification) is useful here. Colposcopy is even better.

    Note any discharge from the penis, vagina or rectum.

    Genital warts or herpes may be due to CSA.

- Digital vaginal examination only if bleeding (may need anaesthesia) or to assess size and smoothness after repeated penile penetration in a pubertal girl.

Diagnostic of blunt penetration are:

    i Laceration or scars in the hymen.

   ii Loss of hymenal tissue.

Supportive only:

    Hymenal orifice 10–15 mm in prepubertal girl.

    Notches or bumps with scarring

    Signs of friction due to intercrural intercourse

    Labial fusion.

4. Anus: lying on left side, legs curled up, gently separate buttocks for half a minute. If the anus is lax and dilated from the beginning, this is abnormal.

    i Note any injury, perianal swelling ('tyre') or haematoma, fissures, skin tags, warts.

   ii The anus may 'twitch' (normal) or gape open within half a minute, several centimetres of rectum often becoming visible = "reflex anal dilatation" (RAD). This sign is found in constipation as well as buggery. Persistence of RAD is suggestive of the latter. It is believed by some to be due to internal sphincter laxity secondary to retrograde penetration as in anal intercourse, which may be commoner in boys than girls.

  iii Digital examination is contentious, and is to look for or confirm constipation, routinely by some police surgeons, but few paediatricians.

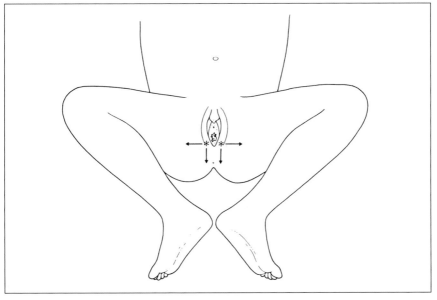

Figure 3.3 Examination position: gentle traction between thumb and index finger at posterior edge of labia to show irregular torn hymen

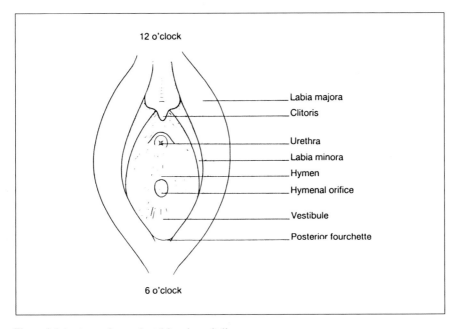

Figure 3.4 Anatomy of pre-pubertal female genitalia

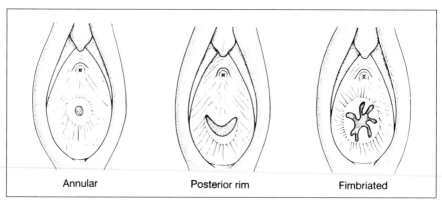

Figure 3.5 Variations in configuration of the hymen. (From the Report of the Royal College of Physicians (1991) on the Physical Signs of Sexual Abuse in Children pp 8 and 12

Diagnostic of blunt penetration
Scar or laceration extending beyond the anal mucosa onto the perianal skin in the absence of an adequate explanation.
Supportive only:
  Lax anus without explanation.
  RAD >1 cm.
  Acute changes (erythema, swelling, fissures, venous congestion and bruising).
  Chronic, of repeated anal intercourse (funnelling, thickened anal verge, increased elasticity and weakening of the anal sphincter).

Diagnostic dilemmas

- No physical sign, on its own, is diagnostic of CSA.
- Absence of physical signs does not exclude sexual abuse, especially as time often allows regression of dilatation and healing.
- Masturbation and oral sex may leave no sign.
- Pitfalls include lichen sclerosis of perineum, Crohn's disease of rectum, rectal tumours, haemolytic uraemic syndrome affecting the anus, nappy rash.

Investigation

To safeguard against invalidating forensic samples, the chain of evidence must be maintained. The person taking a sample, passing it on, or processing it, must record the time, date and next person to whom it is entrusted.

1. Forensic swabs from vagina, rectum, mouth for sperm and acid phosphatase.
2. Photographs.
3. Bacteriology swabs for gonorrhoea, trichomonas (both highly suggestive of CSA), chlamydia (suspicious).
4. Blood of perpetrator (and child if chronic abuse) for syphilis, hepatitis B and HIV testing.

5. Pregnancy test if appropriate.
6. Consider examination of the perpetrator(s) for sexually transmitted disease, penile or vulval warts.

Diagnosis is based on any one of the following:

1. Allegation by child and strong circumstantial evidence.
2. Allegation by child and signs found consistent with the diagnosis (vaginal dilatation, anal dilatation, torn foreskin or vaginal frenulum etc).
3. Sexually transmitted disease (STD).
4. Pregnancy.
5. Gross physical signs – with follow up, disclosure or 6 may follow.
6. Admission by perpetrator (rare, because it is widely known to be a criminal act).

Action

1. Calculated non-precipitate action: arrange a case conference whenever a highly suspicious history is obtained with or without clinical or forensic evidence of CSA.
   A child protection plan, therapy for the child and family are the agenda items.
   Criminal investigation and prosecution may follow.
   It is better to be returned to a possibly abusing household than to remove the child with insufficient evidence that will not stand up in court. Further investigation may reveal more, when removal may be indicated.
2. Consider removal of the child, to a place of safety, or requesting the alleged perpetrator quit the home if:

   i   The perpetrator is named by the child and lives in the same house; the child may be in real physical danger.
   ii The child is likely to be made to change testimony if allowed home.
   iii The injury is recent and severe.

3. Treat potential sexually transmitted disease in rape with a single dose of intramuscular procaine penicillin with probenecid. If seen within 72 h of intercourse, prevent pregnancy with 'morning after' pill (Ovran, Schering PC4). Prescribe the usual antibiotics for STD bacterial isolates.
   Specific antihepatitis B immunoglobulin 0.06ml/kg as soon as possible after exposure.
4. Consider referral to a child psychiatrist.
5. Reassure the child, that she is believed and not responsible for possible familial consequences, and that the injuries are, of themselves, unlikely to have any long-term physical sequelae.
6. An indecisive investigation still needs follow-up, as disclosure may follow later, particularly if the abuse continues.

Further reading

Chadwick D L (1989) *Color Atlas of Child Sexual Abuse*. Chicago:Year Book Medical Publishers
Her Majesty's Stationery Office (1988) *Diagnosis of child sexual abuse: guidance for doctors.* London: HMSO.

Her Majesty's Stationery Office (1991) *Working together Under the Children Act 1989*. A guide to the Arrangements for Inter-agency Co-operation for the Protection of Children from Abuse. London: HMSO
Meadow R (1989) *ABC of Child Abuse*. London:British Medical Journal
Royal College of Physicians of London (1991) *Physical Signs of Sexual Abuse in Children*. London:RCP

SUDDEN INFANT DEATH SYNDROME (SIDS)

Definition

Sudden and unexpected death in a previously healthy infant 1 week to 2 years old, in whom a carefully performed autopsy fails to reveal an adequate explanation.

A distinction must be drawn with sudden unexpected death due to unrecognized but treatable overt disease, accidents, and infanticide by suffocation.

Incidence

One in 500. Commonest cause (50%) of deaths in this age group.

Timing

Peak at 6 weeks to 6 months, winter>summer, early hours of the morning.

Mechanisms

1. Apnoea: Final common pathway of many disease processes, may be obstructive, central (brainstem) or mixed. Lung collapse associated with end expiratory apnoea, as in pertussis.
2. Hyperthermia: increased in prone sleeping and overwrapping, especially during a viral infection.
3. Infection with minor symptoms may lead to 1 and/or 2.
4. Metabolic: hypoglycaemia from inborn errors, e.g. MCAD deficiency, in total probably 2–5% of cases.
5. Toxins: botulism is implicated in 5% of cases in the USA.
6. Homicide 1%.

Risk factors

Prematurity, multiple birth, prone and hyperthermia, single parent, maternal smoking, multiple siblings. Boys > girls, low birthweight (bronchopulmonary dysplasia and < 1.5 kg = 7 × increased risk).

Clinical

Blood stained vomit/secretions may occur at death, and not due to injury. Take temperature.

Investigations

Swabs, culture of urine, heart blood, CSF. Blood, urine, skin fibroblasts and liver biopsy for inborn errors.

Management

1. Resuscitation may be attempted if recently found. If brought to hospital, the infant is taken into the Accident and Emergency department, not left in the ambulance.
2. Privacy for the parents. A brief history is obtained. Confirm death and inform parents. Guilt often expressed from feelings of responsibility for it. Unless illness is obvious, suspicious circumstances, or abnormal parental attitude, explain that it appears to be a cot death. They are given the baby to hold. Photograph of the baby taken for presentation to parents later. Time for parents to "say good-bye" essential; they may wish to return later.
3. Explain to the parents

    i Police visit the home to take a statement, and may remove bedding for analysis.
    ii No blame is likely to attach to them, nor inquest held, but the Coroner has a duty to investigate all sudden deaths and must be informed.
    iii Post-mortem is required by law.
    iv Social worker for support. Offer to contact the Foundation for the Study of Infant Deaths parent support group.

4. Support in hospital: someone (it is often the chaplain) to stay with parents at all times.
5. Inform the primary care team, and community vaccination scheme to prevent distress from reminders. Bromocriptine is prescribed to suppress lactation.
6. Continued support: paediatrician with responsibility for SIDS counselling sees at 2 weeks, 6 weeks and up to 2 years after the death.

Recurrence

If one of twins, up to 1 in 40 within the next month. Risk is otherwise 1 in 300 for subsequent siblings.

Subsequent pregnancies

Provide emotional support, apnoea monitor/oximetry (despite lack of proof of efficacy they give reassurance and allow parents to sleep).

Prevention

1. The CONI (Care of the Next Infant) scheme, developed by the Foundation for the Study of Infant Deaths. Health Authorities are invited to establish weekly community nurse visiting for discussion and advice. A symptom diary, weighing scales and chart to record daily weights (recent weight loss may herald SIDS), an

apnoea monitor and room thermometer are provided by the local branch of the Foundation.

2. Encourage parents to seek professional advice for relatively minor symptoms, and use the Baby Check scoring system as a standard.
3. Advise positioning babies on their side or back, and light clothing and coverings if the room is maintained at 18°C. From one month to a year, a vest, nappy and babygrow, and 2–3 layers of blanket suffice, with a light cardigan in cold weather; total Tog rating 9–10.
4. When suffering a viral illness avoid overheating by reducing covers.
5. Stopping parental smoking may confer benefit.

Further reading

Bacon C J (1991) The thermal environment of sleeping babies and possible dangers of overheating. In *Recent Advances in Paediatrics*, **9**, T J David, ed. Edinburgh:Churchill Livingstone, pp 123-136

Couriel J M (1991) Paediatric support after sudden infant death. In *Recent Advances in Paediatrics*, **9**, T J David, ed. Edinburgh:Churchill Livingstone pp 171–185 Essential reading to understand family responses to SIDS and provide practical support.

Culbertson J L, Krous H F, Bendell R D (1989) *Sudden Infant Death Syndrome: Medical Aspects and Psychological Management*. London:Edward Arnold. Comprehensive review of hypotheses of causation, and counselling

Engelberts A C, de Jonge G A (1990) Choice of sleeping position for infants: possible association with cot death. *Archives of Disease in Childhood*, **65**, 462–467

Chapter 4

Behavioural and psychological dysfunction

CRYING

Crying normally increases from birth to a maximum at 2 months of average 2–2.5 hours a day, peak between 6 pm–12 am. A rapid decline then follows.

Three month colic/infantile colic

Definition

More than 3 hours crying for 3 or more days a week. Affects 15–20% at 6 weeks, halved by 3 months; 10% persist to a year old.

Excessive crying, as perceived by the parent, may lead to abuse.

Management of persistent crying for weeks

Inconsistency or uncertainty in the parental approach is likely to exacerbate colic, but is not a primary cause.

Feeding–sleeping–crying diaries are useful to record the pattern and parents' responses and actions.

Interventions found effective:

1. Carrying the infant, and reducing excessive stimulation.
2. Counselling and support to establish routines. Parent support groups such as CRY-SIS
3. Cows' milk protein (CMP) avoidance: 5% may have transient intolerance, so avoidance may be worthy of trial, using a protein hydrolysate (e.g. Pregestimil). Breast fed mothers: try CMP free diet. Improvement seen in a week. Return to CMP if no improvement, and after 1–2 months if successful.
4 Activated dimethicone may help some cases.

Abnormal infant cries

1. Syndromic: Cri du chat is 'mewing', hypothyroidism a growl like a 'record slowing down'.
2. Cerebral:

   i   High pitched cerebral cry in an asphyxiated or meningitic baby.
   ii Cry with bizarre eye movements or apnoea may be the only signs of seizure.

3. Severe intermittent pain: shrill pain cry with pallor, followed by flushing, recurring every few minutes, for one or more hours, in intussusception.
4. Moderate/more persistent pain cry +/- fever: otitis media, urinary tract infection, gastroenteritis (Helicobacter especially painful).
5. Cry with cyanosis: breath holding, reverse shunting across an open ductus arteriosus or intracardiac shunt.

Further reading

Drug and Therapeutics Bulletin (1992) Management of infantile colic. **30**, 15–16

BEHAVIOUR PROBLEMS

Approximately 20% of 3 year olds have behaviour problems.
   If severe, they tend to persist, especially in boys with poor peer relationships.
Factors include:

1. In the child: temperament (difficult, moody, excessive crying), delayed speech and development.
2. Environmental stress: poverty, high rise living, homeless accomodation.
3. Maternal depression, poor marriage.
4. Parenting skills poorly developed: parents themselves neglected or abused, or in care as a child.

   Factors reducing the impact of poor parenting

1. Consistent support and encouragement from another adult.
2. Positive school atmosphere.
3. The child's own positive temperament.

BEHAVIOUR MODIFICATION

The child's behaviour is influenced by the consequence of that behaviour. Thus undesired behaviour is reinforced unless countered. Any consequence which increases the frequency of a behaviour (desired or undesired) is termed a positive reinforcer.
   Examples:

- screaming or vomiting induces the parent to acquiesce.
- repeatedly getting out of bed until allowed to stay up.

- 'inability to sleep' without a parent present.

In the same way, praise for passing a bowel motion into the potty, being dry, completing a meal etc, encourages repeat performances.

Methods of behaviour modification

1. A plan of action must be agreed between the carers. Failure to do so results in 'divide and rule' by the child, who should be instructed about the plan if old enough to understand.
2. Establish a base line
   The behaviour(s) to be modified is charted for a period, e.g. 1–2 weeks.
3. Techniques used

   i 'Extinction' means complete and immediate ignoring of the unwanted behaviour, e.g. head banging, temper tantrums in shops. A temporary upsurge in the undesired behaviour is usual, until the child realizes new rules are in force.

   ii 'Shaping' behaviour: gradual change, usually more acceptable to parents, in a series of steps.

Examples:

   a. Inability to get the child into bed at a reasonable hour is treated by bringing bedtime forward by 15 minute steps each night.
   b. Child insists parent cradles him until asleep. Encourage the use of a transitional object such as a soft toy, at first at daytime naps, then night. Withdrawal from the room in steps: sitting on the bed, then next to it, then at the door.
   c. Stop 'rewarding' the child with a milk drink for waking the parent, e.g. reducing by an ounce a night, replace with a dummy.

   iii Cueing: preparation for an activity, e.g. bedtime routine starts with bathtime, making a clear distinction between day and night, which helps establish the desired behaviour.   *Routine*

   iv 'Time out': immediate exclusion from activities, to show disapproval, at every exhibition of the undesired behaviour, e.g. biting or fighting → immediately being sat on a chair or removed from the room for a short period (<5 minutes) before being allowed back in.

   v Positive reinforcement of a desired behaviour: praise and encouragement. Cost effective. From a mental age of 3 years, supplement it by daily filling in of a chart and giving stickers for complying with the desired behaviour, e.g. dry bed, clean pants, or good behaviour in shops.

FOOD AND MEALTIME PROBLEMS

Parental concern, and feelings of rejection, due to real or imagined insufficient intake and food fads, are common.

Presentation by age includes:

1. First 2 years:

   i   Failure to thrive

      a. Breast feeding difficulties, e.g. 'starvation at the breast' as the infant adjusts to a reducing milk supply.
      b. Understimulation, often linked with maternal depression.
      c. Inadequate intake: ignorance, unusual diets (e.g. macrobiotic), hardship, deliberate starvation.

   ii Reluctance to take solids, and hence also to chew. Increased likelihood if weaning is delayed beyond 6 months of age, or reluctance by the baby or toddler to give up the breast.

2. Between 1 and 3 years:

   i   Battles over control between parents and child. Food fads are common. Other family members may exacerbate the situation by increasing anxiety levels or undermining efforts at setting limits.
   ii Disorganized/chaotic meal times.
   iii Interaction of an irritable child on a disorganized mother leads to a cycle of mother offering less food, resulting eventually in a reduction in appetite and failure to thrive.

3. Adolescence: anorexia and bulimia nervosa (see later).

Assessment

1. Growth: determine whether a failure to thrive or feeding problem. Plot all available height and weight measurements. Include birth weight, and allow for parental height where indicated.
2. Feeding charts and food diary: to determine adequacy of intake. Obtain a detailed record of every item of food at meals and snacks. Often intake is more than the parent thought, and may identify snacking as a major cause of not eating at meal times. Disorganization and depression may be reflected in failure to complete a chart or keep a diary.
3. Observation of a meal: ideally at home, alternatively in hospital, to see interaction between mother and child, e.g. excessive distraction with toys or TV, child running from the table, maternal tension etc.

Management

Involvement of dietetician, health visitor, psychological and medical personnel according to severity, and the need for parental support.

Examples of feeding problem interventions:

1. Milk has remained the main food source, so solids are refused. Action: reduce milk intake progressively, if necessary by watering it down. Hunger encourages interest in solid food.

2. Food fad: offer food at meal times, throwing it away if refused, but not offering an alternative. Alternatively introduce a single new item of food daily, with reward charts to reinforce acceptance.
3. Refusal to take from the spoon: allow finger feeding/exploration of food.
4. Inadequate food intake: at first no increase in amount, just aim to empty the plate. Increase size of portions slowly, as large portions can be daunting.
5. Chaotic prolonged mealtimes, the child running around the room. Action: the food is only presented if sitting at the table, so limiting the duration of meal times, and parental attention, as a consequence.

Anorexia nervosa

Definition

Avoidance of eating with failure to gain weight, or weight loss at the time of the expected growth spurt, in an otherwise healthy girl, (ratio girl:boy = 9:1). Associated with vomiting, purging, exercising, feeling fat and fear of it, preoccupation with body weight and calories, amenorrhoea. A paradoxical interest in food and food preparation is often shown.

Bulimia nervosa

Definition

Recurrent binging followed by self-induced vomiting, laxative abuse, or fasting to counteract binging, while maintaining a near normal weight.
   Incidence of each is 1% of adolescents, far less common in children.
   Theories of causation of eating disorders

   i   Family pathology with overprotectiveness, unresolved conflicts; a battle of control between child and parent; 'Peter Pan' avoidance of growing up. Family history of eating disorders.
   ii Environmental: society's pressure to be thin, an idealized view of physical appearance.
   iii Occupational (e.g. dancers, modelling), high achievers.
   iv Sexual abuse.
   v   Genetic (increased incidence among monozygotic twins).

Presentation

   i   Anorexia. Age usually 9–19 years. Emaciated, may previously have been 'plump'. Failure of development, or loss, of secondary sex characteristics. Skin becomes rough, limbs cold.
   ii Bulimia. Late adolescence, history of food battles in early childhood. Recurrent vomiting 'of unknown cause', oesophagitis, dental erosions due to stomach acid.

Differential diagnosis

Abuse, malignancy, inflammatory bowel disease, malabsorption, hyperthyroid or hypoadrenal disorders excluded clinically or by investigation.

Obstacles to diagnosis: reluctance to admit to disorder, and its increased occurrence in cystic fibrosis or diabetes mellitus sufferers when symptoms mimic disease.

Management

1. Hospitalization enables feeding to be supervised, and vomiting to be prevented. Later, social skills training groups to enable expression in words rather than food refusal. Week-ends at home are the start of rehabilitation to cope at home.
2. Behaviour modification: rewards for gaining weight, i.e. privileges gained, e.g. wearing own clothes, watching TV, outings.
3. Family therapy or individual psychotherapy, dynamic or cognitive.
4. Medication: a limited role for antidepressants in bulimia nervosa. Fluoxetine, a 5-hydroxytryptamine uptake inhibitor, has a role in bulimia.

Prognosis

Mortality 0–5% from suicides and starvation. Persistent poor socialization, sexual relationships, menstrual problems, weight preoccupation in 50%. Relapse and depression common.

Further reading

Bryant-Waugh R, Knibbs J, Fosson A, Kaminski Z, Lask B (1988) Long term follow up of patients with early onset anorexia nervosa. *Archives of Disease in Childhood*, **63**, 5–9

Crisp A H (1983) Anorexia nervosa. *British Medical Journal*, **287**, 855–858

SLEEP DISTURBANCE

Most infants sleep through the night by 6–12 weeks, but 20% of 1–2 year olds still wake most nights, reducing to 8% by 4 years old. Over 50% with a sleep problem in infancy still wake at 5 years. Frequent night wakings are related to:

1. Poor feeding interval patterning.
2. Environmental: wet/dirty nappy, covers fall off.
3. Intercurrent illness disturbing an established pattern, or a chronic condition seems to prevent its establishment, e.g. eczema (scratching) or asthma (woken by cough or wheeze).
4. Parenting problems, family stress, e.g. birth of a sibling, house move, new school, abuse.

These factors are modified by cultural expectations, e.g. in Asian families children often sleep in their parent's bed, so are comforted more readily.

Management

Disturbed sleep, secondary to behaviour alone, can quickly be improved, independent of duration. Cueing, shaping and positive reinforcement are used. Extinction, i.e. ignoring, is not popular but works in 3–4 nights. Drugs play little part.

Further reading

Douglas J (1989) *Behaviour Problems in Young Children*. London:Routledge

CLINICAL SLEEP CONDITIONS

Table 4.1 Clinical sleep conditions

	Nightmares	Night terrors*
Age	Peaks at 2 and 7 years	6–12 years
Sex	M = F	M > F
Sleep stage	Rapid eye movement	Stage 4
Recall	Complete next morning	None

*Sleep walking and sleep talking are similar forms of parasomnia

Management

Explanation usually suffices.

Frequent night terrors and sleep walking may be reduced by diazepam 5–10 mg or imipramine 25 mg.

Alternatively, success is claimed for watching for sweating and increased movement, then waking the child before the terrors ensue. They abate after some weeks of this regimen.

NOCTURNAL ENURESIS

Definition

The involuntary passage of urine during sleep, without underlying physical cause, over the age of 3 years.

Prevalence: 10% at 6 years, 3% at 12 years, 1% of adults. M:F = 2:1, commoner in lower socioeconomic groups.

Causes

Developmental: immaturity of control is common, with more frequent passage of urine by day.

Hereditary: often familial.

Environmental: stress, e.g. family break-up, separation from mother, house moves, birth of a younger sibling, hospital admissions, accidents, operations; punitive handling may prolong the condition. Dry nights on holiday away from home confirm continence is possible.

Examination

- Genital examination for signs of abuse, or an ectopic ureter, e.g. persistent vaginal leakage of urine.
- Spine for hairy patch, lipoma, pigmented patch.
- Neurology; sensation of the saddle area, power of the intrinsic muscles of the feet (S2–4), and plantar reflexes.
- BP, urinalysis, urine culture.

Differential diagnosis

View onset enuresis with suspicion. It may be organic in origin, especially in the absence of a family history, though it does occur in primary enuresis.

1. Emotional factors:
   - i Abuse, marital discord, family illness, new sibling.
   - ii New school, bullying, learning difficulties. Timing may be indicative, e.g. Sunday night – school related problem?

2. Organic:
   - i Urinary tract infection.
   - ii Epilepsy.
   - iii Diabetes mellitus or insipidus.

DIURNAL ENURESIS

Definition

Wetting by day beyond the age control is normally attained.

Prevalence

At 4 years disturbed children are more likely to wet than normal children (17% vs 8%).

Affects 10% of those with nocturnal enuresis, and the sex ratio is reversed (M<F 1:1.5)

Causes

1. Usually due to primary enuresis, i.e. never dry; due to lack of training; small bladder capacity; or incomplete emptying.
2. Urine infection sometimes found, as 'covert bacteriuria', but symptoms improve with antibiotics.
3. Also consider: deprivation; mental handicap; spina bifida; structural, e.g. posterior urethral valves.

Variations

1. Onset of day and night time wetting is associated with

   i Emotional upset.
   ii Organic factors, including:

      a. Progressive neurological spinal lesions, e.g. diastematomyelia.
      b. CNS degenerations.

2. Day time wetting alone, with dry nights, is almost always emotional/developmental, e.g. on the way home from school. Dryness for 1 hour virtually excludes a spinal cord abnormality, urethral valves or ectopic ureter.
3. Day–time urinary frequency (pollakiuria), every 5–10 minutes while awake. A self–limiting condition of younger children, with no pain, and sterile urine. Reassurance and bladder training usually suffice, but an antimuscarinic, e.g. propantheline 1 mg/kg/day in 3–4 divided doses, hastens resolution.

Management of enuresis

Treatment can be offered from 4 years old. From about that age 15% of bedwetters become dry annually without treatment.

1. A non-punitive approach by the parents, and removal of nappies or plastic pants if the child is over 5 years, should be advised. It may be curative by reducing the child's anxiety and bolstering his self-image.
2. Drugs are only recommended for specific situations, from the age of 5 years: where the child or parents need a demonstration that dryness can be achieved, or socially for a holiday, scout or guide camp.

   i Of the tricyclic antidepressants, imipramine is favoured. A course lasts 6–8 weeks, followed by withdrawal within 4 weeks. Maximum benefit is in the first week, but long–term success is only 10–20%, with relapse frequent on stopping treatment. The danger of a younger sibling ingesting accidentally cannot be overstated.
   ii Desmopressin nasal spray, a synthetic analogue of antidiuretic hormone, is a physiological approach to treatment as these children have relative nocturnal polyuria and some may have low ADH levels. It will result in dryness on treatment in 15–50% and improvement in 70%, but relapse after its withdrawal is common, with only 20–40% sustaining continence. It is relatively expensive, but still only about the cost of washing the sheets by machine daily.

3. The behavioural approach

   i From 4 years old a daily star chart plus small rewards. Rewarding each dry night, and then shaping behaviour by a reward for longer periods of up to a week, works for 20%. Give the child responsibility for changing her own sheets.
   ii From 6 years old conditioning using an alarm can achieve long-term dryness in 80% providing the parents are properly advised and supported.

For night time an enuretic alarm with pad and bell (with amplifying booster if unrousable), or a mini dri-nite alarm, are equally effective.

Day time wetting can be detected by a sensor attached to the pants. Tackling both nocturnal and diurnal enuresis at one time is unlikely to succeed, take one at a time.

Attention to detail is rewarded. Demonstrate setting up, and how the alarm works. Check details of use carefully, ensuring the apparatus is tested twice weekly for battery failure. Review every 1–2 weeks for a minimum of 8 weeks continuous trial, maximum 4 months. If still not dry, try again in 6 months.

Relapse responds well to a second course. Overlearning by drinking extra fluids stresses the detrusor muscles and reduces the relapse rate, once 14 consecutive dry nights (the definition of initial success) are attained.

4. Family therapy and self hypnosis are of limited use unless part of a behavioural programme.

Prognosis

Defined as continued success, no relapse in 6 months:

1. Annual spontaneous remission is 15%.
2. Enuresis alarm 80% cure.
3. Drugs:

    i Imipramine 10–20%.
    ii Desmopressin spray: on treatment 70%, up to 40% long-term success.

Reasons for failure: lack of motivation in the child, adverse psychological factors and family stress. A quarter of those with persistent enuresis develop other psychological disturbances.

Essential reading

Blackwell C (1989) *A Guide to Enuresis. A Guide to the Treatment of Enuresis for Professionals.* Bristol:Octagon Communications
Meadow S R (1977) The use of buzzer alarms to cure bed wetting. *British Medical Journal*, **2**, 931–935

Further reading

Devlin J B, O'Cathain C O (1990) Predicting treatment outcome in nocturnal enuresis. *Archives of Disease in Childhood*, **65** 1158–1161

FAECAL SOILING

Definitions

Untrained

Still 3% at 4 years old, 1.5% of 7 year olds. Boys:girls = 5:1. Immaturity and delayed development are the main causes.

Soiling

Involuntary passage of liquid or semisolid faeces. A third are enuretic. Associated with chronic constipation (see Gastrointestinal problems).

Encopresis

Normal stool deposited in pants/anywhere but the toilet, i.e. normal bowel control in an emotionally disturbed child. Marital conflicts, punitive training, disrupted family, and sexual abuse must be considered.

Assessment

Onset, from birth, with delayed passage of meconium, or ribbon-like stool is likely to be organic. After a period of fever or reduced fluid intake, constipation with pain or fissuring may establish fear of defaecation.

Timing: encopresis is most likely between 3 pm and 7 pm. Nocturnal soiling is more likely to be organic.

Family attitudes, punishment and handling the problem of soiling is sometimes abnormal.

Clinical

Growth affected by organic causes and severe abuse.

Neurology of sacral segments S2–4 for sensation.

Abdominal examination: large faecal mass present = retention with overflow, i.e. soiling. If it is otherwise normal, then recent or regular evacuation has occurred.

Rectal examination: easily felt faecal masses are usually present. Examination may be emotionally traumatic and should not be repeated without good reason.

Signs of sexual abuse are rarely specific, but must be looked for.

Investigation

An abdominal X-ray may show constipation not detected clinically.

Management of encopresis using behaviour modification

Using the gastro-colic reflex, reward as for enuresis, ignoring the soiling which is drawing attention. No place for medication. Family therapy may be necessary.

Prognosis

Ninety per cent improved within a year, almost all by adolescence. Persistence of soiling is associated with conduct disorders.

Further reading

Blackwell C (1989) *A Guide to Encopresis. A Guide to the Treatment of Encopresis.* Bristol:Octagon Communications

RECURRENT ABDOMINAL PAIN (RAP) HEADACHE/LIMB PAINS

Definition

Pain recurring at least monthly for 3 months and remaining well between episodes (Table 4.2). Organic pathology is found in 10%, identifiable for further investigation from the history and examination.

Table 4.2 Recurrent abdominal pain (RAP)

Characteristics of RAP	*Indications for further investigations*
Abdominal pain is periumbilical, rarely disturbs sleep. Colicky for a few minutes, or dull continuous ache for hours or days. No radiation	Gross abdominal distension. Loose motions (note: some RAP show intermittent diarrhoea). Pain in the flank, hypochondrium, or suprapubic region. Radiation of pain away from umbilicus. Weight loss. Growth failure.
Headache diffuse, persistent, unresponsive to analgesics.	Nausea, vomiting, eye symptoms, ataxia. Papilloedema, hypertension.
Limb pains similar to headaches.	Presence of swelling, redness, temperature, very localized pain.
Investigations Urine microscopy +/– FBC. Routine abdominal US not justified.	As appropriate.

Incidence

Ten to 15% of children aged 5–15. Accounts for 95% of chronic abdominal pain.

Correlates

1. Psychological stress, i.e. a conversion disorder

   i Home: move, marital discord, separation, family illness/death, poor parent–child relationship.

  ii School: bullying, learning difficulties, behaviour problems.

 iii Sexual abuse.

2. Migraine: familial, personal.
3. Medical (70+ causes for RAP): mainly constipation, occasionally lactose intolerance. See abdominal causes, headache, and limb pains.

Diagnosis

Absence of organic disease, presence of emotional or behavioural symptoms and often a family history. Response to an elimination diet in appropriate cases (see below).

Management

1. All investigations necessary to clarify the diagnosis should be arranged at the first visit. Repeated investigation undermines the physician's stated diagnosis of a non-organic cause.
2. Psychiatric help/school counsellor may be needed if psychological factors are prominent.
3. Emphasize that the pains are real, but not dangerous or indicative of disease.
4. Encourage normal activities and the need to learn to live with the discomfort. Symptom diaries are useful to chart progress; enter associations with foods and activities.
5. Dietary manipulations worthy of trial:

   i   Elimination of specific foods if indicated from diary (commonly cows' milk, eggs, wheat).
   ii Try a lactose free diet for 4 weeks in Black children.
   iii Increasing dietary fibre reduces transit time and pain in some.

6. Failure to improve, or a change in symptoms, may indicate an organic cause.

Prognosis

Improvement in 60–80%.
   RAP: as adults, 50% have persistent headache, and other non-specific symptoms, with a higher incidence of irritable bowel, and peptic ulcer.

Further reading

Apley J (1975) *The Child with Abdominal Pains*, Oxford:Blackwell
Leader (1991) Neurological conversion disorders in childhood. *Lancet, i,* 889–890
Oster J (1972) Recurrent abdominal pain, headache and limb pains in children and adolescents. *Pediatrics*, **50**, 429–436

PSYCHIATRIC DISORDERS

Classification

1. Conduct disorders (40% of total): persistent antisocial behaviour ('juvenile delinquency') = behaviour that is illegal. Deprived, from large disrupted families. Early and persistent school failure is common, e.g. truanting.

2. Emotional disorders (40% of total): neurotic behaviour, reactive to stress or a phase of development causing anxiety or depression, e.g. related to school, during puberty, or a distressing family event. Lack of confidence and depression in adolescence may lead to suicidal thoughts. Examples: school refusal, psychosomatic illness, anorexia nervosa.
3. Mixed disorders (20%).

Psychotic disorders are rare in childhood: autism in infancy, schizophrenia in later adolescence.

Chronic illness, e.g. epilepsy, diabetes mellitus, physical handicap cause increasing behaviour problems in adolescence.

Non-communication in early childhood

1. Shy and withdrawn: should be appropriate to age and environment, e.g. pre-school child starting playgroup. Otherwise consider stress (family, school), abuse (physical, sexual, emotional), depression, physical illness, or mental handicap.
2. Specific language disorder: frustration is often prominent.
3. Hearing difficulty: the change in behaviour may also be progressive or fluctuant, reflecting the severity of the sensory impairment.
4. Elective mutism: situation-related, e.g. speaks to the parent, not teachers. Commoner in girls. Increased association with abuse. Alternatively, an expression of anger in older children.
5. Autism: a triad of deficits in communication, social interaction and imagination.

Further reading

Hall D M B, Hill P (1991) Shy, withdrawn or autistic? *British Medical Journal*, **302**, 125–126

School absence: medical and psychological aspects

Loss on average is 5 days per year, girls>boys; 90% are due to illness.

Causes

1. Respiratory, especially influenza.
2. Other infections, infestations, and exanthema of childhood.
3. Injuries.
4. ENT disorders, asthma.
5. Truancy and school refusal.

Truancy compared to school phobia

The main difference is that in school refusal the parent knows where the child is, often at home (Table 4.3)!

Table 4.3 Truancy compared to school phobia

	Truancy	*School refusal*
Frequency	2–5% of school absences	1% of school absences
Sex	Boys>girls	Equal
Social class	4 and 5	All equally
Family	Large, maternal depression, often single. History of truancy/schooling problems	Conforming, no excess marital problems
Parents	Rejecting	Overprotective
Attainments	Underachieving	Usually average/good
Disturbance	Conduct disordered, antisocial	Anxious, phobic
Clinical	'Loners', minor impediments of appearance, speech, hearing	Dread of school, somatic complaints with school days. Refusal to go, or sent home because of physical symptoms
Location	Streets, arcades, with other truants	At home with parent or relative
Management	1 Educational guidance centre, remedial help 2 Education Supervision Order supervised by the Education Welfare Officer	1 Maintain school attendance. Firm resolute handling 2 Family therapy, antidepressants. Frequent review is most effective
Prognosis	Poor. Increased adult antisocial behaviour. Criminality may persist into adult life	Good. Majority return to school. Neurotic disorders in adolescence

Further reading

Hersov L (1985) Persistent non-attendance at school: truancy and school refusal. In *Progress in Child Health, Vol 2*. Edinburgh:Churchill Livingstone pp 55–62

Hyperactivity and attention deficit

Definition

Short attention span, distractible, impulsive, clumsy, and with language delay. May be 'pervasive,' i.e. at home and school, or 'situational' in one or the other. Antisocial behaviour is increased. Commoner in boys, ratio 3:1

Incidence

From <1% in UK to 7% in USA and Sweden. Variation between centres may be acceptance or otherwise of the diagnostic label.

Reported associated and exacerbating factors

Socioeconomic difficulties, parental alcohol, environmental lead exposure.

Assessment

Reports from parents and school, or the use of hyperactivity scores based on questionaires, are essential.

Neurological examination may reveal minor abnormalities ("soft signs") of tone, coordination, and praxis.

Differential diagnosis

Family disruption, conduct disorders, depression, anxiety, learning disorder, chorea, Gilles de la Tourette's syndrome.

Management

1. Counselling, behavioural reduction in inappropriate reactions by and to the child by parents and teachers.
2. Reduction in extraneous stimulation during learning tasks.
3. Methylphenidate (an amphetamine) is favoured outside the UK in a dose of 10–15 mg twice daily. Improved behaviour and concentration are usually reported. Side effects include temporary growth impairment and appetite supression.

Prognosis

Behaviour and school problems tend to persist, though motor difficulties improve.

Depression

Definitions

1. Major depressive episode = persistent negative mood (despair), feeling worthless, inappropriate guilt, no enjoyment in life. Minimum duration for diagnosis is 2 weeks. Delay in diagnosis is common.
2. Adjustment disorder = less severe depression, due to life event. May occur during the period of adjustment.
3. Dysthymia = chronic low grade depression.
   Risk factors: loss of a parent through death or divorce, neglect or abuse, or a previously affected family member.

Incidence

Two to 8% of older children and adolescents.

Clinical

Behaviour: irritable, difficult, aggressive ('masked depression'), social withdrawal, school performance deteriorating. Suicidal thoughts and activity.

Physical symptoms: poor appetite, loss of interest, tiredness. Weight loss, pain in the chest or abdomen.

Differential diagnosis

Altering the adverse factor improves mood in neglect/abuse, physical illness, and marital unhappiness, but is generally ineffective in depression.

Management

Family and individual therapy, often with tricyclic antidepressants, for major depression. Recovery within 6 – 18 months is usual. Over half relapse in 5 years and the likelihood of depression in adult life is high.

Controversy

Depression in the prepubertal child, its extent and severity, is increasingly accepted as a real entity.

Further reading

Kazdin A E (1990) Childhood depression. *Journal of Child Psychology and Psychiatry*, **31**, 121–160
Rutter M, Izard C E, Read PB (1985) *Depression in Young People*. London:Guildford press

INFANTILE AUTISM AND OTHER PERVASIVE DEVELOPMENTAL DISORDERS (PDD)

In addition to autism, PPD includes

1. Rett syndrome (girls only, deterioration in development in infancy, with autistic features, a characteristic ataxia with hand-washing movements).
2. Asperger's syndrome (schizoid personality, normal intelligence, indulge in monologues, difficulties in imaginative understanding, e.g. of metaphors; loping gait and clumsiness).

Autism

Definition

Pervasive deficit in social interaction, communication, activities and interests, manifest in the preschool years. Functioning is usually at a retarded level, despite 'islands' of ability.

Incidence

1:5000, boys:girls = 3:1

Associations

1. Structural abnormalities of cerebellum on MRI in 50%.
2. Autistic features in some with fragile X syndrome and in Rett syndrome.
3. Manifestation of tuberous sclerosis.

Manifestations

1. Qualitative impairment in reciprocal social interaction:
   Lack of awareness of the existence or feelings of others, no/abnormal sensitivity to pain and discomfort, no/impaired imitation, social play, and ability to make peer friendships.
2. Qualitative impairment in verbal and non-verbal communication:
   No/impaired communication verbally, abnormal voicing, refers to self as 'you', perseveration of thought (lengthy monologues), eye avoidance, lack of imaginative play.
3. Restricted repertoire of activities and interests: stereotyped body movements, a preoccupation with parts of objects, desire for sameness may result in rage if an established routine is not followed, obsessional about a single interest.

Differential diagnosis

Hearing impairment and mental retardation in younger children, schizophrenia in the older child.

Management

1. Behaviour modification to encourage socialization, language acquisition, self-help skills, reduce self-mutilation and aggressive outbursts.
2. Haloperidol for stereotyped behaviour and overactivity may help.

Prognosis

Persistent severe impairment in social relationships, emotional and cognitive development in 60%, with further deterioration in adolescence in 20%. Many require long-term institutional care.

Psychomotor epilepsy develops by adolescence in 35%.

Better outcome if the IQ at diagnosis is >50, and if communicative speech develops by 6 years of age.

Further reading

Rapin I (1991) Autistic children: diagnosis and clinical features. *Pediatrics* **87**, 751–760
Wing L (1988) *Aspects of Autism: Biological Research.* London:Royal College of Psychiatrists

Further general reading

Graham P (1986) *Child Psychiatry. A Developmental Approach.* Oxford:Oxford University Press

Chapter 5

Adolescence

The time in life with the lowest mortality and morbidity from disease (Table 5.1).
The adolescent has special needs and problems peculiar to this age.

Table 5.1 Mortality in adolescence: rate per million population

| | | 10–14 years | | | 15–19 years | |
		M	F		M	F
Accidents, poisoning and violence	1st	124	56	1st	512	141
Malignancy	2nd	49	39	2nd	77	53
Suicides	9th	1	3	3rd	40	12
Congenital abnormalities	3rd	21	17	6th	26	22

ADOLESCENT ISSUES

Excessive risk-taking characterizes many adolescent actions which result in hospitalization and death, as well as coming into conflict with the law. Failure to appreciate fully the consequence of actions and the disinhibiting effects of alcohol and drugs, each play a part.

DETERIORATION IN DISEASE DURING ADOLESCENCE

1. Operated cardiac abnormalities: palliative procedures resulting in strain on the heart, which progressively fails as pubertal growth makes greater demands.
2. Cystic fibrosis: puberty associated with deterioration in respiratory function, the major cause of death, mean age early 20s.

Further reading

Penketh A R L, Wise A, Mearns M B, Hodson M F, Batten J C (1987) Cystic fibrosis in adolescents and adults. *Thorax*, **42**, 526–532

CONDITIONS APPEARING FOR THE FIRST TIME

1. Acne
2. Orthopaedic disorders, e.g. scoliosis, Osgood-Schlatter disease, slipped femoral epiphysis, patella dislocation: see Orthopaedics.

Transfer of adolescents with chronic disease to adult clinics, e.g. for diabetes mellitus, cystic fibrosis and haemophilia, is determined by the maturity and wishes of the patient. Generally it is better for emotional and physical growth to be completed, avoiding disruption at a potentially turbulent time. The epileptic and handicapped may have special difficulties in adjusting and finding appropriate follow-up clinics.

SEXUALITY AND SEX–RELATED DISEASE

1. Among 16 year olds in the UK, 30% report having had intercourse, Black> Whites>>Asians.
2. Risk factors for early sexual activity include early puberty, socioeconomic deprivation, school failure, smoking, mother or sibling a teenage parent, and a permissive society.
3. Cervical cancer risk is related to age at first coitus, multiple sexual partners and male partners who have had multiple partners, and sexually transmitted viral infections.
4. Contraceptive advice is increasingly being sought. This is rarely the province of the British paediatrician, though often proffered by our North American counterparts.

Teenage pregnancy

Risk factors

One in 7 females has first coitus before leaving school. Pregnancy is a risk in younger teenagers, due to occasional encounters and lack of contraception, especially in lower socioeconomic groups. A small sub group deliberately become pregnant to give meaning to their lives and provide a means of escape from home and school.

Incidence

Progressive increase in pregnancies from 6.8 per 1000 16 year olds in 1969 to 8.7 in 1986.

Abortion

Legal abortion can be requested by an under 16 year old without parental permission. 3400 were performed in 1989 in under 16 year olds compared with 37 000 between 16 and 19 years of age.

Prognosis

Increased morbidity and mortality for mother and baby is now attributed mainly to socioeconomic factors and a lack of antenatal care. Below 15 years old, there is still a relatively higher risk of cephalopelvic disproportion, anaemia, toxaemia, hypertension, vaginal infections, and delivery of a low birthweight infant.

Schooling usually stops in the fifth month, and should continue at home or in special units. Over half fail to return to school after delivery, and have few skills to offer, perpetuating their poorer socioeconomic circumstances.

Sexually transmitted disease

Incidence

Highest in young adults, 20–24 years, closely followed by the 15–19 year old age group.

Risk factors

Include:

    i Lack of protected intercourse and appreciation of the risk the individual is exposed to.

    ii Teenage genitals are particularly vulnerable to infection.

Organisms

Chlamydia and gonorrhoea are the commonest organisms. HIV is increasing. Herpes simplex type 2 is usually asymptomatic. Genital warts (a papilloma virus infection) increase the likelihood of cervical cancer. Cervical smears for carcinoma in situ should be discussed and even offered annually to sexually active adolescents.

Vaginal discharge

Symptoms

Dysuria and/or pruritus, or none.

Character

1. Clear mucoid is normal, but with pruritis suggests threadworms.
2. Purulent:

    i Genital herpes: vesicles and systemic upset may be present.

    ii Bacterial, usually streptococcal and gonococcal: pruritus, dysuria, or asymptomatic.

    iii Foreign body: toilet paper or objects used for stimulation, abuse or contraception.

3. Cheesy: Candida.
4. Frothy: Trichomonas.

Assessment

1. Sexual abuse or sexually active? The younger the age the higher the suspicion.
2. Speculum examination for foreign body and genital herpes identification.
3. Identify pathogen by culture, or sellotape swab for thread worm and treat appropriately.

Vaginal bleeding

1. 'Physiological': painless irregular bleeding is usually due to anovular cycles which are common in the first 2 years after menarche, after illness or stress.
2. Other causes, may be painful:

    i   Vaginal: trauma or foreign body.
    ii Uterus, ovaries and tubes: intrauterine contraceptive device, oral contraceptives, abortion, ectopic pregnancy, or polycystic ovaries.
    iii Either site: sexually transmitted disease (STD), polyps, malignancy, or bleeding disorders.

Lower abdominal/pelvic pain

In addition to gastrointestinal disorders and primary dysmenorrhoea, consider endometriosis, pelvic inflammatory disease, adhesions, ectopic pregnancy, ovarian cysts/torsion/tumour.

Assessment of bleeding and pain

1. History of menstruation, sexual activity and contraception, or possible abuse, and symptoms of hyperthyroidism, should be elicited.
2. Pelvic examination requires bimanual palpation.
3. Investigations may include FBC, swabs for STD, pregnancy test, coagulation, thyroid function, pelvic ultrasound, and laparoscopy.

Further reading

Grant L M, Demetriou E. (1988) Adolescent sexuality. *Pediatric Clinics of North America*, **35**, 1271–1289
Strasburger V C (ed) (1989) Adolescent gynecology. *Pediatric Clinics of North America*, **36**.

BEHAVIOURS WITH POTENTIAL FOR INJURY AND ADDICTION

Injury and suicide

The commonest cause of death in adolescence is injury. These are:

i Unintentional (road traffic accidents, accidents at work). Failure to wear protective gear (e.g. crash helmets, safety belts), excessive speed, and the increasing use of alcohol contribute to the above expected incidence of death and injury from 15 to 24 years.

ii Intentional: suicide and non-fatal deliberate self harm (NFDSH)/parasuicide. Most often a response to an acute crisis, usually family related in younger teenagers, or mental disturbance in older adolescents.

Incidence

Increasing. In the Oxford region 2.8/1000 males, 0.6/1000 females completed (i.e. killed themselves) in late adolescence. Unusual under 16 years.

Risk factors

i Feelings of depression and hopelessness, family disorganization, social problems, alcohol, frank psychosis.

ii Imitation of peers and media reports of completed teenage suicide.

iii Gender: NFDSH attempted in 6 × as many females as males, but males are 5 × more likely to complete, and within a year of the first attempt. Males are more violent (firearms, hanging, jumping), females prefer poisons or medication.

Intervention

i After an attempt: a child psychiatric evaluation in all cases, and in attempted and completed suicides, community support for peers to prevent imitation.

ii Prevention: identifying depression, social withdrawal, a family history of suicide or alcoholism.

Murder is rare in the UK, whereas in New York State it is the second commonest cause of death in 15–19 year olds.

Substance abuse

Often a manifestation of depression, inadequate social functioning, and a way of coping with overwhelming feelings.

Experimentation ('sensation seeking') is common, but continued use is most likely in the vulnerable person.

First experience is about 12 years old, building up to a peak at 15–17 years, males more than females.

Risk taking behaviours involving drugs, sniffing, alcohol, tobacco, in association with poor education, are linked to unwanted pregnancy, and with increased risk to the fetus as a result.

Trends in smoking and drinking show a decline over the last decade. Illicit drug use is steadily increasing in the UK, the reverse of the trend in the USA.

Volatile substance abuse

Mainly in early teens, boys>>girls. Annual UK mortality 100, rising.

Prevalence

Up to 10% of secondary school children experiment. 0.5–1% persist.

Substances

Glues (toluene), cleaning fluids (chlorinated hydrocarbons), acetone, petrol, and butane (non toxic) are commonly 'sniffed'.

Clinical

    i Acute. Confusion, sedation. Hallucinations are common. Complaints of bronchial irritation, nasal obstruction. Cardiac arrhythmias and disturbed liver function. Airway freezing from a butane spray may cause laryngospasm and death.

   ii Chronic.10% become chronic, leading to poor school performance, cerebellar signs, occasionally dementia. Progressive renal damage. Subsequent alcohol abuse is common in this group.

Diagnosis

Tell-tale smell, presence of glue on the face and clothing; chronic abusers may have a facial rash.

Further reading

Ashton C H (1990) Solvent abuse. *British Medical Journal*, **300**, 135–136
Leader (1988) Complications of chronic volatile substance abuse. *Lancet*, ii, 431–432

Drugs

Prevalence in 14–16 year olds: >25%, M>F. Most are not regular users. Dependence is rare at this age.

1. Types of drugs: Increasing use – Cannabis, cocaine and its purified form 'crack'. Phencyclidine (angel dust) may be increasing. Reducing – amphetamines except 'ecstasy', LSD, opiates by injection.

2. Trends in the UK for 14–16 year olds: increased × 4 over the last 10–20 years.
3. Reasons teenagers themselves perceive for experimenting with drugs: mainly peer and social pressure, while escapism and family tensions are less important.

Tobacco

Prevalence

Half a million smokers between 11–15 years old; 20% will die from tobacco related disease.

Although recent trends show improvement, 40% of children smoke before leaving school. Boys smoke more cigarettes than girls, but in 1988 more 15 year old girls smoked regularly (19% F, 15% M).

Consequences of adult smoking (% of all cases): low birthweight (25%), heart disease (30%), early childhood deaths from respiratory diseases (40%), bladder cancer (50%), emphysema (85%), lung cancer (90%).

Alcohol

Alcohol related: drunkeness, drugs, smoking, pregnancy, suicide, fighting, absence from school or work; criminal and driving convictions rise throughout adolescence. At all ages M>F, tends to peak at 18–20 years, then decline; fortunately, heavy teenage drinking is not directly predictive of middle–aged alcoholism!

Education: sex, drugs, alcohol, tobacco

Successful approaches require a multifactorial approach involving school, parents, ministers, community leaders, the media.

Altering attitudes at the stage at which they are formed is the aim. For smoking this is about 11–12 years. If deterred beyond 16 years the battle may be won!

A programme could include:

1. Facts about disease transmission, e.g. HIV by unprotected intercourse, sharing needles; advice on reducing multiple partners.
2. Confront feelings of invulnerability that allow risk-taking behaviours, e.g. talks by AIDS sufferers.
3. Role modelling by prominent sportspersons saying 'no' to drugs, smoking, alcohol.
4. Environmental support by promoting group activities with health orientated goals.
5. Parenting skills improved by discussion, their behaviour altered to provide suitable role models.

Overall, the efficacy of available education programmes is disappointing.

Further reading

Holland W W, Fitzsimmons B (1991) Smoking in children. *Archives of Disease in Childhood*, **66**, 1269–1274
Stout J W, Rivara F P (1989) Schools and sex education: does it work? *Pediatrics*, **83**, 375–379
Strasburger V C (1989) Adolescent sexuality and the media. *Pediatric Clinics of North America*, **36**, 747–773

EDUCATION: GENETIC COUNSELLING

Planning for adult relationships and possible parenthood by sufferers and siblings of those with congenital abnormalities and genetic disease should include comprehensive counselling.

Examples:

1. Offspring of a parent with congenital heart disease have a 10% risk of being similarly affected.
2. Genetic disease

   i At risk groups are offered screening, e.g. Blacks for sickle cell trait, Cypriots for thalassaemia carrier, Ashkenazi Jews for Tay-Sach's disease to determine status and advisability of screening potential partners.
   ii Sibling with a condition, e.g. cystic fibrosis or haemophilia: assess whether the teenager is a carrier and the family informative, explain the relative risks of meeting another carrier.

3. Chromosomal mosaicism/translocation carrier of Down's syndrome requires discussion about antenatal diagnosis.

Chapter 6

Nutrition and nutritional disorders

FEEDING INFANTS

The desirable choice in almost all babies is breast feeding, achieved in 80–90% initially in the UK. By 3 months about half are still doing so, at 6 months only 25–35%.

Physiology of the neonatal gut

See Neonatal gastrointestinal problems.

Physiology of breast feeding

1. Oestrogen, progesterone and placental lactogen cause enlargement of the alveoli and lactiferous ducts of the breast.
2. Prolactin release: induced by suckling (can be induced even in the non-parous). Stimulates milk secretion.
3. Oxytocin: neural release induced by baby's cry, and tactile from suckling. Causes milk 'let down' reflex, and uterine contractions, (which may even be painful), hastening involution.
4. Ovulation is inhibited in 90% of women during normal intensive breast feeding.

'Sociology' of breast feeding

1. In the developed world, attitudes towards breast feeding relate positively to: mother being breast fed herself, of higher social class, better educated, and from a wealthier area (e.g. the South of England).
2. Reasons for avoiding breast feeding: inconvenience, uncertainty of volume taken, embarrassment, unfounded fear of losing breast shape. Greater encouragement in schools and the media may improve rates.

3. The developing world's vulnerability to advertising by milk companies has resulted in an agreed code of practice. The dangers of infection and malnutrition among impoverished people, who can ill afford these products, are self evident.
4. To encourage breast feeding worldwide the WHO/UNICEF statement '10 steps to successful breastfeeding' exhorts:

    i Have a written breast feeding policy, known to all health care staff.
    ii Train the staff in the skills necessary to implement this policy.
   iii Inform all mothers of the benefits and management of breast feeding.
   iv Help mothers initiate breast feeding within half an hour of birth.
    v Show them how to breast feed and maintain lactation even if separated from their infant.
   vi Newborns to have nothing other than breast milk unless medically indicated.
  vii Mother and infants to stay together throughout the 24 hours.
 viii Encourage breast feeding on demand.
   ix Give no artificial teats or pacifiers to breastfeeding infants.
    x Foster the establishment of breast feeding support groups and refer mothers to them on discharge from hospital.

Common reasons for failure of breast feeding

1. Pain from cracked nipple, engorged breasts, breast abcess.
2. Failure to fix: baby sick, weak, premature, nasal obstruction, cleft lip and palate. Poor positioning at the breast, nostrils occluded, inverted nipples.
3. Inadequate milk: mother anxious, tired, sick, offered conflicting advice, stress of test weighing. Infrequent, rigidly spaced feeds, complementary bottle feeds.

Contraindications to breast feeding

1. Maternal drugs: absolute – antimitotic, lithium, tetracycline, phenindione. The concentration of other drugs in breast milk are insufficient to cause concern.
2. Maternal illness: chronic disease and malnutrition, open TB in the first month of treatment, until mother is non-infectious and the baby protected by vaccination and chemoprophylaxis.
3. Confirmed or very likely HIV +ve and HTLV-2 infected mothers.

Characteristics of the various milk feeds (Table 6.1)

1. Calories: higher density required for prematures less than 1.5 kg.
2. Fat levels similar, though more steatorrhoea with cows' milk (50% versus 20%). Maternal unsaturated fatty acids reflect her diet, i.e. can be very variable. Humanized types contain vegetable or animal fats, which may cause the stool to be grey-green.

Table 6.1 Comparison of human, cow, and modified milks

Contents per 100 ml	Human	Cow	Modified	LBW*	Soy	Hydrolysat
Calorie	70	67	65	80	65	69
Carbohydrate (g)	7	4.5	7	8	7	9
Fat (g)	4.2	3.9	3.5	4.5	3.2	2.6
Protein (g)	1.4	3.4	1.8	2.4	2.2	2.4
Casein: whey ratio	3:7	8:2	4:6			
Sodium (mmol/l)	6	20	10	30	10	14
Calcium: phosphate ratio	2:1	1:1	1:1	1.5:1	1.2:1	
Renal solute load (mosmol/l)	90	225	127		230	338

*LBW = low birthweight

3. Carbohydrate: lactose, with added maltodextrin/glucose for LBW milks as prematures have a limited ability to absorb lactose.
4. Protein: in human and cows' milk the lactalbumin content is similar (0.7 g/dl), but better nitrogen retention occurs with the human casein:whey ratio.
5. Renal solute content is 3–4 times higher in cows' milk, reflecting sodium content and urea production. Note high osmolality of soy and hydrolysates.
6. Phosphate content is much higher in cows' milk (95 mg/100 ml) than human (15 mg/100 ml) with a lower calcium:phosphate ratio.
7. Vitamins and iron: lacking in both human and cows' milk, added to the various modified milks but additional supplements required for rapidly growing premature and LBW infants.

Modified cows' milk formula

Close to human in protein, carbohydrate and sodium. Often contains high levels of unsaturated vegetable fats, added iron and vitamin D. Intermediate levels of calcium and phosphate (30–60 mg/100ml for each).

Premature infant formula milks

These supply:

1. Extra calories (80 kcal/100ml) and protein (2 g)
2. More sodium (30 mmol/l) for growth and renal leak.
3. Calcium and phosphate quantity similar to other modified milks. Deficient bone mineralization from low intake may need supplementation (see Metabolic bone disease of prematurity).

Improved growth in length, head circumference and weight, and bone mineralization compared with breast fed babies. Shorter hospital stays result.

Hazard: risk of necrotizing enterocolitis although greater than with breast milk, is greatly reduced when given as a complementary feed to mother's breast milk.

Soy milk and hydrolysates

Free of milk protein, lactose, usually sucrose, and gluten. Suitable for post-enteritis lactose intolerance, cows' milk protein intolerance (but may develop soy intolerance).

Soy formula is unsuitable for the premature and LBW. Soy milk sold in supermarkets and health stores contains no calcium, vitamins or iron, and is unsuitable for the under 5s.

Hazards of cows' milk feeding

1. Psychologically less satisfying.
2. Greater likelihood of infection during preparation, and lack of the anti-infective properties found in fresh breast milk: macrophages, immunoglobulin IgA, lysozyme, interferon, lactoferrin inhibiting the growth of iron-dependent *E. coli*; bifidus factor in breast milk encourages the growth of lactobacillus.
3. Biochemical disorders, now unusual in modified cows' milk formulae (MCMF): hypocalcaemia, hypernatraemia, raised urea and metabolic acidosis from high protein load and sulphur containing amino acids. The hyperosmolality may cause thirst, crying and so overfeeding.
4. More saturated fats than breast milk, unless a MCMF.
5. Cows' milk protein intolerance: post-enteritis, acute colitis, occult bleeding resulting in anaemia.
6. Acute anaphylaxis/allergy, eczema.

Goats' milk

As a substitute in cows' milk protein (CMP) intolerance or in an attempt to avoid eczema (of unproven benefit). Folic acid supplement and pasteurization against brucellosis is advised.

Feeding regimens

Bottle: 60 ml/kg day 1, increasing by daily 30 ml increments to 150 ml in the term infant, 180–200 ml/kg in the premature and small for dates infant.

Term infant

In the first week offer 4 hourly, 6 feeds in 24 hours. The overnight feed may be omitted on attaining 4 kg.

The premature infant

1. i Mother's breast milk:
       If <1.5 kg give mineral supplements of sodium 4 mg/kg/day, and potassium diphosphate 15 mg/100 ml of feed.

Protection against necrotizing enterocolitis (NEC) is only slightly reduced if used together with low birthweight formula milk.

ii Mature donated breast milk maintains IQ but is nutritionally inadequate in the very premature, and LBW formula milk 150 ml/kg/day is advised if mother's own milk is not available.

2. Mode of feeding

i Nasogastric is more physiological than the nasojejunal route, which is more prone to NEC, and only indicated for recurrent apnoea due to aspiration.

ii From 1–2 h old, give hourly, or continuous feeds in the extremely low birth-weight, to avoid gastric distension and aspiration.

iii As suckling is weak, and aspiration possible, bottle or breast feeding is often delayed until around 1.2–1.5 kg or 33–34 weeks' gestation.

iv The 'joey' principle of nursing the tiny prem between the breasts often enables earlier commencement of nutritive as well as 'comfort' suckling.

3. If not breast fed, LBW milk for those under 1.5 kg birthweight, until 1.8 kg attained.

4. Discharge home, regardless of the actual weight, when these criteria are fulfilled: (i) birth weight regained; (ii) gaining weight; (iii) taking feeds orally no more than 3 hourly × 8 in 24 h.

5. Supplements for less than 2 kg birth weight from week 3–24 of life: vitamin E and folic acid for the first 3 months, ACD, B_6 and iron supplements for the first 6 months of life.

Weaning

1. Weaning is the introduction of solids, recommended between 3 to 6 months old. Solids are more energy dense than milk, and too early introduction has been associated with obesity. Delayed introduction beyond 6 months old may result in difficulty in establishing mixed feeding.

By the time a litre of milk is consumed solids should be gradually added to the diet, continuing with breast or modified cow/soy milk.

'Door stop' cows' milk is introduced after 12 months to avoid iron and vitamin deficiencies. Background: fresh cows' milk and tea chelate iron. When ingested with low iron containing foods → poorer weight gain, and more behavioural, developmental and educational problems.

Skimmed milk is too low in fat and should not be given under 5 years old, though semi-skimmed is permitted after 2 years old.

2. Childrens' vitamin drops (A,C,D) daily from a month to 2 years, up to 5 years in vegetarians and dark skinned babies.

3. Vegetarian weaning requires an adequate milk intake, as:

i Other protein sources lack the balance in amino acids babies need.

ii Energy density may be too low: fats (avocado, margarine, butter) can be added.

Complementary foods provide balance, e.g. cereals with legumes; dairy products with seeds, nuts and cereals; greens with legumes. Vitamin D and B_{12} supplements are advised for vegans. Malnutrition has been seen in macrobiotic, Rastafarian and fruitarian diets.

Other exclusion diets may result in deficiencies in calcium and iron.

Further reading

Lucas A, Cole T J (1990) Breast milk and neonatal necrotising enterocolitis. *Lancet, ii,* 1519–1522

Lucas A, Morley R, Cole T J, Gore S M *et al.* (1990) Early diet in preterm babies and developmental status at 18 months *Lancet,* 1477-1481

Wharton B (1990) Milk for babies and children. No ordinary cow's milk before 1 year. *British Medical Journal,* **301**,774–775

PRINCIPLES OF FLUID AND ELECTROLYTE THERAPY, AND NUTRITION

Minimum fluid requirements, oral or intravenous, per 24 hours

100 ml/kg for the first 10 kg bodyweight.
50 ml/kg for next 10 kg body weight.
20 ml/kg thereafter.

Calories

Always calculate to expected weight in failure to thrive, not actual weight, to avoid underestimating caloric needs for growth.

First year:

0–3 months: term infants 110 kcal/kg/day (460 kJ/kg/day), prematures up to 140 kcal/kg/day (580 kJ/kg/day).

After 4 months: 95 kcal/day (400 kj/kg/day)

Thereafter give 1000 kcal + 100 kcal × age in years

Ratio 40% carbohydrate, 40% fat, 20% protein.

Minerals

Sodium, potassium, chloride 2 mmol/kg/day.
Calcium, phosphate each 5 mmol/kg/day.
Elemental iron 1–2 mg/kg/day from 21 days old.
Fluoride as 1 ppm in tap water, or toothpaste started at the eruption of the first tooth.

Indications for the parenteral route

1. Failure to absorb via the gut: stomach pooling, ileus/obstruction.
2. Repeated aspiration/risk of aspiration in apnoea or repeated seizures.
3. Suspected inborn error exacerbated by protein load (usually milk).

Total parenteral nutrition (TPN)

Indications

Inability to use the gut for so long (usually >10 days) that survival and health are compromised.

1. Surgical: intestinal atresia, resections, omphalocele.
2. Burns.
3. Necrotizing enterocolitis.
4. Protracted diarrhoea.
5. Extreme prematurity, especially with respiratory distress syndrome. Partial parenteral nutrition (carbohydrate and Vamin), introduced by day 2–3 of life, minimizes catabolism.
6. Severe uncontrolled inflammatory bowel disease.

Contraindications

1. Acute phase of illness with hypoxia, acidosis or hypotension.
2. Elevated serum bilirubin >200 µmol/l in the newborn.
3. Serum urea >8 mmol/l.
4. Platelets <20 × 10⁹/l.

Requirements in infancy, the commonest time for TPN

1. Fluids: 60–160 ml/kg in the first week, 150–200 ml/kg thereafter.
2. Calories: 125 kcal/day (60 kcal maintenance + 75 kcal growth) as:

   i Nitrogen: 3.5 g/kg/day = 50 ml of 7% Vamin/kg/day.
   ii Carbohydrate: glucose 6 mg/kg/min = 8 g/kg/day = 80ml of 10% glucose solution. Maximum 18 g/kg/day as a 15% solution.
   iii Fat is nitrogen sparing: e.g. Intralipid 1–3 g/kg/day.

   Slow introduction over 3–4 days of (i) and (iii) is necessary to avoid hyperammonaemia +/– acidosis, and hyperlipidaemia respectively.
3. Minerals: normal requirements for maintenance and growth, reduced for calcium and phosphate otherwise they may cause precipitation in the infusate. Iron comes from the top up blood transfusion often required.
   Trace mineral supplement must be given to prevent deficiency.
4. Vitamins: see below.

Hazards (In addition to electrolyte and acid-base distubances)

- Overload with cardiac failure, persistent ductus arteriosus.
- Infection, catheter thromboses etc, extravasation necrosis.
- Cholestatic jaundice in neonates, hypoxaemia from lipid deposition in the lungs.

Minerals: selected rare deficiency syndromes

Copper

1. In malabsorption and unsupplemented total parenteral nutrition.
- Pancytopenia.
- Bones show changes like scurvy and child abuse.

2. Congenital deficiency. Menkes kinky hair syndrome XL. Due to unavailability of ingested copper. Progressive neurodegeneration despite i.v. treatment.

Zinc

1. Congenital. Need for high intake in acrodermatitis enteropathica AR, in which deficiency → malabsorption, anaemia and failure to thrive.
2. In malnutrition. Impaired growth and delayed puberty have been reported.
3. Premature infants who are breast fed or receiving prolonged parenteral nutrition → failure to thrive, with characteristic weeping excoriating eczema of face.

VITAMINS

Deficiency of vitamins, essential co-factors in enzyme activity, continue to be of worldwide concern (Table 6.2). Studies in developing countries have shown prophylactic vitamin A improved survival of young children by 30%. Debate continues on the usefulness of multivitamin tablets in improving IQ test scores in British and American schoolchildren.

Vitamin supplementation in special situations

1. K_1 once only. Infants born to mothers with intention to breast feed, the asphyxiated, emergency caesarian sections, all infants entering special care baby unit. In effect, offered to all babies.
   Controversy: i.m. administration association with childhood leukaemia postulated, oral recommended until further research clarifies the issue.
2. Prematures: vitamin E, folic acid for 3 months.
3. Malabsorptive states: the fat soluble drugs A, D, E, K.
4. Haemolytic states, e.g. sickle cell, spherocytosis: folic acid.
5. Metabolic diseases, e.g. in galactosaemia, galactomin, a synthetic milk, requires full vitamin and mineral supplementation.
6. Total parenteral nutrition: Multibionta or Solivito + Vitlipid contain essential requirements.

Prescriptions

- Calculate from daily requirement: calcium and phosphate 5 mmol/kg/day, elemental iron 1–2 mg/kg/day.
- Calcium effervescent tablet (Sandocal) = 10 mmol Ca^{2+}

Table 6.2 Vitamins: selected abnormalities

Vitamin	Deficiency state and clinical findings
A	Children with protein-energy malnutrition in India, Brazil, and the Middle East. 1 Increased incidence of respiratory and diarrhoeal illness 2 Night blindness, photophobia $\rightarrow$ xerophthalmia (dry cornea), Bitot's spots (grey conjunctival patches) $\rightarrow$ keratomalacia (ulcer, perforation) $\rightarrow$ blindness 3 Growth failure 4 Dry, scaly, hyperkeratotic skin
B_1 Thiamine:	Infantile form in breast feeding mothers eating milled rice 1 Wet beri-beri: cardiac failure, sudden death 2 Dry beri-beri: polyneuritis, aphonia 3 Thiamine dependence in an inborn error: maple syrup urine disease
B_2 Riboflavin:	Malabsorptive states or malnutrition $\rightarrow$ smooth purple tongue, cheilosis (swollen, cracked lips)
B_3 Niacin:	Corn (maize) is high in leucine, blocks tryptophane $\rightarrow$ niacin 1 Pellagra: triad of diarrhoea, dermatitis (skin erythematous and bullous on exposed areas) and dementia 2 Hartnup disease: amino-acid transport defect of gut and kidneys, mimicks pellagra
Biotin:	Deficiency due to a rare inborn error (IE) or total parenteral nutrition (TPN) 1 IE $\rightarrow$ fits, developmental regression, deafness 2 TPN $\rightarrow$ dermatitis, lethargy
B_6 Pyridoxine	Dependency and deficiency states, anorexia, isoniazid administration for TB (excessively rare in children) 1 Dependency: convulsions in infants, EEG normalizes with i.v. pyridoxine 2 Deficiency: peripheral neuropathy, hypochromic anaemia, dermatitis
B_{12} Cobalamin	Malabsorption, resection of stomach or terminal ileum, Crohn's disease. Rarely it may be due to congenital absence of intrinsic factor or carrier protein transcobalamin II. Signs: megaloblastic anaemia, eventually posterior and lateral spinal column disease
C	Dietary lack. Hydroxyproline incorporation into collagen is impaired, resulting in deficient osteoid, bleeding into gums, and under periostium. 1 The pain results in pseudoparesis and frog-legged position in infants 2 Rickety rosary, anaemia, lethargy and weakness A therapeutic trial of vitamin C is diagnostic, 200 mg daily
D	See Metabolic problems
Folic acid	Malabsorption, e.g. coeliac, cystic fibrosis $\rightarrow$ megaloblastic anaemia. In haemolytic anaemias

- Calcium Sandoz syrup 15 ml = 8.1 mmol Ca^{2+}
- Phosphate 15 mg/100 ml of feed, or as 1 mmol/kg/day
- Ferrous sulphate syrup paediatric BP 5ml = 12 mg elemental iron
- Sodium iron edetate (Sytron) 5ml = 27.5 mg elemental iron

Table 6.3 Vitamin doses

Normal daily requirements	*Treatment of deficiency*
A 500–3000IU	5000 IU. In xerophthalmia 25000 IU
C 30 mg	200 mg daily until improved
D 400 IU	1500 IU for 4–8 weeks

Prematures: add vitamin E 15 mg, folic acid 50 μg for the first 3 months

Chronic hypervitaminosis

1. Vitamin A: raised intracranial pressure, hyperostosis of long bones.
   As isotretinoin treatment, for acne vulgaris, it is teratogenic.
2. Vitamin D: hypercalcaemia → failure to thrive, floppy, constipation, polydipsia, polyuria. Nephrocalcinosis, excessive calcification of metaphyses and base of skull. See William's syndrome.

Further reading

Benton D, Buts J-P (1990) Vitamin/mineral supplementation and intelligence *Lancet, i*, 1158–1160
West K P, Pokhrel R P, Katz J, LeClerq S C *et al* (1991) Efficacy of vitamin A in reducing preschool child mortality in Nepal. *Lancet, ii*, 67–71

FAILURE TO THRIVE

Interchangeable with growth failure – see Short Stature in Growth problems and Food and Mealtime problems in Behavioural and psychological dysfunction.

PROTEIN ENERGY MALNUTRITION (PEM)

Definitions

Marasmus or wasting = <60% of median reference weight for median reference height, the reference being an international standard, e.g. National Centre for Health Statistics data. Mid upper arm circumference <110 mm identifies infants with an increased mortality rate (Table 6.4).

Kwashiorkor = <80% median reference weight + oedema +/– depigmentation, and hair changes. Restricted to the Tropics, aflotoxins have been incriminated in its causation.

Incidence

1. Developing world: 15 million deaths annually from malnutrition and associated infections.
   Factors include: low income; poor housing; climatic: drought and flood; poor sanitation; no clean water supply; poor parental education and health knowledge;

poor/no control of infectious diseases (lack of immunizations); inappropriate feeding practices with illness, e.g. stopping breast feeding; inadequate access to health services.

2. Developed world:

   i Carer responsible through neglect (the commonest cause of short stature in the UK), macrobiotic, fad or unsupervised elimination diets.

   ii Disease: malabsorption from cystic fibrosis, coeliac disease.

   iii Anorexia nervosa has up to 100000 sufferers in the UK alone.

Precipitation and exacerbation of PEM by:

1. Parasitic infestations with *Strongyloides stercoralis* or *Ascaris lumbricoides* → anorexia. Hookworm is the commonest cause of iron deficiency world-wide.

   Protozoal: *Giardia lamblia* → protracted diarrhoea and malabsorption; amoebiasis causes protein losing enteropathy and bleeding.

2. Reduced caloric intake → villous atrophy and reduced disaccharides → malabsorption, achlorhydria.

3. Achlorhydria allows secondary bacterial diarrhoea → perpetuation of the cycle.

4. Reduced immunity commonly results: infections → hypercatabolic states, subsequent death from TB, pneumonia, measles.

5. Abnormalities of pancreatic enzymes, and fatty liver exacerbated by aflotoxins in the diet, are common.

Table 6.4 Characteristics of marasmus and kwashiorkor compared

	Marasmus	*Kwashiorkor*
Dietary deficiency	'balanced'	Protein>carbohydrate
Age peak	6–12 months	12–24 months
Weight % of median for age	60%	60-80%
Height relatively preserved	-	+
Oedema, low albumin	-	+
Depigmentation skin and hair	-	+

Common to both: Depression, lethargy, anaemia, hypovitaminosis A, villous atrophy, disaccharide deficiency, reduced pancreatic enzymes, fatty liver.
Marasmic kwashiorkor, a mixture of the two, is also seen.

Management

1. Dehydration and electrolyte (especially K^+, Ca^{2+}, phosphate, Mg^{2+}) deficiencies to be made good. Transfuse if haemoglobin <4g/l.

2. Feeding is introduced slowly to avoid secondary lactose intolerance and reactive hypoglycaemia. Start with half strength milk. Once full strength feed is tolerated introduce high energy feeds until the target weight is achieved, usually within 4–6 weeks.

3. Infections and infestations identified and treated.

4. Deficiencies of iron, vitamin A and K, made good. Zinc may be important.

Prognosis:

Mortality 5% at best, often higher if mismanaged, or too rapid early feeding.

Further reading

Hendrickse R G (1991) Kwashiorkor: the hypothesis that incriminates aflotoxins. *Pediatrics*, **88**, 376–379

Williams C D (1933) A nutritional disease of children associated with a maize diet. *Archives of Disease in Childhood*, **8**, 423

STUNTING

Definition

Less than 90% of median height for age. An adaptive response to early malnutrition, which has survival value though mortality is still greater than in unaffected children.

Pathophysiology

1. Acute malnutrition → loss in weight = wasting.
2. Chronic or repeated incidents of infection, subnutrition → reduced growth velocity → stunting.
3. Catch-up growth occurs as nutritional intake increases, but may be incomplete, especially among under 2 year olds. Recovery of growth in height occurs when a critical ratio of 85% weight for height is achieved.

Prevalence

1. Developing world. A sign of poverty which affects 30–40% of <5 year olds. Monitoring children's height or growth velocity is an index of the basic nutrition and health needs in that community.
2. Developed world. Social and emotional deprivation are commonly associated with short stature; also found with adverse intrauterine factors, e.g. infection, alcohol, and toxaemia; common in cerebral palsy, and globally retarded children.

Further reading

Costello A M De L (1989) Growth velocity and stunting in rural nepal. *Archives of Disease in Childhood*, **64**, 1478–1482

Waterlow J C (1988) *Linear Growth Retardation in Less Developed Countries*. Nestlé Nutrition Workshop Series. Volume 14. New York:Raven

OBESITY

Definition

In practice = weight for height >120% of the mean (50th centile) for age and sex.

More exact = >85th centile for age for triceps skin fold thickness or >120% of the Body Mass Index (called Quetelet's index in which weight/height^2 = body mass) for the mean height and weight for that age; 90% = underweight, 110–120% = overweight.

Incidence

3% of schoolchildren in the UK.

Aetiology

Most (99%) is exogenous, i.e. caused by overeating. This may be absolute, or relative, i.e. a lower metabolic rate increases susceptibility if physically inactive. Poor self esteem, depression, and social isolation may precede or follow. Only 1% are pathological/organic.

Factors favouring obesity

1. Family obesity: genetic factors and eating habits.
2. Low social class: faulty diet, excess fat intake.
3. Single child with a single parent.
4. Large family.

Best predictor at 2 years: birth weight and maternal weight. Early stimulation of an excess of fat cells in infancy leading to irreversible obesity is no longer considered plausible.

Clinical clues

Exogenous obesity from overeating tends to tall stature, advanced bone age, early puberty, symmetrical fat distribution. Remain tall as adults if tall and obese before puberty.
Pathological obesity is usually associated with short stature and characteristics pointing to the diagnosis.

Causes of pathological or organic obesity

1. Endocrine

   i Hypothyroidism: high upper segment to lower segment ratio.
  ii Growth hormone: normal proportion for bone age, frontal bossing, hypoglycaemia in infancy.
 iii Pituitary tumour (Froehlich syndrome) with hypogonadism is usually due to a craniopharyngioma or germinoma of the hypothalamus.
 iv Cushing syndrome has trunkal obesity, wasted limbs, rapid onset, growth arrest.

2. Hypothalamic disturbances with progressive obesity

i Prader-Willi: long face, fish hook mouth, small genitals, low intelligence, pathological appetite from 2–3 years old.
   Absent growth spurt, death in adults from bronchopneumonia. Pickwickian syndrome. 50% have deletion on chromosome 15.

ii Laurence-Moon-Biedl AR: polydactyly, mental retardation, retinitis pigmentosa.

3. Chromosomal

Down's syndrome, XXY.

4. Immobility

Mental retardation, spina bifida, muscular dystrophy.

5. Achondroplasia

6. Drugs

Prednisolone, valproate.
Investigate: as dictated by clinical history and findings.

Treatment of exogenous obesity

1. Indications.

   i After 6 months old if crossing centiles and parents obese encourage reduction in weight gain, but not weight loss. Infants need a pint of milk a day and ACD vitamin drops.

   ii Motivated children. Little danger of anorexia in the truly obese teenager, more in the slightly overweight.

2. Principles in children

   i Aim for weight loss. Eat less. Inpatient start: only if difficulty in establishing the diet or proof needed that it can be achieved.

   ii Diet: 3.4–4.2 mJ = 800–1000 kcal/day, 40% as protein.

   iii Educate: healthy eating = nutritive foods, avoid added sugar and fats.

   iv Empty mouth between meals, i.e. avoid snacking. If necessary give raw carrots, celery, low calorie drinks.

3. Enlist school's help or advise packed lunches.
4. Activities: must be regular, otherwise often fail due to lack of fitness.
5. Group support, and frequent clinic visits supervised by dietician.

Prognosis

Infancy: 10% of obese infants become obese adults.

Children: the older the child at onset of obesity the more likely they will be obese adults, e.g. 40% at 7 years, 70% at 10–13 years. Boys have a better prognosis than girls.

Adults: increased mortality from hypertension and diabetes mellitus if 'apple'-shaped, i.e. fat over abdomen, compared with 'pear' shaped fat distribution on buttocks and thighs.

Further reading

Griffiths M, Payne P R, Stunkard A J, Rivers J P W, Cox M (1990) Metabolic rate and physical development in children at risk of obesity. *Lancet*, i, 76–79

Table 6.5 Special diets and their indications

Diet	Indications
1 Cows' milk avoidance (use soy/protein hydrolysate)	Post infective cows' milk intolerance. Allergy. Allergic colitis. Use in the hope of avoiding eczema is probably illusory.
2 Colouring and preservative free	Hyperactivity/allergy
3 Oligoantigenic*	Uncontrolled by medication: epilepsy, migraine, hyperactivity, eczema, vaginal discharge
4 Ketogenic	Uncontrolled epilepsy

* Egger J, Carter C M, Soothill J F, Wilson J (1989) Oligoantigenic diet treatment of children with epilepsy and migraine *Journal of Pediatrics, 114*, 51-58

Further reading

Bentley D, Lawson M (1988) *Clinical Nutrition in Paediatric Disorders.* London:Bailliere Tindall

Chapter 7

Growth

Major determinants include nutritional balance, psychological well-being, and genetic influences. Racial differences determine body proportions more strongly than height (Africans longer legs, and Asians a longer trunk, than Caucasians).

Endocrine factors

Growth Hormone (GH)

Secreted in pulsatile manner in quiet sleep through the night. Tall children secrete more in amplitude than short, and deprived, children. The latter may have a reversible deficiency of GH.

Insulin-like growth factors (IGF) also called somatomedins

GH stimulates the liver, other organs and tissues to produce IGF, which act locally to promote growth of cartilage and most dividing cells. Reduced in GH deficiency.

Rare inherited disorders:
    i Of IGF production in Laron dwarfism.
    ii Absence of IGF receptors in the African pygmy.

Thyroid hormone

Essential for postnatal growth, and modulating IGF activity. Lack results in reduced limb growth, with preservation of infantile body proportions, delayed bone age and puberty; rarely and paradoxically, precocious puberty.

Sex steroids

Anabolic, account for half the growth in puberty. They advance growth, bone age (see below) and puberty.

    Excess leads to rapid growth, skeletal maturation, premature epiphyseal fusion and short adult stature.

Glucocorticoids

Suppress growth when in excess, probably by GH suppression and inhibition of IGF production.

Table 7.1 Three distinct phases of somatic growth in children: the infancy–childhood–puberty (ICP) model

Phase	Growth pattern	Determinant
1 Infancy	1 Rapid growth of infancy is the deceleration of the fetal growth rate	Nutrition
2 Childhood	2 Slow deceleration from one year old, except for the mid childhood adrenal spurt	Growth hormone
3 Puberty	3 Pubertal growth spurt	Sex steroids + growth hormone

Growth

From the ICP model (Table 7.1), small for dates babies who fail to catch up, or those infants who receive inadequate nutrition, are doomed to remain short; obese infants who remain so are likely to be tall as adults.

Some linear growth milestones

1. The rate of growth is maximal in utero, so by term a third of adult height has been achieved, 75 cm by a year.
   Deceleration in growth continues throughout childhood, except for a mid-childhood growth spurt between 6 and 9 years, attributed to adrenarche.
2. By the onset of puberty girls average 140 cm, and boys average 150 cm due to 2 extra years before the pubertal growth spurt.
   The onset of puberty in girls is associated with early growth acceleration, as oestrogen is a potent stimulus to growth hormone secretion, compared with testosterone, which has to be present in larger amounts, i.e. acceleration is relatively later in boys' puberty.
3. Growth during puberty adds about 22 cm for girls and 25 cm for boys.

Recording and interpreting growth measurements

Single measurements are plotted on 'distance' charts, showing how a child compares with the rest of the population. During puberty the 'tempo' of growth may vary between children a great deal.
   Growth velocity = the rate of growth over a fixed time interval. When compared with standards for that child's age a low velocity is found where growth is falling away, and high velocity when it is accelerating. To maintain adequate growth, velocity must oscillate about the 50th centile. A single value on or little above the 25th centile is acceptable, but not if it continues over successive years. Changes in

growth will be evident, if on the 3rd centile as slowing, and on the 90th as a rapid increase.

As velocity is independent of actual height, a velocity chart shows change in growth rate more rapidly than on a longitudinal growth chart, enabling action to be taken earlier (Figure 7.1).

Peak height velocity (PHV) is the maximum rate of growth achieved during puberty (Figure 7.2):

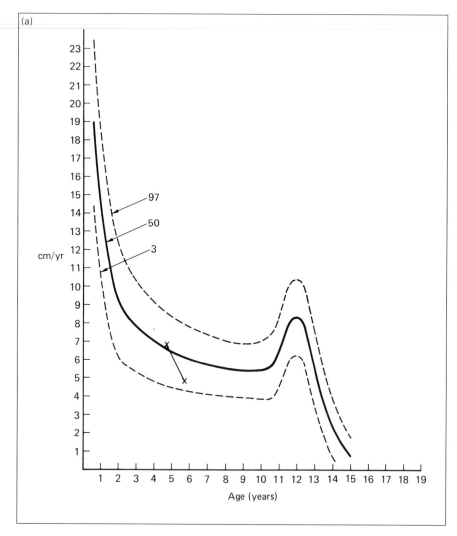

Figure 7.1: A comparison of growth plotted on a velocity chart (a) compared with a linear growth chart (b). A fall from the 50th centile for velocity during the early stages of Crohn's disease indicating a problem before it shows as a fall off on the distance growth chart

1. Girls about 12 years old, breast stage 3, peak before menarche, gain 6–11 cm in the year PHV achieved.
2. Boys about 14 years old, 12 ml testes, relatively later on in puberty. Gain 7–12 cm in their PHV year.
3. Early maturers tend to have greater PHV than late maturers.

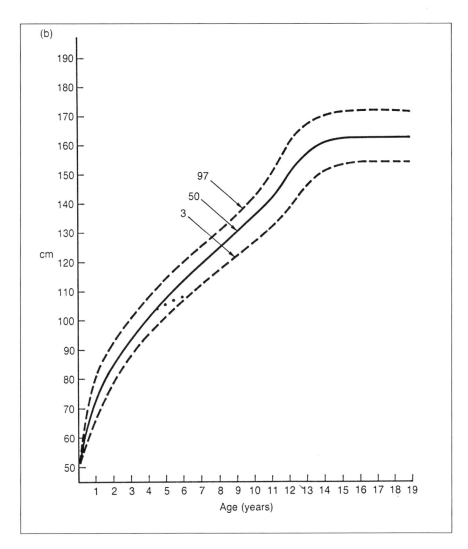

Figure 7.1: *Cont'd*

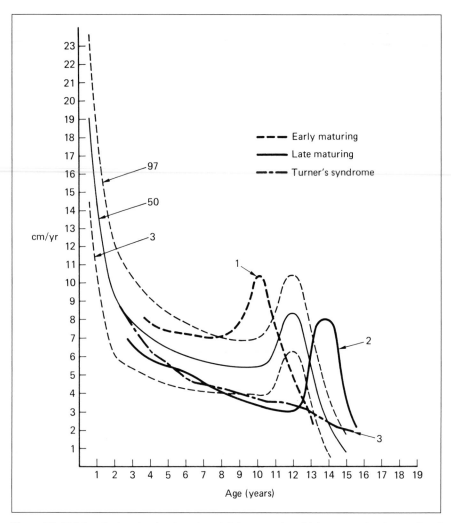

Figure 7.2: Height velocity, showing 1. early and 2. late maturing girls' progress. 3. Absent pubertal PHV in untreated Turner's syndrome, preceded by growth failure from 4 years old.

Hazard of interpretation of growth measurements

1. Growth is non-linear, e.g. many children have a growth spurt in spring, reduced growth in the autumn.
2. Errors in measurement are additive over periods of less than a year.
3. Minimum reliable period between measurements is 6 months.

Decimal age is favoured for rapid calculation of growth rates, and works in tenths of a year, not months.

Example: Girl born on 5th July 1983 = 83.507.

1. Say she is measured on 29th May 1990, = 90.405.

Age is 90.405 - 83.507 = 6.90 years.
2. Reviewed 31st December 1990 at age 90.997-83.507 = 7.49 years.
   Increase in height found was 3.2 cm, in 0.59 years (7.49-6.90).
   Velocity = 3.2 /0.59 = 5.4 cm/year.
   Plot velocity on the chart at the midpoint in time (7.49 + 6.90)/2
   = 7.20 years.
3. Conclusion: 25th centile, satisfactory velocity for a single estimation.

The concept of 'bone age'

By the use of standardized X-rays estimate the maturity of each epiphyseal centre of the left hand and wrist to derive a score. The age at which the score is on the 50th centile is the bone age of that individual. Tanner and Whitehouse (UK) and Greulich and Pyle (USA) are the standard systems which quantify how much growth has occurred and how much is to come.
   Menarche = 12–13 years.
   Final end point is adult, fused epiphyses, at 16 years.
   'Normal' bone age approximates to within a year of the chronological age.
   'Delayed' bone age implies potential for more growth than expected from chronological age. Not necessarily all that growth potential will be achieved.
   Final adult height is likely to be reduced in any condition if diagnosis and treatment are excessively delayed, as the epiphyses inexorably, slowly, close.

Examples

1. In constitutional delay, bone age is within the 3rd–97th centile lines on the chart for the height at bone age, but not necessarily chronological age (Figure 7.4).
2. In growth hormone deficiency as growth velocity falls progressively the bone age falls below the centiles (Figure 7.3).
3. Accelerated bone age: bone age advanced beyond chronological age by sex steroids results in prematurely fused epiphyses, shortened final adult stature, e.g. adrenogenital syndrome.

Growth Points

- Increased early nutritional intake causes more rapid growth in height. Bone age is concordant.
- The normal deceleration in growth in late childhood may result in low growth velocity of <5cm/year prior to the onset of puberty. Constitutional delay and late onset of puberty is commoner in boys as a reason for seeking medical advice, who see their peers tower above them.
- The earlier the onset of puberty the earlier the growth spurt, the fusion of epiphyses and therefore the shorter the final adult height.

- The more delayed the onset of puberty the smaller the peak height velocity and the final adult height.

Catch-up growth

It is the acceleration in growth following removal of a retarding effect: e.g. malabsorption, corticosteroids, or following institution of effective treatment such as thyroid or GH replacement. Cannot make up for years in bone age lost.

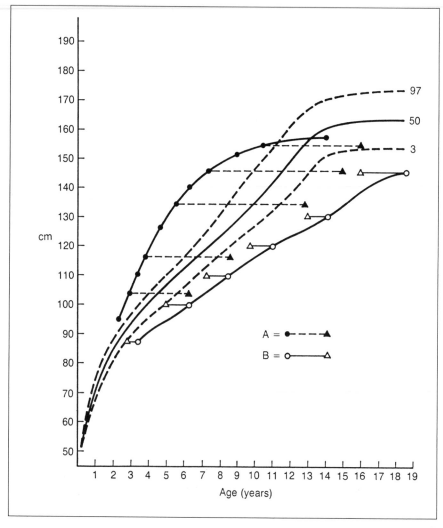

Figure 7.3 Linear growth chart showing children with growth disorders and how bone age outside the centiles acts as a warning sign. A = congenital adrenal hyperplasia B = growth hormone deficiency.

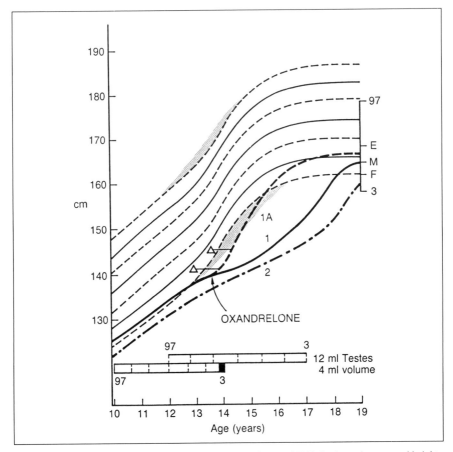

Figure 7.4 Chart of constitutional growth delay. M (mother) and F (father) are the parental heights, E the estimated mid-parental height and the bar the 3rd and 97th centiles.

Boy 1 had only 2–3 cms growth in the year prior to a 3 month course of oxandrolone H, which resulted in a sustained pubertal spurt, as testes were 4 ml at its initiation and increased to 10 ml, allowing the spurt to continue, Final height was close to expected. The continuous line shows the slower, smaller spurt if left untreated, which theoretically can result in a shorter final height, as the older one is at peak height velocity (PHV) the smaller the PHV is.

Boy 2 is small and shows the common pattern of delay with social deprivation.

Comparing childrens' height with their parents'

To obtain an approximation to the mid-parental percentile. (The 3–97th centiles for offspring of these parents are approximately 10 cm either side of this mid point).
1. Boys: plot mother's height on the right hand margin height grid, add 13 cms (4 inches) and mark it in. Now plot father's height, and take the mid point between the two marks. This is the mid-parental height centile. It may be above father if mother is less than 7 cm shorter as in Figure 7.4.

2. Girls: plot father's height, deduct 13 cm and mark it on the right hand margin height grid. Now mark in mother's height. The mid parental height is the mid point. This may be above father's height if mother is 13 cm taller.

GROWTH DISORDERS

Short stature

Social deprivation is the single most important cause of short stature in the UK.

Many organic causes have no specific treatment, but full explanation leads to realistic expectations of growth and final height.

Probably 1 in 10 below the 3rd centile need treatment for short stature, others for conditions in which growth is incidentally impaired.

Societal implications: employment and marital prospects are significantly reduced in short adults (women < 5' (152.4 cm), men <5' 2" (157.5 cm)).

Causes of short stature or failure to thrive

Common

1. Nutritional disorders:

     i Undernutrition.
    ii Malabsorption: intestinal infection, tropical infestation. Individually uncommon: coeliac, cystic fibrosis, Crohn's disease, Hirschsprung's disease.

2. Constitutional: individual and familial short stature.
3. Deprivation, disordered feeding behaviour: see below.
4. Intrauterine growth retardation (IUGR).

     i Permanently impaired growth potential in toxaemia starting before 34 weeks' gestation.
    ii Damaged in utero by alcohol, drugs, infections.
   iii Genetic (Noonan's, Aarsog's syndrome) or chromosomal effect (Down's, Turner's syndrome).
    iv Low birthweight and dwarfed, sporadic conditions, e.g. Russell-Silver syndrome.

5. Systemic diseases:
   Heart: especially cyanotic congenital lesions.
   Lung: asthma (c. 10% have growth delay), cystic fibrosis.
   Renal: shrunken kidneys, renal tubular acidosis, uraemia, diabetes insipidus.
   Haem: sickle cell, thalassaemia.
   Mental retardation.
   Diabetes mellitus, poorly controlled or onset in early childhood.
6. Chronic infection: malaria; or with organ impairment, e.g. pyelonephritis.

Uncommon

1. Endocrine: hypothyroid, hypopituitary, Cushing's syndrome.

2. Iatrogenic: steroid excess.
3. Metabolic: rickets, diabetes insipidus, renal tubular acidosis, hypercalcaemia, storage disorders, e.g.mucopolysaccharidoses.
4. Skeletal dysplasias: achondroplasia, Albright's hereditary osteodystrophy, hypophosphatasia.

Some inherited syndromes associated with short staure

- Aarsog's syndrome: XL dominant, short, hypertelorism, round face, small nose, stubby fingers, shawl scrotum, cryptorchid.
- Achondroplasia: AD, 80% are due to a new mutation. Short limbs, large head, normal trunk, spinal deformity with cord compression, occasional hydrocephalus.
- Albright's hereditary osteodystrophy:
  1. Parathormone levels normal or high due to end-organ unresponsiveness = Pseudohypoparathyroidism = Albright's with low Ca^{2+}
  2. Pseudopseudohypoparathyroidism = Albright's with normal Ca^{2+}. Both are XL dominant, short, obese, short 4th, 5th metacarpal, mental retardation, calcified basal ganglia and subcutaneous tissues, exostoses. Tetany/fits from hypocalcaemia may need large doses vitamin D.
- Hypophosphatasia: AR, alkaline phosphatase of bone and liver deficient, pyrophosphate accumulates preventing normal calcification. Neonatal deaths, respiratory difficulties as chest wall is extra pliant, if milder–rachitic, cranial synostosis.
- Noonan's syndrome: AD, variable penetrance, short, mental retardation, webbed neck, pectus excavatum, small penis, cryptorchid, delayed puberty. Normal chromosomes.
- Russell-Silver syndrome: sporadic, low birthweight, short, triangular facies, small jaw, low set ears, clinodactyly 5th finger; asymmetry of body size or limb length is usual.
- Spondylo-epiphyseal dysplasia: usually X linked, short trunk, squat neck, narrowed and calcified intervertebral disc spaces.

Assessment of failure to thrive and short stature

The approach to both short stature, and failure to thrive in infancy, is similar. Height or weight or both are affected, sometimes with abnormal behaviour and delayed development a consequence of the primary cause. The definition includes those below the 3rd centile for age, and those with decelerating growth velocity towards a stature inappropriate for the family.

In older children the commonest referral is for constitutional delay in growth with exaggeration of the natural slowing of growth before the onset of puberty, at the time that peers are at their peak height velocity, causing alarm in the family, and despondency in the (usually) boy.

Essential information

- Timing and duration of growth failure, and any associated symptoms.
- Birthweight and gestational age (growth retarded?).

- Previous heights from clinic, school (give clues to duration of problem).
- Parental heights, their onset of puberty, menarche (for familial short stature and/or delay).
- Social factors include family constitution, maternal depression, ability to cope, emotional and physical abuse; check food intake, anorexia or food avoidance.

Examination

- Accurate height of child, and parents, using Harpenden stadiometer, weight, head circumference.
- Sitting height to determine disproportion between trunk and limbs (achondroplasia, spondyloepiphyseal dysplasia), and limb length if asymmetrical (e.g. Russell-Silver syndrome).
- Skin: lipomata and cafe au lait patches in Turner's syndrome.

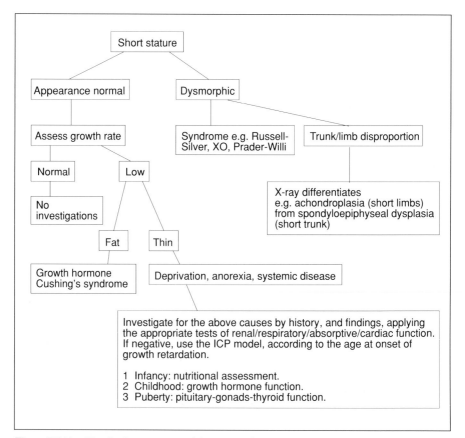

Figure 7.5 Algorithm for the assessment of short stature (after Brook)

- Assess pubertal rating, testicular volume with Prader orchidometer. Do BP, check fundi, acuity and visual fields.
- At this stage an algorithm (Figure 7.5) can be useful in deciding on whether and what investigations are in order.

If significantly below the 3rd centile in height, or low velocity (<25th centile over one year or <5cm/year over 3 years old), or symptomatic do:

1. Urine culture, routine urinalysis.
2. Full blood count, ESR, folate, Ca^{2+}, phosphate, alkaline phosphatase, creatinine, T4, bone age.
3. Consider if jejunal biopsy, TSH, cortisol, growth hormone, (usually as full pituitary function test including sex hormones), chromosomes, skull X-ray, head CT are indicated from the examination or initial investigations.
   Review 6–12 monthly and repeat growth velocity measurement in those below 25th centile.

Interpretation

1. Normal looking – do bone age of the left wrist:

   i Normal growth velocity – family history aids interpretation:
   a. Constitutional delay in growth and puberty (CDGP). Height and bone age delayed 2–4 years and a family history of delayed menarche or shaving.
   b. Familial short stature – normal timing of puberty, normal bone age.
   c. Intrauterine growth retardation (IUGR) – low birthweight, normal family growth pattern; bone age is variable.

   ii Low growth velocity – below 25th centile after correcting for skeletal maturation.

   a. Deprivation/growth hormone (GH) deficient – short, bone age usually delayed, growth hormone response is below normal, euthyroid.
   Deprivational failure to thrive and short stature
   Symptoms
   Food intake is variable: excessive or apparently voluntarily small.
   Thirst may be marked.
   Coeliac like, large bulky offensive stools, apathetic.
   Blue, cold extremities.
   Puberty considerably delayed.
   Appear much younger than actual age, may have frozen watchfulness or be over-affectionate to strangers.
   Investigations and treatment
   Social enquiry is essential. Bone age is usually retarded, growth hormone level low on stimulation tests, reverting to normal in a few weeks in a caring environment. Social work and psychiatric intervention is warranted, and long–term fostering may be required.
   Feeding disorders represent 80% of non-organic cases of failure to feed. With treatment over half can recover. Infant characteristics: fussy, difficult and demanding, difficulties in fixing, control of lips, tongue and swallowing. Maternal characteristics: conflicting advice received, disorganized,

often unsupported emotionally, alcohol, lower intelligence, psychological disturbance.

Treatment:

Analysis of feeding routine determines behavioural guidelines, e.g. regularity of feeds? enough time? excessive noise/distraction techniques? sitting on lap or fed on the run? maternal anxiety is preventing the child from self-feeding?

b. Systemic disease affecting the rate of growth. Investigations as indicated by symptoms and signs of malabsorption, cardiac, renal, hypothyroidism, intracranial tumour, metabolic disorder etc.

c. Turner's syndrome without the usual stigmata. The rate of growth suboptimal for family may be the only finding.

2. Distinguishing features of facial appearance or body proportions.

i   Normally proportioned: chromosomes for Turner's syndrome.

ii   Disproportionately short trunk or short limbs: eg spondylo-epiphyseal dysplasia or achondroplasia.

Investigations include skeletal survey, calcium, phosphate, serum alkaline phosphatase for rickets, hypophosphatasia.

Treatment

1. Constitutional growth delay in boys: with testes >4 ml will respond to 3–6 months of oxandrolone 2.5 mg daily, the self sustained acceleration merging later with the natural pubertal growth spurt. Alternatively, advance the onset of puberty with 3 months of human chorionic gonadotrophin by monthly injection.
2. Familial short stature: explanation and reassurance.
3. IUGR: results with GH disappointing, see GH replacement.
4. Deprivation: improve environment, and psychological wellbeing; may need foster care.
5. GH deficiency: see GH replacement.
6. Turner's syndrome: GH and oxandrolone in combination.
7. Short limbs: GH may have a place. Consider limb lengthening surgically in achondroplasia, hypochodroplasia (also Turner's, late/inadequate treatment of GH deficiency or adrenogenital syndrome).
8. Psychological adjustment. Help is indicated while waiting for treatment to be effective or if none is available. Important to relate to the child as for chronological age. Resulting problems include: underperforming or being bullied at school, and as a short adult difficulty in finding employment and marriage.

Growth hormone replacement

Indications and regimen

1. Absent or reduced GH or GH releasing hormone secretion

i   Idiopathic.

ii Secondary to disease, trauma, irradiation for leukaemia, tumour.

Dose 15–24 IU/m²/week, higher in puberty, as a daily evening (mimicking physiological secretion) subcutaneous injection, until growth ceases. Growth response is proportional to the amount of GH administered.

In skeletal dysplasias, e.g. achondroplasia or renal failure, as little as 4 cm a year is still useful.

2. Impaired peak GH levels in small, otherwise normal children. Response is variable, and may be poor, especially if intrauterine growth retarded, where the bone age advances in tandem with no improvement in the final height.

Controversy concerning normal short children about the 3rd centile centres on the doubtful ethics of treating them, with finite resources (annual cost £5000), and defying otherwise acceptable genetic height.

3. Turner's syndrome. Relative growth hormone end organ unresponsiveness needs a larger dose of GH to be effective, combined with a small dose of androgen for the best response. Start from 4–5 years old, at the time growth begins to fail.

Prognosis for final height in GH deficiency and Turner's syndrome is related to early diagnosis.

Further reading

Brook C D G, Hindmarsh P C (1990) The management of short stature. In *Recent Advances in Paediatrics vol 9*. p 61-74 T J David ed. Edinburgh:Churchill Livingstone

Parkin J M (1989) The short child. In *Clinical Paediatric Endocrinology*, 2nd ed. C G D Brook ed. Oxford:Blackwell pp 96–117

Skuse D H (1985) Non-organic failure to thrive: a reappraisal. *Archives of Diseases in Childhood*, **60** 173–178

Stanhorpe R., Preece M A, Hamill (1991) Does growth hormone treatment improve final height attainment of children with intrauterine growth retardation? *Archives of Disease in Childhood*, **66**, 1180–1183

Tall stature

Culturally perceived as less worrying than short stature.

Distinguish between accelerated growth and simple tallness by obtaining serial measurements to obtain growth velocity.

1. Accelerated childhood growth resulting in stunted adults, unless treated: precocious puberty, adrenogenital syndrome, adrenal tumours, hydrocephalus.
2. Most tall children presenting are from tall families, usually girls worried about excessive adult height. Kyphosis is a problem in a small proportion.

To make an accurate prediction the height of the child and parents, plus child's bone age, are needed. (Tanner J M, Landt K W, Cameron N, Carter B S, Patel J (1983) Prediction of adult height from height and bone age in childhood. *Archives of Disease in Childhood*, **58**:767–776.)

Causes of tall stature

1. Constitutional, familial, isolated, obesity.

2. True precocious puberty (unless treated may result in a stunted adult).
3. Chromosomal: XXY, XYY
4. Endocrine

   i Thyrotoxicosis.
   ii Congenital adrenal hyperplasia (unless treated may result in a stunted adult), adrenal secreting tumours, some Cushing's syndrome.
   iii Gonadal secreting tumours.

5. Hydrocephalus (unless treated may result in a stunted adult).
6. Metabolic: Marfan's syndrome, homocystinuria.
7. Sotos' syndrome, Beckwith syndrome.

Assessment of tall stature

- Birth weight heavy in Beckwith syndrome and Sotos' syndrome.
- Mental development may be abnormal in XXY, hydrocephalus, homocystinuria, Beckwith, and Sotos' syndrome.
- Facial appearance: long in Sotos' and Marfan's syndromes. Lens dislocation in Marfan's syndrome and homocystinuria.
- Signs of precocious puberty in congenital adrenal hyperplasia.
- Limbs disproportionately long in length in XXY, Marfan's, and homocystinuria.

Differentiating features and management

Reduce pressure on the tall child produced by the adult (parents, teachers and others) misconception that emotional and intellectual maturity equate with size.

Relationship problems for girls with boys may be an indication for treatment.

May be at greater risk of sexual abuse if puberty is also advanced.

1. Normal looking

   i Normal growth velocity
Familial or isolated.

Increased growth hormone secretion. Normal bone age.

Do a final adult height prediction: subjectively, the family may consider it excessive if >200 cm for boys, >180 cm for girls, and request treatment. Give testosterone or ethinyloestradiol respectively when 10 cm short of target height, (in girls, about a bone age of 12 years, ethinyloestradiol 0.1 mg daily for 2 years reduces by 5 cm) or until epiphyseal fusion is complete.

Long-acting somatostatin analogues may become clinically useful, and avoid potential sex hormone side effects, e.g. oestrogens in Marfan's syndrome may worsen aortic root laxity.

   ii Increased growth velocity
>97th centile in 6 months or >75th centile for 1–2 years.

   a. Precocious puberty: secondary sexual characteristics may not be evident at first, if due to virilizing congenital adrenal hyperplasia or tumour, or Cushing's syndrome or gonadal tumour. Treat according to aetiology. See precocious puberty.

   b. Hyperthyroidism: clinical signs, advanced bone age.

c. Obesity: usually clinically obvious, slightly advanced bone age, end up normal height for the family.
d. Growth hormone excess: tall for parents, prepubertal, CT scan may show enlarging pituitary adenoma.

2. Looks abnormal

i Long limbs

a. Arms = Marfan's syndrome (disorder of fibrillin, carried on chromosome 15) and homocystinuria.
Family history (though Marfan's may be sporadic).
Examination: thumb sign +ve = thumb protrudes when flexed across the palm, wrist sign +ve = overlap of thumb and fifth finger when they encircle the other wrist.
The span of upper limbs to each middle finger tip > height by 4 cm or more, or decreased upper:lower body ratio, normally <1.0 in Caucasians, 0.9 in Africans.

Complications of Marfan's syndrome and homocystinuria compared:
1. Skeletal
Joints: hypermobile in Marfan's. Stiff and enlarged in homocystinuria.
Scoliosis: common to both, as are hernias.
2. Cardiovascular
Heart: mitral and aortic valve incompetence in both. Ascending aortic dilatation only in Marfan's.
Vascular: thromboses only seen in homocystinuria, responsible for the mental retardation, strokes and myocardial infarctions.

Table 7.2 Management of Marfan's syndrome and homocystinuria

System	Disorder	Effect, age of appearance	Management
Cardiovascular*	Aortic aneurysm Mitral valve	Dissection from adolescence Incompetent in childhood	Annual US if at risk. Graft aorta, aortic valve. Antibiotic prophylaxis for dental procedures
Eye	Lens subluxation	Poor vision, from childhood myopia, retinal detachment	Glasses, ophthalmic supervision
Orthopaedic	Scoliosis Spondylolisthesis Patella dislocation	Childhood Adolescence (Marfan's) Adolescence (Marfan's)	Brace Fusion
	Thickened stiff joints in childhood in homocystinuria		
Neurological (homocystinuria only)	Thrombosis causing mental handicap and strokes	Late childhood to adult life, rarely in infants	Pyridoxine and a low protein diet

* Aortic aneurysms in Marfan's alone, M>F, tendency identified by excessively distensible aortic root on US, while myocardial infarcts due to thromboses occur in homocystinuria.

3. Ocular

Eye lenses: sublux upwards and out in Marfan's, down and inwards in homocystinuria. Myopia, retinal detachment common to both.

Diagnosis

Marfan's syndrome: at least two systems must be affected. US of aortic root shows more distension than normal in those at risk of aneurysmal dilatation. Genetic counselling often identifies other affected family members.

Homocystinuria AR in urinary amino acids.

Prognosis Cardiovascular complications are more common in males with Marfan's syndrome, account for 95% of deaths and reduce life expectancy by 40%. Half homocystinurics are mentally handicapped.

b. Legs = Klinefelter's syndrome XXY: chromosomes, counselling.

ii Unusual appearance

Sotos' syndrome (cerebral gigantism), compared with the Beckwith, also called the Beckwith-Weidemann, syndrome (BWS). Both sporadic, large from birth, early excessive growth but normal adult height, frequently mental slowness. BWS has distinctive features: macroglossia, macrosomia, exomphalos, neonatal hypoglycaemia due to hyperinsulinism. Sotos' syndrome produce large head, hands and feet. Management in BWS is mainly special schooling needs, after the initial problems.

Further reading

Hindmarsh P C, Brook C G D (1989) Tall stature. In *Clinical Paediatric Endocrinology*, 2nd edn, C G D Brook ed, Oxford: Blackwell, pp128-142.

McClain L G (1989) The tall athlete and Marfan syndrome: need for clinical differentiation. *Journal of Adolescent Health Care*, **10**, 564–566.

Further general reading

Growth disorders (1986) *Clinics in Endocrinology and Metabolism*, **15** (3) London:W B Saunders

Rallison M L (1986) *Growth Disorders in Infants, Children and Adolescents*. New York:Wiley

Chapter 8

Puberty and growth

PHYSIOLOGY

1. Initiation of puberty:

   i Awakening or release from inhibition of neurons in the medial hypothalamus that secrete gonadotrophin releasing hormone (GnRH) from the hypothalamus, mainly at night.

   ii Decreased sensitivity to negative feedback of increased gonadotrophins.

2. Girls are more sensitive to GnRH and release gonadotrophins more readily and therefore at an earlier age than boys, and may explain why precocious puberty is commoner in girls.

Assessment of pubertal stage

Stages 1 to 5, 1 is prepubertal, 5 mature adult

3. Sequence of events at puberty

Girls   i Breasts and pubic hair appear at 11 (9–13) years.

          ii Breast stage 2 to menarche: median of 2 years.

          iii Menarche 13 (11–15) years.

          iv Complete in 1.5–6 years, mean 4.2 years.

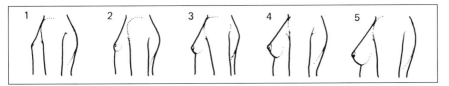

Figure 8.1 Breast stages 1 to 5.
Stage 2 is the breast bud.
Stage 3 is like a small adult breast
Stage 4 the areolar and nipple stand proud of the breast
Stage 5 nipple and breast have the same shape

From Tanner J.M. (1962) Growth at Adolescence 2nd edn. Oxford: Blackwell Scientific by kind permission of the author and publishers.

Boys i Testes 4 ml at 10–14 years, 12 ml at 12–17 years.

       ii Pubic hair at 12 + years, usually after testes or penis begin to enlarge.

       iii Complete in 2–4.5, mean 3.5 years.

4. Growth in puberty

Sex steroids and growth hormone (GH) are synergistic in growth promotion. The sexes differ in their timing of response.

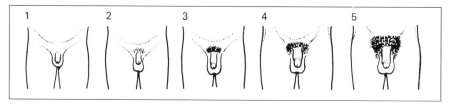

Figure 8.2 Genitals and pubic hair stages 1 to 5.
Stage 2 the scrotum reddens and enlarges, the testicles enlarge (4 ml)
Stage 3 penis lengthens, scrotal skin thins, testes larger.
Stage 4 the glans enlarges, penis broader. Testes grow, and scrotum larger and darker. Stage 5 is adult.

From Tanner J.M. (1962) Growth at Adolescence 2nd edn. Oxford: Blackwell by kind permission of the author and publishers.

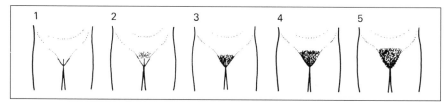

Figure 8.3 Pubic hair stages 1 to 5.
Stage 2 has a few long downy hairs around the base of penis or the labia majora.
In stage 3 it spreads sparsely across the pubes.
Stage 4 is adult type, but smaller in area than stage 5 when it also spreads to the medial aspect of the thighs.
Axillary hair is graded 0 = none, 1 = a few hairs, 2 moderate spread, 3 = adult (no illustration)

From Tanner J.M. (1962) Growth at Adolescence 2nd edn. Oxford: Blackwell by kind permission of the author and publishers.

Girls' oestrogen secretion is at a peak as the rate of growth falls: peak height velocity occurs at breast stage 2 to 3, average age 12 years old.

Slow growth in girls in early puberty is abnormal. GH failure is likely.

Boys show a progressive increase in testosterone with growth, which is slow initially. Their growth spurt is late, at genital stage 3 to 4, average 14 years.

DISORDERS OF PUBERTY

Precocious puberty

Definition

Onset of pubertal changes before 8 years in girls, 9 years in boys. 5 times more common in girls, 80% 'non pathological', whereas 80% boys have a significant cause.

Pathophysiology

Ninety per cent are girls, probably because they have a lower threshold to GnRH for pulsatile release of LH and FSH from the pituitary.

Hamartomata of the hypothalamic-pituitary region are common in true precocious puberty. Usually benign in girls, these tumours are rarely so in boys.

The commonest cause of early pseudopuberty is congenital adrenal hyperplasia (CAH). Despite treatment of virilizing conditions like CAH or removal of a secreting tumour true puberty may be triggered due to maturation or 'priming' of the pituitary.

Causes of precocious puberty

(Initial difference is from premature isolated thelarche and isolated pubarche)

1. True puberty (synchronous)

   i Idiopathic central precocious puberty.
   ii Central precocious puberty secondary to:
     Hypothalamo-pituitary tumours and infections.
     Raised intracranial pressure.
     Cranial irradiation.
   iii Primary hypothyroidism.

2. Pseudopuberty (asynchrony, pituitary gonadotrophin independent)

   i McCune-Albright syndrome.
   ii Adrenal disorders:
     Cushing's syndrome, congenital adrenal hyperplasia, primary tumours.
   iii Gonadal disorders:
     Ovarian cyst, ovarian tumour (granulosa cell, thecoma, luteoma) Leydig cell tumour.
     Gonadotrophin-independent precocious puberty (testotoxicosis).
   iv Ectopic gonadotrophin producing tumours.
     Dysgerminoma, hepatoblastoma, teratoma, chorionepithelioma.
   v Exogenous sex steroids.

Warning signs of probable abnormal puberty

A lack of harmony, or asynchrony, between age, growth, and pubertal changes.

Girls

   i Breasts developing with little virilization: differentiate between self limiting premature thelarche, true precocious puberty or autonomous oestrogen excretion e.g. follicular ovarian cyst.
   ii Breast and pubic hair is likely to be true precocious puberty, only rarely McCune-Albright syndrome (cafe au lait spots, fibrous dysplasia of long bones, precocious puberty), or ovarian tumour (onset often at 4 years, deeply pigmented areola, abdominal pain early on).

   iii Vaginal bleeding at too early a stage of breast development: taking contraceptive pill accidentally or deliberately administered, sexual abuse, foreign body.

   iv Significant pubic hair, lack of breast development ie lack of consonance.

      a. Fine hair: adrenarche, or premature ovarian failure (e.g. Turner's syndrome).

      b. Coarse hair: CAH or virilizing tumour.

Boys

   i Bilateral enlargement of testes in true precocious puberty or testotoxicosis (familial, cyclical sex steroid production from the gonads despite absence of LH, FSH pulsatility, variable GnRH test response. Cause unknown).

   ii Small testes, virilized in congenital adrenal hyperplasia (CAH) and adrenal tumour.

   iii One testis irregular, enlarged, the other small: Leydig cell tumour or adrenal cell rest in CAH.

In boys and girls

Hypothyroidism may present inadequate virilization (pubic hair) for the stage of testicular or breast development.

Clinical

First distinguish from normal variations in early pubertal development:

- Premature thelarche: onset <3 years, small breasts (B2, B3), absent pubic/axillary hair, pink vaginal mucosa, normal growth and bone age, resolves by 8 years old. Follicular cyst (small, seen on ultrasound) increases circulating oestradiol. The oestrogen may be exogenous – foods (chicken neck, veal, beef) or contraceptive pill. Unless of long standing, needs follow-up for possible precocious puberty.
- Premature adrenarche: onset >6 years, scant pubic hair (PH2, rarely PH3), axillary hair or smell, normal genitals/breasts for age, slightly advanced growth and bone age. Due to early rise in adrenal androgens.
- Gynaecomastia: breast (usually B2) in boys in stage 2–3 of puberty. Resolves in 1–3 years, rarely needs surgery. Pathological in Kleinfelter syndrome, partial androgen insensitivity, prepubertal boys with 11-hydroxylase deficiency.

Investigations

1. Height and bone age, usually advanced in true and pseudopuberty.
2. Gonadotrophins:

   i Gonadotrophin releasing hormone (GnRH) test to assess whether pubertal or prepubertal levels of FSH and/or LH.

   ii FSH alone is raised if a follicular cyst.

   iii Human chorionic gonadotrophin (hCG) or LH like activity in gonadotrophin secreting tumours (do US/CT/MRI of liver).

   iv Low FSH, LH in thelarche, adrenarche.

3. Serum sex steroids: if elevated and FSH, LH low = gonadal/adrenal tumour or enzyme defect.
4. Urinary steroids + serum 17-hydroxyprogesterone for adrenal enzyme defects.
5. T4 for hypothyroidism: enlarged testes + absent hair in boys, isolated breast development in girls.
6. Pelvic ultrasound:

   i Multicystic ovary and enlarged uterus with endometrium in true precocious puberty.
   ii A few cysts in an ovary + small uterus in premature thelarche.
   iii Ovarian asymmetry and tumours, adrenal enlargement due to adenoma, carcinoma.

7. CT/MRI of pituitary fossa and region for hamartomas, tumours, hydrocephalus.

Table 8.1 Differential diagnosis of precocious puberty (PP)

Disorder	Gonadotrophins	Serum sex steroids	Gonadal findings on palpation/ultrasound
Central PP	Pubertal (pubertal GnRH test)	Pubertal	Normal testes Enlarged uterus Multicystic ovaries
Gonadotrophin–independent PP (testotoxicosis/ McCune-Albright)	Prepubertal (low GnRH response)	Pubertal, or higher	Normal pubertal testes Enlarged uterus Symmetric ovaries
Secreting tumours	1 Prepubertal with supressed GnRH response, unless LH/hCG secreting 2 Gonadotrophin secreting: LH and/or hCG	i Leydig→ testosterone. ii Granulosa-theca cell > oestradiol raised Pubertal or higher levels still Positive pregnancy test	One testicle much larger or unilateral ovarian mass Testes moderately enlarged

hCG = human chorionic gonadotrophin

Management

1. Psychological support

Preparation for menarche; dealing with aggression and masturbation in boys. School help in placing in an older class if able to cope. Sexual abuse a danger.

2. Delay sexual development

   i Gonadotrophin releasing hormone analogues (GnRH-A) 'down regulate' by hyperstimulation in true precocious puberty.
   ii Cyproterone actate or medroxyprogesterone acetate supresses sex steroid production in the rare gonadotrophin independent precocious puberty (testoxicosis) and are useful in the initial stimulating phase of GnRH-A treatment.

3. Growth prognosis after treatment

   i True precocious puberty: unaltered in girls, i.e. reduced adult height c. 3rd centile or below, but better in boys.

   ii Improved in CAH, gonadal/adrenal tumours after the virilizing effect is removed, though true precocious puberty may follow the priming effect of the androgens, and may also need treatment.

Further reading

Leader (1986) *Precocious puberty. Lancet* ii, 80–82

Delayed puberty

Presentation

1. Complete absence of signs of puberty by 14 years in boys or girls.
2. Arrest in the normal progression of puberty.
   NB: Puberty rarely begins spontaneously after 18 years old. Growth in height is synchronously delayed, and may almost stop if the testes are small, <10 ml.

Other warning signs of developing endocrinopathy (central or peripheral)

1. Remaining in one pubertal stage for >18 months is suspicious.
2. Large testes, and inadequate virilization, in hypothyroidism.
3. Growth velocity of only 2 cm per year in early puberty.
4. No growth spurt with breast stage 2 or if 10 ml testes present.

Causes of delayed puberty

Common

With normal LH, FSH levels:

1. Constitutional delay of growth and puberty (CDGP) is physiological, frequency 1 in 200. The delay is synchronous for both height and bone age which is delayed 2–4 years. Often familial, and up to 20 years old before final height is attained, it is appropriate to that predicted from the parents' heights.
2. Deprivation.
3. Chronic disease: severe asthma, sickle cell, anorexia nervosa, coeliac, Crohn's disease, cystic fibrosis, diabetes mellitus, renal failure.
4. Excessive physical training (ballet, athletics).

Uncommon

1. Central: hypogonadotrophic hypogonadism, normal or low LH, FSH

   i Idiopathic; familial with anosmia = Kallman's syndrome XL, AR or AD; multiple deficiencies but principally GH.

   ii Secondary to hypothalamo-pituitary disease.

2. Peripheral: gonadal, hypergonadotrophic with raised LH, FSH levels

   i   Gonadal dysgenesis in normal XX, XY individuals, and XO, XXY disorders.
   ii Gonadal failure: chemotherapy, irradiation, autoimmune, anorchia, orchitis, injury.
   iii Inborn errors: complete androgen insensitivity (testicular feminization).

Assessment

1. Constitutional delay growth pattern (CDGP) from early age. Age of menarche and shaving in family may provide further evidence of CDGP.
2. Previous growth: related to the onset of deprivation (often early childhood), or the chronic disease. In asthma and sickle cell anaemia childhood linear growth may be low normal, but the pubertal spurt delayed. Tall stature suggests XXY.
3. Psychological issues: vandalism, aggression, glue sniffing, may mask depression about immature appearance.
4. Systemic symptoms and signs of disease, especially occult inflammatory bowel disease, coeliac disease. Midline defects or reduced ability to smell in Kallman's syndrome.
5. Neurological signs (fundi + visual fields)?
6. Abnormal appearance (Turner's /Kleinfelter's syndrome)?

Investigations

Majority require only a bone age and T4.
   If in doubt, look for:

Both sexes

LH, FSH elevation = gonadal failure. Normal or low in CDGP and chronic disease or hypogonadotrophic hypogonadism for which a CT or MRI scan of the pituitary area may be indicated.

Boys

1. Human chorionic gonadotrophin test. Testosterone rises on stimulation in constitutional delay, but not if hypogonadotrophic hypogonadism.
2. GnRH test: reliability poor. If still in doubt, wait for signs of puberty!

Girls

1. Ovarian ultrasound for bioassay of sex hormone function (presence, size and number of follicular cysts).
2. Chromosomes.
   Some girls with Turner's syndrome may have no external stigmata.

Management

1. Treatment should always include psychological support.
2. If clear cut CDGP and boy has 4 ml testes, and is emotionally disturbed by poor growth, give oxandrolone for 3–12 months; this primes GH secretion, and growth is sustained when the testes achieve 10 ml in volume.

   Both CDGP and partial hypogonadotrophic hypogonadism (PHH) show normal harmony of growth and development, so may need to induce puberty for 2–3 years then observe after stopping treatment to see if: (i) normal progression = CDGP, or (ii) regression = PHH.
3. Treatment principle in hypogonadotrophic hypogonadism (central) and hypergonadotrophic hypogonadism (peripheral) is to replace the missing hormone, introducing it gradually to imitate physiological puberty, so minimizing the psychological trauma of rapid induction.

   i   To virilize boys give testosterone i.m.
   ii Girls are initially given ethinyloestradiol alone, then cyclically with a progesterone agent to induce menstruation.
   iii Pulsatile GnRH therapy can be used in adult life to induce fertility in hypogonadotrophic hypogonadism. Hypergonadotrophics cannot be fertile, although girls could accept a donor egg.

Further reading

Stanhope R, Preece M A (1988) Management of constitutional delay of growth and puberty. *Archives of Disease in Childhood*, **63**, 1104–1110

End of Chapter 8

Table 9.3 Drugs for hormone replacement

	Dose	*Frequency and route*
Cortisol	20 mg/m²/24 h	2–3 × daily, oral
DDAVP	0.05–0.15 ml	2 × daily, intranasal
Ethinyloestradiol	initially 2–5 mg	1 × daily, oral
Fludrocortisone	0.15–0.25 mg/m²/day	1 daily, oral
Growth hormone	15 IU/m²/week	1 daily, subcutaneously
Human chorionic gonadotrophin	1500 units	once weekly i.m.
Oxandrolone	1.25 or 2.5 mg (or 0.05 mg/kg)	1 daily, oral for 3–12 months
Testosterone	100 mg i.m.	6 weekly, then 4 weekly, then 2 weekly, over 12–18 months

Further reading (Chapter 9)

Brook C G D (1989) *Clinical Paediatric Endocrinology*, 2nd edn. Oxford: Blackwell

Hughes I A (1986) *Handbook of Endocrine Tests in Childhood*, Oxford: Butterworth-Heinemann, useful for revision

Styne D M (1988) *Paediatric Endocrinology for the House Officer*, Baltimore: Williams and Wilkins, a practical (North Amercian) approach.

Chapter 9

Endocrine problems

PITUITARY AND HYPOTHALAMUS

Embryology and physiology

1. Pituitary:

Origin of the lobe	Communication from the hypothalamus
anterior lobe: oral ectoderm.	via the pituitary portal system.
posterior lobe: neuroectoderm of the diencephalon.	via the magnacellular neurones.

2. The hypothalamus controls pituitary secretion of releasing factors and inhibiting factors (Table 9.1).

Table 9.1 Hypothalamic hormones and responding effects on pituitary hormone release

Hypothalamus	Anterior pituitary
Acidophilic cells secrete:	Growth hormone (GH): acts via insulin like
Growth hormone releasing hormone (GHRH)	growth factors (IGF)
Somatostatin	Inhibits GH release
Prolactin release inhibiting factor	Prolactin
Basophilic cells secrete:	LH released acts on the ovary, or Leydig cell of
Gonadotrophin releasing hormone (GnRH) acts	testes to produce testosterone. FSH released acts
on anterior pituitary to release the	on the ovary, or Sertoli cells to induce
gonadotrophins luteinizing hormone (LH)	spermatogenesis. They secrete inhibin and
follicle stimulating hormone (FSH)	activin which modulate FSH release.
Thyrotrophin releasing hormone	Thyrotrophin stimulating hormone (TSH)
Corticotrophin releasing factor	Adrenocorticotrophic hormone (ACTH)
Supraoptic + paraventricular nuclei	*Posterior pituitary*
Magnocellular neurons (1% change in serum	Vasopressin
osmolality is sufficient to cause secretion)	

Important pulsatile modes of release

All anterior pituitary hormones are secreted in this way, probably so too the respective releasing/inhibitory factors.

1. GH: mainly 90 minutes after onset of sleep and subsequent sleep cycles, in sleep stages III, IV, with a dominant periodicity of 3 h. Greatly increased during puberty, due to the effect of sex steroids on GHRH.
2. GnRH: pulses vary in amplitude and frequency with different stages of development and point in the menstrual cycle. Continuous high levels of GnRH or analogue cause reversible supression, called 'down regulation', and used therapeutically in precocious puberty.
3. FSH, LH

   i After birth high levels of GnRH stimulate production of FSH and LH to pubertal levels for 6 months in boys, 2–4 years in girls. They then fall, except in hypogonad states, e.g. Turner's syndrome.
   ii As puberty approaches, 60–90 minute cycles develop, first in sleep, then also by day. The sex steroids produced provide negative feedback.

4. ACTH: Circadian rhythm, peak at 0700, nadir at midnight.

GROWTH HORMONE DEFICIENCY (GHD).

Incidence may be as high as 1in 4,000

1. Congenital

   i   Idiopathic: GHD +/– other anterior pituitary hormones.
   ii Inherited GHD is familial AD or AR.
   iii Developmental: pituitary aplasia, hypoplasia, associated with midline defect, cleft lip and palate.
   iv Craniopharyngioma.

2. Acquired

   i   Post traumatic: breech, sphenoid fracture.
   ii Infective: post meningitis, TB.
   iii Tumour: pituitary adenoma, pinealoma, optic chiasma glioma.
   iv Irradiation.
   v   Infiltration: Langerhans cell histiocytosis.

3. Transient

   i   Peripubertal.
   ii Psychosocial.
   iii Primary hypothyroidism.

Clinical

1. Neonatal hypoglycaemia.
2. Impaired linear growth:

i A single measurement 3 standard deviations below the mean.

ii If repeated after 6 months a growth velocity <25th centile or <5cm/year.

3. Onset:

i Congenital: short stature noted from 2 years old.

ii Growth arrest or reduced velocity in transient suppression and acquired GHD.

4. Skin fold thickness is increased, i.e. overweight from reduced gluconeogenesis.
5. Midface underdevelopment, dental malocclusion.
6. Small penis and scrotum.
7. High pitched voice.

Investigations of short stature when GHD is suspected

1. Bone age (usually, but not always, delayed).
2. Blood for FBC, electrolytes, urea and creatinine, chromosomes in girls to exclude Turner's syndrome. Urine for specific gravity/osmolality, pH, protein and blood.
3. Growth hormone assay: 'classical' insulin tolerance test (ITT).

In peripubertal years, if bone age >10 years then prime with the appropriate sex hormone (sustenon or ethinyl eostradiol) to avoid overdiagnosis of GHD.

Usually done as a triple stimulation test which assesses both anterior and posterior pituitary function:

i.v. insulin + thyroid releasing hormone (TRH) + gonadotrophin releasing hormone (LHRH). Blood glucose should fall below 2.2 mmol/l, or symptoms of hypoglycaemia occur.

Beware of inducing severe hypoglycaemia if hypoadrenal. Check the 9 a.m. cortisol if panhypopituitarism is suspected. Omit insulin if less than 175nmol/l.

Death, mainly from hyperosmolar i.v. glucose given for hypoglycaemia following ITT, usually in preschool children, has prompted advice from the Chief Medical Officer. Use other less hazardous tests (e.g. clonidine, arginine, glucagon) if GHD alone is suspected.

Results are obtained and tabulated as follows:

Time (min)	Blood glucose (mmol/l)	GH (mU/l)	Cortisol (nmol/l)	TSH (mU/l)	LH (U/l)	FSH (U/l)
0	x	x	x	x	x	x
15	x	x				
30	x	x	x	x	x	x
60	x	x	x	x	x	x
90	x	x	x	x		
120	x	x	x	x	x	x

 Prolactin is often measured, but is rarely of direct relevance in children. Raised in suprasellar lesions and interruption of the portal vessels delivering prolactin inhibiting factor from the posterior pituitary, e.g. craniopharyngioma, and after radiation.

Interpretation

   i Growth hormone <15mU/l = partial, <7mU/l = severe deficiency. Physiological tests over 12–24 h may be more revealing of disordered secretion.

      A low growth velocity is the most sensitive of all tests for GH deficiency, and arguably no further test is required.

   ii Plasma Cortisol: failure to rise 2–3 × above basal level = ACTH deficiency, or suppression where the basal level already high, e.g. in glucocorticoid administration.

   iii Thyroid stimulating hormone: normal resting up to 3 mU/l, peak of 10–30 mU/l at 30 minutes. High basal, sometimes with an exaggerated peak = hypothyroidism.

   iv Gonadotrophin releasing hormone (LHRH): prepubertal peak in LH of 3–4 U/l, and FSH up to 2–3 U/l. Absent response = gonadotrophin failure or simply prepubertal/delayed puberty. High basal and peak values in primary gonadal failure, e.g. Turner's or Kleinfelter's syndrome, and inappropriately high for age in precocious puberty.

Treatment and prognosis

1. Human growth hormone: see Growth for details of administration.
2. Other hormone replacements may be indicated (thyroxine, cortisol, sex steroids, antidiuretic hormone).
3. Psychological adjustment – avoid overprotection and infantilizing of the short child, especially at school.

   Earlier identification and institution of human growth hormone should improve the final height prognosis; previous disappointing results may have been due to late diagnosis and inability to make up for growth lost.

Further reading

Shah A, Stanthorpe R, Matthew D (1992) Hazards of pharmacological tests of growth hormone secretion in childhood. *British Medical Journal*, **304**, 173–174

HYPOPITUITARISM

Short, pale, narrow face, sexual infantilism.

Investigation

1. Triple stimulation test.
2. Thyroid, LH and FSH levels are reduced, despite stimulation, in panhypopituitarism.
3. Diabetes insipidus biochemistry may be due to a hypothalamic tumour.
4. Neuroradiology of the pituitary area for ballooning of the sella, clinoid erosion, or calcification in a suprasellar mass.

Treatment

Treatment is of the associated hormone deficiencies (see end of chapter for doses).

THYROID DISORDERS

Biochemistry of thyroid disorders

Normal range: TSH 0.3–5.0 µU/l (70–100 µU/l for 2–5 days after birth).
Plasma total T4 = 70–150 nmol/l, free T4 = 9–25 pmol/l.
Plasma total T3 = 1.2–2.8 pmol/l, free T3 = 4–8 pmol/l.
Prematures tend to have low T4, T3 levels for the first 4–8 weeks.

As cheap, reliable methods of assessing free T4 and TSH are increasingly available, the relevance of absent, low or high thyroid binding globulin (all X linked) resulting in low or high total T4, T3, but normal free T4, T3 and a normal TSH, is now limited. The immunometric assay of TSH supercedes radioimmunoassay, and is very sensitive. Thus, low values <0.1 µU/l are indicative of hyperthyroidism, even though apparently euthyroid, e.g. early Graves' disease, or an autonomous solitary nodule (rare in children).

Inherited disorders in order of site of action:

   i Familial thyroid unresponsivness to TSH (very rare) – no goitre.
      Goitre present at birth, or develops insidiously:
  ii Decreased thyroid iodide trapping
 iii Defective iodide organification (commonest inborn error): peroxidase deficiency, usually in association with Pendred's syndrome (1:30 000 schoolchildren) of deafness, goitre and mild hypothyroidism; may not present until puberty.
 iv Enzyme deficiency: inability to deiodinate iodotyrosines.
  v Abnormality of thyroglobulin synthesis, storage or secretion.
 vi Peripheral resistance to thyroid hormone, elevated T4, normal TSH.

Congenital hypothyroidism

Incidence

1 in 3500 in UK, M:F = 1:2

1. Commonest cause: sporadic absence, ectopic and/or hypoplastic due to maldescent during fetal development.
2. Rarely: panhypopituitarism, familial inborn errors of thyroid metabolism, ingestion of goitrogens or drugs by mother after the 8th week of gestation.

In hyperthyroid mothers: no contraindication to breast feeding by taking antithyroid drugs, as levels are very low in breast milk.

Clinical

1. Goitre – points to goitrogen (iodide in maternal asthma remedies, thioureas, greens of the brassica family) or inborn error (AR inheritance is usual, so ask for the family history, and Irish tinker origin).
2. Signs most prevalent in the first 3–6 months:

    i Newborn: prolonged physiological jaundice, transient hypothermia.
    ii Feeding difficulties, respiratory distress with feeds, and constipation; a hoarse cry slow to start = the 'flat battery' sign.
    iii Posterior fontanelle remains open, >1cm.
    iv Floppy, lethargy, mottled cold limbs, supraclavicular fat pads.
    v Anaemia (pale) and carotinaemia (yellow tinge to skin).

3. Becoming more evident as the months pass:

    i Facial puffiness, large tongue, umbilical hernia, reduced growth in length, high upper to lower segment ratio as measured from the symphysis pubis, delayed closure of the anterior fontanelle (closure usually by 18 months).
    ii Mental retardation.

Screening

The aim is early identification to reduce mental handicap which may result from treatment delay beyond 6 weeks of age.

Blood spot using the Guthrie card, for TSH level. Normal value is <10 μU/l by the end of the first week of life. Level >50 μU/l is diagnostic, and repeat estimations are arranged for values >20 μU/l.

NB: *Infants with TSH deficiency are not detected by this method, and clinical vigilance is still necessary.*

Investigation

1. Low T4, T3. A low free T4 indicates true hypothyroidism, not thyroid binding globulin deficiency.
2. TSH

    i High in primary hypothyroidism.
    ii Normal or low

        a. Secondary = pituitary: reduced TSH.
        b. Tertiary = hypothalamic: reduced thyroid releasing hormone (TRH). Requires a TRH test to distinguish between them. If a low TSH is confirmed, GH and ACTH activity should be measured as TSH is rarely an isolated deficiency.

3. X-ray shows delayed ossification, and fragmentation of epiphyses.
4. Scan: [123]I or ^{99m}Tc uptake is low in hypothyroidism. Size and (ectopic?) site of the gland is shown.
5. Goitre present: radioisotope scan is followed by perchlorate within 2 h.

    i Excessive discharge of isotope confirms the peroxidase organification defect.
    ii If normal, biopsy and thyroid synthesis studies define the abnormality.

Diagnosis

Primary hypothyroidism = TSH >50 μU/l and a T4 <75nmol/l or free T4 <9 pmol/l; 95% are now identified by screening before any clinical signs are noted.

Treatment

Thyroxine 100 mg/m²/day, 25–50 μg/day in the first year. Monitor free T4, growth and bone age.

Excessive treatment leads to advancement of bone age, possible craniostenosis and later to reduced adult height as epiphyses prematurely fuse.

Due to faulty feedback suppression, TSH may remain high for years, so probably best ignored.

If diagnosed by TSH screening at birth, review at 1–2 years old to exclude transient neonatal hypothyroidism due to maternal ingestion of goitrogens or TSH-receptor blocking antibodies acquired transplacentally from mother with autoimmune thyroid disease.

Acquired hypothyroidism

Causes

1. Iodine deficiency is the commonest cause world wide, occasionally goitrogens (drugs, vegetables, milk from cows fed Brassica).
2. Autoimmune (Hashimoto's) thyroiditis: commoner in girls, usually after puberty. Family history in 40%. Gradual onset. Commoner among diabetics, Down's and Turner's syndromes.
3. Thyroglossal duct cyst containing the active thyroid gland removed at surgery.
4. TSH deficiency: pituitary tumour.

Clinical

1. Behaviour good, school work and application excellent!
2. Family history

   - of thyroid disorders, goitres in autoimmune thyroiditis (Hashimoto's or Grave's disease) and enzyme defects.
   - of perceptive deafness in Pendred's syndrome.

3. Initial history and/or signs of thyrotoxicosis in 10% with Hashimoto's.
4. Goitre:

   i Symmetrical enlargement: iodine deficiency, adolescent (simple) goitre, goitrogens, Pendred's. May be symmetrical and small in Grave's disease.
   ii Irregularly enlarged, firm (bosselated) in Hashimoto's.
   iii Solitary nodule suggests autonomous hyperthyroidism or malignancy, not hypothyroidism.

5. Growth failure with infantile proportions. May be the only sign for years.

6. Usual manifestations of hypothyroidism, and occasionally also precocious puberty with scant or no pubic hair.

Investigations

1. Low free T4, elevated TSH, and in Hashimoto's antimicrosomal antibodies and antithyroglobulin antibodies.
2. Low free T4 and TSH points to pituitary or hypothalamic cause; consider CT.
3. Bone age delay is proportional to the duration of hypothyroidism.
4. ^{123}I scan prior to surgery of a thyroglossal cyst will identify if it contains the only active thyroid tissue.
5. Biopsy the nodular goitre, and 'cold' nodule on scan, for carcinoma.

Management

Thyroxine indicated:

    i As for congenital hypothyroidism
    ii Euthyroid with a cosmetically distressing goitre. Size usually diminishes adequately over many months.
    iii Biochemical hypothyroidism only.

Adolescent goitre (simple colloid goitre)

A diffuse soft euthyroid goitre, often familial. No bruit, non tender. Usually regresses spontaneously. Biopsy shows colloid only, not the diffuse lymphocytic infiltration of Hashimoto's. Years later may progress to euthyroid multinodular goitre.

Graves disease

Definition

Autoimmune hyperthyroidism, with eye involvement, and rarely the pretibial skin. Rare in early childhood, increasing in adolescence.

Pathophysiology

Thyroid stimulating immunoglobulin (TSI) acts on the TSH receptor. Autoimmune, due to interaction of T- and B-lymphocytes, in both Graves and Hashimoto's (a family history of either is often obtained). Five times more common in girls. Mucopolysaccharides and lymphocytes infiltrate orbital, skin and subcutaneous tissues.

Clinical

1. School performance and behaviour deteriorate.
2. Accelerated growth velocity, hyperphagia, +/- weight loss.

3. Beta-adrenergic stimulation: tachycardia, bounding pulse, palpitations, sweating, tremor.
4. Smooth goitre often with bruit, eye signs, and rarely pretibial myxoedema.

If the goitre is painful, subacute (de Quervain's) thyroiditis is likely, occurring after coxsackie, mumps or adenovirus infection, and causing transient hyperthyroidism.

Investigations

TSH <0.1 µU/l and thyroid stimulating antibodies present. Total T3 and free T3 are raised proportionally more than total T4 or free T4. (Transient rise, then fall in T4 over 2–3 months occurs in subacute thyroiditis before recovering).

Management

1. Medication. Complete remission in 70%. Carbimazole in high dose for the first 2 months. Administer for 1–2 years, occasionally up to 6 years. Rashes in 2% occur early, and usually respond to antihistamines. Granulocytopenia at 1–2 months, usually recovers following withdrawal. Substitute with a thiourea drug. Propranolol for thyroid storm may be life saving. Subacute thyroiditis responds to aspirin, rarely needs steroids.
2. Surgery. For medical treatment failures, depending on local surgical expertise. Postoperative hypothyroidism and transient (usually) hypoparathyroidism may occur.
3. Radioactive iodine. Consider in older adolescents who fail, or will not comply with, the medical regimen. Rarely used in the UK.

Neonatal hyperthyroidism

Definition

Due to transplacental maternal thyroid stimulating immunoglobulin (TSI). Rare, occurs in 1% of the infants at risk whose mothers have Graves disease with high TSI titres.
TSI has a half life of 2 weeks and the condition is therefore self-limiting.

Clinical

Symptoms: onset at birth may be delayed up to 7 days by maternal antithyroid drugs. Irritable and hungry but with poor weight gain and diarrhoea. Tachypnoea from cardiac failure.
Signs: exophthalmos, palpable goitre present, rapid pulse, supraventricular tachycardia, cardiac failure.

Investigations

Free T4, T3, TSI titres raised.

Management

Untreated, cardiac involvement may cause death.
Propranalol (2 mg/kg/day) controls symptoms, carbimazole (1 mg/kg 8 hourly) and Lugol's iodide solution 1 drop 8 hourly act additively. Stop treatment after 4–6 weeks.

Further reading

Fisher D A (1989) The Thyroid Gland. In *Clinical Paediatric Endocrinology* 2nd edition, (C G D Brook, ed). Oxford:Blackwell, pp 309-337.

GONADAL DISORDERS

Normal fetal sexual differentiation

(Endocrine causes of impaired virilization are marked by an asterisk.)

1. Female

In the absence of Y chromosome the undifferentiated gonads and external genitalia become female. By fetal week 20 primordial follicles are appearing.

2. Maleness

All the following steps are necessary to complete development in the fetus.

  i   Testicular development is thought due to surface testicular antigen, the histo-compatability-Y (H-Y) antigen, on the Y chromosome. This induces the primordial gonad to differentiate into a testis at 8–10 weeks' fetal life.
 ii   The testes' Sertoli cells produce anti-Mullerian duct hormone to inhibit Mullerian duct development which otherwise become uterus and fallopian tubes.
iii   The Leydig cells produce testosterone (T) due to placental chorionic gonadotrophin (hCG) stimulation. T is essential to the persistence of the Wolffian ducts which form the vas deferens and epididymis.
        *After delivery, hypopituitarism → low LH output → low testosterone which results in a small penis <2.5 cm stretched length.
 iv   Testosterone is produced by the testes and adrenals. *Inadequate or excessive production will cause inadequately virilized boys, or virilized girls, as in the enzyme deficiencies that characterize congenital adrenal hyperplasia.
  v   Peripheral metabolism of testosterone. The external genitalia tissue to be (sex skin) must contain the enzyme 5 alpha reductase (5ARD) to reduce testosterone to dihydrotestosterone (DHT). *DHT is essential for the external genitalia to develop from the genital tubercle. Absence of either 5ARD or DHT may be complete or partial, resulting in the androgen insensitivity syndrome.

Ambiguous genitalia

1. Female virilization = normal ovaries and Mullerian structures, XX chromosomes

i Virilized external genital

a. Congenital adrenal hyperplasia: 21-hydroxylase, 11 β-hydroxylase, and mildly in 3 β-hydroxysteroid dehydrogenase (3β-HD) deficiency.
b. Maternal androgens: progesterone taken before week 13 of gestation, or androgen secreting tumour.

ii Enlarged clitoris only: in some dysmorphic syndromes; a lipoma or haemangioma; prematures or low birthweight.

2. Male inadequate virilization

Chromosomes: one Y (rarely, XX with H-Y antigen), one or more Xs

i Undescended testes: normal, XXY, or anorchia.
ii Testes present, though not necessarily palpable, +/– scrotal growth, in XY individuals. Due to:

   a. Testosterone enzyme biosynthetic abnormalities: 3β-HD, 17 α-hydroxylase, 20,22 desmolase.
   b. Peripheral metabolism of androgens is abnormal: The androgen insensitivity syndrome (AIS): complete as in testicular feminization, or partial, leading to intersex.

   Testicular feminisation, X linked.
   Complete = normal female phenotype, little sex hair, blind ended vagina, inguinal herniae may contain testes. Risk of testicular malignancy indicates their removal after puberty.
   Incomplete = micropenis, chordee, bifid scrotum (may contain gonads), perineal hypospadius.

   5-alpha reductase deficiency (5ARD) AR. Clinically like incomplete AIS, until puberty when virilisation and deepening of the voice occur.

iii Associated with dysmorphic syndromes.
iv Leydig cell hypoplasia (see pathophysiology).

3. Abnormal gonadal differentiation

i Mixed gonadal dysgenesis.
   Rudimentary testis one side, streak ovary the other, or mixed testes with Mullerian structures. Incompletely virilized, i.e. external genitalia abnormal, XY or XO/XY genotype.
ii True hermaphrodite: phallus, urogenital sinus; menstruation possible. Ovotestes in XX individuals are commonest.

Management of intersex

1. Neonatal emergency

(See end of Neonatal problems for initial assessment).

    i Delay gender assignment.

   ii Delay naming, and avoid 'androgenous names', e.g. Francis, Lesley.

2. Investigation

As dictated by family and maternal history, e.g. maternal progesterone ingestion, early deaths (inborn error?). Look for masses in the scrotum, labia, or groins.

Table 9.2 Implications if external genitalia look ambiguous

Number of gonads palpated		*Investigations*
No gonads =	female virilized: CAH likely or male inadequately virilized	Chromosomes, plasma 17-OH progesterone, 11-deoxycortisol
1 gonad =	abnormal gonadal differentation (streak ovary, testis, one of each)	Chromosomes, pelvic US, hCG test, laparotomy and gonadal biopsy
2 gonads =	male inadequately virilized:	Chromosomes, hCG test*, skin biopsy of labia
	1 Testosterone synthesis abnormal	for androgen binding
	2 Androgen receptor defect	Sinogram of urogenital sinus
	3 5 alpha reductase deficiency (5 ARD)	

*hCG test = prolonged stimulation for 3 days, serum before and 4th day for testosterone, dihydrotestosterone and androgen metabolites to distinguish the biosynthetic abnormalities from 5-ARD deficiency

3. Surgery and sex of rearing

    i Virilized females may need clitoral reduction and vaginoplasty, and if due to CAH, mineralocorticoids and glucocorticoids.

   ii In males, gender ultimately depends on the appearance and ability to construct acceptable external genitals. Acceptable appearance required by school age, complete reconstruction may wait until puberty.

Abnormal testes should be removed because of the potential for malignant change. Cryptorchid boys whose testes cannot be brought down need not have them removed if the testes produce testosterone after hCG stimulation.

4. Psychological aspects

    i Girls with CAH tend to be 'tomboys' but appear otherwise comfortable as females. So too testicular feminization with complete androgen insensitivity. However, in 5-ARD raised as girls, 'changing gender' is a common response by the individual to pubertal changes.

   ii Sex of rearing should be determined by 18 months, to avoid confusion, the exception being 5-ARD where change in sex at puberty is accepted by the boys.

iii Counselling parents at diagnosis and before surgery, and the individual at puberty.

5. Endocrine replacement in CAH

Oestrogens for breast development in testicular feminization.

6. Genetic counselling

For familial and genetic conditions.

Further reading

Savage M O (1989) Clinical aspects of intersex. In *Clinical Paediatric Endocrinology*, (C G D Brook, ed). Oxford: Blackwell, pp 38-54.

Disorders of the penis

Micropenis

1. Idiopathic.
2. Hypothalamic: Kallman or Prader-Willi syndrome.
3. Hypopituitarism: Growth hormone or gonadotrophin deficiency.
4. Gonadal: Down's, Noonan's XXY, Smith-Lemli-Opitz.
5. End-organ: androgen insensitivity.

Investigation

Chromosomes, pituitary function, and hCG with testosterone levels.

Macropenis

1. Precocious puberty.
2. Congenital adrenal hyperplasia (small testes).
3. Priapism, e.g. sickle cell.

Investigation

Pituitary function, bone age, 17-OH progesterone.

Hypospadias (1 in 500)

1. Often familial, chordee associated.
2. Renal anomalies common if scrotal or perineal.
3. Cryptorchidism in 10%, consider inborn error and virilised as in CAH.

Investigations

Chromosomes, US.

Management

No circumcision. Operation at 3 years.

Epispadius

Epispadius is rare.
Extrophy of the bladder is often associated.
Incontinence is a major problem.
Surgery can be offered from 6 months old.

Undescended testes

Incidence

Full term newborn 3%, 1 year 1% (in prematures it is proportional to gestation, as testes begin to descend after 28 weeks).

Clinical

Small scrotum suggests undescended testis. If absent feel along the line of descent. Sit boy up or ask him to squat on heels when testis should descend. Maldescent is lateral to the normal line.

Investigation

Bilateral impalpable testes need chromosomes and hCG stimulation. A positive response indicates laparotomy to bring them down. If no response, observe.

Prognosis

Risks of indirect inguinal hernia and torsion reduced by preventive surgery.
Infertility is likely in the undescended (even if only unilateral), not maldescended, but prospects are probably improved by surgery before 2 years old.
Malignant change is increased in undescended testes. Bringing them down allows examination, but may not alter the incidence.

Foreskin facts

- Non retractile until 3–5 years old.
- Ballooning during micturition is a sign of phimosis, and an indication for circumcision.
- Balanitis may be recurrent: circumcise if more than 5 episodes.

Circumcision

Controversy: claimed 10–fold reduction in the incidence of urinary tract infection in infancy following circumcision in the neonatal period.

Further reading on the pros and cons

Poland R L (1990) The question of routine neonatal circumcision. *New England Journal of Medicine*, **332**, 1312–1315
Schoen E J (1990) The status of circumcision of newborns. *New England Journal of Medicine*, **332**, 1308–1312

ADRENAL CORTEX PROBLEMS

Physiology

Regulation by ACTH through negative feedback. Fetal adrenal gland is the same size as the kidney, and weighs the same as the adult adrenal organ.

Important in utero function as the 'fetoplacental unit': Pregnenolone (produced in the placenta) is converted to dehydroepiandrosterone (DHE) by the fetal adrenal. DHE returns to the placenta to become oestrogen, and helps maintain the pregnancy. Low levels in toxaemia, placental sulphatase deficiency and congenital adrenal hypoplasia.

Mode of action: steroids are lipophylic, therefore diffuse through membranes to the nucleus where they link to receptor proteins. These act on DNA to produce messenger RNA which form proteins that change cell function.

Causes of hypoadrenalism

Neonatal

1. Congenital adrenal hyperplasia.
2. Congenital hypoplasia: X linked; AR; sporadic; with anencephaly.
3. Haemorrhage: asphyxia, intravascular coagulation → adrenal haemorrhage.
4. Maternal steroid administration.

Older infants and children

1. Iatrogenic: steroid administration.
2. Waterhouse-Friderichsen syndrome.
3. Hypopituitarism.
4. Congenital adrenal hyperplasia.
5. Addison's disease: autoimmune, TB.

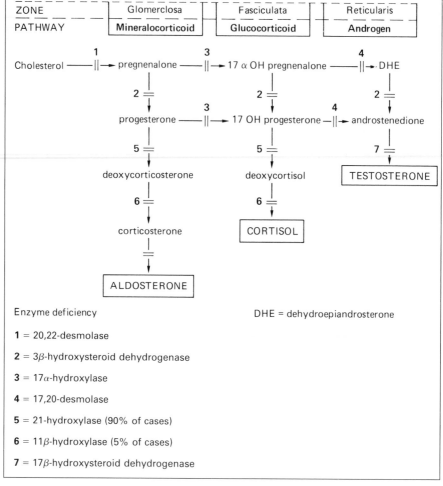

Figure 9.1 Highly simplified outline of adrenal steroid production and some of the more important enzyme deficiencies interrupting it.

Congenital adrenal hyperplasia

Incidence

1 in 6000

Aetiology

Autosomal recessive disorder due to deficiency in one of the five enzymes control-ling cortisol biosynthesis; 90% due to 21-hydroxylase deficiency of whom 70% are salt losers. Trait carried close to the HLA locus on chromosome 6. Asymptomatic (cryptic) cases found in affected families.

Clinical

1. Newborn

- *Commonest cause of gender confusion in the female*: clitoromegaly, labial fusion, cryptochid hypospadic 'male'. Deeply pigmented genitals occur within 2–3 weeks.
- Salt losing crisis at 2–3 weeks old: vomiting (in males confused with pyloric stenosis), failure to thrive, sweating, dehydration, diarrhoea, collapse and coma, rapidly followed by death.

2. Later:

- Pseudopuberty: hair, enlarged penis, small testicles. Isolated pubarche, isolated clitoromegaly (effective treatment may initiate true precocious puberty).
- Excessive growth in height.
- Amenorrhoea, infertility follow.
- The 11 β-hydroxylase deficiency accounts for 5%. It also causes virilization and accelerated growth, prepubertal gynaecomastia and precocious puberty. Hypertension and hypokalaemia develop due to increased mineralocorticoid.

Investigations

1. Blood 17-hydroxyprogesterone (17-OHP), or 11-deoxycortisol for 11-beta hydroxylase defect. Renin will be raised if mineralocorticoid is deficient.
2. Chromosomes if cryptorchid.
3. Routine biochemistry: low sodium, glucose, raised potassium, urea, metabolic acidosis.
4. Urine: increased sodium excretion, gas chromatography for rarer steroid abnormalities.
5. Ultrasound of pelvis, contrast X-rays of vagina and kidneys to exclude other intersex malformations.

Management

1. Early

  i Normal saline i.v. followed by cortisol as hydrocortisone 20–25 mg/m^2/day equally divided into 3 doses.
     Monitor for hypoglycaemia. Ensure adequate glucose intake.
  ii Salt retaining 9 α-fludrocortisone 0.1 mg/day +/– salt supplement 2–3 g/day until semisolids are introduced. Check BP regularly for hypertension caused by the 9 α-fludrocortisone.
  iii Surgical assessment. Clitoroplasty if large. Always rear girls as such regardless of severity of virilization.
  iv Genetic counselling.
  v Psychological support to parents and the child.

2. Later

i Adequate cortisol replacement to ensure controlled growth, avoiding Cushingoid side effects.

Hydrocortisone 12–15 mg/m²/day as 2 doses, more in the morning to mimic diurnal variation, or equivalent as prednisolone (or dexamethasone once growth ceases). Increase at times of stress.

Monitor with serial 17-OHP estimations in blood or saliva, plus blood testosterone if prepubertal.

ii Salt retaining steroid to continue indefinitely if deficient.

iii Surgery: vaginoplasty in puberty.

3. Antenatal diagnosis

An affected fetus will share the same tissue HLA type as a previously diagnosed sibling. Chorionic villous biopsy for DNA studies and sex identification in informative families at 10 weeks. The 17-OHP level is raised in amniotic fluid.

4. Prenatal treatment

Dexamethasone until diagnosis confirmed, ideally from 3 weeks' gestation so that as female external genitalia begin developing androgen suppression may reduce need for reconstructive surgery. Despite early treatment and continuing steroids in the female fetus, results are disappointing.

Further reading

Hughes I A (1988) Management of congenital adrenal hyperplasia. *Archives of Disease in Childhood*, **63**, 1399–1404

Adrenal crisis and the Waterhouse-Friderichsen syndrome

Adrenal crisis

Definition

Acute adrenal insufficiency is characterized by salt loss, metabolic acidosis, hypoglycaemia, circulatory collapse.

Causes

Table of causes of hypoadrenalism, plus acute illness, surgery, trauma, salt loss from excessive sweating or diuretic therapy in a child with hypoadrenalism.

Symptoms

Usually sudden onset, may be preceded by fatigue, irritability and nausea, abdominal pain. Confusion and coma follow.

Waterhouse-Friderichsen syndrome (WFS)

Definition

Bacterial or viral toxaemia causing purpura, and circulatory collapse with bilateral adrenal haemorrhages; usually a post-mortem diagnosis. Low cortisol levels are found in those that die.

Differential diagnosis

Shock due to the overwhelming sepsis of WFS is quicker in onset than that due to adrenal insufficiency. Disseminated intravascular coagulation from other causes.

Management of adrenal crisis and WFS

1. Saline and hydrocortisone 200 mg/m^2 i.v. immediately.
2. Support blood pressure: plasma expanders, dopamine, coagulation factors.
3. Antibiotics if sepsis suspected.

Controversy

'Prophylactic' exogenous glucocorticoid fails to demonstrate protection against WFS, and experimentally may precipitate a Schwartzmann reaction. Nevertheless, it is recommended by some, and early use may inhibit tumour necrosis factor release.

Chronic adrenal failure (Addison's disease)

Definition

Mineralocorticoid and glucocorticoid deficiency due to adrenal damage. Rare.

Symptoms

Fatigue, nausea, vomiting, weight loss, salt craving.

Signs

1. Pigmentation of skin over joints and pressure points, persistent 'tan' in children, not as florid as adults.
2. Symptomatic hypoglycaemia, at higher levels than usual.
3. Postural hypotension >10 mm mercury, increase in pulse of 20/minute. Failure to excrete a water load.
4. Associated conditions
   i Candidal infection of nails and mouth in mucocutaneous candidiasis with immune deficiency syndrome.
   ii Degenerative brain disease in adrenoleukodystrophy.

Investigation

1. Anaemia, serum hyponatraemia, hyperkalaemia, mild metabolic acidosis, low fasting blood glucose.
2. Persistently raised ACTH levels and low cortisol even after prolonged (3–5 days) synacthen administration.
3. Look for adrenal calcification on X-ray and autoimmune antibodies.

Management

1. Hydrocortisone 200 mg/m^2/day stress dose in emergency, 20 mg/m^2/day as replacement. Mineralocorticoid replacement with 9 α-fludrocortisone.
2. 5% dextrose and normal saline as for CAH if dehydrated.
3. Increase steroid at times of illness, surgery.
4. Medilert or SOS bracelet to be worn.

Adrenocortical excess

Cushing syndrome = both exogenous glucocorticoid administration in pharmacological doses and endogenous overproduction.

Causes

1. Cushing disease: basophilic microadenoma of the pituitary producing ACTH causing bilateral adrenal hyperplasia. Usually >7 years old.
2. Adrenal cortical adenoma or carcinoma. Virilization commonly occurs; feminizing tumours are rare.
3. Ectopic ACTH secretion (excessively rare): Wilms tumour, islet cell tumour.

Clinical

1. Catabolic: growth failure, arrest in bone age, osteoporosis (note: adrenal carcinomas can cause virilization, precocious puberty, with small testicles in boys, advanced bone age and increased growth velocity).
2. Appearance: trunkal obesity, thin, wasted limbs, myopathy, Cushingoid facies, buffalo hump, striae, acne, hirsutism.
3. Hypertension, systemic common, rarely intracranial.
4. Immunosuppression.
5. Metabolic: hyperglycaemia, salt and water retention, hypokalaemia, metabolic alkalosis, calciuria and renal calculi.
6. Peptic ulceration.
7. Emotional lability, obsessional behaviour.
8. Polycythaemia.

9. i In exogenous hyperadrenalism: adrenal suppression.
   ii In Cushing disease: hyperpigmentation from ACTH excess.

Differential diagnosis

1. History of steroid administration. Halogenated creams in infants with extensive eczema.
2. Biochemistry of hyperadrenalism:
   i Loss of cortisol circadian rhythm.
   ii Testosterone raised in virilizing tumours.
   iii Dexamethasone suppression test differentiates obesity from Cushing disease, and both from Cushing syndrome.
      a. Low dose: suppression of urinary 17-hydroxycorticosteroids (17-OHCS) and free cortisol by 50% in simple obesity.
      b. High dose: suppression of urinary 17-OHCS in Cushing disease but not in Cushing syndrome from autonomous adrenal secretion or ectopic ACTH producing tumour. CAN SUPPRESS PITUITARY IF HIT HARD ENOUGH.
3. CT and MRI of head and abdomen are of limited help in locating a tumour. Laparotomy may be needed.

Management

1. Iatrogenic steroid excess requires slow reduction in dosage over several weeks or months, often in small decrements if the underlying disease is still active, to avoid rebound, e.g. rheumatoid.
   Consider alternative therapy if side effects are severe, e.g. cyclophosphamide in a nephrotic with vertebral collapse.
2. Cushing disease: transphenoidal microadenomectomy.
3. Adrenalectomy: for carcinoma or adenoma of the adrenal.
4. Replacement glucocorticoid and mineralocorticoid, perioperatively and subsequently if persistent adrenal insufficiency becomes apparent.

ADRENAL MEDULLARY DISORDERS

Pathophysiology

Adrenaline and noradrenaline produced from the chromaffin cells which are also located along the sympathetic chain. Any of these may be sites of tumour transformation when the breakdown products vanillylmandelic acid (VMA), and homovanillic acid (HVA) will be found in excess in the urine.

Phaeochromocytoma

Definition

Chromaffin tumour secreting noradrenaline and adrenaline; 5% occur in childhood, 10% are malignant. Rare cause of hypertension, which is usually constant.

Symptoms

Headache, vomiting. Attacks of palpitations, flushing, pallor, sweating, or anxiety are unusual compared with adults.

Signs

Hypertension and associated retinopathy, cardiomegaly.

Associations

Multiple endocrine neoplasia syndromes (familial, parathyroid adenoma and medullary thyroid carcinoma), neurofibromatosis. Tumours may be bilateral in familial cases.

Diagnosis

1. Plasma noradrenaline is reliable, whereas 24 hour urinary VMA excretion has 10% false negatives.
2. Selective arteriography and venous catecholamine sampling may still be superior to US, CT or radioisotope meta-iodo-benzyl-guanidine (MIBG) scanning to localize a tumour which may be in the abdomen or chest.

Management

1. Alpha and beta-adrenergic blockade, especially of blood pressure, using phenoxybenzamine and propranolol.
2. Surgical removal of tumour.

Neuroblastoma

Neural crest tumour. Variety of presentations, few due to catecholamines, mainly compression or size and metastases (see Oncology for details and screening in infancy).

Multiple endocrine neoplasia syndromes

Familial, hyperplasia or neoplasia of groups of endocrine cells/organs (rare).
MEN 1 = Anterior pituitary, pancreatic islet cells, and parathyroids.
MEN 2 = Phaeochromocytoma, parathyroids, medullary thyroid carcinoma.
MEN 3 = Multiple mucosal neuromas of lips and tongue, Marfan's appearance, phaeochromocytoma, medullary thyroid cancer.

Table 9.3 Drugs for hormone replacement, and
Further reading see page 244

Chapter 10

Diabetes mellitus

Causation

In children almost always from lack of insulin due to islet cell destruction (as opposed to surgical removal, e.g. for nesidioblastosis).

Types

1. Insulin dependent diabetes or type 1 = acute onset, ketosis prone; islet cell antibodies (ICA) and family and human leucocyte antigen (HLA) associations.
2. Non-insulin dependent diabetes or type 2 presents in the obese over 40s with a more gradual onset, no ICAs or HLA relationships.
3. A rare familial, autosomal dominant type 2 form may present in childhood, maturity onset diabetes in the young (MODY).

Epidemiology

Incidence: has doubled over last 20 years in UK to 1:5000 annually.
   Prevalence: 1 in 500 Caucasians and 1 in 2000 Asians under 16 years old.
   Peak onset 10–13 years, but becoming more frequent under 5 years old.
   Boys>girls. Winter>summer, suggesting infection is important in pathogenesis.
Mumps and coxsackie B implicated in some cases, but no one virus consistently.

Genetic factors

1. At diagnosis 15% have an affected first degree relative.
2. Human leucocyte antigens (HLA) DR3, DR4. Absence of aspartate at position 57 on DQ found in 95% (versus 20% in the population).
3. Life-time risk for diabetes is 36% in an identical twin, 10% in a sibling. By 16 years old the risk in a non-identical twin or sibling is 6% overall (HLA identical = 13%, one HLA haplotype in common = 5%, no HLA groups in common = 1.6%).

Pathogenesis

1. Autoantibodies to islet cells in 60–70% at diagnosis (sibling controls 1–5%) may have been present for several years. These indicate the immune system is the mediator of:

2. Lymphocytic infiltration of islets by activated thymus derived (T) cells, relentlessly destroying beta cells.
3. Viral infection/stress which appears to 'precipitate' diabetes, when 80% of islet cells have already been destroyed.

    The mechanism invites intervention strategies, e.g. cyclosporin to supress the immune system and preserve islet cell function; toxicity contraindicates administration to children, at present.

Diabetic microangiopathy or 'triopathy' of retinopathy, nephropathy, neuropathy manifest 10–15 years after diagnosis. Factors influencing their appearance include:

1. Relative sparing in prepubertal children, but the longer the duration of disease the more likely they are.
2. Early good control; the appearance of retinopathy may be delayed.
3. Indifferent control of hyperglycaemia; progressive development of tissue damage until it reaches a point of no return after which improved control cannot retrieve the situation.

NB: 10–15% remain free of microvascular disease after 40 years, the reason for 'sparing' is unknown.

Symptoms

Duration is usually for less than a month: polydipsia, polyuria, thirst, lethargy, weight loss, some pruritus vulvae or balanitis, with a 'flu-like illness; suspected of urinary tract infection or onset enuresis.

    May progress to dehydration, coma and death if symptoms are ignored; under 5s are particularly at risk.

    Vomiting, abdominal pain (± ileus) and rapid respirations in ketoacidosis.

Diagnosis

Random blood glucose >11mmol/l, glycosuria. Ketonuria typically present.

Differential diagnosis

1. Glycosuria.

   - Low renal threshold, normally 9 - 10 mmol/l.
   - Raised blood glucose: stress, corticosteroids, raised intracranial pressure.
   - Renal: Fanconi's syndrome (see renal diseases).

2. Polyuria. Inability to concentrate urine: low urinary osmolality characteristic in diabetes insipidus, nephrogenic or neurogenic, and chronic renal failure with hypertension, uraemia.
3. Ketosis. Common in prebreakfasted, or ill child with vomiting or infection. A feature of the periodic syndrome is ketosis with vomiting which is probably migraine related.
4. Coma. Trauma, drugs, epilepsy, encephalitis, hypoglycaemia (see neurology).
5. Pneumonia a possibility to consider with rapid breathing.
6. Ileus suggests a surgical emergency, but unlikely in the absence of rebound tenderness.

Management of acute hyperglycaemia/ketoacidosis:

1. Newly diagnosed
Mild to moderate ketosis and dehydration in the majority.

i Day 1: soluble insulin 0.25–0.5 u/kg subcutaneously immediately and repeat before each main meal. Some insulin should be given overnight.

ii Day 2: 2/3 previous day's insulin total as 2/3 intermediate, 1/3 short acting (total 0.5–1 u/kg), twice daily, divided 2/3 of total prebreakfast, 1/3 before the main evening meal.

2. Precoma or coma

Coma is mainly due to hyperosmolality. Too rapid rehydration may result in osmotic disequilibrium, which, with hypoxia is thought to cause cerebral oedema, the commonest cause of death in children with diabetes.

Lowering blood glucose by 2–4 mmol/h is optimal.

A nasogastric tube is passed if vomiting or gastric dilatation occurs. Carefully exclude an abdominal emergency.

Monitor fluid input–output, blood glucose, gases, electrolytes and urinary ketones hourly for the first 4 h.

i Fluid resuscitation of dehydration and electrolyte depletion

  a. Weigh, assess severity. A deficit of 10–15% fluid loss is usual, needing i.v. access.

  b. If shocked give plasma, 20 ml/kg over 1/2 h.

  c. Calculate rehydration volume = deficit + daily maintenance.
Daily maintenance = 100 ml/kg first 10 kg, 50 ml/kg next 10 kg, 20ml/kg thereafter.

  d. Rate of administration = 1/4 of the total in the first 4 h, 1/4 the next 8 h, 1/2 the next 12 h.
Example: 18 kg child, 10% dehydrated
Deficit = 1800 ml, daily maintenance = 1400ml
Total = 3200 ml in the first 24 h.
Rate = 800 ml in first 4 h = 200 ml/h, then 100 ml/h next 8 h, 130 ml/h thereafter.
For a 50 kg child, volumes would be 5000 ml + 2250 ml

  e. Constitution of rehydrating fluids:
- normal saline (0.9%) i.v. for 1–2 hours,
- then 0.45% saline until the blood glucose falls to 13 mmol/l,
- when 0.18% saline + 4% dextrose is commenced.

  f. Potassium, 2–3 mmol/kg in the first 24 h, is added early unless anuric.

ii Bicarbonate may be given if pH <7.1. The formula is: mmol HCO_3^- required = 0.1 × base deficit × bodyweight in kg. Infuse over 1–2 h to avoid further lowering of pH in the brain by CO_2 ($H_2CO_3^- \rightarrow H_2O + CO_2$) crossing the blood–brain barrier.

iii Insulin. Soluble insulin 0.1 u/kg/h by continuous i.v. infusion, (remember to saturate insulin binding sites on the plastic tubing by running some of the

infusate through first) or intramuscularly, until blood glucose <14 mmol/l
and the child is orientated. Subcutaneous insulin can then be started, continuing at half the previous rate, for an hour, to avoid rebound hyperglycaemia.
Double the dose after 2–3 h if no fall occurs in blood glucose.

   Sliding scale for subcutaneous insulin once i.v. stopped:
   >20 mmol/l = 0.5 u/kg, 15–20mmol/l = 0.4 u/kg,
   10–15 mmol/l = 0.3 u/kg, 5–10 mmol/l = 0.2 u/kg.
   Commence oral fluids after 12–24 h. Water first, then change to 100 ml
      milk + 10 g glucose (= 15 g carbohydrate) if it is retained.

3. Infection

Infection as possible precipitant requires a chest X-ray, urine and blood culture,
swabs, haemoglobin, WBC. Consider antibiotics.

Continuous management of diabetes

1. Target is 'normoglycaemia' before meals = 4–10 mmol/l while accepting an
   inevitably high post-prandial blood glucose.
2. Diabetic balance = triad of food–exercise–insulin. Too much or too little of one
   without adjustment of the other two results in deterioration in control.
3. Avoid conflict: the desirability of early 'strict' control to stave off complications
   (see pathogenesis) can result in negative attitudes and non-cooperation engen-
   dered by too rigid an approach.
4. Aim is a normal life style.

Food plan

1. The diet should contain sufficient protein for growth (2 g/kg/day), mainly carbohydrate (50%) as 10 g carbohydrate exchanges, some fat (30%); lowering of
   serum cholesterol and triglycerides is an ideal, but compliance is low if too
   restrictive.
   Total daily kilocalories = 1000 +100 per year of age.
2. Calculate daily carbohydrate as 100 g plus 10 g for each year of life. Distribute
   breakfast + morning snack (1/3), lunch + afternoon snack (1/3), evening meal +
   bed time snack (1/3). It is essential to maintain a regular intake throughout the
   day to avoid hypoglycaemia.
   'Glycaemic index' is an attempt to quantify how soluble fibre in foods affect
   blood glucose, e.g. low index for red kidney beans and lentils, high index for
   honey, mashed potatoes. In practice no consistent effect seen, so largely abandoned.

Exercise

Improves self image, avoids obesity, reduces insulin requirements and eases management. Must be taken account of in the food plan. May use sugar to avoid hypos,
but a starchy snack beforehand is better.

Insulin

All newly diagnosed children receive synthetic human insulins. Some are already established on highly purified animal insulin. All 100u/ml.

  i Short acting (soluble) for emergencies, acute hyperglycaemias, covering one and up to two meals.

      Action in 30 minutes, maximal 1–3 h, maximum duration 6–8 h, e.g. Actrapid, Humulin S, Velosulin.

  ii Intermediate acting for background insulin requirements, usually with soluble insulin.

      Action in 2 h, maximal 7 - 15 h, maximum 22 h, e.g. Humulin I, Insulotard, Monotard MC (isophane).

  iii Fixed mixtures of soluble:isophane varying from 1:9 to 2:3 (e.g. Humulin M1–M4 range) are only occasionally used as they lack flexibility on a day-to-day basis.

Hypoglycaemia

Due to imbalance between food, insulin dose, exercise. Most feared complication of diabetes by children and parents. A controlled 'hypo' is often arranged after initial stabilization to identify that child's symptoms and to show parents how to cope.

Desirability of 'good' control may lead to overinsulinization. An excess of deaths in the USA of young adults on continuous insulin infusion may have resulted.

Causes include:

1. Lack of substrate, i.e. missed or delayed meals, carbohydrate intake inadequate prior to bedtime or prolonged vigorous exercise.
2. Excess insulin due to delayed insulin absorption from fatty, fibrotic injection site, or excessive insulin administration.
3. Alcohol alters carbohydrate metabolism.
4. Change from highly purified animal to synthetic human insulin may be associated with reduced neuroglycopaenic symptoms.

Neuroglycopaenic symptoms: blurred or double vision, headache, lethargy, clumsy, confusion, convulsion, coma. Brain damage or death may, rarely, result.

Sympathetic symptoms: hunger, weak, anxious.

Signs: cold clammy skin, pallor, tachycardia, normal BP.

Confirmation: blood glucose finger prick test-strip. Check result by laboratory analysis of venous blood to avoid a potentially tragic error due to contamination of finger by sugar.

Management

Conscious: offer sugary drink.

Coma: 10–20 ml 50% glucose i.v., then oral carbohydrate or 10% glucose infusion; alternatively, glucagon 1 μg or 30 μg/kg i.m. is especially useful at home for parental administration.

10% glucose 5ml/kg

Continued management

During recovery insulin requirements fall, as child returns to normal activities and enters the 'honeymoon phase' of partial recovery of islet cell function which may last many months, as reflected in residual C peptide secretion.

Adolescence often sees an increase in requirements to a total of 1–1.5 u/kg/24 h, and increasing non-compliance.

'Brittle' diabetes occurs in 1%, with frequent ketoacidosis and hospitalization due to home mismanagement and emotional factors. Residential schooling may be necessary.

Injections

Children over 8 years old are encouraged to give their own injections.

Sites on arms, legs and abdominal wall are rotated to avoid fat deposition (lipomatosis).

Reluctance may be helped occasionally with an injector gun or metal tube which hides the needle from sight.

Continuous subcutaneous insulin infusion for adolescents—enthusiasm for this has been replaced by the injection of soluble before each main meal using a pen injector coupled with an injection of intermediate or long–acting insulin for background glucose control. Greater flexibility and convenience are claimed, and may improve 'control' and thus prognosis.

Surgery and diabetes

1. The planned admission. Admit the previous day, assess control by a premeal blood glucose profile, adjust the evening dose if necessary. Nil by mouth from midnight. Before the premed establish a 5% glucose infusion and give half the usual morning dose as soluble insulin.
2. Emergency and planned, once glucose infusion has started. Hourly monitor blood glucose by finger prick, giving insulin according to the sliding scale. Carbohydrate by mouth as for other patients on recovery.

School and the outside world

The class teacher is advised, using the British Diabetic Association school pack. The dietician advises the school catering staff.

Whenever unaccompanied outside the home, older children must carry a 'I have Diabetes' card, Medilert or SOS bracelet or chain, and a supply of glucose.

Travel: adjust the insulin injection to local time. If making an early start, bring breakfast forward and give the usual dose.

Psychological adjustment

Family functioning prior to diagnosis is predictive of likely emotional difficulties. Denial of diabetes is common in adolescence.

Enhancing self-image is helpful, e.g. by group activities with other young diabetics, BDA camps and Outward Bound schemes.

Monitoring by regular 3–monthly out-patient visits

Crude measures include:

1. Hypoglycaemic episodes and symptoms prior to meals. Hunger at the appropriate time suggests good control, although children running persistently high blood glucose feel 'hypo' at normal levels.
2. Growth and sexual maturation. Weight loss is a sign of poor control or infection. Relatively tall at diagnosis, final height is slightly reduced (1–3 cm) from the predicted, unless control is very poor. This is the Mauriac syndrome = short, obese, with hepatomegaly.
   Sexual maturation may be delayed proportional to the duration of diabetes. Especially noticeable in girls, they also tend to overweight in adolescence. Irregular menses or even cessation is also a sign of poor control.
3. Surveillance of microangiopathy:

   i Retinal fundoscopy from adolescence.
   ii Blood pressure, proteinuria/microalbuminuria.
   iii Chiropody.

Methods of patient/parent monitoring diabetes

1. Blood glucose.

   i Using BM Glycaeme or Dextrostix, aim to maintain in the 3–10 mmol/l range.
   ii Daily/alternate days, 1–4/day to produce a 'profile', or at times of suspected hypoglycaemias or hyperglycaemias.
   iii Occasionally indicated overnight (0300 hours) to distinguish if prebreakfast hyperglycaemia is due to:

   - waning insulin, i.e. larger evening dose required.
   - secondary to normal growth hormone surge in sleep, the so called 'dawn phenomenon'.
   - Somogyi phenomenon of hypoglycaemia causing rebound hyperglycaemia through counter regulatory hormones.

   iv Good for education and home emergencies.

   Little proof that blood glucose monitoring alone improves control, and it can lead to reduced compliance and falsification of records.

2. Urine

Traditional–Clinitest or test strip 2–4× a day, single voiding, provides a rough guide. Absence of glycosuria = <12.5 mmol/l blood glucose.
   Poor control = <25% no glycosuria, >20% showing 2% glycosuria.
   Ketones should be tested for even when self-monitoring using blood glucose, as ketoacidosis can occur in children without gross hyperglycaemia.
   Recent innovation–Testing for microalbuminuria (a laboratory test at present) is predictive of nephropathy; improved diabetic control reduces the leak.

3. Glycosylated proteins

The incorporation of glucose is proportional to the circulating glucose levels. Fructosamine and haemoglobin are most commonly used. Glycosylated HbA_{1c} reflects control in the last 1 to 3 months. Most paediatric diabetic clinics report average values are 1.5× upper limit of normal. Thus if the normal non diabetic = <8%, poor control is >12%. Glycosylated fructosamine reflects the last 2 weeks, estimation is cheaper than HbA_{1c} and should be used for children with haemoglobinopathies.

Improved control is seen where special diabetic clinics have been established in District General Hospitals as well as specialist centres, by coordinating paediatrician, diabetic liason nurse, dietician, chiropody and dentist. Eye supervision is required after 10 years old.

4. The adolescent clinic

Bridges the gap between paediatric and adult clinics, aiming to reduce the drop out from supervision which is common at this stage.

Prognosis

Retinopathy: onset after 8 years of poor control. Risk increased if HbA_{1C} is in the poor control range.

Life expectancy after diagnosis of type 1: average 29 years but 40% live more than 40 years.

Further reading

Baum J D, Kinmonth A -L (eds) (1985) *Care of the Child with Diabetes*. Edinburgh: Churchill Livingstone

Bonnici F (1989) Clinical management of diabetes mellitus. In *Clinical Paediatric Endocrinology*, C G D Brook (ed). Oxford: Blackwell, pp. 599–617

Home P J, Thow J C, Tunbridge F K E (1989) Insulin treatment: a decade of change. *British Medical Bulletin*, **45**, 92–110

Johnston D I (1989) Management of diabetes mellitus. *Archives of Disease in Childhood*, **64**, 622–-628

Younger D, Brink S J, Barnett D M, *et al.* (1985) Diabetes in youth. In *Joslin's Diabetes Mellitus* 12th edn. Philadelphia: Lea and Febiger, pp. 485–519

Chapter 11

Developmental and neurological problems

NORMAL DEVELOPMENT

Skills are assessed in four areas of development:

- Gross motor activity.
- Fine motor and vision.
- Hearing and speech.
- Social behaviour and play.

1. Development normally advances synchronously between these areas.

   Mental retardation often involves impaired or delayed fine motor and social behaviour, as well as language, while motor milestones may be normal.

   Global retardation = delay in all four areas.

   A single impairment, such as severe visual handicap, can affect the acquisition of all other skills. If this is not allowed for the handicap will appear global, even though intelligence, hearing, speech and motor skills may be potentially normal.

   Out of synchronization examples indicating a potential problem:

   i Isolated slow speech due to hearing impairment or constitutional developmental delay.
   ii Delayed walking from hypotonia or Duchenne muscular dystrophy.

2. Standing normally follows sitting sequentially and is pathological if an infant unable to sit 'wants' to stand on being pulled to sit. Rigid extension of back and legs is due to a neck extension reflex and a sign of cerebral palsy. Well articulated words but 'nonsense' language, suggests autism.

Variations

1. The range of normal within which a milestone is achieved may be wide, e.g. walking 12–21 months in boys, 10–18 months in girls.
2. Familial variation examples:

   i Bottom shuffling – infant does not crawl and lifts legs to 90° when attempts are made to get him to take weight on his legs, and he then walks late, about 22 months.

    ii Familial slow speech is commoner in boys.

3. Prematures' developmental abilities should be up to corrected age allowing for gestation, and is often nearer actual age.
4. Knowledge of normal deviations is an essential part of any developmental assessment, e.g. language development.

Table 11.1 Normal language deviations

	Age (years)
Echolalia and jargoning	less than 2.5
Non-fluency ('clutter', not true stutter)	3 to 3.5
Pitch control (ability to modulate voice)	3
Omission of words ('telegrammatic' speech)	up to 4
Unintelligible due to immature sounds	up to 3.5
Sounds s, th, r are often not articulated even after starting school	

Table 11.2 Developmental abilities and warning signs at ages often used in assessment

6 weeks old

Social	Smiles, coos responsively, elicited, and by history
Hearing and speech	Stills to mother's voice. Startles to sudden noise
Vision	Follows face in 90° arc. Stares intently.
Gross motor	Primitive reflexes present. Head in line with trunk when lifted from prone by examiner's hand under the belly. Lifts head for a few seconds when sat up

Warning signs
Failure to elicit any of the above.
Asymmetry/absence of Moro, abnormal primitive reflexes (see cerebral palsy).
Persistent squint at any age.

6–9 months old

Social	6 months: enjoys bath, playing 'boo' (H). Chews on biscuit (H) 9 months: shows objects to mother, pats mirror image
Hearing and speech	Responds to own name. By 6 months 'ma, da' By 9 months double syllable babble 'mama, dada', and understands 'no' (H)
Fine motor and vision	Change in grasp from palmar (6 months) to index approach, pincer grip (9 months). Transfers at 7 months from hand to mouth. Mouths objects. Foot regard, no longer looks at hands. Fixes on pellet of paper, follows a fallen object
Gross motor	By 6 months bears some weight on legs when standing, and is rolling over. In prone: head up, weight on hands. Supine: flexes head and trunk as pulled to sitting position. From 7 months sits unsupported. At 9 months: crawls and pulls to stand. Saving reflexes: see below

Warning signs
Absent or slow social responses.
Reduced responses and vocalization, absence of babble.
Any squint. Persistent hand regard after 6 months.
Absence/asymmetry of voluntary hand grasp, saving reflexes; persistent primitive reflexes.

Table 11.2   *cont'd*

12 months

Social	Comes when called, lets go on request, finds hidden object. Waves bye-bye, gives toys on request. Holds out arm for sleeve
Hearing and speech	Understands some words, uses mamma, dadda with meaning
	Shakes head for 'no'
Fine motor and vision	Casts (throws) objects, watches them fall
	Picks up crumbs from carpet (H)
	Pincer grasp, bangs 2 bricks together
Gross motor	Bottom shuffling common, may walk like a bear. Cruises round holding onto furniture, walks one hand held.
	Pivots when sitting, reaches behind (backward saving reflexes)

Warning signs
No frequent tuneful babble by 10 months.
Holds objects close up to the eyes.
Immature grasp, asymmetry of grasp, and of saving reflexes.
No sitting or weight bearing.

18 months

Social	Cup: lifts, drinks, puts down. Spoon-feeds self (H). Pulls at dirty nappy.
	Domestic mimicry of dusting, sweeping etc (H)
Hearing and speech	Points to 3 parts of the body on request, obeys single commands. Says 6 words, jargons, echoes speech
Fine motor and vision	Neat pincer picking up threads, pins. Scribbles using fisted grasp. Turns pages 2 or more at a time
	Builds tower of 3–4 × 1" (2.5 cm) cubes
Gross motor	Walks well, carries toys, climbs stairs (H), climbs into chair (H)

Warning signs
Drools, no words. Fails to understand commands.
Absent pincer grasp, persistent casting.
Not walking: consider blood creatinine phosphokinase in boys.

2 to 2½ years

Social	Plays alone, tantrums, demanding. Dry by day. Puts on shoes, socks and pants (H). Turns doorhandles. Uses spoon and fork (H)
Hearing and speech	Phrases of 2–3 words, gives name. 'Naming' games. 50 words+
	Has inner language, e.g. demonstrates 'give dolly a drink' on request
Fine motor and vision	Turns one page at a time, imitates a straight line in both vertical and horizontal, and a circle. Unscrews lids
	Build a tower of 6–8 × 1" cubes
Gross motor	Runs, kicks ball, jumps on the spot. Pushes trike with feet (H)
	Walks downstairs 2 feet per tread

Warning signs
Lack of understanding of speech, no phrases by 30 months.
Unsteady on his feet.

Table 11.2 *cont'd*

3 to 3½ years

Social	Uses toilet unassisted except wiping bottom (H). Dress and undress with minimum assistance. Knows some nursery rhymes (H). Handles knife and fork (H) Plays with peers.
Hearing and speech	Gives full name, sex. Counts to 10 by rote. Uses plurals. Understands prepositions (on, under, behind etc) Asks who? where? (H). 3–5 word sentences (H)
Fine motor and vision	Mature pen grasp, copies + and 0. Correctly matches two or more colours. Threads large beads. Tower of 9 × 1" (2.5 cm) cubes
Gross motor	Stands on one leg for a few seconds. Peddles trike (H) Stairs - adult style of ascent (H). Jumps off bottom step

Warning signs
No phrases.
Persistent daytime wetting/soiling.
Clumsy (motor coordination and/or vision disorder).

4–5 years

Social	Wipes own bottom (H). Eats using a knife and fork (H) Dresses unsupervised except for tie, laces. Imaginative play Plays in groups, takes turns, shares toys, obeys rules (H)
Hearing and speech	Gives name, address, age. Counts up to 10 by 4 years, 20 by 5 years. Knows three coins. Grammatical speech. Transient 'stammer' from urgency to speak is common. Asks meaning of abstract words
Fine motor and vision	Matches 4 colours, copies cross, square, and, by 5 years, a triangle. Imitates a bridge with 3 bricks, builds 3 steps with 6 cubes at 4 years, 4 steps with 10 cubes at 5 years. Draws a recognizable man
Gross motor	4 years: climbs trees, and ladders, enjoys ball games (H) By 5 years: hops, may skip, jumps off 3 steps. Catches a ball

Warning signs
Socially isolated, bullied.
Unintelligible or ungrammatical speech.
Unable to give name or address (parents may not have told address).

H = by history, otherwise by observation or eliciting the activity.

Further reading

Sheridan M D (1978) *Children's Developmental Progress*. NFER
Lingam S, Harvey D R (1988) *Manual of Child Development*. Edinburgh:Churchill Livingstone

Disorders of development and special needs

Definitions of terms commonly used in developmental assessment

Impairment An abnormality of body function or structure.
Disability Reduced ability to perform a task or function.
Handicap A continuing impairment or disability of body, intellect or personality likely to interfere with normal growth, development, the capacity to learn, and the achievement of normally realistic goals.

Examples of some developmental impairments

1. Permanent and serious: mental handicap, specific speech and language disorders, cerebral palsy, muscular dystrophy, autism.
2. Developmental delay: skills improve with maturation. Examples:

   - Mild global backwardness.
   - Delayed speech and language.
   - Clumsiness.
   - Specific learning disabilities, e.g. reading, writing, spelling, (defined as a difficulty not due to poor teaching, dullness, physical or sensory defect).

Incidence of some handicapping conditions

Mental retardation 30/1000.
Severe learning difficulties 4/1000.
Cerebral palsy 2/1000.
Autism 3/10000.
Severe deafness 2/1000.
Blind/partially sighted 1/1000.

Causes of delayed development

1. Deprivation: determine by history and observation.
2. Idiopathic: constitutional, familial. Affects one field only, e.g. speech, walking, with catch-up later.
3. Mental handicap: many areas, often global delay.
4. Specific abnormality: blind, deaf, cerebral palsy, muscular dystrophy.
   See special needs and mental handicap for assessment and management.

   Always be aware of dangers of arrested/deteriorating development.
Common causes include:

1. Abuse/emotional deprivation.
2. Intercurrent acute or chronic illness.
3. Uncontrolled seizures, the effect of drugs in their management.

Unusual causes:

1. Hydrocephalus: structural, post-infective or post-traumatic.
2. Hypothyroidism, lead poisoning.
3. Degenerations affecting the brain.

Causes of speech and language delay

1. Deprivation: determination by social history/observation.
2. Developmental delay often with a family history: frustration often manifested by the child.
3. Deafness: all other functions normal.

4. Global delay signifies mental handicap.
5. Autism: abnormal behaviour and relationships.

Further reading

Hall D M B (1989) Assessment of the Slow Preschool Child. *Archives of Disease in Childhood*, **64**, 295–300

Benefits of early detection

1. Minimize disability, examples: in deafness early introduction of amplification may improve the prognosis for speech; surgical removal of a cataract before 6 months preserves sight.
2. Reduces secondary disabilities, e.g. behaviour disorder secondary to slow speech, by advising the parents on appropriate management, reduces frustration from communication difficulties.
3. Genetic investigation and counselling may prevent the birth of a similarly affected infant.

DEVELOPMENTAL ASSESSMENT

Most serious defects are suspected or detected by parents, nursery staff or teachers.

Taking a history reveals the reason for presentation, whether due to parental concerns (important and should not be dismissed) or professional (parents may deny any problem).

1. Further details of the problem or illness. At what age did the parents became concerned. Is the condition progressive, static or improving? Continuous or intermittent?
2. The pregnancy: bleeding, infections, drugs, and their timing in gestation; toxaemia and the length of gestation, birthweight, difficulties in labour and delivery; was resuscitation required?
3. Concerns in the first weeks often requiring admission to the special care nursery, e.g. hypoglycaemia, jaundice, apnoea, feeding difficulties, needing to be woken for feeds.
4. Previous illness, and the response to it. Medication likely to alter development, concentration; exposure to environmental hazards.
5. Developmental history. Parental recall for past achievements is poor except for smiling, walking, and talking, especially if slow. Enquire what he does now. Be precise with the aid of a table of normal milestones.
6. School: days lost through illness or refusal; changes of school. School performance may require discussion with the teacher as well as parents.
7. A family history may reveal abnormal or unusual patterns of development. Neurological and non-neurological conditions in relatives, and consanguinity, to be noted.
8. Social and emotional problems may have great bearing.

Observation in the following order facilitates evaluation

Preschool child

1. Play, spontaneous speech.
2. Posture, walking, fine motor coordination with toys (also tests vision).
3. Performance: offer in turn, showing what the task is, bricks, crayons, colour matching according to the level of ability. Observe understanding, concentration, visual acuity.
4. Comprehension of language: to point to parts of the body, to objects in books on request, to pick up named objects, and carry out commands appropriate to age.

At school age add

Reading, arithmetic functions (+, −, ×, /,), writing name, age, address, short story, or drawing a picture of a favourite activity. These activities also demonstrate his application, concentration, and organizational skills.

Allow for strange environment, immaturity, possible language barrier, and the effects of disability, e.g. deafness.

Sensory testing, neurological and physical examination follow, and, if appropriate, investigation (see mental handicap).

Sensory screening: what to know

Vision

Visual acuity: 1 month = 1/15th adult, 8 months = 1/4 adult (6/24), 3–5 years = adult (6/6).

Incidence of visual problems

Registered blind 1/2500 children. At school entry 6/1000 have a severe defect, and 27/1000 moderate defects (mainly squints).

Colour blindness: 6% of boys have green defect (deuteranomaly).

At risk

1. Retinopathy of prematurity in the low birthweight <1500 g.
2. Familial squint and myopia, choroidoretinal degenerations, cataracts.
3. Associations, e.g. with mental handicap, cerebral palsy, Down's syndrome, CHARGE association.
4. Metabolic disorders: galactosaemia, Lowe's syndrome.

Delayed visual maturation

Uncommon, sporadic, noted by parents as a failure of visual fixation within the first 4 weeks. May take some months to develop, but normal thereafter. Absence of abnormality on history, examination, or electroretinogram, allows an expectant approach.

Sensitive periods within which action must be taken for function to be preserved:

1. Visual cortex appreciation: remove cataract by 6 months old.
2. Binocular vision is normally established by 6 months: 'patch' occlusion of a squint or amblyopia up to 5–8 years old helps, though some argue that after 3 years of age it is already too late.

Testing for common defects

Acuity
1. Infants: a newborn should fix on mother's face or a 10 cm red ball at 20–30 cm, and by 10 weeks old follow through a 180° arc. At a year, 1 mm sugar balls (hundreds and thousands) are followed or grasped, but now discredited as an exact test. The objective test is forced choice preferential looking, at variable sized black and white gratings.
2. From 3 years: the Snellen chart is the standard. Test at 6 metres, or 3 metres using a mirror. Single letter card matching tests (5 or 7 letter Stycar) are less accurate.

   Abnormal result: 6/12 or worse, or a difference between the eyes of two lines or more.

   Registration: Blind = <3/60 in the better eye, partially sighted = 4/60 to 6/24 in the better eye.

Squint
Non-paralytic squints are often inherited, and refractive or astigmatic.
   Paralytic: nuclear agenesis, tumour or pressure.

1. Manifest squint: use the corneal reflection test, examine eye movements by moving an interesting small object (not a light) horizontally, obliquely and vertically. A paralytic squint is likely if either eye fails to complete a movement in a particular direction. The corneal reflection remains stable throughout in pseudosquint due to a wide bridge to the nose, or epicanthic folds.
2. Latent squint is detected by the cover-uncover test, occluding each eye in turn. Not an essential test. Hold a small toy at 30 cm from the eyes, then cover one eye with a card or the parent's hand. Repeat at 6 metres with a picture as the visual target. A light is unsuitable as it cannot be focused on.

Manifest squint	= a squinting eye that moves to fix on an object when the other is covered.
Alternating	= each eye will move in turn when covered.
Latent	= the eye squints if covered, and swings back to its original position when uncovered.

A useful test of vision is the response to covering the good eye!

Refractive errors   Myopia can be progressive during childhood, so regular testing is necessary especially in affected families.

Amblyopia   The suppression or failure to develop a clear visual image by the brain due to refractive error, a difference in refraction between the eyes, squint, or cataract. Still rarely identified before 3 years old by which time acuity is usually already permanently diminished.

Management

1. Multiprofessional assessment: cause, severity and remedial action, e.g. glasses, soft contact lenses, surgery.
2. Parents receive counselling, genetic advice.
   For the more visually disabled, further management considerations:
1. The severely visually impaired have less opportunity to practise and develop gross motor, fine motor and social skills, and with poor sound localization, show speech delay. To avoid mislabelling, the Reynell Zinkin developmental scales for young visually handicapped children should be used. On average, an otherwise normal but effectively blind child performs at half their chronological age.
2. The parents need to teach their infant the location of parts of their own bodies, and where a sound comes from in space.
3. The child has to be shown how they can explore and manipulate objects and toys for themselves, instead of having them thrust into their hands, which leads to fear and fisting.
4. Discourage self-stimulating behaviours such as eye poking, rocking.
5. Promote visual attention if noted to fixate on light reflections in a mirror. Use visual lures, e.g. Christmas tree decoration 6 cm shiny ball, pentorch inside a translucent finger puppet.
6. Home visits by the advisor from Royal National Institute for the Blind. A local peripatetic teacher liaises with the schools/special schooling. Sunshine Homes are residential schools which accept blind children, who require Braille, from 3 years old.
7. Learning ability assessment: size of type needed, lighting, low vision aids, need for proximity to blackboard, or use of a whiteboard with black marker pen for enhanced visual contrast.
8. Mobility assessment, and ability safely to cross the road.

Hearing

Normal speech development requires adequate hearing. A loss of more than 30 dB for any length of time in early childhood may delay or prevent this aquisition, depending on severity.

Incidence

1/1000 children are profoundly deaf (usually sensorineural or mixed) requiring special educational provision, 2/1000 are moderately deaf needing hearing aids only.

40/1000 school age children are mildly affected, usually conductive from secretory otitis media, and benefit from being close to the teacher in class.

At risk

1. Parental observations and concerns. Delayed language development. Behavioural and educational difficulties.
2. Family history of deafness (50% of congenital cases are genetic).
3. Child is low birthweight, has cerebal palsy, or a malformation, e.g. cleft palate.
4. History of recurrent otitis, or of meningitis/encephalitis.

Causes of deafness

Middle ear disease (common); exclude wax and foreign body first!

1. Secretory otitis media: post-otitis media, allergy, air pollution.
2. Barotrauma: blow to the ear, pressure changes in aircraft.
3. Facial malformations, e.g. cleft palate, absent/defective ossicular chain, e.g. Treacher-Collins syndrome.
4. Down's syndrome, Turner's syndrome.

Sensori-neural deafness (uncommon or rare)

1. Genetic (60%): isolated AR or AD or as part of a syndrome, e.g. Waardenburg.
2. Perinatal difficulties (10%), especially in the low birthweight and premature (asphyxia, hyperbilirubinaemia, congenital infection).
3. Infection:

   i Congenital (10%), e.g. rubella, cytomegalovirus, toxoplasmosis.
   ii Acquired (10%), e.g. measles, mumps, meningitis, encephalitis.

4. Trauma: injury to the base of the skull.
5. Toxins: ototoxic levels of aminoglycosides.

Behavioural clues: failure to quiet to mother's voice, babble ceases (in some profoundly deaf it may continue for months) or becomes monotonous. Behaviour problems, poor speech development or school progress in the older child.

Hearing tests

1. Infancy to 3 years
For screening purposes the minimum level should be 30–40 dB. A sound level meter, to monitor the voice level, is desirable.

From 6–9 months: the distraction test.
Sounds presented at 45° behind the ear:

High frequency: Manchester rattle, 'ss' sound, cup and spoon around its rim.
Low frequency: 'ooo' or 'hum'.

From 2½ years: auditory discrimination of consonant sounds.

 i McCormick toy discrimination test, consists not of phonetically balanced sounds but similar sounds: 14 toys in seven pairs, e.g. plane/plate, duck/cup, tree/key, cow/house, fork/horse, spoon/shoe, lamb/man. Each toy is named, the child is then invited to identify by pointing or looking at a named toy while the examiner's mouth is covered to prevent lip reading.
 ii Performance test: Kendal 'go' game at different sound intensities, puts men in boat on command 'go' or 'sss'.

2. From 5 years: pure tone audiometry 'sweep' at 20 dB, at 500 Hz, 1, 2, and 4 kHz.

Grades of hearing loss

Mild 25–35 dB, moderate 40–60 dB, severe >60 dB, profound >90 dB.

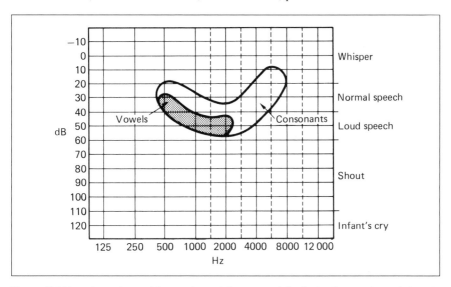

Figure 11.1 Normal speech sound frequencies, and the pattern of distribution in normal speech (note the banana shape)

Management

1. Assess severity, cause, language development and educational abilities, and any associated behaviour difficulties.
2. In secretory otitis media the use of antibiotics and decongestants are of doubtful value. If loss is persistent consider grommets, +/-adenoidectomy.
3. Counsel parents on behaviour, safety hazards in traffic, genetics.
4. *Even the profoundly deaf have some hearing*, mandating the provision of oral training and hearing aids appropriate to the deficit. Makaton and finger signing are adjuncts, or the main method of communication.
5. Inform the local peripatetic teacher of the deaf, in moderate or severe loss, and the local education authority about schooling needs.

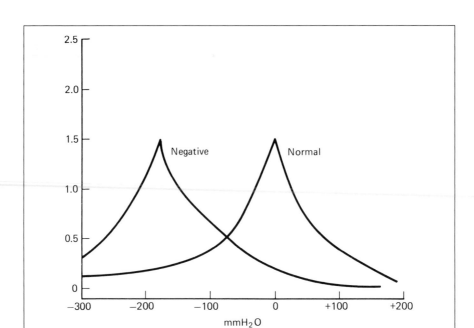

Figure 11.2 Tympanogram, showing one normal ear and one retracted, mobile ear drum showing negative pressures but no fluid in the ear. Hearing is therefore not significantly affected.

Further reading

Feilder A R (1989) The management of squint. *Archives of Disease in Childhood*, **64**, 413–418
McCormick B (1986) Hearing screening for the very young. *Recent Advances in Paediatrics*. R Meadow (ed) Edinburgh:Churchill Livingstone, pp 185–199
Tweedie J (1987) *Children's Hearing Problems: Their Significance, Detection and Management*. Bristol:Wright

Mental Handicap

Definition

Reduced intellectual function with greater dependence on others for personal and social needs than expected for age.

Incidence

Educationally subnormal, moderate (ESN(M)) = IQ 50–69
= 20/1000 children.
Educationally subnormal, severe (ESN(S)) = IQ <50
= 4/1000 children.

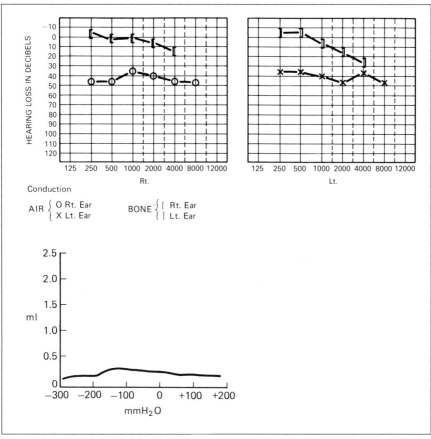

Figure 11.3 Audiogram. The commonest abnormality, showing a conductive hearing loss in both ears, confirmed by normal bone conduction. The tympanogram has no peak, indicating fluid is present in the middle ear.

Causes of mental handicap

1. In children found to be ESN(M)

    i   Normal variation: at the lower end of the normal bell shaped distribution.

    ii   Familial, social and polygenic factors. Children of manual workers × 9 non-manual.

    iii   Fragile X in 20% of males.

    iv   Trauma, cerebral palsy, meningitis, brain malformation in 5%.
        About 90% have no specific 'pathological' condition.

2. ESN(S): 75% are likely to have a recognizable pathology and 75% are prenatal (i–iii):

    i   Down's syndrome 30%, fragile X, other chromosome anomalies 20%.

    ii   Genetic: <5%
        a. Individually rare: e.g. inborn errors of metabolism (only 1% of the total).

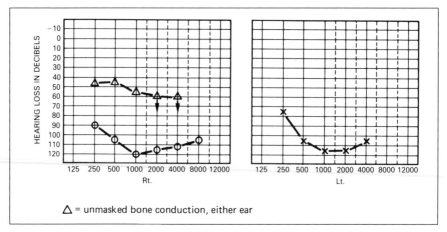

Figure 11.4 Audiogram. Severe bilateral sensorineural hearing loss. Note that bone conduction thresholds measure down to a maximum of 60 dB. A *false* air-bone gap appears in severe loss.

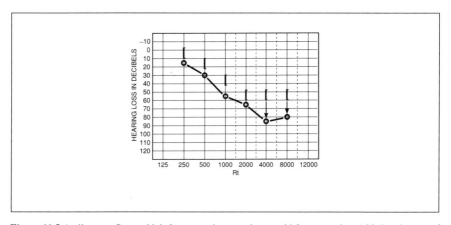

Figure 11.5 Audiogram. Severe high frequency loss, moderate mid frequency loss 'ski slope' curve of birth asphyxia or hyperbilirubinaemia.

   b. Syndromes: usually sporadic but occasionally familial, e.g. hydrocephalus, craniostenosis.
   c. Recognizable genetic syndromes: e.g. Noonan's, dystrophia myotonica, tuberous sclerosis.
iii Prenatal: 20%, congenital infection, alcohol, drugs, intrauterine growth retardation, structural brain abnormalities, e.g. absent corpus callosum, porencephaly.
iv Perinatal: 10%, premature delivery, hypoxia, brain damage, intraventricular haemorrhage, hypoglycaemia, jaundice
 v Postnatal: 10%, CNS infection, trauma including non-accidental injury, status epilepticus, hydrocephalus, craniostenosis, metabolic, e.g. hypernatraemia, hypothyroidism, hypoglycaemia, lead poisoning.

Many ESN(S) children also have epilepsy and/or cerebral palsy, and sensory handicaps.

Aids to diagnosis

Timing of presentation

1. At birth due to antecedent history (ii–iii) or findings (i).
2. Parental suspicions (see Developmental screening).
3. Detected at follow-up of (iv), (v).

Pointers to mental handicap from the history

1. Abnormal behaviour: excessively 'good', has to be woken for feeds, unresponsive, suspected of deafness.
2. Abnormal motor patterns: floppy/stiff, preservation of primitive reflexes, later hyperactivity and repetitive stereotyped behaviour, e.g. turning on taps, rocking, running in circles.
3. Failure to thrive, feeding difficulties.
4. Delayed milestones of development.

Presence of a good 'handle' (see Genetics)

- Facial, e.g. Down's facies, William's, Prader-Willi, de Lange.
- Limbs, e.g. broad thumbs and toes in Rubinstein-Taybi syndrome.
- Association of abnormalities, e.g. CHARGE.
- Microcephaly and short stature, e.g. Seckel's bird headed dwarf.

Pitfalls (differential diagnosis)

1. Normal variation, familial patterns of development.
2. Lack of stimulation: inexperience, ignorance, deprivation, parental depression, abuse.
3. Sensory disorder: deaf, partially sighted.
4. Medical disease: malabsorption, acute illness.
5. Autism.
6. Degenerative disease, i.e. initially normal development.

Investigation

1. For genetic disease: Wood's light for skin manifestations of tuberous sclerosis (TS), blood for calcium, amino acids, thyroid function, urine for organic acids, mucopolysaccharides if indicated, serology for TORCH, urine for cytomegalovirus.
2. Chromosomes for suggestive stigmata, and fragile X examination in physically normal ESN(M) boys, especially with a family history, or if the mother is intellectually 'slow'.

3. Skull X-ray for calcification due to TS and congenital infection. CT scan for suspected TS or structural abnormality, e.g. with cerebral palsy, seizures.
4. EEG only if seizures are present.

Management

1. Counselling and support of parents and siblings from the District Handicap Team (see Services for the handicapped).
   Aims are:

   - To help come to terms with handicap.
   - Enlist active participation in therapy.
   - Anticipatory guidance to prevent or minimize difficult behaviour. Identification of a syndrome, e.g. de Lange's, Prader-Willi, Williams' enables more accurate prediction of associated problems, levels of functioning, and prognosis. This 'labelling' may be welcomed by some parents by removing uncertainty.

2. Assessment, needs, therapeutic programmes for stimulation (e.g. Portage scheme), speech, physiotherapy, self-help skills (see CP).
3. Notify Education Authority for instigation of a Statement of Special Needs, seeking parental permission first.
4. Behaviour modification for behaviour difficulties, e.g. head banging, self-mutilation, masturbation in public.
5. Medication: for seizures; in uncontrollable hyperactivity try chlorpromazine, haloperidol (beware of its extrapyramidal side effects requiring an anticholinergic), and the paradoxical action of amphetamines.

Prognosis

1. Life expectancy is reduced for ESN(S), especially in early childhood, due to respiratory infection, seizures, and associated congenital anomalies, e.g. cyanotic congenital heart disease in Down's syndrome.
2. Psychological problems in 50% of ESN(S); 30% of ESN(M) also have behavioural and emotional difficulties.
3. Majority of ESN(M) can be independent, in sheltered workshops, 'niche' employment (gardeners, labourers) in better economic times. Otherwise likely to attend a Local Authority occupation centre, often living in sheltered accomodation. ESN(S) require constant supervision, with the family, or in a residential home or hostel sooner or later.

Prevention

1. Antenatal diagnosis: for mothers >35 years old (Down's), a family history of untreatable, but detectable in utero, inborn error, or heritable brain malformation likely to show on US.
2. Education: dangers of alcohol abuse; avoid delaying child-bearing too long.
3. Effective universal immunization against rubella.

Further reading

Blasco P A (1991) Pitfalls in developmental diagnosis. *Pediatric Clinics of North America*, **38**, 1425–1438
Illingworth R S (1987) Pitfalls in developmental diagnosis. *Archives of Disease in Childhood*, **62**, 860–865

Services for the handicapped child in the UK

These involve health, education, and social services. Coordination is through joint working groups and a statement of each individual's needs.

Health services are coordinated by the NHS District handicap team—a multidisciplinary group of professionals led by the community or hospital based paediatrician, often based at an assessment centre.

The district handicap team's (DHT) role is to investigate and assess children referred with physical and neurological disabilities.

- The information acquired is pooled at a case discussion.
- Diagnosis, treatment plan, advice and support for the family are planned and a written record made.
- The findings and plans are discussed with the parents, and they may be given a written report too.
- The DHT arranges and coordinates treatment, is a resource centre for information, aids, training, support and advice.

Education

The 1981 Education Act sees any child with a learning disorder as one with greater educational difficulties than the majority of children of their age, or to have a disability which prevents or hinders them from making use of the educational facilities generally provided for children of their age.

Size of the problem

Twenty per cent of school children have a special educational need at some stage in their school careers.

Six per cent of all children under 15 years have a chronic physical disability, and 10–15% have psychological disturbances, affecting school performance.

Learning difficulties increase × 3 (from 5/1000 at 7 years to 16/1000 by 16 years), and maladjustment × 8 (from 0.6/1000 to 5/1000 over the same period).

Chronic disability includes asthma, diabetes, bleeding and behaviour disorders, as well as mental handicap, cerebral palsy, spina bifida, and sensory disorders.

Educational need, not category of handicap, determines placement in an ordinary school, a remedial unit in an ordinary school, or special or residential school.

The Warnock report recommended integration into ordinary schools, with special provision, so long as the parents agree and the placement is not detrimental to the other children in the school. The ability to provide from within available resources is the limiting factor, e.g. classroom amplification equipment, remedial help for specific learning difficulties.

A 'Statement of Special Educational Needs' empowers and obliges the local education authority to assess all children notified to them who may have special needs. From the age of 2 years, and younger if the parents request, a multidisciplinary assessment is done. The parents' views must be sought throughout, and a copy of the report given them. If they object to the recommendations they may appeal, ultimately to the Secretary of State for Education. Annual reviews continue to 13 years old when plans must be made for future education or employment.

Social services

Provide: social work support, placement in day care, or residential care; arrange respite care for the family to have time off from caring.

Advise on entitlements for handicapped people in UK :

i   Attendance allowance from 6 months old, if in need of frequent attention to body functions or continual supervision to avoid danger to themselves or others by day and/or by night.
ii Invalid care allowance for the carer who has to stay at home.
iii Mobility allowance. Aged over 5 years and unable/virtually unable to walk.
iv Severe disablement allowance if >16 years and unable to work.

The Joseph Rowntree Family Fund disburses money for specific items of related need, e.g. washing machine, tumble drier.

Further reading

Blackman J A (ed) (1991) Development and behavior: the very young child. *Pediatric Clinics of North America*, **38**.

Chamberlain M A (1987) The physically handicapped school leaver. *Archives of Diseases in Childhood*, **62**, 3–5

Colver A F, Robinson A (1989) Establishing a register for children with special needs. *Archives of Disease in Childhood*, **64**, 1200–1203

NEUROLOGICAL PROBLEMS

Neurological examination

As with developmental assessment, observation of spontaneous activity will demonstrate most aspects of function, and potential disabilities will become evident.

Age, allowing for gestation, determines our expectations of ability to assume body postures, control movements, and perform tasks.

Posture in infants

Observe, place in supine, pull to sit, stand, suspend and then return baby to the couch in prone.

1. Supine: with the head in the midline, look for asymmetry of movement (hemiplegia), difficulty in raising limbs against gravity (floppy). Tendency to stiff

extension occurs in dystonia and spasticity, and the child may exhibit spontaneous upgoing toes.

2. Pull to sit: response is graded against that expected for age. Is head lag excessive? and lack of flexion at elbow? (see floppy baby); are saving reflexes and sitting balance present? (see reflexes).
3. Stand: ability to take weight is usually present from birth to 3 months, and 'bouncing' on the feet at 4–6 months. Failure to do so suggests developmental motor retardation, hypotonia, hypotonic CP; alternatively, is there rigid extension suggestive of early CP?
4. Horizontal suspension. Normal: arching of back and head above the horizontal from 4 months. If head and limbs hang down, consider hypotonia, or hydrocephalus.
5. Vertical suspension: limbs normally are flexed up to 6 months old. Look for 'scissoring' of the legs in spastic/dystonic CP, or the flexed hips and extended knees of the bottom shuffler.
6. Prone: arched back, extended neck may be excessive in hydrocephalus. Assess ability to take weight on the forearms or hands and the position of the hips, progressing from fully flexed (term infant) to fully extended and rocking on the abdomen by 6–7 months.

Already mobile

1. Crawling: reciprocal pattern, present by 9–12 months? or any asymmetry due to palsy, dislocated hip?
2. Look at, and listen to, the walking pattern (assessment of gait: Orthopaedics).
   - i Limp: hemiplegia, joint disease, length asymmetry.
   - ii Stumbling, broad based: ataxia, ataxic or dyskinetic cerebral palsy.
   - iii Up on tip-toe: spastic cerebral palsy [CP], contracture of heel cord in muscular dystrophy; talipes; behavioural.
   - iv Waddling or lurching gait: dislocation of hip(s), muscular dystrophy, polymyositis, old polio, peripheral neuropathy.
   - v Steppage gait = foot drop: damage to sciatic nerve, peroneal muscular atrophy, lead, thallium poisoning.
   - vi Pes cavus: Friedreich's ataxia, spinal cord injury, spina bifida, diastematomyelia, spinal tumours.

Upper limb function

Observation for:

1. Posture: especially asymmetry, e.g. hemiplegic posture, 'waiter's tip' position of Erb's.
2. Accessory movements
   - i Chorea is rapid involuntary, non-stereotyped movements of face and extremities, present at rest, worse with stress and effort. Demonstrate 'dinner fork' hands on extending the arms in front, pronation of arms and hands when extended above the head. Causes include anticonvulsants, benign familial chorea, post streptococcal chorea, Wilson's disease, Huntington's chorea.

    ii Tremor at rest: Fine = hyperthyroidism, familial or constitutional.

   iii Action tremor (picking up toys, finger-nose-finger test) in physiological tremor and cerebellar lesions.

    iv Athetoid slow involuntary writhing movements of the proximal limbs in cerebral palsy.

    v Habit tic, e.g. allergic salute of rubbing nose with back of hand.

3 Weakness and floppiness: level may be central, spinal, peripheral nerve, neuromuscular junction or muscular (see floppy infant).

4 Grasp and manipulative skills (Figures 11.6 and 11.7). Influenced by maturation, motor strength and coordination, and visual defects. Observe play with a toy, threading beads, pencil grasp and control.

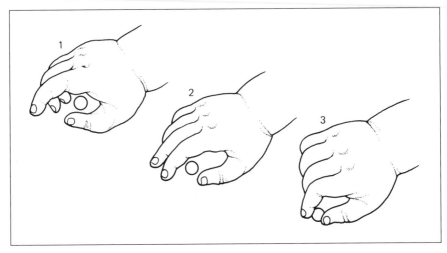

Figure 11.6 Normal development of grasp
    1. Raking movement at 6 months
    2. Scissor movement between thumb and middle phalanx of index finger
    3. Pincer grasp

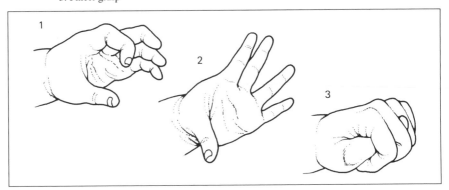

Figure 11.7 Abnormal hand postures when attempting to grasp
    1. Spastic
    2. Athetoid
    3. Mana obscena, unable to remove thumb from between middle and ring fingers

Cranial nerves examination

I Smell

By history

II

a. Acuity: see Development
b. Visual fields:

> *Distraction*: hold attention to the front with a toy, introducing a second object from the periphery of vision with the other hand, or by an assistant, into each quadrant in turn. Child should turn to fix on it.
> *Confrontation*, in older children, examiner half a metre away, his arms abducted fully. Child instructed to look at examiner's nose and point at the finger wiggled. Repeat, with the contralateral eye of child and examiner covered with their respective hand. The examiner's free hand is used to wiggle a finger, and the child confirms seeing the signal by saying 'yes'. All four quadrants are tested.
>   This method only detects gross defects, e.g. homonomous hemianopia in association with a hemiplegia.

II, IV, VI: Eye movements

  i Observe for ptosis (hydrocephalus, tumour, migraine, myasthenia gravis) and pupil size asymmetry in Horner's syndrome (birth trauma).
 ii Nystagmus:
    Ocular=   pendular or roving: poor macular vision due to gross visual disturbance, e.g. cataracts, retrolental fibroplasia, albinism, severe astigmatism, optic nerve compression/glioma.
    Vestibular= vertical and horizontal varies with head position, e.g. mumps labrynthitis, otitis media. Worse looking away from lesion.
    Cerebellar= Increased looking laterally, eyes drift back, e.g. encephalitis, phenytoin, hydrocephalus, tumour.
    Brainstem= vertical nystagmus or affecting only one eye or only when head held in a certain position. Tumour, demyelinating disease, or cerebellar malformation likely. Drugs, alcohol and cerebellar abnormality cause nystagmus on looking down ('downbeat').
    Congenital= conjugate, purely horizontal, whichever way the child looks. Normal/near normal vision, neurology otherwise normal. Improves with age.
 iii Conjugate deviation of the eyes:
    downwards: hydrocephalus, kernicterus.
    sideways : towards the lesion if acute, e.g. seizure, abscess, bleed.
             : away if established, e.g. hemiplegia.
  iv Lateral deviation, ptosis, dilated pupil = III cranial nerve lesion.
   v Medial deviation = VI cranial nerve.
    False localizing sign of raised intracranial pressure.

Involvement also of VII = brainstem lesion/tumour.
 vi Head tilt, if corrected may reveal vertical squint.
     Head tilt is also a sign of posterior fossa tumour.
 vii Corneal reflection: see Vision testing.

V

Corneal reflex with a wisp of cotton wool or by gently blowing at the eyes.

VII

Asymmetry on crying, laughing, baring teeth.

 i   Acquired lower motor lesions: otitis media, mastoiditis, Bell's palsy, trauma, hypertension, tumour.
 ii Congenital nuclear agenesis in Moebius' syndrome, includes the VI nerve, bilaterally.
 iii Absence of muscle at one corner of the mouth is associated with congenital heart defects.
 iv Symmetrical weakness in myopathies is elicited by asking the child to puff out his cheeks, and bury his eyelids.

VIII

See Hearing tests.

IX, X

Nasal speech, weak 'g','k'; testing for the gag reflex is left to last.

XII

Tongue deviates to the affected side.
   Bulbar nerves: affected by cerebral palsy; infections, e.g. encephalitis, polio, TB; toxins: tetanus, diphtheria, botulinum; parainfection: Guillain-Barre; phenothiazines; brainstem tumour; myasthenia gravis.

Deep Tendon Jerks

1. Normally brisker in the neonate. To elicit hyper-reflexia at the knee start tapping the shin from the ankle up. Hyper-reflexia may also show as a crossed adductor response (contralateral hip adducts as a knee jerk is elicited).
2. Increased in decerebration, cerebral palsy, hysteria, degenerations of the CNS, isolated cord segment.
3. Decreased by drugs, in mental retardation, Down's syndrome, cerebellar disorders, lesions from spinal cord to muscle.

Table 11.3 Time of expected appearance and disappearance of reflexes and their diagnostic implications

Moro	From birth, for 4–5 months. Persists in dystonic phase of cerebral palsy (CP)
Stepping	From birth for 8 weeks. Persists in CP, with 'scissoring' of the lower limbs, as the feet touch the floor when the body is held vertical
Positive support	First 3 months. Excessive and persistent, rising onto the toes, in CP
Asymmetric tonic neck	From week 1 for 6 months. Never obligatory unless CP or raised intracranial pressure
Palmar grasp	From birth for 3 months. Persists in CP/returns in brain injury
Plantar grasp	From birth until ready to walk, about 12 - 18 months

Saving/parachute responses are necessary for balance*:

Downward parachute	With examiner's hands under armpits, allowing the body to fall vertically makes the legs extend. Appears from 4–6 months
Forward parachute	Face down, holding the trunk at 45^0 to the horizontal. Swinging down towards the couch causes the arms to extend. From 4–6 months
Lateral saving	Swing trunk from side to side causes the ipsilateral arm to extend laterally. Elicited from 6 months
Backward saving	Gently allow the infant to fall backwards from the sitting position. The arms extend to the side and back, from 10 months

* Presence of lateral saving but apparent inability to sit is indicative of lack of opportunity or stimulation.

Cutaneous reflexes

1. Plantar reflex (S1) is flexor in the first week, becoming extensor until walking at 12–18 months. Stroke the outer border of the foot to avoid eliciting the plantar grasp response.
2. Abdominal (T7–12) and cremasteric reflexes (L1) elicited from 4 months.

Skin

Look for axillary freckling and café–au–lait patches (>5 × 1 cm diameter) of neurofibromatosis, the ash leaf lesions and shagreen patches of tuberous sclerosis.

Head circumference

See large heads and microcephaly.

Retinal Fundoscopy

Patience! Best done sitting baby/toddler up or propped looking over mother's shoulder. May require sedation. Dilate if in doubt. Discs are normally pale compared with adults.

Cerebral Palsy (CP)

Definition

A non-progressive disorder of the developing brain affecting movement and posture. It is a group of conditions with various causes and neurological dysfunctions.

Aetiology and incidence

1. Antenatal (60%): most CP is due to an early prenatal abnormality. 'Difficult birth is merely a symptom of deeper effects that influenced the development of the fetus' (Freud, 1897).
2. Low birthweight (10%): <1.5 kg at birth have a tenfold risk. Incidence increasing with increased survival of these infants; 70% of diplegia, hemiplegia and quadriplegia related to complications of pregnancy and prematurity.
3. Familial and genetic (10%), e.g. Joubert's syndrome (AR abnormal eye movements, hyperventilation in infancy, mental handicap, ataxic cerebral palsy later. Cerebellar vermis aplasia.)
4. Post-neonatal (10%): infection, trauma, hypoxia often in already vulnerable children.
5. Birth asphyxia. Only 10%. Relatively few asphyxiated newborns develop CP. This accounts for the unchanging incidence of CP of 2/1000 live births.
6. Grading of severity: mild 30%, moderate and severe 70%.

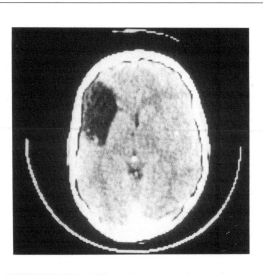

Figure 11.8 A congenital right hemiplegia with large left frontoparietal porencephalic cyst.

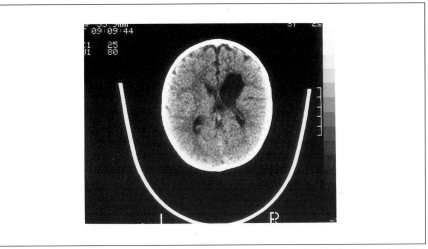

Figure 11.9 Hemiplegia in a very low birthweight infant with marked periventricular leucomalacia right ventricle frontal horn, bilateral frontal cortical atrophy.

Nomenclature of part affected, and aetiology

Diplegia = legs>arms: periventricular leucomalacia in premature, hypoxic-ischaemic insult (HII) to cortex at the 'watershed zones' between major blood vessels.

Hemiplegia = half the body, arm>leg: congenital, birth injury, HII, brain malformation (e.g. cyst), child abuse, meningitis, prolonged seizure (Figures 11.8 and 11.9).

Double hemiplegia (quadriplegia)= arms>legs: mainly congenital (Figure 11.10). Apparent monoplegia (one limb) and paraplegia (lower limbs only) is usually a hemiplegia or diplegia respectively.

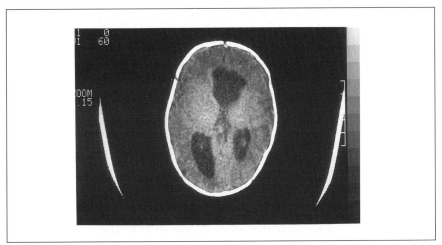

Figure 11.10 Double hemiplegia with a semilobar holoprosencephaly (a single ventricle in the frontal half of the brain).

Motor pattern, aetiology

Spastic (70% of cases) = increase in tone found in the diplegias and hemiplegias.

Dyskinesia (15% of cases)= constant change in tone: associated with hypoxia, hyperbilirubinaemia.

> dystonia = writhing movements resulting in prolonged abnormal body postures.
> athetosis = continuous slow writhing movements of the limbs.
> chorea = sudden jerky movements of fingers, hands, limbs.

Ataxia (5% of cases) = incoordinate movement, often with hypotonia: in hydrocephalus, congenital malformation of the cerebellum.

Ataxic diplegia (10% of cases) = mixed CP: usually seen with hydrocephalus.

Hypotonia = reduced tone which may persist or precede any of the above motor patterns.

Clinical presentation

1. 'Floppy infant' especially in ataxic CP.
2. Delayed motor development.
3. Strong hand preference begining under a year (hemiplegia).
4. Failure to thrive.
5. Older child presents with prolonged bottom shuffling (diplegia) or gait abnormality, e.g. toe walking (diplegia, hemiplegia), wide based with arms abducted (ataxic CP).
6. Persistent drooling with speech delay.

The motor pattern may initially be hypotonic, and progress through dystonia to a spastic or dyskinetic CP with choreoathetosis.

Preservation of primitive reflexes in spastic and dyskinetic CP–Moro, tonic neck reflex (TNR), palmar grasp, stepping 'scissor' gait.

Reflexes always indicating abnormality: (i) obligatory ATNR (ii) an ATNR more marked on one side (iii) poor arm extension on eliciting the parachute reflex in hemiplegia.

Affected side underdeveloped in hemiplegia: compare nail and foot size on the two sides of the body.

Common associated abnormalities: mental handicap, epilepsy, squint. Hearing deficits are commoner in dyskinetic CP.

Immobility causes windswept posture, kyphoscoliosis, dislocation of hips (especially with tight adductors, e.g. diplegia), and constipation.

Contractures are due to sustained spastic pull, e.g. tight heel cords, and immobility. Lack of physiotherapy contributes.

Investigation and differential diagnosis

Cranial ultrasound for prematures, and neonates with abnormal neurology, has become routine. Echodensities, ventricular dilatation, and periventricular cysts may be predictive of cerebral palsy (see Neonatal problems).

CT may show cysts, or atrophy, often asymmetrical in hemiplegia. Calcification from intrauterine infection and tuberous sclerosis is well seen. Identifies tumour, some degenerative diseases, allows recognition of specific inherited syndromes, e.g. Joubert's syndrome.

Metabolic investigations for degenerations, e.g. Tay-Sach's, metachromatic leukodystrophy and Wilson's, immune function in ataxia telangiectasia, and nerve conduction in Friedreich's ataxia are indicated for progressive disease.

Assessment of disability in activities of daily living, mobility and schooling.

1. Self-help skills in dressing, toileting, washing: increase independence or manageability by adaptations to clothes (e.g. using velcro fastenings), and the home, e.g. suction pad under plates, grab handles for toilet, bath aids, lift.
2. Mobility:
Ability to crawl or walk using rollator, crutches, or plastic splints, or sit in a wheel chair either hand powered or motor driven.
   The DHSS can provide special large, stable trikes.
   Assess ability to negotiate streets, board public transport, or drive an adapted vehicle.
3. Educational setting

   i Pre-school: ordinary or observation nursery.
   ii School: ordinary or special according to child's abilities and local resources. Explore transport needs, access, stairs, adapted furniture, ability to use adapted computer keyboards.

Associated disorders requiring assessment

- 60% are mentally handicapped.
- Squint found in 30%. Visual abnormalities in 20% (refractive errors, amblyopia, optic atrophy, hemianopia).
- Hearing loss 20%. Speech and language are often delayed or abnormal.
- Learning difficulties and behaviour problems are common.
- Regurgitation and reflux with oesophageal ulceration secondary to disordered gut motility in severe CP can be troublesome, and is termed the Sandifer syndrome. Treatment includes H_2-antagonist, cisapride, or surgical fundoplication.

Management

Aim: the maximum independence and self-dignity possible for that disabled person.

1. Therapy
Stimulation of motor, sensory, language, cognitive and social skills equally. Therapists to set realistic goals for speech, self help, mobility, and coordinate to minimize disruption of the family. Global stimulation gives the best results, physiotherapy alone only results in small gains.

   Physiotherapy
   A therapist's skills are:

   i Advice on handling, bathing, sitting, walking, using transport, and aids to mobility, e.g. rollators, wheelchairs, crutches.

   ii To prevent secondary deformity from contractures, e.g. seating correctly prevents scoliosis and kyphosis; taking weight on the legs using a standing frame helps develop the acetabulae and prevent subluxation/dislocation of the hip and equinus deformity of the foot.

   iii Support and counselling role.

   iv To work with orthopaedic surgeons in planning operations and maximize any benefit from them.

Speech therapy (ST)

   i Help in drooling (behavioural techniques, drugs, eventually may advise surgical relocation of the salivary duct towards the pharynx), feeding difficulties, learning to chew; may use videofluoroscopy for analysing these disorders.

   ii Conventional ST.

   iii Sign language, e.g. Makaton, for the child who understands but has limited expressive speech.

   iv Advice on communication aids (e.g. Bliss symbol board, Cannon communicator, computers) and voice synthesizers.

Occupational therapy

   i Hand skills in dressing, use of toys or tools, writing.

   ii Adaptations to the home e.g. bath aids, lifts, ramps, extensions.

Portage scheme and workers
Named after the city in Oregon, USA where it was developed. The parents select a desired goal, e.g. to eat using a spoon/dress/build a tower of bricks during once weekly visits by the lay worker who is supervised by a professional (usually a psychologist). Daily routines for the child and parents are worked out aimed at achieving these goals by small steps.

2. Medication

   i For symptomatic epilepsy.

   ii Drugs to reduce spasticity, e.g. baclofen, diazepam, and in dystonic CP some with normal intelligence respond to L-dopa.

3. Counsel, support, genetic advice for the parents. Introduction to the local toy library.

4. Schooling: integration into mainstream school for those of normal intelligence. Aids to learning and remedial help, as indicated from the assessment.

5. Orthopaedic assessment of shoes and splints; brace or surgery to correct kyphus and scoliosis; surgery to lengthen heel cords, to cut hip adductors in the non-weight bearing child at risk of dislocation from adductor spasm.

Prognosis

Initial motor and mental abilities are the most important determinants.
   Diplegias: if still dystonic by 3 years, walking is unlikely.
   Hemiplegias: most walk by 2–3 years unless severely mentally handicapped. Normal intelligence in a third. Seizures are common (50%) especially in the retarded.

Double hemiplegias and quadriplegias: often severely mentally handicapped, frequent seizures.

Dyskinesias walk 2–3 years after learning to sit. Often intellectually more able than they appear and may be 'locked in', e.g. communication by eye pointing only. Seizures are uncommon.

Further education to 19 years for the majority. Employment opportunities for the handicapped school leaver are limited.

Needs of disabled young adults

Independence through adapted housing, shops and places of entertainment to cater for wheelchairs. Physically handicapped and able bodied (Phab) clubs help them meet their peers on equal terms.

Further reading

Scrutton D (1984) Management of the motor disorders of children with cerebral palsy. *Clinics in Developmental Medicine no 90*. Oxford:Blackwell

Spina Bifida

Definition

A failure of closure of the neural tube by 28 days of fetal life.

Anencephaly is the open head end of the neural tube. The infant is stillborn or survives a few hours.

Encephalocele is a protrusion of the brain, usually occipital, through a defect in the skull. Hydrocephalus is a frequent association.

Meningocele is a sac from arachnoid and dura elements, contains CSF, but no neural tissue. When arising from the head, hydrocephalus may follow surgical removal of the sac. If it arises from the spine the spinal cord beneath may be dysplastic, with associated minor foot or bladder problems.

Myelomeningocele

Definition

A cystic lesion of the meninges on or in which is the open flattened spinal cord. The commonest form of spina bifida, most are thoracolumbar in the UK.

Incidence

Highest in the Irish and Welsh. In the UK the incidence was 1–2/1000, which fell to 0.6/1000 in the 1980s. This phenomenon is only partly explained by antenatal detection and termination.

Clinical findings below the level of the lesion

1. Motor weakness. Spastic or flaccid or mixed paraplegia.
2. Sensory loss. Anaesthesia and poor circulation result in injury and pressure sores.
3. Sphincter function. Loss of normal bowel and bladder sensation and voluntary control occur if the level is above S2. Urinary incontinence and patulous anus with constipation and soiling are common.

Associated problems in infancy

1. Meningitis. Ventriculitis is usual, with brain damage. Closure of the defect reduces the risk of Gram negative infection, but see shunt infections, below.
2. Hydrocephalus occurs in 80%, from aqueduct of Sylvius abnormalities or the Arnold Chiari malformation which is usually present (cerebellar vermis elongated downwards, displacement of the 4th ventricle and a kinked medulla into the upper cervical canal).

   Ataxic diplegia is the most commonly associated CP, further handicapping the child.

   Squint, laryngeal stridor and blindness may occur due to raised intracranial pressure.
3. Urinary tract abnormalities:

   i Neurological.

       a. Absent/reduced function in S2–S4 = weak, flaccid bladder either small, dribbling, or distended with overflow. Some vesico-ureteric reflux but the kidneys are relatively protected.

       b. Spastic isolated cord at S2–S4 = reflex bladder with incomplete emptying due to incoordinate detrusor and external sphincter activity. High intra-vesical pressures develop, causing reflux and hydronephrosis. Urinary tract infection follows; without intervention uraemia is common by late childhood.

   ii Structural: horse shoe and duplex kidneys are common.
4. Others: Skeletal: Skull lacunae, extra/bifid ribs. Congenital heart disease.

Management (aims as for CP)

1. Selective skin closure of the defect has come to be considered ethically acceptable.

Criteria for skin closure

    i Paraplegia below L2.
    ii Hydrocephalus with >2 cm cortex present.
    iii Skin closure possible without extensive flaps.
    iv No kyphoscoliosis.
    v No other serious congenital malformation.

2. Shunt (ventriculo-peritoneal preferred) for hydrocephalus is usually required after closure. Complications include blocked shunt, and infection with *Staphylococcus aureus*; if a ventriculo-atrial shunt is inserted, shunt nephritis may occur.

3. Urinary tract: monitor function regularly every 1–2 years. Treat symptomatic urinary infection. If persistent, rotate antibiotic prophylaxis to reduce the tendency for resistant strains to emerge. If the bladder is difficult to empty by manual compression, catheterization is needed to preserve renal function.
4. Continence

   i Intermittent bladder self catheterization from 7 years for those with the bladder capacity to remain dry for 2–3 hours. Learnt within 1–2 days by the child, or parents of a younger child. Soft plastic catheter for boys, metal reusable catheter for girls.

   ii Chronic indwelling catheter works well in other cases, provided the balloon does not slip out.

Regular enemas +/- abdominal straining reduce bowel leakage.
5. Orthopaedic supervision of deformities, bracing for walking, selective surgery to enable shoes to be worn for walking.
6. Schooling, counselling, education as for CP.

Counselling, prevention and antenatal diagnosis

Recurrence risk of 1 in 20 after one affected child, 1 in 8 after two.

Folic acid pre- and peri-conceptional supplementation reduces recurrence. Whole population supplementation to reduce the chance of a first occurrence has been suggested.

Antenatal screening for alpha-fetoprotein of maternal blood and selective amniocentesis have combined with ultrasound examination of the fetus to reduce the number of liveborn infants to a handful, the result of unbooked pregnancies or parental request.

Prognosis beyond 5 years old

Survival

1. Natural history without surgery = 15%.
2. Non-selective surgery = 50% (i.e. if all children are treated).
3. Selective sugery = 90–100% (about 50% of children are eligible). Criteria for surgery are based on the children found to survive after non-selective surgery.

Degree of handicap

1. Operated on:
   Normal intelligence in 70%. Physical handicap is mild to moderate in 20%, severe in 50%; 30% are severely handicapped physically and mentally.
2. Non-operated survivors:
   Similar intellectually and in upper limb function to operated cases, provided hydrocephalus is appropriately dealt with, but all are wheelchair bound and doubly incontinent.

Further reading

Menzies R G, Parkin J M, Hey E N (1985) Prognosis for babies with meningomyelocele and high para-
  plegia at birth. *Lancet*, ii, 993-995. Comment by an ethical working party follows this article
Brocklehurst G (ed) (1976) *Spina Bifida for the Clinician* Spastics International Medical Publications,
  London:Heinemann

Spina bifida occulta

Deficient posterior arch L5–S1 is a normal radiological finding up to 10 years old, but an overlying lipoma, tuft of hair, or birth mark anywhere along the spine may be associated with:

1. Sinus or dermoid cyst – may connect between skin and meninges.
2. Diastematomyelia – split cord, with dura or bony spur between the two halves. Traction of the cord on the dura/bone may cause progressive damage as the spinal cord and the vertebrae grow at different rates.

Seizures

Prevalence: 5–7% of all children have a seizure, but only 5 per 1000 are epileptic (Table 11.4).

Recurrence risk of epileptic seizure after a first generalized seizure is 50% within a year, and 90% after a second. If focal the risk is higher.

A close relationship between age, seizure type, prognosis, and sometimes family history, characterize many of the convulsive disorders of childhood.

It is essential to distinguish specific situations, e.g. febrile convulsions or hypoglycaemia, and non-epileptic events, e.g. breath holding, from recurrent, usually unprovoked, seizures consistent with epilepsy.

Table 11.4 Frequency per 1000 and categories of seizures from the National Child Development Study

Epilepsy	4
Febrile convulsions	23
Seizure with CNS infection	1
Breath-holding, faints, temper tantrums	18
Single afebrile seizure in <5 years old	21

Febrile convulsions

Definition

A seizure as the temperature is rising from an infection not directly involving the CNS, between the ages of 6 months and 5 years. Duration usually 5 minutes or less, rarely over half an hour and/or multiple.

Management

If no obvious focus, always obtain urine for culture. LP if less than 18 months, unless reviewed regularly by an experienced paediatrician, or if signs of meningism are present.

Prognosis

1. Recurrence of FC is age related: under a year a 50% chance; 90% occur within 2½ years.
2. Risk of developing epilepsy:
   Score 1 for each of the following factors: 0 or 1 = 2–3%, 2 or 3 =13%

   i Family history of epilepsy.
   ii Complex FC: >20 minutes, focal, recurrence within 24 h.
   iii Abnormal development or neurology before the FC.

   Of the 0.5% of children who develop epilepsy half never had a recurrence after the first FC.
3. Even after prolonged FC lasting >30 minutes evidence of damage is rarely found at follow-up.

Prevention of recurrence of febrile convulsion

1. Paracetamol regularly as soon as pyrexial. Remove clothing. Tepid sponge is relatively ineffective. Avoiding shivering which worsens the situation.
2. Diazepam rectally once pyrexial, 5 mg under 3 years, 10 mg if older, given by parents, twice daily for a maximum of 48 h.
3. Oral, continuous prophylaxis is only given exceptionally, for regardless of treatment only 4% of the total develop epilepsy.
   Given until 2 years fit free or 6 years old, whichever is the sooner. Phenobarbitone has behaviour and learning side effects, valproate the danger of hepatotoxicity. Drug levels need monitoring. Efficacy poor.

Immunization: simple febrile convulsion is not a contraindication to DTP nor is modification of MMR required, but parents must be warned of the normal response and need for an antipyretic; supply and instruct on the use of rectal diazepam.

A classification of childhood epilepsy

1. Partial = focal onset in a part of one cerebral hemisphere.

   i Simple: no loss of consciousness.
   Focal motor seizure or focal sensory seizure.
   Benign focal epilepsy of childhood.
   ii Complex: with loss of consciousness, may follow simple onset.
   Psychomotor epilepsy, includes temporal lobe epilepsy.
   iii Secondary generalization: common, start as simple or complex and progress to generalized tonic and/or clonic seizure.

2. Generalized, from the onset. Important to establish it is not a secondary generalization of a complex partial, from the history or by observation.

   i Absence seizures: petit mal, atypical absence seizures.
   ii Myoclonic seizures: infantile spasms, Lennox-Gastaut syndrome, juvenile myoclonic epilepsy.
   iii Tonic, tonic-clonic seizures: grand mal, reflex epilepsy (photosensitive, sound or touch sensitive).

3. Unclassifiable: neonatal
4. Reactive febrile convulsions, acute metabolic/toxic episode.

Seizures by age (see Figure 11.11 and Table 11.5)

Familial factors

Present in idiopathic, petit mal (40%), benign Rolandic epilepsy (40%) and about 30% of temporal lobe epilepsy. Common in febrile convulsions, and when also linked with epilepsy may indicate a poorer prognosis.

The gene locus has been found for benign familial convulsions on chromosome 20 (AD rare, severe with complete recovery), juvenile myoclonic epilepsy of Janz on chromosome 6 (AD onset in adolescence, myoclonic jerks on waking, other seizures may precede them. Valproate best).

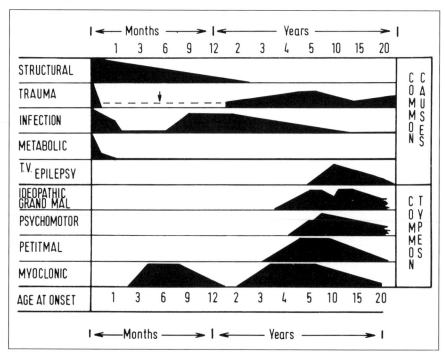

Figure 11.11 Approximate age of onset, subdivided into provocative causes and types. In trauma, the arrow and dotted line indicate child abuse in infancy.

Causes of seizures or coma (aide memoire: A-E-I-O-U, C-'DPT')

A = apoplexy from hypertension, or intracranial bleed.
E = epilepsy.
I = infection:

    i acute: febrile convulsion, meningitis, encephalitis
    ii chronic: TORCH, subacute sclerosing panencephalitis

O = oxygen lack (hypoxia) secondary to cardiorespiratory disease.
U = uraemia, and other metabolic disturbances:

    i Transient: hypoglycaemia, hyponatraemia, Reye's syndrome, hypernatrae-
       mia, hypocalcaemia, hypomagnesaemia, pyridoxine deficiency.
    ii Persistent: inborn errors, e.g. PKU, hyperammonaemias.

C = Congenital brain malformation: hydrocephalus, cyst.
D = Drugs, drug withdrawal, brain degenerations.
P = Pseudoseizure: hysterical, Munchausen by proxy.
T = Trauma, accidental/nonaccidental;

    i Tumour, other space occupying lesions – clot, abscess.
    ii Toxins: lead poisoning.

Assessment of the child with convulsions

Diagnostic approach

Further differentiation into idiopathic or symptomatic epilepsy follows from history, examination and investigation. Thus, the idiopathic label is a diagnosis of exclusion, and often has a genetic background with a good prognosis for spontaneous remission. Complex partial seizures, on the other hand, are usually symptomatic, with a moderate prognosis and may benefit from surgery.

1. History
    i Eye witness account is essential.
    ii Child's recollection of aura suggests psychomotor epilepsy.
    iii School record: impaired attention +/- performance, in subclinical seizures or petit mal.
    iv Diagnostic pointers to a symptomatic cause:

        a. Prenatal or perinatal abnormality predisposing to damage.
        b. Previous developmental delay or neurological abnormality.
        c. Similarly affected sibling if inborn error/environmental poison, e.g. lead/ drugs, or abused.

2. Clinical
    i Nutritional state: failure to thrive in abuse, metabolic or degenerative disease.
    ii Head circumference: reflects brain growth/hydrocephalus.
    iii Skin.

Table 11.5 Seizures by age

Type	Age (Peak)	Frequency (per 1000)	Aetiology	Clinical	EEG	Drug	Prognosis
Neonatal	0–4 weeks	5	Hypoxic-ischaemic, IVH, trauma, metabolic, infection, malformation, drug withdrawal	Tonic, clonic (rare in prem) myoclonic and 'subtle'	Not diagnostic	Various	Variable: see Neonatal problems
Infantile spasms	3–12 months (5)	0.2	1 Cryptogenic (30%) = normal development, examination, and CT 2 Prenatal: tuberous sclerosis, congenital brain malformation, congenital infection 3 Perinatal: hypoxia, birth injury 4 Postnatal: meningitis, encephalitis, trauma, PKU, severe hypoglycaemia	Lightning flexion of trunk, arms extended and abducted or flexed and adducted, often in runs followed by a cry, on waking or going to sleep	Hypsarryhthmic	ACTH,S, Cl	Normal: 30% of the cryptogenic. Mental handicap 80%. Epilepsy 50% Mortality 5–10%. Spasms go in 50% by 5 years, often to be replaced by Lennox-Gastaut syndrome
Lennox-Gastaut	1–8 years (1–4)	0.4	1 Same as infantile spasms. 2 Pre-existing severe seizure in 60%	Nocturnal onset. Sequence is stare, jerk, fall; status epilepticus is common. Control difficult	Slow spike-waves at 2–3/s, multifocal abnormalities	V,Cl,S Ketogenic diet	Episodes of minor epileptic status common. IQ and development deteriorate. Mental handicap 80%
Febrile convulsion	6 m–5 years	20–30	Lowered seizure threshold, often familial	As temperature rises, GTCS 1–5 mins. Occasionally tonic, focal, rarely akinetic.	Normal	D,V,P	Epilepsy 2%
Petit mal	3–16 years (4–8)	1	Genetic. 12% of parents and sibs also affected, and 45% an abnormal EEG	Sudden unconsciousness, no loss of posture. Eyes stare, eyelid flicker, chewing, for 15 s. No postictal drowsiness	Diagnostic 3 s spike and wave synchronous in all channels	E,V	Resolves in 90% Grand mal may follow

Type	Age		Cause/Genetics	Clinical features	EEG	Drugs	Prognosis
Benign focal epilepsy (benign rolandic)	3–13 years (7–10)	2–3	Genetic or idiopathic	Nocturnal onset, half face, arm, may spread to GTCS. Boys>girls	High voltage spike in Rolandic area	C	Spontaneous remission by 16 years old
Juvenile myoclinic	10–16 years	1	Genetic, (carried on chromosome 6), and idiopathic cases	Usually soon after waking, initial sudden jerk of limbs and face. Frequently followed by clonic-tonic with brief loss of consciousness. Half have absences like petit mal	Fast 4–6 s multiple spike-wave. Photosensitive	V	Spontaneous remission in adolescence
Photosensitive	8–14	0.1–0.5	Genetic, girls>boys. May be part of other epilepsies	GTCS due to flashing lights, TV, video games. Usually <5 mins.	Photic stimulation gives photoconvulsive response.	V	Spontaneous remission in adult life
Grand mal	Any age (6–10)	4–6	Idiopathic, genetic in some. 50% have GTCS as part of other epilepsies	Prodome of pallor, irritability. Forced expiration→cry, GTCS. Variable amount of clonic activity. Cyanosis, salivation, urinates. Lasts 1–15 mins usually. Focal weakness may follow. Post-ictal sleep, headache	Spike-wave or polyspikes. May be normal interictally	C,V,P,PT	Seizure free on medication for 70%. Remission in 75%, after drug withdrawal if fit free on medication for 2 years
Psychomotor	Any age (5–10)	2	1 Scar: mesial temporal sclerosis following prolonged febrile convulsion <4 years old 2 Injury: trauma, meningitis. 3 Malformations: hamartoma/vascular. 4 Tumour: 'indolent glioma'. 5 Familial. 6 Idiopathic	Aura: abnormal/frightening, rising from the abdomen upwards, then quiet, motionless, +/– automatisms, e.g. fumbling, lip smacking, swallowing, looking frightened, laughing, mumbling. Visual, auditory, or olfactory hallucinations. Secondary generalization →GTCS Duration 1–15 mins	Focal spike with phase reversal at focus in temporal lobe, or other part of brain, correlating to symptoms. May develop 'mirror focus' on contralateral side.	C,PT,V	30% each: 1 Fit free off medication. 2 Some fits but independent 3 Institutionalized care for psychoses, antisocial acts and/or mental handicap. Poor prognosis: Early onset, daily fits, left sided focus, low IQ, hyperkinetic rage. Deaths: up to 10% by 10 years

GTCS=Generalized tonic-clonic seizure, C=carbemazepine, Cl=clonazepam, D=diazepam, P=phenobarbitone, PT=phenytoin, V=valproate

- bruising in abuse.
- ophthalmic division, port wine stain in Sturge-Weber.
- café au lait patches, axillary freckles in von Recklinghausen.
- ash leaf depigmented patch, shagreen patches, adenoma sebaceum in tuberous sclerosis.
- linear streaks in incontinentia pigmentii.

iv Fundi: papilloedema, pigmentation, e.g. rubella, toxoplasmosis, toxocara; haemorrhages from pressure/trauma.
v   Blood pressure: raised in cerebral oedema, renal failure, nephritis.
vi Neurology: assess abilities appropriate to age, note focal signs.

3. Investigations

i   First convulsion: investigate only if <6 months old, or an ill child, or a suspicion of symptomatic epilepsy.
ii Electroencephalogram (EEG) (Figures 11.12–11.18) is diagnostic in petit mal and subacute sclerosing panencephalitis; confirmatory if spike with phase reversal in focal epilepsy, or diffuse spike-wave abnormalities of infantile spasms and grand mal. The mid-temporal spike of Rolandic epilepsy should be distinguished from the anterior temporal spike of temporal lobe epilepsy. If the diagnosis is still in doubt, video + EEG (+/– telemetry) or ambulatory monitoring may record an epileptic event. Note that non-fitting children may have focal spikes or spike-waves.

EEG is not indicated in uncomplicated febrile convulsions

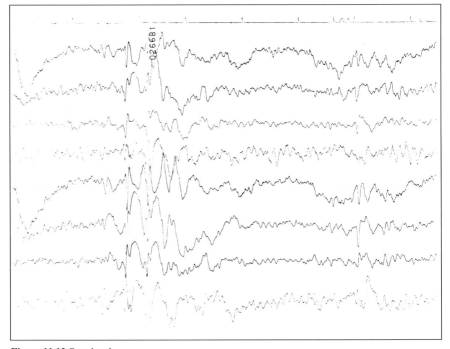

Figure 11.12 Grand mal.

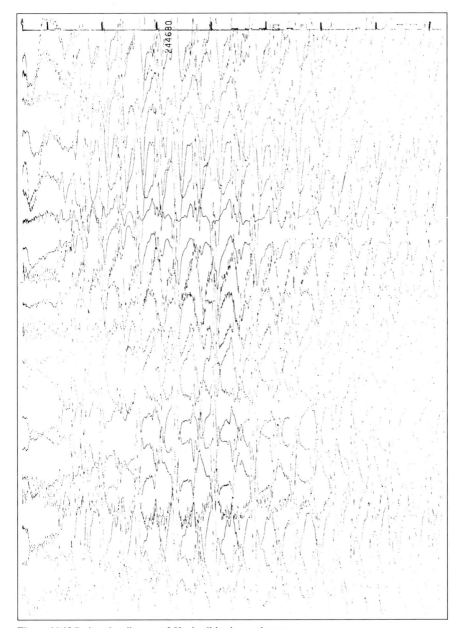

Figure 11.13 Petit mal, spike-wave 3 Hz, in all leads, synchronous.

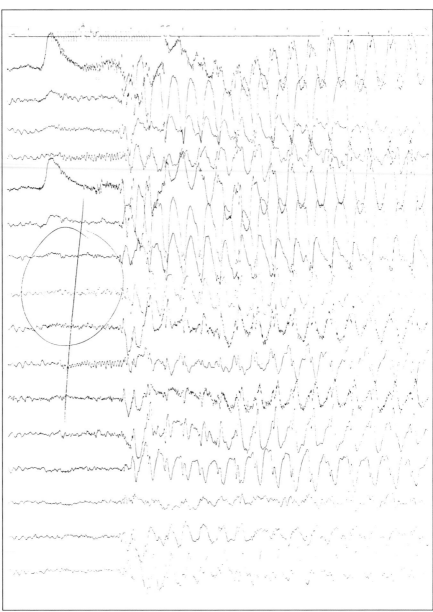

Figure 11.14 Photosensitive epilepsy. Look at the top line which is a 1 second time marker with the flash rate (20/sec) superimposed.

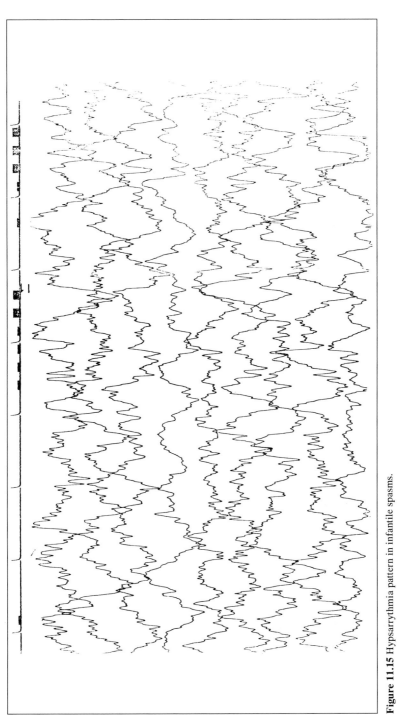

Figure 11.15 Hypsarrythmia pattern in infantile spasms.

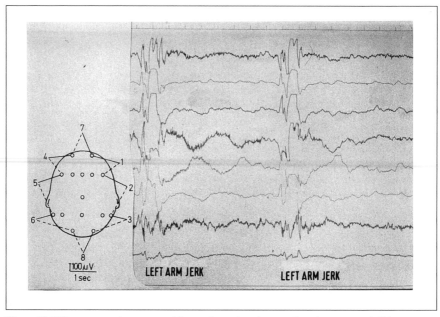

Figure 11.16 Burst-supression pattern with myoclonus, in subacute sclerosing panencephalitis.

iii Lumbar puncture: in an ill child, or after a febrile convulsion with mening-
    ism. As the latter sign is not reliably present in meningitis under 18 months,
    have a low threshold to LP: if irritable, drowsy, high pitched cry, or a rash is
    present.
iv Blood: blood glucose at the time of seizure; serum electrolytes, calcium,
    urea; microbiological culture, serology, TORCH if signs indicate; for inborn
    errors, lead level.
v Urinalysis: blood and protein in renal hypertension.
vi Radiological investigations

   a. X-ray skull for trauma, calcification, erosion, suture separation etc., abdo-
      men for lead if suspected.
   b. CT: urgent if in coma without adequate cause, or signs of raised intracra-
      nial pressure are present. If in doubt, CT before LP. Absence of papil-
      loedema is no guarantee. Structural abnormalities are uncommon if the
      neurology and EEG are normal.
      A third of CT scans are abnormal in seizures (but only 8% in primary
      generalized epilepsy) and two thirds if the CNS examination is abnormal.
   c. MRI is especially useful in posterior fossa and spinal lesions.
      Also consider in the 25% with complex partial epilepsy, as 70% of them
      have structural abnormalities which may be suitable for surgery and possi-
      bly missed by CT, e.g. neuronal migration defects, hippocampal sclerosis.
   d. Photon emission tomography (PET) further defines function.

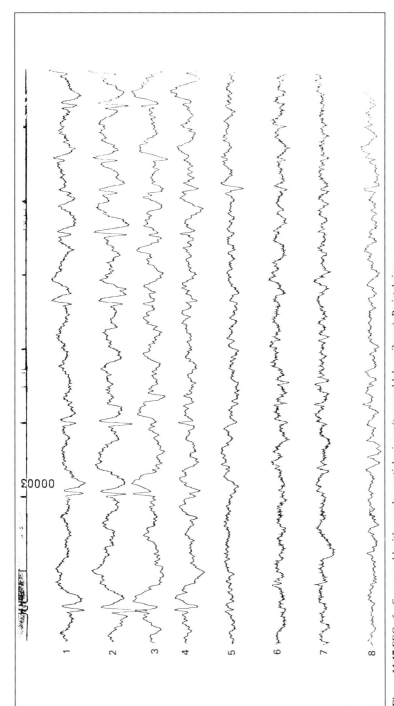

Figure 11.17 EEG of a five year old with complex partial seizure (temporal lobe epilepsy). Parietal ring. Right sided leads 1–4 show focal spike-wave abnormality, with phase reversal between leads 2 and 3.

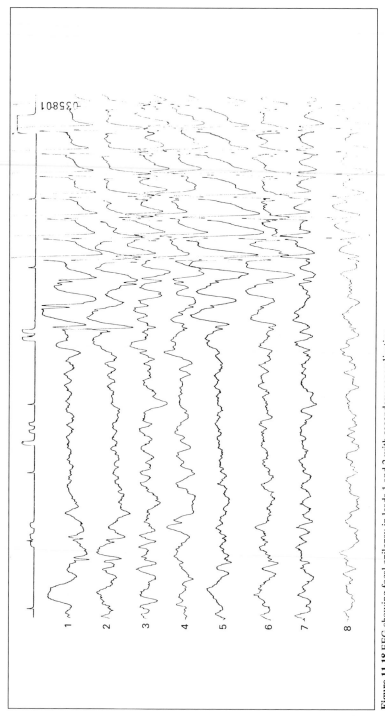

Figure 11.18 EEG showing focal epilepsy in leads 1 and 2 with secondary generalization.

Management of epilepsy

Discussion of relative risks of recurrence and long term prognosis help allay fears. Many parents believe their child is dying during the first observed seizure, and all fear recurrence.

i Medication

Start after second or third seizure.
  Time between seizures <12 months.
  Administration once or twice a day is sufficient as half lives are long. Up to 20% suffer side effects.
  Number of drugs: monotherapy effective in 80%, 10–15% need two, only 5% require three (or none if no benefit and still fitting).
  Progressive regimen if convulsions persist:

   a. Introduce first line drug, at smallest dose normally required, up to maximum dose if required.
   b. If still convulsing review the diagnosis, add the next best drug, then slowly withdraw the initial drug. Optimize this dose.
   c. Next step is to use 2 first line drugs, then a first and second line drug. Once stable consider withdrawal of one of these drugs.
   d. Penultimate step is an add-on drug, unless specifically indicated early, e.g. vigabatrin in infantile spasms.
   e. Finally surgery.

Special considerations re individual drugs:

   a. Valproate often relegated to second line drug under 2 years because of hepatotoxicity (risk 1 in 50 000, check liver function before commencing).
   b. Carbemazepine is preferred before phenobarbitone and phenytoin for less impairment of cognitive function and performance.
   c. Add-on drugs: vigabatrin, a GABA transaminase inhibitor, may be added in poorly controlled children over 3 years old. In complex partial seizures 50% remit, and up to 90% of infantile spasms and tuberous sclerosis. Lamotrigine, a folate antagonist, may help Lennox-Gastaut and other atypical absence attacks.
   d. Steroids/ACTH given early may improve the prognosis in infantile spasms.
   e. Ketogenic diet, or a hypoallergic diet, may help refractory epilepsy, particularly if associated with migraine.

ii Parental advice

Reassure. Frequently voiced concerns include death during seizure, and cerebral tumour as the cause of seizure.
  Avoid fostering an overprotective attitude.
  Advise avoiding precipitants, e.g. flashing lights, alcohol, hypoglycaemia, overtiredness.
  Give antipyretics for fever.

iii Protection

If fits are frequent enough to warrant medication no bicycling on roads, no rope climbing in gym, and closely supervised swimming and bathing until seizure free for 6 months.

Avoid contact sports. Wear a head protector if prone to heavy falls.

In photosensitive epilepsy, sit at 45° to, and 3 m from TV which should have a back light to reduce contrast. Computer screens have no flicker so are safe.

iv Psychological support

Especially in psychomotor epilepsy where behavioural disorders can be disruptive and attention seeking. Sometimes pseudoseizures and epilepsy coexist, requiring psychiatric guidance on management.

v Surgery

Indications:

- In partial epilepsy with a defined focus.
- Unresponsive to treatment for >2 years.
- Causing significant handicap.

Best done at adolescence. Removal of mesial temporal sclerosis, hamartoma or 'indolent glioma' of temporal lobe leaves 50–70% of cases seizure free, and most of the remainder with fewer seizures.

Educational and social effects of epilepsy

66% attend normal school. Most have primary generalized epilepsy, and are one standard deviation below the mean in reading and maths at 16 years old. Cognitive and specific learning difficulties are more common and 34% attend special school mainly for poor educational progress.

Disturbed behaviour, e.g. overactivity, distractability, aggression, impulsiveness, is found in 30–40%, but as it is not specific to epilepsy the concept of an 'epileptic personality' is invalid. Behaviour and psychiatric disorders occur in up to 75% with complex partial seizures. Drug monotherapy may be beneficial.

Poor self-esteem and social isolation are common.

Deterioration over time is linked with continued seizures, and side effects of medication, especially phenobarbitone.

Uncontrolled epilepsy

History of forgetting or repeated dosing is common; obtain blood for drug level (and measles antibody if suspicious of SSPE). If unhelpful, consider CT and degenerative disease enzyme estimations. Exclude Munchausen by proxy!

1. Drug related:

i Low serum level. Non-compliance, inadequate medication or reduced drug level due to liver enzyme induction.

ii Normal or high serum level. Intoxication from drug excess or idiosyncratic reaction. May be the wrong drug for that type of seizure.

2. Psychological stress.
3. Structural abnormality, e.g. hydrocephalus, glioma.
4. Degenerative diseases: e.g. subacute sclerosing panencephalitis (SSPE), Tay-Sach's disease.

Withdrawal of anticonvulsants

After 2 years of being fit free consider slow withdrawal over 12 months; 60% obtain a permanent remission.

Remission is more likely if neurology and EEG are normal from the outset.

Driving and the adolescent

To apply for, and hold a driving licence, a sufferer must have been seizure free for 2 years, or if nocturnal only, for 3 years.

If adolescent and considering driving, he may prefer to stay on medication. If offering the opportunity of withdrawal, point out that a single seizure counts as a recurrence. Epilepsy after 5 years old bars holding a public service vehicle or heavy goods vehicle licence.

Conditions confused with epilepsy

Generally conditions requiring explanation and reassurance.

1. Early childhood

i Breath holding, onset 6 months to 3 years.
ii Benign paroxysmal vertigo, onset 1–3 years.
iii Night terrors onset 18 months to 4 years.
iv Sleep walking 3 years old onwards.

Breath holding is precipitated by a stimulus, e.g. sudden anger/fright/pain followed by a cry, and cyanosis if breath is held in expiration, or pallor if primarily vasovagal with asystole. Limp and unconscious for a few seconds, he then may become stiff with clonic movements, followed by rapid recovery. ECG shows slowing before EEG. Medication is unhelpful. Prognosis excellent. Rarely, Munchausen by proxy instigated by suffocation, e.g. against the breasts, when ECG and EEG slow together.

Benign paroxysmal vertigo is also sudden, pallid, but fully concious, with vomiting, nystagmus and unsteadiness lasting 5 minutes. Ear infection is a common antecedent. Recurs 1–4 times a month, for up to 4 years.

Night terrors occur in sleep, then waking screaming and failing to recognize parents. Terrified, becoming calm within minutes, followed by natural sleep, with no recollection the following morning. Sleep walk is semipurposeful, and the child usually wakens.

2. Later childhood and adolescence

    i Hyperventilation.

   ii Hysterical fits: girls>boys.

  iii Vasovagal. May be postural or valsava induced, e.g. by vomiting in a migraine attack.

  iv Narcolepsy: onset 10–20 years old.

Assessment Self-induced (i) may be a response to anxiety, and not deliberate. Explanation with advice on rebreathing into a paper bag is usually sufficient. On the other hand (ii) is more complex, with apparent loss of consciousness, posturing, +/- jerking, but no incontinence or post ictal drowsiness. (iii) usually occurs on standing still or about to have an injection. Faintness, blurred vision and awareness of falling, prior to loss of consciousness for a few seconds, makes epilepsy unlikely. Elicit an attack using a tilting X-ray table. In (iv) a sudden irresistible sleep urge by day may be accompanied by cataplexy, sleep paralysis or hypnogogic hallucinations. The EEG is diagnostic, with rapid eye movement onset to sleep (the reverse of the usual progression), from which the patient can be roused, unlike epilepsy.

Further reading

Joint Working Group (1991) Guidelines for the management of convulsions with fever. *British Medical Journal*, **303**, 634–636

O'Donohoe N V (1988) *Epilepsies of Childhood* 2nd edn. Postgraduate Paediatrics Series. Woburn:Butterworths

Pellock J M (ed) (1989). Seizure disorders. *Pediatric Clinics of North America*, **36**:2 Philadelphia: W B Saunders

Stephenson J B P (1990) *Fits And Faints*. London:MacKeith Press/Blackwell Scientific

Table 11.6 Anticonvulsants, dosage, side effects

Drug	Daily dose	No. per day	Weeks for drug to equilibrate	Side effects
Carbemazepine	10–20 mg/kg*	2	1	Drowsiness, dizziness, rashes, GI upset, leucopenia, hyponatraemia
Clonazepam	50–200 μg/kg	1	1–2	Drowsiness, ataxia, salivation
Diazepam	0.1 mg/kg			Respiratory depression with phenobarbitone
Ethosuximide	30–50 mg/kg	1	1–2	GI upset, headache, ataxia
Phenobarbitone	3–10 mg/kg	1	2–3	Sedates, hyperactive, poor concentration, rickets
Phenytoin	4–8 mg/kg	2	2	Cerebellar ataxia, gum hypertrophy, hairy, coarse face, rickets
Valproate	20–60 mg/kg	1–3	1/2	GI upset, weight gain; hepatitis in first 1–2 months, especially with polypharmacy in preschool age; pancreatitis, hair loss
Vigabatrin	1–2 g per day	2		Excitation, agitation, psychosis

* Start at 5 mg/kg for 4 days, then 10 mg/kg; avoids oversedation, which can occur even at low dosage in some children.

Status epilepticus

A seizure of more than 30 minutes or repeated seizures with failure to regain consciousness between them.

Management of seizures including status epilepticus

1. Stabilize: airway, breathing, check BP. Oxygen by face mask.
2. Establish i.v., take blood for blood count, glucose, anticonvulsant level, glucose, electrolytes, calcium, consider liver function tests, drug screen, blood culture, blood gases.
3. Check blood glucose using stick method. Give glucose 25% i.v. 1 g/kg if <4 mmol/l.
4. Drugs (Table 11.7)

   i At time 0 - 10 mins
      Diazepam i.v./rectal: acts in 1–2 minutes, may repeat after 10 minutes. If fits stop but then recur, repeat and consider infusion of diazepam. Lorazepam is an alternative first drug, and acts for 16 h.
      Clonic movements persist: paraldehyde i.m. Add phenytoin i.v. to prevent recurrence.

   ii At 10–20 minutes
      Phenytoin i.v. over 5–10 minutes (with ECG monitoring for ventricular arrhythmias) acts within 15 minutes, or
      Phenobarbitone i.v. acts in 15–45 minutes. Watch for respiratory depression, hypotension. Consider intubation.
      Paraldehyde i.v. acts rapidly, and is safe if suitably dilute.

   iii At about 30 minutes
      Chlormethiazole (Heminevrin) infusion for 2 h or more.

   iv More than 30 minutes
      Thiopentone general anaesthesia for 2 h or more, with EEG monitoring if available.

Prognosis

Most severe in the preschool. Mortality 10%, mental retardation 50%, hemiplegia 20%, subsequent epilepsy common.

Table 11.7 Drugs for status epilepticus

Chlormethiazole (Heminevrin) infusion 5 mg/kg/h to max. 20–30 mg/kg/h
Diazepam: i.v. 0.3 mg/kg or rectal 0.5mg/kg. Infusion: 0.1 mg/kg/h (50 mg in 500 ml dextrose saline)
Lorazepam i.v. up to 0.1 mg/kg, maximum 4 mg
Phenobarbitone: i.v. /i.m. 20 mg/kg
Paraldehyde:

   (i)   i.m. 0.1 mg/kg, or 1 ml/year at 1–5 years, 5 ml + 0.5 ml/yr over 5 years
   (ii) rectally at 0.3 ml/kg/dose
   (iii) slow i.v. infusion, 5% solution in normal saline, 0.2 ml/kg/dose

Phenytoin: i.v. 15–18 mg/kg slowly over 20 minutes

COMA

Definition

A state of unrousable unconsciousness.

Causes of coma by frequency

Common

1. Neurological: epilepsy, head injury from accidental trauma or child abuse.
2. Infective: gastroenteritis, septicaemia, meningitis, encephalitis. Parainfection, e.g. exanthema, post-vaccination.
3. 'Metabolic': poisoning (alcohol, drugs, medication, glue), hypoglycaemia, diabetic ketoacidosis, acid-base disturbances.

Uncommon

1. Anaphylaxis, stings, bites.
2. Metabolic: electrolyte disturbances, hepatic coma, e.g. Reye's syndrome, renal or adrenal failure, inborn errors (amino acids, organic acids, urea cycle etc).
3. Anoxia and ischaemia including cardiorespiratory arrest, hypotension at operation or postoperatively.

Rare

1. Hypertensive encephalopathy.
2. Hysteria.
3. Neurological: intracranial vascular accidents, tumour, e.g. cerebral leukaemia, degenerations of the nervous system.

Stages of coma

The sequence of progression is reflected in the Lovejoy coma scale used in Reye's syndrome.

1. Lethargy, drowsy. Normal neurology, response to pain and respiratory pattern.
2. Disorientated, delirious. Hyperreflexia, hyperventilation.
3. Obtunded. Bilateral hemisphere dysfunction, e.g. drugs, metabolic, meningitis.
   Posture: decorticate = arms flexed at elbows. Pupils reactive. Hyperventilating.
4. Coma. Midbrain temporal lobe herniation and brainstem compression, e.g. trauma, abscess, clot.
   Posture: decerebrate = extended arms and legs, often asymmetrical. Pupil(s) fixed, dilated (false localizing sign). Hyperventilation or Cheyne-Stokes respiration.
5. Deep coma. Brainstem dysfunction, e.g. drugs, posterior fossa mass, clot.
   Posture: decerebrate progressing to flaccid. Pupils may be reactive if due to drugs, otherwise fixed, dilated. Cheyne-Stokes or apnoea.

Assessment

1. History: access to drugs, trauma, infectious contacts. Continue as for epilepsy.
2. Posture: see above. Also look for asymmetry of movement, may be hemiplegia.
3. Abnormal movements: myoclonic jerks suggest anoxia or metabolic cause; multifocal seizures an infective or metabolic encephalopathy.
4. Respiratory pattern.
   Cheyne-Stokes is unusual in children.
   Hyperventilation: blood gases are useful in interpreting the cause.

   - i   Central due to brainstem damage.
   - ii Metabolic acidosis: diabetes, uraemia, salicylate poisoning.
   - iii Respiratory alkalosis: early salicylate poisoning, hepatic failure.
   - iv Mixed respiratory alkalosis/metabolic acidosis: Reye's syndrome.

5. Eyes: remember normal fundi do not exclude raised intracranial pressure.

   - i   Fixed dilated pupils: anoxia, oedema, atropine or glutethimide poisoning.
   - ii External ophthalmoplegia but reactive pupils: poisoning.
   - iii Pinpoint pupils: pontine damage, opiates, pilocarpine.
   - iv Unilateral fixed dilated pupil: pressure on third cranial nerve, a false localizing sign, from temporal lobe herniation.

6. Motor system

   - i   Increased tone, hyperreflexia, upgoing toes in meningitis, raised intracranial pressure, hypoglycaemia, Reye's syndrome.
   - ii Reduced tone, usually downgoing toes if metabolic or drugs.

Investigations

Blood and urine for toxicology, and as for epilepsy.

Management

1. Establish airway, give oxygen.
2. Reduce intracranial pressure if present clinically (Table 11.8).
3. Monitor, including the Glasgow or Adelaide Coma Scale (Table 11.9), maintain fluid balance, turn, eye care.

Irreversible coma must be distinguished from metabolic causes, poisoning and hypothermia.

Head injury

Concussion and vomiting are common. Indications for hospitalization include: focal neurological signs, drowsiness/coma, skull fracture, significant head trauma but CNS appears normal at present.

Beware 'lucid interval', followed by deterioration, in subdural haemorrhage, which commonly occurs in children without a skull fracture.

Table 11.9 Assessment of conscious level using the Glasgow coma scale

Best motor response		Verbal response*		Eye opening	
Obeys*	5	Orientated	5	Spontaneous	4
Localizes	4	Confused conversation	4	To speech	3
Abnormal flexion	3	Inappropriate words	3	To pain	2
Extensor response	2	Incomprehensible sounds	2	Nil	1
Nil	1	Nil	1		

Table 11.8 Medical reduction of intracranial pressure

Indication	Treatment
Acute cerebral oedema	1 Mannitol 50%, 0.5 ml/kg in 30 mins. Then 0.25 ml/kg 2–3 hourly or as indicated by intracranial pressure (ICP) monitoring 2 Mechanical hyperventilation reduces cerebral blood flow, maintain P_aCO_2 between 3.3–4.0 kPa 3 Sedation, pain relief, careful nursing to prevent surges in ICP.
Tumour, encephalitis	Dexamethasone 2 mg 4-hourly.

Score of 3-7 severe head injury, 8-11 moderate head injury.
*Under 5 years old responses are assessed similarly, but in place of obeying commands observe for normal spontaneous movements. Verbal responses are: best response previously known or likely for age scores 5, confused or incomprehensible words, or spontaneous irritable cries if not yet talking score 4, cries to pain score 3, moans to pain score 2.

Management

1. If severe: secure airway, assume neck may be fractured by avoiding head turning. Assess for other injuries. X-rays skull, cervical spine.
2. Assess in all cases:

    i Consciousness: Glasgow coma scale.
    ii Scalp wounds, blood/lacerations to tympanic membranes.
    iii CSF rhinorrhoea, bruising of both eyes or over a mastoid are signs of fracture. Antibiotic cover for CSF rhinorrhoea.
    iv CNS status: pupils, asymmetry of movement, toe reflexes.
    v Vital signs: Blood pressure (BP), pulse, respiration. Raised BP + bradycardia = brainstem cone.

3. Post–traumatic epilepsy in 10% (reduced to 6% with prophylactic phenytoin in one series) of survivors of severe head injury. Onset within one year.

Prognosis

Applying the worst score from the Glasgow coma scale, <3 = 50% die, 4 to 5 show moderate brain damage in 50%, while >5 80–90% have a good recovery, some with minor deficits.

Toxic encephalopathy

Definition
Depressed consciousness, often preceded by fever, associated with seizures, due to non-inflammatory brain swelling.

Pathology
Fatty degeneration of the liver and kidneys is common.

Causes
Most critical are Reye's syndrome and lead encephalopathy. The differential diagnosis is that of coma.

Reye's syndrome

Definition
Characterized by acute liver dysfunction, brain swelling, and hypoglycaemia which may be profound in <2 year old. Associated coagulation disorder is common.

Incidence
30–60 annually in the UK, and declining.

Pathophysiology
Outbreaks associated mainly with influenza B and varicella infection.

Inborn errors of protein and fat metabolism are implicated in sporadic/familial cases.

Some may be due to giving aspirin in the prodrome, and has resulted in a ban on this drug's use under 12 years old.

Clinical
Prodrome of a flu-like illness 7–10 days before, is followed by progressive stages of deterioration:

Stage 1: Vomiting++, lethargy, drowsy, upgoing toes
Stage 2: Disorientated, aggressive, hyperventilation. Enlarging liver, no jaundice
Stage 3: Coma, hyperventilation, decorticate posture (cortex dysfunction)
Stage 4: Coma, decerebrate, III cranial nerve palsy and pupils dilated (midbrain pressure symptoms)
Stage 5: Coma, flaccid, respiratory arrest despite improving liver function (foramen magnum impaction).

Investigations

Elevated blood ammonia and liver enzymes, bilirubin rarely raised, hypoglycaemia common, respiratory alkalosis + metabolic acidosis. EEG changes reflect stages. Electron microscopy. Diagnostic: mitochondrial changes, loss of glycogen. Abnormalities of urinary and blood amino acids and organ acids in Reye-like presentation of inborn errors.

Management

Avoid LP if history and investigations are suggestive. Intracranial pressure monitoring determines the intensity of medical brain decompression and possible need for surgical brain decompression.

Fluid restrict, maintain blood glucose, give platelets and fresh frozen plasma for coagulation defects.

Prognosis

Early recognition (before stage 3) and >2 years old have good prognosis. Mortality 45% overall. Survivors usually recover, some have learning or severe handicap.

Lead encephalopathy

Now rare in the UK due to legislation against lead-containing paints. Imported in some Asian cosmetics (surma) and patent medicines. Low level exposure from water drawn through lead pipes, and crops and dust contaminated by petrol exhaust fumes.

Pathophysiology

1. Acute illness: vomiting, ataxia, lethargy, then coma, and seizures, due to free circulating lead affecting the bone marrow, brain, and kidneys.
2. Chronic exposure leads to deposition in bones. Note that abdominal pain, constipation, peripheral neuropathy, and blue lead line on gums are rare compared with adults.

Assessment

Consider in any child with

> Pica, anaemia, irritability/slowed development – usually precede acute encephalopathy by 4–6 weeks.
> Raised intracranial pressure.

Investigations

1. Blood lead level is diagnostic. Urinary coproporphyrins are increased and a useful sceening test in an emergency.
2. X-ray of long bones: lead lines at the metaphyses; abdomen: rarely radiopaque flakes in intestines.

3. Haemolytic anaemia and basophilic stippling of red cells.
4. Urine: proteinuria, glycosuria, generalized aminoaciduria occasionally. *Fanconi*

Management

Avoid LP. Medical brain decompression is instituted.

Chelate lead with dimercaptosuccinic acid (DMSA), 10–30 mg/kg/day for 5 days, orally (supercedes dimercaprol and calcium EDTA. The latter mobilizes bone lead and may temporarily worsen the condition).

Environmental health officer is involved urgently in identifying the source, and the child is not returned home until it is removed.

Prognosis

Residual learning difficulties, distractability, and mental retardation proportional to severity and duration of exposure.

Further reading

Cole G F (1991) Acute encephalopathy of childhood. *In Paediatric Neurology* (E M Brett ed). Edinburgh:Churchill Livingstone pp 667–699. A useful chapter on mechanisms and management.

FLOPPY INFANTS

Systemic causes must first be excluded as they are the most common.

1. Acutely ill, usually infectious disease.
2. Failure to thrive/maternal deprivation.
3. Malabsorption: coeliac disease, cystic fibrosis.
4. Hypothyroidism.
5. Metabolic: rickets, scurvy, hypercalcaemia, renal tubular acidosis, inborn errors.
6. Congenital lax ligaments: Marfan's, Ehlers-Danlos syndromes.

Next establish the level of the lesion (Table 11.10)

Assessment of neurological hypotonia in infancy

Antigravity movement is a useful discriminator between central and peripheral causes:

1. Present in non-paralytic causes (cerebral palsy, perinatal encephalopathy and mental retardation).
2. Absent in paralytic causes (anterior horn cell, peripheral nerve, neuromuscular junction and muscle disorders).

Clinical

Lies in 'frog posture' in supine, pull to sit demonstrates gross head lag, in ventral suspension dangles like an inverted U.

Table 11.10 Hypotonia, level of lesion, conditions, and signs associated with them

Level	Conditions	Signs
Central		
1 Cortex	1 Encephalopathy	1 Reflexes exaggerated, upgoing toes; hypotonic cerebral palsy present or may result
	2 Congenital brain malformation	2 Specific features of face, hands, ears etc, enable identification, e.g. malformation syndromes, Down's, Prader-Willi
	3 Non-specific mental retardation	3 Non-specific hypotonia, normal reflexes
	4 Degenerative	4 Initial normal development. Look for, e.g. macular changes (Tay-Sach's), hepatosplenomegaly (mucopolysaccharidoses). Do WBC enzymes, urine metabolic screen
2 Basal ganglia	Dyskinetic cerebral palsy	Dystonia, choreoathetosis, preserved primitive reflexes
3 Cerebellum	Ataxic cerebral palsy	Ataxia, decreased reflexes
Peripheral		
1 Spinal cord	1 Transection or transverse myelopathy	Flaccid paralysis below the lesion, a sensory level present, bladder dilated. Spasticity may develop later
	2 Myelodysplasia	Vertebral anomalies, overlying skin markers, hypotonia, absent reflexes, club feet
2 Anterior horn cell	Werdnig-Hoffmann (AR)	Fasciculation of the tongue, finger tremor, symmetrical hypotonia, absent reflexes, alert intelligent expression. Prognosis: respiratory death <2 years old
	Polio or coxsackie	Abrupt onset, usually asymmetrical weakness, flu-like prodrome, CSF lymphocytosis
3 Peripheral nerve	Guillain-Barré polyneuritis	Ascending weakness, absent reflexes. Delayed conduction velocity, CSF protein raised
4 Neuromuscular junction	1 Myasthenia gravis	Transient in infant of myasthenic mother, or persistent. Facial weakness, suck, swallow and cry weak. Neostigmine test
	2 Botulism	Clinically similar, may progress to respiratory failure, even SIDS[*]. Toxin in food/absorbed from gut clostridia
5 Muscle	1 Congenital myopthy (various types)	Floppy from birth, slowly or non-progressive. Muscle biopsy may differentiate types
	2 Dystrophia myotonica (AD)	Respiratory difficulties may be lethal. Poor suck, ptosis, fish mouth, floppy. Mental handicap. Shake mother's hand–slow release is highly suspicious. EMG ('dive bomber' noise) and muscle biopsy diagnostic
	3 Glycogen storage disease type II (AR)	Progressive, floppy, cardiac failure, macroglossia. Globular heart on X-ray, abnormal ECG. Absent acid maltase in WBCs and liver
	4 Congenital muscular dystrophy	Floppy, progressive weakness. EMG and biopsy, elevated creatine phosphokinase

[*]SIDS = sudden infant death syndrome

Investigation

Dictated by history and clinical findings.

1. Non-paralytic: CT, chromosomes.
2. Paralytic:

    i CSF pleocytosis: polio/coxsackie. Elevated protein alone: Guillain-Barre (GB) or transverse myelitis (TM) or tumour. If in doubt, a myelogram or MRI will detect the latter.

    ii Nerve conduction studies distinguish between GB and TM by slowing in GB. Neostigmine 0.04 mg/kg i.m. restores muscle power in myasthenia.

    iii EMG identifies denervation in Wernig-Hoffmann and polio, low amplitude in dystrophy, and 'dive-bomber noise' pattern in myotonia.

    iv Muscle biopsy with special stains is diagnostic in dystrophies.

Management

Physiotherapy: to prevent contractures, encourage motor development, general stimulation and for respiratory infections, which may be life threatening.

    Genetic counselling: for a family history of similarly affected individuals, consanguinity, or after finding an inheritable cause.

Onset of hypotonia with weakness after infancy

Diminished reflexes and hypotonia.

1. Spinal cord

    i Compression.
    ii Chronic spinal muscular atrophy.

2. Peripheral neuropathy

    i Guillain-Barré syndrome.
    ii With ataxia: Friedreich's ataxia.
    iii Peroneal muscular atrophy (Charcot-Marie-Tooth).

3. Juvenile myasthenia gravis.
4. Muscles: muscular dystrophies, dermatomyositis.

Clinicopathology

1. Spinal

    i Cord compression caused by tumours, dermoid cysts, extradural and intradural abscess, injury, or diastematomyelia.

        Signs: A sensory level +/- hyperaesthesia at the level of the lesion, localized tenderness over the vertebrae, a paravertebral mass, cutaneous signs of trauma, spina bifida or neurofibromatosis.

    ii Chronic spinal muscular atrophy.

        Degeneration of anterior horn cells, like Werdnig-Hoffmann. Usually AR.

2. Peripheral nerve

i Guillain-Barré syndrome

Definition   The commonest peripheral neuropathy.

A segmental demyelination, onset 2 weeks (1–28 days) after an upper respiratory/GI illness due to a viral exanthema, glandular fever, or herpes group infection.

Clinical   Symmetrical ascending paralysis, often acute, also affecting the arms. Painful parasthesiae may accompany the onset.

Flaccid paralysis, areflexia, downgoing toes. Muscles painful on palpation.

Glove and stocking sensory impairment. Bladder may become atonic. Systemic hypertension can occur due to autonomic involvement.

Speech, swallowing and respiration may be affected.

Ptosis, and papilloedema occasionally.

Often very irritable, and moody for weeks after recovery. Intelligence is usually unaffected.

Progression   Maximum weakness about 10 days after onset. Recovery begins 1–2 weeks later, is variable, with relapses and remissions over weeks to months.

Investigations   CSF protein 0.1–0.3 g/l, no cells. Motor nerve conduction velocity is initially normal, slowing as the weeks go by. Serology for glandular fever, hepatitis, mycoplasma.

Differential diagnosis   Poliomyelitis (CSF lymphocytosis), transverse myelitis (stable motor and sensory level), botulism (toxin antibodies), polymyositis/dermatomyositis (raised CPK), cerebellar tumour (with papilloedema do CT), spinal mass (local pain, flexed curve to the affected part of the spine due to associated muscle spasm; needs a myelogram). Nitrofurantoin, vincristine, isoniazid, heavy metal poisoning and acute porphyria are even rarer causes.

Management   Passive exercises, chest physiotherapy. Monitor respiratory function; if <25% of predicted, cyanosis, disturbed blood gases, consider mechanical ventilation.

Plasma exchange is beneficial in some cases. *↖ immunoglob when unable to walk*
    steroids if chronic course

Prognosis   Full recovery in 80%, not related to severity of attack but to starting recovery within 18 days of onset. Mortality <5%.

ii Friedreich's ataxia

See ataxias

iii Peroneal muscular atrophy (AD)

Definition   The commonest inherited neuropathy with onset often <10 years old. Characterized by a high stepping gait, pes cavus, weak dorsiflexion and eversion and absent reflexes at knee and ankle. Wasting of peroneii → inverted champagne bottle appearance. Upper limbs are less involved.

Pathology Peripheral nerves are thickened; demyelination predominates over remyelination, shows as 'onion bulb' on nerve biopsy. Motor nerve conduction velocity is reduced in the common peroneal nerve.

Management Supportive, genetic counselling.

Prognosis Almost normal adult life.

3. Juvenile myasthenia gravis (MG)

Definition

Very rare, autoimmune production of antibodies to the acetylcholine receptor at the neuromuscular junction. Neonatal and juvenile MG share the same mechanism.

Clinical

Ptosis, progressive weakness during the day. May be precipitated by infection, or stress. Differential is depression, polyneuritis, and ophthalmoplegic migraine. Neostigmine test is diagnostic. Thymomas, found in adults, are rarely present in childhood.

4. Duchenne muscular dystrophy

Definition

The absence of the muscle protein dystrophin results in a progressive degeneration of striated muscle with fatty infiltration causing hypertrophy. Creatine phosphokin-ase elevated ×10 normal.

Incidence

1 in 5000 males.

Genetics

Spontaneous new mutation in a third, the majority are inherited as a sex-linked recessive condition. The carrier state and affected individuals can be identified by DNA analysis in informative families, allowing antenatal diagnosis.

Clinical

Late walkers, hypertrophied calves, onset of weakness from 2 years onwards with a slow, awkward gait. Climbing up their own legs = Gower's sign.

Begins to waddle, to become a Trendelenburg dip of the hip, and show excessive lumbar lordosis. Contractures of the heels develop, so he walks on his toes.

Proximal muscle groups affected most, ends up with just diaphragm and fingers in late teens. A third have an IQ <75. ECG is abnormal in the majority.

Management

Mobility must be maintained as long as possible.

1. Lightweight calipers from waist to foot and release of heel contractures with minimal bed rest for any reason can prolong this phase, to about 12 years.
2. A wheelchair from which he can transfer himself to bed and toilet is followed by an electrical wheelchair and total dependence in activities of daily living.
3. Kyphosis and scoliosis are dangers. A spinal brace or spinal surgery preserves the chest shape. Respiratory infections become potentially lethal. Loss of weight heralds the final phase. Death in late teens is usual.
4. Schooling: the level of activity determines when a boy has to transfer to a special school for the physically handicapped.
5. Home adaptation: ramps, hoists or adaptation of downstairs rooms into bedroom and bathroom.

Genetic counselling

Of family with taking of blood for DNA studies from the child, female siblings and mother at diagnosis to prevent unwanted sufferers.

Prognosis

Death in late adolescence or early adult life.

Dermatomyositis

Definition

A rare, autoimmune disease with a characteristic butterfly skin rash, violaceous upper eyelids and proximal muscle weakness; oedema may be present. A vasculitis affects the gut.

Clinical

Low grade fever, aches and pains, appear 'malingering'. Dysphagia, abdominal pain, bleeding from upper and lower gastrointestinal tract. Not associated with malignancies.

Diagnosis

ESR usually raised. CPK often elevated, not as high as in Duchenne. Antinuclear factor may be positive. EMG shows mixed myopathic and denervation pattern. Inflammatory cells surround muscle fibres in the biopsy.

Management

Steroids, physiotherapy.

Prognosis

25% mortality without treatment. Now 90% recover, few deaths.

ATAXIA

Definition

A disturbance of coordination and motor rhythm in volitional activities affecting posture, limb movement, eye movements and speech.

Types

- Acute
- Acute intermittent
- Progressive
- Chronic

Differentiation from other conditions with involuntary movements

1. Acute chorea (see rheumatic fever)
   Writhing, jerky movements of limbs and face occur spontaneously and interrupt normal volitional movements.

   - Interfere with eating, dressing, talking, and writing and cause clumsiness, with consequent 'getting into trouble' at home and at school.
   - Increased by emotion, disappear in sleep.
   - Weakness. Marked hypotonia with characteristic 'dinner forking'.
   - Normal tendon reflexes.
   - Mood very labile.
   - Duration 2–3 months, may recur.

2. Others: chorea is not usually difficult to distinguish from tics (which can be demonstrated at will), the obscenities uttered in Gilles de la Tourette syndrome, and progressive conditions like Wilson's disease, or Huntingdon's chorea (family history).
3. Drug induced extrapyramidal reactions may confuse unless a history of ingestion is obtained (e.g. metaclopramide, haloperidol, chlorpromazine). Diphenhydramine reverses these effects.

Acute ataxia

1. Intoxication: phenytoin, piperazine ('worm wobble'), alcohol, DDT, lead.

2. Acute cerebellar ataxia: 1–5 years old, post chicken pox, during coxsackie, Echo, polio, infectious mononucleosis, mycoplasma. Sudden onset, ataxia + hypotonia, lasts 1–8 weeks, recovery is complete. CSF may show up to 100 lymphocytes.
3. Myoclonic encephalopathy: dancing eyes, myoclonic jerking of face, limbs. Present at rest, thus differs from cerebellar ataxia. Most cases are idiopathic, or post coryzal, and rarely an occult neuroblastoma. Response to ACTH may be dramatic. Mild mental retardation ensues in 50%.

   Investigation: requires urinary homovanillic acid and vanillyl mandelic acid estimation, US or body CT looking for suprarenal calcification, skeletal survey, chest X-ray, bone marrow.

Acute intermittent ataxia

Causes

1. Seizure: minor epileptic status, and post ictally.
2. Benign paroxysmal vertigo: see conditions confused with epilepsy.
3. Migraine: basilar type with loss of vision or flashing lights, tinnitus, slurred speech.
4. Metabolic, all very rare AR conditions:

   - Arginosuccinic aciduria: urea cycle defect → ataxia, mental retardation, fragile hair. See Metabolic problems for management.
   - Hartnup's disease: tryptophan transport defect →mental disturbance and retardation, double vision, pellagra-like rash. Give nicotinamide.
   - Maple syrup urine disease: see metabolic problems.

Progressive ataxia

1. Posterior fossa tumours

Headache, vomiting, head tilt, neck stiffness, papilloedema common.
Fits are *rare*; 55% of all childhood tumours are infratentorial. Exclude Chiari malformation, or a cyst by CT. No LP!

Clinical signs relating to tumour sites

   i   Cerebellar astrocytoma gives unilateral ataxic signs, with falling to or veering to the affected side.
   ii Medulloblastoma is midline, in the roof of the 4th ventricle → early obstructive hydrocephalus, trunk and limb ataxia, with a tendency to fall forward or back.
   iii Ependymoma arises from the floor of the 4th ventricle. Early hydrocephalus. Infiltrative,with cranial nerve palsies and stiff neck.

Management

Surgery may cure a cerebellar astrocytoma, but medulloblastoma cannot be completely removed and needs irradiation; 5 year survival 40%. Ependymoma less malignant than medulloblastoma.

2. Posterior fossa subdural or epidural collection, cerebellar abscess

Urgent recognition alters prognosis. Occurs after trauma or failure to respond to antibiotics, and a CT is needed.

3. Friedreich's ataxia (AR)

Definition

A degeneration of the spinal cord dorsal columns and cerebellum. Ataxia, loss of position and vibration sense, areflexia, and scoliosis result. Sensory nerve conduction velocity is reduced, whereas motor nerve conduction velocity is usually normal.

Progression

Onset usually in late childhood, with loss of ability to walk from adolescence onwards. Diabetes mellitus and cardiomyopathy appear in adult life, the latter causing early death.

4. Metabolic (all rare)

Abetalipoproteinaemia, ataxia-telangiectasia, Refsum's syndrome: AR, phytanic acid oxidase deficiency → onset 4–7 years old, loss of appetite, ataxia, dry scaly skin, progressive deafness, retinitis, peripheral neuropathy. Diet low in phytates is beneficial.

Chronic ataxia

1. Ataxic cerebral palsy

See cerebral palsy

2. Hydrocephalus

Pathophysiology

Obstruction, overproduction, or failure of absorption of CSF.

   i Obstruction to CSF pathways at foramen of Munro, 3rd ventricle, aqueduct of Sylvius, or foramina of the 4th ventricle, caused by:

a. Congenital malformations

Aqueduct stenosis: sporadic, or rarely X-linked.

Arnold-Chiari malformation of downward elongation of cerebellar tonsils through the foramen magnum, and frequently associated with spina-bifida.

Dandy-Walker syndrome: 4th ventricle outlets absent → massive ballooning, with a large posterior fossa, evident clinically or on skull X-ray.

b. Inflammatory disease: congenital cytomegalovirus or toxoplasmosis infection, meningitis, intraventricular/intracranial bleeds, TB.

c. Tumours: see Progressive ataxias.

ii Overproduction of CSF: very rare, due to choroid papilloma.

iii Failure of CSF absorption by the arachnoid granulations: 'gumming up' after bleeds or infection also occurs, but the main mechanism is obstruction.

Symptoms

Vomiting, headache (see below), failure to thrive, drowsiness, shrill cry, developmental delay (especially motor), or mental regression which can be severe.

'Cocktail party' personality = facile social manner and an acquired stock of phrases, appearing more intelligent than is the case. May be found in the spina-bifida with a shunt.

Clinical

- Large head, failure of anterior fontanelle to close and wide sutures (or sprung if acquired after infancy). Percuss lightly holding the child's head with the other hand immediately opposite to feel a vibration or fluid thrill.
- Distended scalp veins.
- Bulging fontanelle – its absence is not a reliable sign.
- Sunsetting sign, lid retraction.
- Eyes: papilloedema is unusual in infants; retinal haemorrhages appear if acute, and optic atrophy if long standing; presence of choroidoretinitis in congenital infection.
- Ataxia: titubation of head, unsteady trunk, intention tremor, staggering gait, hypotonia and hyporeflexia.
- Ataxic cerebral palsy in some cases: hypotonia with increased reflexes, upgoing toes.
- Acute signs: slow pulse rate, elevated BP, slow irregular respirations.

Differential diagnosis of a large head

1. Is the CNS normal? If so, is it

   i Normal variation
   ii Familial (measure parents' and siblings' heads)
   iii Disproportionate growth in a premature, failure to thrive, rickets, achondroplasia, or haematological disease, e.g. sickle cell or thalassaemia.

2. Abnormal CNS present.

i   Hydrocephalus, subdural haemorrhage or effusion must be differentiated, by US if the fontanelle is still open, or by CT.

ii   Abnormal boat-shape in craniostenosis of the sagittal suture (seen on X-ray) with minimal CNS signs.

iii   Cerebral glioma is likely to have localizing signs (see below), identified by CT.

iv   Megaencephaly may be idiopathic or due to neurofibromatosis, inborn errors such as mucopolysaccharidoses or Tay-Sach's disease.

v   Sotos syndrome presents as developmental slowness, high forehead, large hands and feet, initially tall for age +/- precocious puberty.

Management

- Conservative treatment with observation or isosorbide as long as no significant mental deterioration, onset of stridor, or visual impairment, occurs. Intracranial pressure monitoring is rarely needed to clarify.
- Surgery is dependent on the rate of increase, and underlying cause, e.g. a high CSF protein (>1 g/l) will cause a shunt to block. In tumours consider removal, or palliation with a shunt alone.
- Commonest shunt used now is ventriculoperitoneal. Major danger is infection (*Staph. aureus*), usually acquired at the time of insertion.

MICROCEPHALY

Prenatal onset: small head at birth – congenital infection, alcohol, syndromes.

Progressive failure to grow: postnatal, e.g. cerebral hypoxia/injury, post-meningitis, craniostenosis.

DEGENERATIONS OF THE CNS

Most die in childhood.

Rare except for HIV.

Presentations variable, may include all or some of the following:

Poliodystrophy: Grey matter involvement = personality changes, seizures and early onset of dementia (e.g. Tay-Sachs, Neimann-Pick, Gaucher's disease).

Leucodystrophy: White matter involvement = cortical blindness, deafness, motor skills impaired through weakness or spasticity, ataxia, peripheral neuropathy (e.g. metachromatic leucodystrophy, Schilder's disease):

1. Eye signs: cloudy corneas in mucopolysaccharidoses; cherry red spot in Tay-Sachs and Neimann-Pick disease; optic atrophy in leucodystrophies.
2. Organomegaly, e.g. large liver and tongue in some glycogenoses; liver, spleen and bones in mucopolysaccharidoses (MPS); liver and spleen in Gaucher's disease.

Causes of CNS degeneration

1. *Metabolic*: a variety of storage disorders due to:

    i Absence of lysosomal enzymes, e.g.

        a. Leucodystrophies: aryl sulphatase = metachromatic leucodystrophy.

        b. Poliodystrophy: hexosaminidase A = Tay-Sachs disease, sphyingomyeli-nase = Neimann-Pick.

    ii Abnormal copper metabolism, e.g. Wilson's disease AR, Menkes syndrome XL: kinky sparse hair, fits, low serum copper and caeruloplasmin.

    iii Presently unknown, e.g. Huntington's chorea,

2. *Infection*: HIV, subacute sclerosing anencephalitis (SSPE) post measles.
3. *Immune disorder*: ataxia-telangiectasia AR.
4. Sex associated.

    i Sporadic: Rett's syndrome = girls only, regression at 1 year old, hyperventilation episodes, hand wringing, jerks, seizures, spastic CP by 4 years.

    ii XL: Lesch-Nyhan syndrome: see Metabolic problems.

Investigations

1. Urinary amino acids, dermatan and heparan sulphate (MPS)
2. Blood for white cell enzyme studies (e.g. Neimann-Pick), hexosaminidases (e.g. Tay-Sachs), uric acid (e.g. Lesch-Nyhan syndrome), caeruloplasmin (e.g. Wilson's), HIV antibody.
3. CSF: measles antibodies for SSPE.
4. Bone marrow aspirate: abnormal cells of Gaucher's, Neimann-Pick.
5. Liver biopsy, muscle biopsy: glycogen storage disorder.
6. Skin fibroblast culture: various inborn errors of metabolism detected.
7. Electrical tests: EEG burst-supression pattern is characteristic in SSPE. Motor nerve conduction velocity and visual evoked responses reduced in some leucodystrophies. Electroretinogram responses reduced in poliodystrophies.
8 MRI: demyelination in leucodystrophies well shown.

Genetic counselling

Most conditions are AR, some AD (e.g. Huntington's), rarely X-linked (e.g. Lesch-Nyhan). Accurate diagnosis is therefore essential.

    Fetal studies: chorionic villus biopsy for DNA studies (e.g. Huntington's), for enzyme testing and fetal sexing.

    Blood testing for carrier state, e.g. Tay-Sachs, allows siblings to be counselled.

Management

1. Bone marrow in MPS, zidovudine in AIDS. Gene therapy may be possible for other degenerations in the future, but at present none is available.
2. Counselling family. Parent support groups/societies.
3. Activities and goals depend on the age of onset and rate of deterioration.
4. Respite/hospice care.

Prevention

1. Safer sex.
2. Immunization: SSPE is rare after measles vaccination.
3. Premarital counselling in at risk groups, e.g. Ashkenazi Jews and Tay-Sachs.
4. Antenatal diagnosis.

HEADACHE

Major causes

1. Acute: infection, hypertension.
2. Neurological: migraine, raised intracranial pressure, post-traumatic, intracranial bleed.
3. Tension.
4. Local: sinusitis, dental caries.

Migraine and tension headaches

Recurrent headaches affect 15–20% of children, peak incidence 12 years.

Migraine

Definition

Headache with two of the following: unilateral headache, visual aura, nausea or vomiting, family history.

Prevalence

3% of children, 10% of adolescents.

Pathophysiology

Hypotheses:

    i Vascular vasoconstriction (aura) followed by vasodilatation (headache).
    ii Primary neurogenic (spreading depression of Leao).

Neither is confirmed as the primary mechanism.

Clinical

Onset from 2 years old, may appear as pallor and vomiting alone, and only later is headache verbalized by the child. Other manifestations include recurrent abdominal pain, and slurred speech and ataxia in basilar artery migraine.

Table 11.11 Migraine and tension headache differences

	Migraine	*Tension*
Character	Throbbing	Sharp, or dull ache
Site	Hemicranial, bifrontal	Often generalized, vertex, or unclear
Frequency	Paroxysmal or isolated attacks at intervals	Continuous or many hours every day for days/ weeeks/months at a time
Aura	Eyes–spots, scotoma, bright light. Ears–tinnitus	None
Associations	Nausea, vomiting, photophobia	Dizziness, depression, light headed
Neurological symptoms and signs	Transient ataxia, 'pins and needles' hemiplegias, aphasia, dysarthria, opthalmoplegia	Normal
Preference	Lie down in a dark quiet room	Continue normal activities
Family history	Migraine, car sickness	Not usual
Precipitants	Frequent: hunger, exercise, foods*, acute stress, sunlight, perfumes.	Frequently denied, schooling/family problems
Sleep	May wake child from sleep	Prevents sleep occasionally
Medication	Paracetamol; if nausea and vomiting add metoclopramide. If very severe: ergotamine	Ineffective

* Foods include: oranges, chocolate, cheese, yoghurt, colourings, preservatives.

Examination

Café-au-lait patches for neurofibromatosis, press over sinuses to elicit tenderness of sinusitis. Teeth for caries.

Cranial nerves, especially visual fields; fundoscopy; auscultation over skull and eyes for bruit from arterio-venous malformation/aneurysm.

General examination must include blood pressure, and if abuse is suspected, the genitals.

Differential diagnostic points

1 Migraine from tension (see table 11.11)
2 Sinusitis always has rhinorrhoea.
3 Raised intracranial pressure headache is worse lying down, coughing or straining, and associated with early morning waking.
4 Facial muscles tensed due to refractory error (eye testing has usually already been done!) and dental malocclusion with pain at meal times.

Investigation

Not warranted if normal examination and diagnosis is clear-cut. Indications for further investigations (after Hockaday J M (1990). Management of migraine. *Archives of Disease in Childhood*, **65**, 1174–1176):

1. Inappropriately large head in a preschool child.
2. New neurological symptoms or physical signs. Increase in frequency and severity of headaches.
3. Failure

   i to return to full normal health between attacks.
   ii of simple analgesia to relieve headache.

4. Deterioration: in developmental progress or growth velocity; personality or behavioural changes.

Management

1. Reassure. If tension headache, gently probe for causation. If incapacitating or associated with school refusal, child psychiatric involvement is helpful.
2. Medication: paracetamol is safe, and ergotamine may be used over 12 years of age, but is likely to be replaced by sumatriptan, a highly selective 5HT agonist. Vomiting can be troublesome if persistent so try prochlorperazine 250 µg/kg 2 or 3 times daily. Although useful metoclopramide in the preschool child can cause severe extrapyramidal reactions.

Prophylaxis in migraine

1. Avoid stressful situations.
2. Avoid precipitants. Dietary manipulation; trial of the hypoallergic diet if severe/hemiplegic migraine.
3. Medication if >2 attacks per month: flunarazine (a class 4 calcium channel blocker) is promising (not available in UK at present). Little better than placebo are pizotifen (0.5–1.5 mg daily) or propranolol (1–2 mg/kg/day), but worth a trial for 2–3 months, by which time the headaches may have remitted.

Prognosis

Tendency to recur for 2–4 years, then remit up to adult life.

Further reading

Barlow C F (1984) *Headaches and Migraines in Children.* Spastics International Medical Publications. Oxford: Blackwell
Hockaday J M (ed) (1988) *Migraine in Children.* London:Butterworth

RAISED INTRACRANIAL PRESSURE

Causes

Within the confines of the skull, too much blood, tissue (tumour, abscess) or CSF. In the relatively pliable child's skull the sutures widen or are 'sprung', thus signs appear relatively later than in the adult.

Rapid rise as with bleed/ trauma/ malignant tumour or abscess leads to more severe manifestations.

Clinical

1. Headache

Vertex or frontal, worse on lying down, relieved by vomiting. Present at night, on waking, ease up after breakfast; mild and sporadic to begin with. Crying and coughing raise pressure, so both are avoided.

2. Other symptoms

Vomiting may be projectile, and without headache is unlikely to be due to raised pressure.

Drowsiness is a feature of rapidly rising pressure.

Convulsions are unusual at presentation, unlike adult.

3. Signs

Absence of papilloedema is no guarantee.

    i False localizing signs:

        a. Third nerve palsy (dilating pupil, followed by ptosis, divergent squint) with contralateral hemiplegia in uncal herniation syndrome due to temporal lobe swelling.

        b. Sixth nerve palsy due to its long intracranial course, and, rarely the seventh cranial nerve.

    ii Bradycardia, hypertension, stridor/ Cheyne-Stokes respiration.

   iii Neurological patterns: see Coma and Reye's syndrome.

INTRACRANIAL TUMOURS

Second commonest malignancy of childhood.

Peak age 5–9 years, mainly infratentorial; rare under 1 year when half are supratentorial. Brain secondaries from other sites are rare.

Sites: 45% cerebellar, 25% cerebrum, 10% ependymomas, 10% brainstem, 10% midline, e.g. craniopharyngioma, pituitary, optic nerve.

Pathology

Gliomas (75%)

Tumours of glial (supportive) cells. Medulloblastoma (see ataxia) is rapidly growing, made up of small round cells. Gliomas of brainstem and pons are also rapidly growing, whereas those of the optic pathways are usually associated with von Recklinghausen's disease and are slow growing with a good prognosis.

Astrocytomas: (20%)

Astrocytes are usually benign and slow growing, infiltrative, with a tendency to become cystic.

Craniopharyngioma (rare)

Derived from squamous cells of Rathke's pouch, i.e. a developmental, slow-growing benign tumour producing its effects by compression.

Clinical

Principal symptoms and signs are the result of three mechanisms:

1. Raised intracranial pressure.
2. Brain shifts.
3. Local infiltration.

Signs

- Hydrocephalus: bulging fontanelle, or if sutures are already fused, a 'cracked pot' note on skull percussion.
- Cerebellar involvement:
    Unilateral – incoordination on the same side.
    Midline – incoordination both sides. Signs are intention or action tremor, dysdiadokokinesis, unsteady gait, hypotonia, hyporeflexia, nystagmus, slow dysrhythmic speech.
- Occiput tilted to the side of the tumour due to nerve traction or to correct a strabismus from a sixth nerve palsy.
- Stiffness and neck pain.

- Cranial nerve palsies: infiltration (brainstem gliomas) pressure effects producing false localizing signs (cerebellar astrocytomas).
- Pituitary abnormalities, visual field defects, optic atrophy in craniopharyngioma, optic nerve gliomas. The latter also presents with unilateral or asymmetrical nystagmus.
- Focal seizures in supratentorial gliomas: a rare cause of focal seizures in childhood, but must be considered if they are intractable or hemiplegia develops.
- Seeding in medulloblastoma and brainstem glioma → cord compression with paraplegia/spinal nerve root infiltration with root pains, areflexia, spinal tenderness.

Investigation

Skull X-ray may show pressure effects: sutures splay >3 mm in infant, sprung in older child; digital markings (also found in normal children), enlargement of the pituitary fossa, erosion of the clinoids.

Suprasellar calcification in craniopharyngioma.

CT is not as good as MRI at demonstrating posterior fossa abnormalities and spinal tumours or cysts.

Treatment

Surgery and irradiation according to site and malignancy of tumour. Chemotherapy pre-irradiation may improve results in under 3 year olds. Growth may be affected after pituitary irradiation, so requires pituitary function tests and follow up.

Prognosis

5–year disease free survival (and as a % of all childhood brain tumours in brackets): cerebral astrocytomas 25% (25%), cerebellar astrocytomas 95% (20%), medulloblastomas 50% (20%), brainstem tumours and ependymomas 20% (10% each), craniopharyngioma 80% (5%) with 10% postoperative mortality.

BENIGN INTRACRANIAL HYPERTENSION

Definition

Headache +/– diplopia, 6th nerve palsies, blurred vision, vomiting. Papilloedema and haemorrhages may be present. Follows recurrence of otitis media, steroid withdrawal, minor head injury.

Pathophysiology

Intra- and extracellular oedema, mechanism unknown.

Investigations

CT scan normal. LP diagnostic (>140 mm CSF), often therapeutic!

Treatment

LP. Dexamethasone is used if the intracranial pressure is elevated for prolonged periods of weeks or months, as vision is at risk.

Prognosis

Some children are left with minor deficits.

INTRACRANIAL BLEEDING

1. Trauma, accidental and non-accidental. Immediate danger of subdural and extra-dural haematomas. Chronic subdural collections may follow.
2. Spontaneous subarachnoid haemorrhage: rupture of arteriovenous malformation or aneurysm in 60%. Sudden onset, severe headache, meningism, apyrexial.

Prognosis

Mortality 20%, influenced by avoiding LP!

Further reading

Brett E M (1991) *Paediatric Neurology* 2nd edn. Edinburgh:Churchill Livingstone

Faerber E N (1986) Cranial computed tomography in infants and children. *Clinics in Developmental Medicine No 93*. Oxford:Blackwell

Fenichel G M (1988) *Clinical Pediatric Neurology. A Signs and Symptoms Approach*. Philidelphia:Saunders

Stephenson J B P and King M D (1989) *Handbook of Neurological Investigations in Children*. London:-Wright

Weiner H L, Urion D K, Levitt L P (1988) *Pediatric Neurology for the House Officer*. 3rd edn. Baltimore: Williams and Wilkins

Chapter 12

Respiratory disease

Disorders of the respiratory tract are the commonest illnesses in the under fives, among whom there are 57000 acute admissions to hospital and 700 deaths annually in the UK.

Risk factors

1. The respiratory residua of neonatal intensive care, e.g. subglottic stenosis and bronchopulmonary dysplasia, have become increasingly prominent causes.
2. More likely and severe in the very young, exacerbated by poverty and parental cigarette smoking.

Pathophysiology of respiratory disease in the growing child

1. Immunity

Initial lack of specific antibodies in the infant and preschool children may result in a respiratory tract infection every 2–4 weeks in the winter months, often brought home from school by an elder sibling. Breast feeding gives some protection against respiratory tract infection in the first year of life.

The lymphatic system is very reactive: glands in the neck and hilar regions readily enlarge; tonsils and adenoids are at their largest at 6–8 years (previously peak age for their removal!).

2. Lung development, airway size and resistance, respiratory failure

  i Airway development is complete at birth (16 generations), but the alveoli continue to divide, mainly in the first year, to complete 24 generations. The powers of recovery from damage to the lungs are therefore greatest during that period. However, the collateral channels (pores of Kohn, canals of Lambert) are not developed before 4 years old, preventing diffusion and contributing to hyperinflation, CO_2 retention and segmental collapse in obstructive airway problems.

ii Peripheral airway resistance in infancy and early childhood is relatively high under 5 years old, and the lungs have less elastic recoil, making the work of breathing greater.

iii Airway resistance in disease: as resistance to flow is related to the reciprocal of the fourth power of the radius, narrowing can rapidly become critical in the small airways of infants and small children by restricting air movement in or out. Mechanisms:

a. Intraluminal obstruction by inflammation or structural narrowing. As the air flow speed increases past the obstruction a wheeze may occur.

b. The trachea and extrapleural bronchi have C–shaped cartilages, allowing dynamic airway compression (DAC) of the posterior membranous segment from surrounding hyperinflated lung in bronchiolitis or asthma (Figure 12.1). The abnormally soft cartilage in tracheomalacia also allows DAC.

c. Interestingly, the spiral smooth muscle in infants' airways extends further down the bronchioles than in older ages, yet they usually fail to respond to β-sympathomimetics.

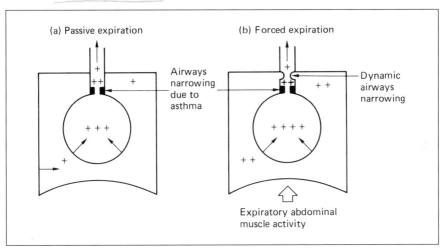

Figure 12.1 Expiration is normally a passive process. If the small to medium airways are partially obstructed the abdominal muscles are used to force the air out. A positive pressure gradient from alveoli to the mouth is established. At the point where the pressure is less than the surounding pleural pressure the airways will be compressed. Now, the airflow across this point becomes fixed and the rate of exhalation is independent of effort.

iv Mechanical factors contributing to respiratory failure

a. The chest wall is more pliable in infancy, demonstrated by:
Sternal recession: in upper airway narrowing (epiglottitis), and lung collapse (e.g. respiratory distress syndrome).
Sternum prominent (pigeon chest): in air trapping, e.g. bronchiolitis.

b. The infant diaphragm has less type 1 slow twitch, high oxidative fibres and tires more easily than in older children and adults, who have more of these muscle fibres.

c. Mucus plugging of small airways.

3. Investigations

X-rays

 i Chest. The thymus is large, jib–shaped or with a wave sign in infancy. It may 'disappear' radiologically in shock or cyanotic heart disease.
 ii Sinuses, age of appearance: mastoids 6 months, maxillary 1–2 years, sphenoid 3 years, frontal 5 years.
Sites for the onset of sinusitis are therefore age related.
 iii Barium swallow for oesophageal reflux/tracheoesophageal fistula/double aortic arch.

Blood gases, oxygen saturation

 i Ventilation-perfusion imbalance leads to hypoxaemia, defined as a P_aO_2 <7 kPa (50 mmHg). Pulse oximetry is often used to monitor oxygen saturation continuously, which should be maintained at 95%, equivalent to P_aO_2 13 kPa (90 mmHg).
 ii Low carbon dioxide occurs in hyperventilation, mild asthma, or early salicylate poisoning.
 iii Carbon dioxide elevation = respiratory failure (or rapid bicarbonate administration). In infants and children this equals a P_aCO_2 >6.0 kPa (45 mmHg), except in asthma when a 'normal' P_aCO_2 >5.4 kPa (40 mmHg) indicates respiratory failure as the P_aCO_2 is initially subnormal due to increased alveolar ventilation (and dead space).

Causes of respiratory failure must be due to obstruction, restriction, diffusion defect, or depression of the respiratory centre (Table 12.1).

Table 12.1 Causes of respiratory failure

Obstructive	*Restrictive*	*Diffusion defect*	*CNS depression*
Upper epiglottitis, stenosis, aspiration, laryngospasm, Robin anomaly, choanal atresia	Pneumothorax Pulmonary oedema Hypoplastic lung Diaphragmatic hernia Ascites	Intersitial pneumonitis Pulmonary oedema Interstitial fibrosis	Drugs Trauma Encephalitis Asphyxia
Lower Pneumonia, aspiration, lobar emphysema	Small chest Muscle/nerve weakness		

Respiratory function tests

See asthma.
Combined study: pneumogram = monitoring respiratory and heart rhythm and rate, blood oxygen tension/saturation. In near-miss cot deaths and cyanotic episodes it is used to determine the type of apnoea (see Neonatology) or bradypnoea, or abnormal cardiac rhythm. Add EEG or video surveillance in cases with neurology or when smothering abuse is suspected.

Others: sweat test, immunoglobulins, bacterial or viral antibodies, and precipitins for fungi, pH monitoring for acid reflux, drug levels, as indicated.

Examination

1. Appearance: pale, normal or cyanosed in air?
2. Listen for audible sounds

   i Stridor: mainly inspiratory if the narrowing is above the glottis. If below the glottis, expiratory wheeze or stridor may also be heard.

   ii Rattle: mainly an inspiratory sound, often easily transmitted and felt by a hand on the chest wall = secretions in the pharynx or trachea.

   iii Wheeze: occurs predominantly on expiration, synonymous with asthma but occurs in any partial airway obstruction.

   iv Snoring is due to upper airway pharyngeal obstruction. Sudden cessation of snoring despite visible inspiratory effort is a sign of complete obstruction and urgent need for a surgical opinion.

3. Cough. Preschool children swallow their sputum, and are often sick during coughing bouts due to the muscular effort compressing their stomachs. Abdominal pain from the muscular strain is common. A chronic, productive cough at that age should make one suspect cystic fibrosis/bronchiectasis.
4. Effort due to respiratory distress:

   i Grunting on expiration against a partially closed glottis is seen mainly in infants with respiratory distress syndrome, and older children in pain, e.g. pneumonia with pleuritic involvement.

   ii Infants extend the neck to shorten airway; head bobbing suggests exhaustion. Children with upper airway obstruction lean back, head extended. In lower respiratory obstruction they tend to sit forward and fix the accessory muscles of respiration, leaning on their thighs or the furniture.

   iii Flaring of the alae nasi:

     a. Increased airway resistance: in obstructive airways.
     b. Effort: temperature, parenchymal infection, stiff lungs.

   iv Chest

     a. Intercostal recession: pulmonary disease, as collapse or obstructive airways.
     b. subcostal recession: air trapping.

   v Respiratory rate
     Upper limit of normal:

Neonatal	50/min
Infancy	40/min
1 - 10 years	35/min
>10 years	25/min

5. Finger clubbing:

i Pulmonary causes: cystic fibrosis, empyema, bronchiectasis, tumour.
ii Non-pulmonary causes: cyanotic congenital heart disease, subacute bacterial endocarditis, inflammatory bowel disease, biliary cirrhosis.

6. Ears, nose and throat, and neck examination, are often left to the end of the examination, so I have dealt with them under upper respiratory problems.
7. Chest

i Shape: sternal recession develops in upper airway obstruction or widespread lung atalectasis in the very young with pliant costal cartilage. Barrel shaped/ pigeon chest if hyperinflated.
ii Movement: asymmetry may be visible, due to unilateral hyperinflation or collapse.
iii Tracheal shift confirms (ii).
iv Percussion: gently, as the chest wall is thin. Not of value in the recumbent infant, as the resonance elicited is from the mattress!
v Auscultation:

   a. Harsh bronchial breath sounds over the whole chest are normal in infancy, and in the midclavicular zone in early childhood.
   b. Coarse crackles (crepitations) close to the stethoscope are due to secretions in the bronchi, and often confused with referred sounds from the pharynx which are as if 'at a distance'. Both can also be felt by the palpating hands.
   c. Fine crackles are fluid in the alveoli. Heard in pneumonia, with oedema fluid, and respiratory distress syndrome.
   d. Wheeze: narrowing of the trachea and main bronchi, by inflammation or dynamic airway compression (see above).

UPPER RESPIRATORY TRACT

Improvements in health and health care have resulted in a decline in suppurative middle ear disease, and an increase in concern of the cause and effects of secretory otitis media on behaviour and speech development.

Examination of ears, nose and throat

1. Ears

i Shape: small, round, absent lobes in Down's syndrome.
ii Low set ears = below a horizontal line drawn from the outer angle of the eye, e.g. trisomies 13, 18, 21. In renal agenesis they may also be large and floppy.
iii Between the mouth and the tragus: congenital fistulae, papillomata due to first branchial arch (FBA) maldevelopments. Conductive or sensorineural deafness is a recognized association of the FBA syndrome.
iv Mastoid for swelling and tenderness in otitis media.

Table 12.2 Relation of age to infectious respiratory illness

Age	Illness	Bacteria	Viruses
Neonatal	Pneumonia	*E. coli* ++++ Pseudomonas +++ Group B haemolytic streptococci +++	Respiratory syncitial virus (RSV) +++
Infancy	Pneumonia	Pneumococcus ++++ *Staph. aureus* ++ Chlamydia trachomatis +	Para-influenza, influenza and RSV all ++++ Measles +++ Adenovirus ++ Coxsackie ++
	Bronchiolitis		RSV ++++
	Wheeze related viral infection		RSV ++++. Rhino–, para–influenza, Adeno–, influenza viruses all ++
Preschool	Laryngotracheitis		Para-influenza ++++ Influenza, RSV +++
	Epiglottitis	*Haemophilus influenze* +++	Para-influenza, Influenza Adeno–, RSV all ++++
	Asthma	Mycoplasma pneumoniae ++	Rhino–, RSV, Para– influenza all ++++
	Pneumonia	Pneumococcus ++++ β-haemolytic strep. + *Haemophilius influenzae* +	RSV, Para–influenza, influenza, all ++++
School age	Pneumonia	Pneumococcus ++++ *Mycoplasma pneumoniae* +++	RSV, Para–influenza, influenza all +++
All ages	Otitis media, coryza, pharyngitis	Pneumococcus ++++ Group A β-haem. strep +++ *Haemophilus influenzae* +++	RSV, adeno–, rhino– para–influenza, influenza etc all ++++

Examination of the tympanic membrane (TM)

i Demonstrate procedure to the small child on parent or doll.

ii Invite the child to hold the auriscope jointly with examiner, encouraging trust and a feeling of control.

iii Best view obtained: infant – pull ear lobe downwards.
child – pull pinna up and back.

Common findings

Grey drum, cone of light reflex = normal.
Dull grey + retracted (malleus is pulled in, and retracts posteriorly)
= blocked eustachian tube.
Dull grey, bulging +/– bubbles or fluid level = secretory otitis media.
Pink around rim of TM   = crying.

Uniformly red	= acute otitis media.
Dark, almost black	= impending perforation or blood behind the TM.
Black hole	= perforation.
Bullae on TM (unusual)	= *Mycoplasma pneumoniae*.

2. Nose

  i Shape examples: snub nose in the fetal alcohol syndrome, saddle in Down's syndrome, beak-like in craniofacial dysostosis e.g. Crouzon's disease: oxycephaly, exophthalmos, exotropia, optic atrophy, beak nose, prominent mandible.
 ii Flaring of nostrils in fever, acidosis, asthma, pneumonia, acute abdomen, pain.
iii Discharge: whether purulent, blood stained and unilateral in foreign body obstruction or choanal atresia.
 iv Internal inspection using an auriscope.

   a. Look for nasal septum deviation (common), and at the mucosa which is often pale and swollen in allergic rhinitis.
   b. Scars/ulcers in Little's area due to nose picking and bleeds.
   c. Polyps associated with sinusitis, allergic rhinitis, and also cystic fibrosis. A sweat test is called for.

3. Mouth

See tonsilitis and pharyngitis, and gastrointestinal tract for other abnormalities found on examination.

Causes of acute cough

1. Acute infections

  i Upper respiratory tract infection (URTI): coryza, tonsillitis, pharyngitis.
 ii Laryngitis, epiglottitis.
iii Lower respiratory tract: bronchiolitis, bronchitis, pneumonia.

2. Asthma, wheezy baby syndrome.
3. Pertussis, and pertussis like, e.g. adenovirus, parainfluenza, chlamydia.
4. Foreign body.

Coryza

Usually viral, may be a prodrome to measles or pertussis.

Clinical

Sneezing, nasal discharge, sore throat.
Includes febrile 'cold' with systemic upset.
Duration 1–2 weeks. Sinusitis, otitis media common bacterial complications.

Management

1. *Infants* Treat impaired feeding with 0.9% saline nose drops or topical decongestant 0.5% ephedrine/0.025% oxymetazoline nose drops, and painful distension of the TM with paracetamol elixir, for 2–5 days only; longer may lead to rebound vasodilatation (pseudoephedrine orally may cause hallucinations and is of little value).

2. *Older ages* Paracetamol for fever, consider cough suppressants (e.g. codeine linctus paediatric has a place if it is keeping the child and family awake at night). Antibiotics are only indicated for complications. Antihistamines cause drowsiness, and have no objective benefit.

Tonsillitis

Usually viral (see table).
   Swollen, red tonsils, often with exudate, fever, sore throat and cough.
   The only reliable sign is a red flush on the medial side of the anterior faucal pillars.
   Streptococcal infection is also characterized by high fever, vomiting, cervical lymphdenopathy and pinpoint haemorrhages on the soft palate and fauces.

Pharyngitis

Erythema of pharynx and tonsils, otherwise indistinguishable from tonsillitis.

Differential diagnosis

- Commonly influenza, adenovirus, the prodrome of measles (look for Koplik's spots).
- Glandular fever has a white membrane +/- purpuric spots at the junction of hard and soft palate, adenovirus a yellow exudate.
- Part of the presentation of scarlet fever or typhoid fever.
- Herpangina (coxsackie A) is uncommon: small vesicles surrounded by a red margin on the fauces; they burst and become tiny ulcers. It affects all ages, with high fever and lasts 3–6 days. Not to be confused with hand-foot-and mouth syndrome (coxsackie A 16), which has vesicles on the tongue and buccal mucosae, backs of the hands, buttocks, and occasionally palms and soles.
- Diphtheria is rare, has a characteristic ulceration and grey web-like membrane which bleeds if its removal is attempted, foul smell, and 'bull neck' swelling of cervical glands.

- An easily removed tonsillar membrane is found in Vincent's angina. Do viral and bacterial culture of swabs and microscopic and bacterial examination of membrane tissue.
- Isolation of *N. gonorrhoeae* is highly suggestive of sexual abuse.
- Acute lymphatic leukaemia and agranulocytosis may present similarly, so a blood film, Paul Bunell or Monospot test is done in appropriate cases.
- Candidiasis in an older infant or child, +/- parotid swelling in HIV.

Management

Paracetamol, fluids. Penicillin for 10 days if streptococcal infection is clinically likely. Swabs for confirmation in uncomplicated tonsillitis or pharyngitis are not cost effective and cause delays.

A reduction in rheumatic fever may have resulted from the indiscriminate use of penicillin, but problems of allergy, diarrhoea and unrealistic expectations in the treatment of upper respiratory infection have ensued.

Diphtheria needs intubation, antitoxin (after testing first for sensitivity to horse serum), penicillin i.v., bed rest and serial ECGs for early recognition of potentially fatal myocarditis.

Otitis media

Prevalence

Two out of 3 children by 3 years, 1 in 3 of them having 3 or more. Peak at 6–36 months, declines after 6 years.

Factors

Poverty, day care/institutionalized, male, underlying abnormality, e.g. cleft palate.

Caused by URT viruses and bacteria; important bacteria are *Streptococcus pneumoniae* (30%), *Branhamella catarrhalis* and group A β-haemolytic Streptococcus (20% each), *Haemophilus influenzae*, *Staphylococcus aureus* (5% each).

Clinical

Severe ear pain during an URTI, with fever, hearing loss, and bright red bulging drum.

Infants may scream with pain, pull at the ear, and have constitutional upset.

Myringitis bullosa is a bleb on the TM caused by *Mycoplasma pneumoniae*.

Spontaneous or therapeutic perforation with release of pus relieves pain. Mastoiditis is rare.

Management

    i Antibiotic: Penicillin orally, or parenterally for 1–2 days if very ill, for a total of 7–10 days. Ampicillin has theoretical advantages, not proven clinically, but is worth changing to if no improvement occurs after 1–2 days. Alternatives in penicillin allergy are erythromycin or co-trimoxazole.

ii Antipyretic/analgesic, e.g. paracetamol.
iii Decongestants, local and systemic, and antihistamines, are all of unproven value but often given.
iv Myringotomy for persistent pain and fever, and a bulging drum; rarely necessary, but allows the culture of pus and selection of the most appropriate antibiotic.

Recurrent acute otitis media including the use of grommets

Prevalence

About 30% of children have 3 or more recurrences. If pain is severe, or hearing loss >40 dB persists more than 3–4 months, grommets may be inserted; they are usually extruded after 6–12 months. Tympanosclerosis, with permanently impaired hearing, is a complication of repeated (usually >3) insertion.

Controversy

Although effective in the short term, with improved behaviour, concentration and education, there is little difference in these outcomes from the unoperated on prolonged follow-up.

Beware

Cholesteatoma is likely where an offensive smelling, thin, chronic discharge from a postero-superior or attic perforation (may be difficult to see) is detected.

Secretory otitis media (SOM)

Prevalence

Affects up to 40% at 1 year, falling to 15% by 6 years.

Pathophysiology

Related to, but not necessarily caused by, infection, and eustachian tube malfunction (regularly in cleft palate, Down's syndrome). Negative middle ear pressure develops, and increased secretion from the lining cells of a fluid–thin, or thick and viscid, grey or amber. The TM has impaired mobility and hence conductive deafness is common.

Risk factors include mouth breathing, institutionalization, deprivation, and passive smoking.

Clinical

The TM may be bulging, showing bubbles of fluid behind the drum, or be retracted.

Behaviour disturbance, (often due to deafness and subsequent frustration in communication), slow speech development, and intermittent deafness are each complained of and can be identified.

Investigation

1. Tympanometry is a test of mobility of the TM, using positive and negative air pressure transmitted via a snugly fitting ear piece. It requires no patient cooperation.
2. Free field testing using an audiometer, emitting pure tones, screens hearing.
   See Deafness for illustrations of 1 and 2.

The Rinné test (bone better than air conduction) is a simple if not wholly reliable screen for SOM producing >30 dB loss. Applicable in cooperative children over 5 years old.

Management

    i Decongestants, antihistamines and antibiotics are of uncertain value. However, nose blowing is important, as negative middle ear pressures are induced by sniffing.

   ii Persistent symptomatic bilateral deafness: grommet insertion (adenoidectomy at the same time may reduce the number of reinsertions). Swimming with grommets in situ is now permitted by most surgeons, providing precautions (ear plugs and swim cap worn, no diving) are taken.

  iii Check that hearing improves after (ii), otherwise a hearing aid for persistent conductive or previously unsuspected sensorineural loss may be required.

Indications for adenoidectomy and tonsillectomy

An appreciation that the tonsils are physiologically large in early childhood with a peak at 6–8 years has resulted in a reduction in unnecessary operations.

Opinion at present favours:

    i Selective adenoidectomy with insertion of grommets for repeated otitis media or serous otitis media causing persistent deafness with impairment of development or education. Contraindicated in bifid uvula or submucous cleft, because of the danger of postoperative palatopharyngeal incompetence.

   ii Tonsillectomy – absolute indications:

       a. Obstructive sleep apnoea. Night time waking, coupled with day time somnolence. Parents note sudden cessation of snoring as the airway becomes obstructed by too large tonsils causing acute hypoxia. Commoner in Pierre Robin and Down's syndromes and the over 18 months old.

          Operationally defined as apnoeas of 10 s each, 30/h in 7 h of sleep.

          Hypoxia and hypercapnia lead to pulmonary hypertension, and finally to cor pulmonalae.

          Adenotonsillectomy is urgently indicated.

b. After a quinsy (some argue this is only a relative indication).

iii Tonsillectomy, relative indications:

a. More than 3 *severe* episodes of tonsillitis per year for 2 years.
b. 5 episodes in 1 year with significant loss of schooling.
c. Recurrent otitis media.

Parents should be informed that the operation improves 60% of cases only. Those with simple repeated upper respiratory infections, allergies, etc should be dissuaded.

Further reading

Grundfast K M (1989) Recent advances in paediatric otolaryngology. *Pediatric Clinics of North America* **36**, number 6
Maw A R (1991) Developments in ear, nose and throat surgery. In *Recent Advances in Paediatrics 9*, (T J David ed) Edinburgh:Churchill Livingstone pp. 93–108

Chronic upper respiratory conditions

Causes of chronic cough

(Typical presentations and management discussed under individual conditions.)

1. Postnasal drip (some authorities doubt this is a clinical entity!): repeated coryza, allergic rhinitis, vasomotor rhinitis, sinusitis. Especially on being exposed to new pathogens by commencing school.
2. Asthma: may be the only symptom–after exercise, or at night.
3. Infection: viral (causing bronchitis in preschool and school ages), tuberculous glands (rare), *Mycoplasma pneumoniae*.
4. Unknown: a large group, possibly post viral.
5. Post-pertussis: usually early childhood.
6. Foreign body.
7. Recurrent aspiration syndromes of early infancy, with feeding and then vomiting.
8. Cystic fibrosis or lung collapse, rarely immotile cilia (Kartegener's syndrome).
9. Extrinsic compression of the trachea or bronchus by enlarged heart, glands, or tumour.
10. Smokers cough and psychogenic cough in adolescence.

Allergic rhinitis

Prevalence   10% of children.

Clinical   Sneeze, rhinitis, and itchy nose causing 'allergic salute' by rubbing the nose with the back of the hand, nasal voice, snoring, halitosis. Aggravated by smoking, or paint fumes.

Investigations   See Immune problems for discussion of the rationale of allergy testing.

1. If suspected by history, skin prick testing may identify the cause.

    i   House dust mite, animal danders (perennial).
    ii   Moulds (perennial + atmospheric changes).
    iii   Pollens (seasonal: trees in spring, grasses in summer).

2. IgE and radioallergosorbent tests (RAST) are less specific, more expensive. Nasal provocation tests are rarely required.

Diagnosis   History confirmed by investigations, or exclusion of the allergen. Alternatively, empirically by the response to prophylaxis. *Vasomotor rhinitis* is a diagnosis of exclusion, when no allergen is found or prophylaxis proves ineffective. Systemic nasal decongestants (pseudoephedrine) may help and submucous diathermy works.

Management
1. Avoid the allergen, e.g. cat. Removal may be warranted, but the response is delayed as it takes at least 2 months finally to remove animal danders from the home.
2. Medication: duration as indicated by symptoms.

    i   Acute: decongestants for 5 days (longer may produce rebound hyperaemia).
    ii   Acute or persistent: antihistamine, e.g. terfenadine.
    iii   Prophylaxis: local application of sodium cromoglycate 4–6 × daily or beclamethasone 2–3 × daily.

3. Anaphylaxis may follow hyposensitizing injections, which are therefore rarely warranted.

Chronic sinusitis

Definition   More than 3 weeks nasal obstruction and discharge, and postnasal drip manifest by laryngitis and cough night>day, often with a headache in older children.

Predisposing conditions   Allergy, cystic fibrosis, Down's syndrome, immotile cilia syndrome, immune disorders.
    Local factors: foreign body, deviated nasal septum, polyps, trauma, swimming, nasal decongestants, infected teeth.

Investigation   X-ray confirmation = sinus opacification, air-fluid level, mucosal thickening about 0.5 cm or more.

Management
1. Humidification, decongestants for 3–5 days only, amoxicillin or co-trimoxazole for 2–3 weeks, plus an antihistamine in allergic cases.
2. Antral puncture and wash out if no improvement in 5–6 weeks in maxillary sinusitis.

The neck

Presentation for assessment of a mass in the neck is common, pits or fistulae relatively uncommon. The precise anatomical site is a useful guide (Figures 12.2 and 12.3).

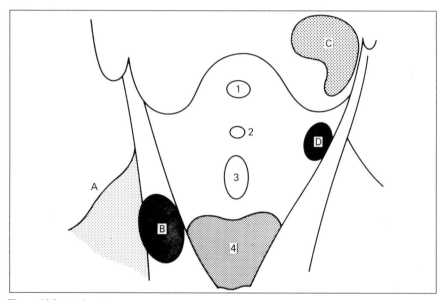

Figure 12.2 Anterior view:
Midline
1 = Submandibular lymph gland.
2 = Dermoid cyst, attatched to the skin, not the deeper structures like a thyroglossal cyst, number 3.
3 = Thyroglossal cyst, moves upwards on tongue protrusion.
4 = The thyroid gland moves upward on swallowing, distinguishing it from upper mediastinal glands that remain fixed.
Lateral
A = cystic hygroma.
B = sternomastoid tumour.
C = Parotid gland.
D = Jugulo–digastric gland.

Cervical adenitis

1. Shotty cervical glands, with some fluctuation in size noted by parents, is common and normal.

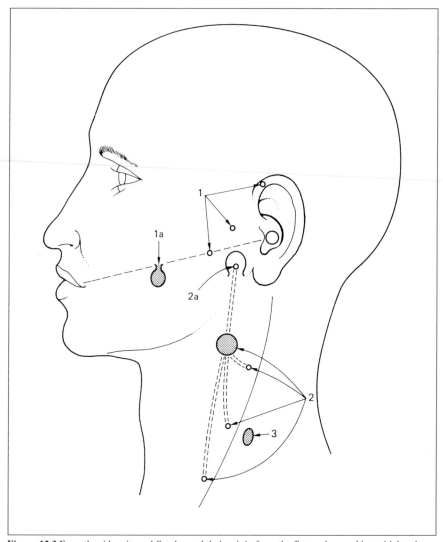

Figure 12.3 From the side, pits and fistulae and their origin from the first and second branchial arches and pharyngeal pouches.
1 = First arch preauricular pits, and the area where they commonly occur together with 1a = first arch skin tag, along the line between the auricle and angle of the mouth.
2 = Branchial cyst and external fistulous openings, anterior to the sternomastoid.
2a= Fistulous internal opening through the tonsil.
3 = Branchial remnant.

2. Painful enlarging gland with fever occurs with suppurative lymphadenitis. Streptococcal infection is most likely. Consider Kawasaki disease.
3. Lymphadenopathy with intermittent fever in viral infections (infectious mononucleosis, adenovirus, cat scratch virus) and psittacosis.
4. Association with eczema, Still's disease, drugs, serum sickness.

5. Progressive enlargement suggests a tuberculous gland, or atypical mycobacter. If tuberculin test is positive and the gland fluctuant remove it surgically and treat.
6. Supraclavicular glands with progressive enlargement over 3 weeks require Mantoux, ESR, FBC and biopsy for malignancy (typically leukaemia, lymphoma, occasionally metastases).

Further reading

Bain J, Carter P, Morton R (1985) *Colour Atlas of Mouth, Throat, and Ear Disorders in Children*. Lancaster: MTP Press (Simple, useful illustrations)
Isaacs D (1987) Why do children get colds? In *Progress in Child Health*, (J A Macfarlane, ed) **3**, pp. 38–46. Edinburgh: Churchill Livingstone

Nose bleeds

Common in mid-childhood, usually from Little's area.
    History of bleeding, or of family members with bleeding tendencies, should be asked for.
Common causes:

1. Trauma, nose picking, (bleeding is aggravated by low humidity).
2. Infection.
3. Allergic rhinitis: chronic nasal discharge, inflamed mucosa.
4. Foreign body: unilateral, purulent/serosanguinous discharge.
5. Bleeding disorders, vascular abnormality.
6. Tumours (rare).

Investigations

Visual inspection, FBC including platelets, and coagulation if appropriate.

Management

1. Applying 'clothes-peg' constriction of the anterior nares between thumb and first finger for 15 minutes is almost invariably effective unless an underlying clotting or vascular abnormality is present.
2. Continued/recurrent bleeding: chemical cautery, followed by electrocautery if unsuccessful.

Stridor

Definition

  i Obstruction to the larynx or upper trachea causing a predominantly inspiratory noise. Stridor predominantly on expiration is suggestive of subglottic narrowing.
 ii Croup is a 'brassy' cough +/- stridor due to acute infection.

Causes of acute stridor

1. Acute laryngotracheobronchitis.
2. Epiglottitis.
3. Foreign body.
4. Measles, glandular fever.
5. Rare but important: diphtheria, retropharyngeal abscess, acute angioneurotic oedema, laryngeal burns.

Indications for intubation

1. Rising pulse and respirations, restlessness and cyanosis = hypoxia.
2. Progressive exhaustion manifest by quieter breath sounds, and shallower respirations.

   Generally blood gas analysis plays no part in management.

Table 12.3 Features of epiglottitis, laryngotracheobronchitis (LTB) and foreign body above the carina

	Epiglottitis	LTB	Foreign body
Age	2–7 years	1–3 years	>6 months–4 years
History	Hours	1–2 days of coryza	Sudden onset, act of inhalation may be missed
Appearance	Pale, toxic, shock Sits, propped on hands behind, neck extended	Anxious/lethargic	Normal
Fever	+++(>38.5 C)	+	0
Voice	Hoarse, weak	Hoarse	May be aphonic
Cough	+	++	+++
Drooling, dysphagia	+++	0	0
Respirations	Laboured	Increased	Variable
Hypoxia	Frequent	Unusual	Variable
Epiglottis	Swollen, cherry red	Inflamed larynx, trachea	
X-ray of neck	Large epiglottis	Normal	May see opaque FB
X-ray of chest	Normal	Inflammatory changes in 50%	If FB moves below carina, lung or lobe may overinflate or collapse
Blood culture	+ve	0	0
Intubated	60–80%	1%	?

Airway assessment and management. Dos and don'ts

1. Epiglottitis

    i Intubation for 1–2 days is the mainstay of treatment so admit to an intensive care unit immediately. To buy time, give nebulized adrenaline, 1 ml of 1 in 1000, diluted to 3 ml, effective for up to 30 minutes.

    ii If the child is well enough, X-rays may be obtained en route, but he must be accompanied at all times by resuscitation equipment and a competent physician.

    iii Avoid excessive handling, leave putting up a drip and blood taking until the airway is secure, unless the child is not distressed or has collapsed already.

iv Acute laryngospasm and complete obstruction may follow pharyngeal stimulation so inspection of the oropharynx should only be done by experienced anaesthetic/paediatric staff as part of the intubation procedure. (An ENT surgeon should be on hand for emergency tracheostomy.) Proceed as follows:

    a. Inhalation anaesthesia without the use of paralysing agents. The larynx may be so swollen that the only evidence of the airway is bubbles of air produced during the child's spontaneous breathing, which is abolished by paralysis.

    b. Oropharyngeal tube is used initially, and changed for a nasoendotracheal tube after secretions have been sucked out and satisfactory ventilation secured.

    c. Antibiotics: ampicillin resistant strains dictate the need for combining it (400 mg/kg/day) with chloramphenicol (100 mg/kg/day) or using a third generation cephalosporin (cefotaxime 100 mg/kg/day) alone, for 5 days.

    d. Extubation 24–48 h later is usually possible. Depending on patient compliance, minimal sedation enables sitting up, and encourages spontaneous coughing to clear secretions.

2. Laryngotracheobronchitis

A progressive spread of the inflammatory process down the respiratory tree, due usually to viral infection. Only 1% of hospitalized cases require intubation.

Clinical

  i Coryza → laryngitis → croupy cough.

 ii Tracheitis: onset of inspiratory stridor after 1–2 days, worse at night.

iii Bronchitis: respiratory effort increases as infection spreads down the bronchial tree.

Sternal indrawing seen, wheeze and coarse crackles heard.

Diagnostic confusion with epiglottitis occurs in the more severe, rapidly deteriorating cases, when the strictures regarding pharyngeal examination in epiglottitis must also apply.

Investigation X-ray of the nasopharynx distinguishes it from epiglottitis.

Management

  i Mist. Although popular with parents, it is of unproven value.

 ii In hospital: minimal disturbance, parental presence for reassurance; oxygen for hypoxia via face mask or nasal prongs, if tolerated, with close clinical observation for further deterioration.

iii Progressive hypoxia needs intubation as for epiglottitis. Adrenaline via a nebulizer has a temporary effect, but is useful while arranging intensive care.

iv No antibiotics are necessary. Steroids advocated by some.

Duration of illness usually 2–3 days, occasionally 2–3 weeks.

Recurrent croup is characterized by a barking, metallic cough, and may follow LTB.

Characterized by mild URTI, followed by sudden onset of croup at night. The child is afebrile and anxious. Better by the next morning.

Often familial, asthma may follow.

3. Foreign body

Infants and toddlers eating hamburgers, ice lollies, small plastic toys, coins, pins etc; older children inhale peanuts, beans, seeds (Table 12.4).

Table 12.4 Characteristics of foreign body inhalation

Level of obstruction	Timing of onset	Symptoms
Laryngeal/tracheal		
i mechanical obstruction	Immediate	Cough
a. large, e.g. coin		Stridor, aphonia, dyspnoea,
b. oedema: small, sharp object		cyanosis
(e.g. egg shell, pin).		
ii Chemical inflammation due to	Hours to days	Wheeze or pneumonia
vegetable fibres, e.g. beans		
Lower respiratory tract	Hours, days, weeks	Wheeze, unresolved infection
obstruction, inert material, e.g.		or lung collapse, chronic cough
smooth plastic or metal,		and haemoptysis
roasted peanut, grass seed		

Management   Any history of choking, cough +/– cyanosis requires laryngoscopy and bronchoscopy.

1. On chest X-ray the FB may be opaque.
2. X-rays on full inspiration and expiration may show a persistently hyperinflated lobe if the FB acts as a ball valve obstruction.
3. These films may be impossible to obtain in small children, who should then be screened. Lung or lobar collapse with swinging of the mediastinum, or splinting of a diaphragm leaf due to ball valve obstruction, may then be seen when not previously visible on X-ray.

Management of other causes of acute stridor

Measles and glandular fever are unlikely to cause serious airway obstruction and can be managed conservatively.

Intubation to secure the airway must be considered in the following:

1. Anaphylaxis and angio-oedema (the latter usually shows as generalized swelling)

Due to allergen exposure in a sensitised child or family with C1-esterase inhibitor deficiency.

i Clear airway. Lay child flat, legs elevated.
ii Give oxygen.
iii Drugs

a. Administer subcutaneous (or deep intramuscular if shocked) adrenaline 10 μg/kg or 0.1–0.2 ml of 1/1000, and i.v. chlorpheniramine 5–10 mg.
b. Repeat adrenaline in 15 minutes if no response, and give aminophylline 5 mg/kg over 10 minutes, continuing the infusion at 1 mg/kg/h. Steroids are not helpful in the acute situation, though i.v. hydrocortisone 100–200 mg is often given.

2. Laryngeal burns

Presumed present if soot is seen in the nostrils after a house fire.

3. Retropharyngeal abscess (rare)

Infants present with fever, drooling, neck hyperextension and a bulge of the posterior pharyngeal wall, pressing on the larynx. Danger of aspiration if it bursts, or erosion of the carotid artery. Incise under anaesthesia. Penicillin and flucloxacillin cover Group A β–haemolytic streptococcus and *Staphylococcus aureus*, the common pathogens.

4. Diphtheria (exceedingly rare)

See pharyngitis and infectious diseases.

Further reading

Kilham H, Gillis J G, Benjamin B. (1987) Severe upper airway obstruction. *Pediatric Clinics of North America*, **34**, 1–14

Causes of chronic stridor

1. Airway narrowing above the larynx:

i Tonsillar hypertrophy.
ii Tongue: Pierre Robin sequence, haemangioma.

2. Small or infantile larynx ('laryngomalacia').
3. Intraluminal narrowing at larynx and below:

i Subglottic or tracheal stenosis, haemangioma, cysts, laryngeal web, laryngeal cleft.
ii Vocal cord paralysis: raised intracranial pressure, recurrent laryngeal nerve damage.
iii Papillomata.

4. Compression of larynx or trachea:

    i Vascular ring.
   ii Tumour, cystic hygroma, retrosternal goitre.

Investigation of chronic stridor

Indicated for persistent stridor or onset after 6 weeks old lasting >2 weeks. Not indicated for recurrent croup from URTI.

1. Barium swallow (see vascular ring), X-rays of neck for cysts, goitre, mediastinal masses.
2. Laryngoscopy with a light anaesthetic, or even none, to watch for vocal cord paralysis or the sucking into the airway of the folds of a small larynx.
3. Bronchoscopy if the lesion is likely to be below the cords, e.g. subglottic stenosis, haemangioma (like a cavernous haemangioma in the skin, it grows in the first 1–3 months, then slowly regresses by 2–5 years old).

Infantile larynx

Commonest cause of persistent inspiratory stridor in infancy.

Pathophysiology Disproportionately small larynx, its walls are sucked inwards more than usual, but there is no pathological softening of cartilage.

Clinical Appears aged 1–4 weeks, worse with URTI and crying, varies with posture. Micrognathia and Harrison's sulci are associated.

Investigation Confirm on direct laryngoscopy an omega shaped, anteriorly placed, small larynx, whose opening becomes slit-like on inspiration.

Prognosis Rarely obstructs, improved by 1 year, gone by 3 years.

Subglottic stenosis

Congenital, and acquired following prolonged intubation for respiratory support in extreme prematurity, just below the true cords.
    Presents as croup if mild, or inspiratory and expiratory stridor if more severe.
    Laryngoscopy confirms. Avoid intubation, which may make matters worse; avoid surgery as widening occurs with growth.

Recurrent respiratory papillomatosis

Papilloma virus 6 and 11 infection found in the preschool age group. It may be acquired, at delivery, from maternal anal warts. Extends from the larynx downwards. Endoscopic removal, using CO_2 laser, repeated as often as necessary. Tracheostomy may be necessary. Lung parenchymal involvement rare, but may cause death.

Vascular ring

Due to embryonic remnants of the paired aortic arches encircling the oesophagus and trachea, and compressing the trachea between them. Tracheal stenosis is a common association.

Clinical
Persistent brassy cough and wheeze in early infancy.

Diagnose by a barium swallow to show indentation of the oesophagus by the aorta, and with a plain X-ray of the trachea, the aberrant vessel compressing the tracheal air column.

Acute cyanotic attacks/cot death 'near miss'

Finding a cyanosed infant or one in a pale, collapsed state, is not uncommon.

Exclusion of aspiration, acute infection (septicaemia, respiratory tract, meningitis), and consideration of intussusception, dehydration, or seizures, is mandatory. Metabolic problems, e.g. hypoglycaemia or inborn errors, may be evident from the initial investigations.

Repeated cyanotic or apnoeic episodes without obvious cause engender considerable parental (and medical) anxiety. Mechanisms proposed include:

1. Gastro-oesophageal reflux (also implicated in recurrent wheeze and stridor in infancy, but inconclusively). Not consistently demonstrated by oesophageal pH monitoring, but may be a cause in some cases.
2. Cardiac irregularity or vasovagal stimulation 'breath holding attacks' leading to hypotension and hypoxia.
3. Intrapulmonary shunting, associated with prolonged expiratory apnoea. Said to be provoked by emotion, pain, and cough, and also described as 'breath holding attacks'. No bradycardia or ECG abnormalities are found. A postulated precursor to sudden infant death syndrome, but controversy surrounds the original cases described (see reference).

Investigation   In addition to those on admission, continuous monitoring of heart rate and blood oxygen level for 24 h. In selected cases, barium swallow, oesophageal pH, or ECG and echocardiography.

Management
1. Monitoring at home with apnoea monitor or pulse oximeter or transcutaneous oxygen monitor. Parents should be instructed in basic resuscitation.
2. Antireflux posture and alginate or cisapride may be worthy of trial.

Further reading

Simpson H, Hampton F (1991) Gastro-oesophageal reflux and the lung. *Archives of Disease in Childhood*, **66**, 277–279
Stephenson J B P (1991) Blue breath holding is benign. *Archives of Disease in Childhood*, **66**, 255-257. Attacks the intrapulmonary shunt hypothesis, see associated articles.

LOWER RESPIRATORY TRACT PROBLEMS

Radiological changes – causes to consider

A. *Recurrent or persistent lung field infiltrates and consolidation*

1. Infection: partially treated bacterial infection, TB, mycoplasma, psittacosis, pertussis, cytomegalovirus, Loffler's syndrome, *Pneumocystis carinii*.
2. Asthma.
3. Aspiration.
4. Foreign body.
5. Left to right cardiac shunt causing recurrent pneumonia.
6. Cystic fibrosis, bronchiectasis.
7. Malignancy: leukaemia (associated infection), lymphoma (recurrent infection and primary process), secondary deposit (nodular), Langerhan's cell histiocytosis (honeycomb).
8. Drug toxicity, e.g. nitrofurantoin, methotrexate.
9. Congenital: lobar sequestration (basal, in contact with the diaphragm), congenital lung cysts.
   Helpful pointers:
   - A history of previous similar episodes (asthma, cystic fibrosis).
   - Recurrent, persistent cough and breathing difficulties, perhaps despite antibiotic (infection, inhalation, congenital).
   - Vomiting/swallowing difficulties (aspiration), inhalation, ingestion of drugs, or findings of generalized/local suspicious lymphadenopathy or masses (malignancy).
   - A pansystolic murmur on auscultation.

B. *Asymmetry of lungfield transradiancy*

Increased transradiancy

(A rotated chest X-ray makes interpretation difficult.)

1. Compensatory hyperinflation due to ipsilateral partial collapse or contralateral collapse in which case the contralateral lung is more opaque than usual.
2. Pneumothorax.
3. Lobar emphysema: foreign body, bronchial compression, congenital.
4. Lung cysts, pneumatoceles.
5. Bronchiolitis obliterans is included in MacLeod's syndrome of absent lung (post Adenovirus or M. pneumoniae infection).

Opaque hemithorax

1. Pneumonia.
2. Aspiration.
3. Complete collapse of a lung.

4. Pleural effusion, empyema.
5. Haemothorax.
6. Diaphragmatic hernia, pulmonary agenesis.
7. Massive tumour.
8. Chylothorax:
    post traumatic/surgery.
    malignant obstruction.

Congenital abnormalities of the lung presenting as asymmetry in transradiancy

1. Lobar emphysema   due to deficiency in bronchial wall cartilage, usually in an upper lobe, creates a ball valve obstruction, hyperinflation of the lobe and compression of the surrounding lung.
   Presentation is usually neonatal with wheeze and respiratory distress, occasionally later, or may be asymptomatic.

2. Lung cysts-pulmonary, bronchogenic (lined with bronchial epithelium, usually mediastinal in position).
   Presentation: (i) Compress surrounding lung tissue or bronchi, have rounded margins, may be fluid filled. (ii) Often become infected. (iii) Pneumothorax occasionally.

Lobar sequestration is intralobular, multicystic, not connected to the bronchial tree, and with systemic blood supply, in contact with the diaphragm, left>>right lower lobe; occasionally the lobe is outside lungs.
   Presentation: cough, unresolved pneumonia, or incidental finding on chest x-ray. A CT demonstrates the consolidation +/- cavitation, and abnormal blood supply.

3. Diaphragmatic hernia usually presents in the newborn period, and is due to a failure of closure of (usually) the left pleuroperitoneal canal (90% cases) in the 10th week of embryonic life. The intestines in the chest prevent normal lung growth. See Neonatal problems for presentation and management.

Treatment: Surgery indicated for most cysts, even if not causing symptoms as they may well develop subsequently. Exclude staphylococcal infection, and hydatid disease in older children.

Pneumothorax

(Also see Neonatal problems.)

1. Trauma to chest wall or oesophagus, and surgery.
2. Assisted positive pressure ventilation.
3. Asthma.
4. Pneumonia with empyema, especially staphylococcal.
5. Cystic fibrosis (usually in adolescence).
6. Marfan's syndrome, Ehlers-Danlos syndrome.

7. Adolescent idiopathic pneumothorax.
8. Congenital lung cysts (see above).

Clinical presentation and management   Often sudden deterioration, unsuspected to be due to pneumothorax. Pain, breathless, cyanosis. Chest X-ray is definitive.

1. A small pneumothorax (<5%) may be left to reabsorb spontaneously, aided by breathing 100% oxygen.
2. Otherwise insert an intercostal drain connected to an underwater seal and apply continuous negative pressure (CNP) at 10 cm H_2O. 1–3 days of CNP are usually required for it to seal off.
3. Treat the underlying condition, give adequate analgesia, avoid respiratory depression.

Mediastinal masses (Figure 12.4)

Anterior

1 Lymph nodes:
   TB, leukaemia.
   lymphoma
2 Thymus: normal, tumour.
3 Goitre.
4 Dermoid.
5 Cystic hygroma.

Middle

6 Lymph nodes:
7 Bronchogenic cyst.
8 Post stenotic dilation of pulmonary artery (anterior) and aorta (posterior).
9 Pericardial fluid.

Posterior

10 Achalasia.
11 Duplication.
12 Anterior meningocele.
13 Paraspinal tumour:
   neuroblastoma
   ganglioneuroma
14 Hiatus hernia

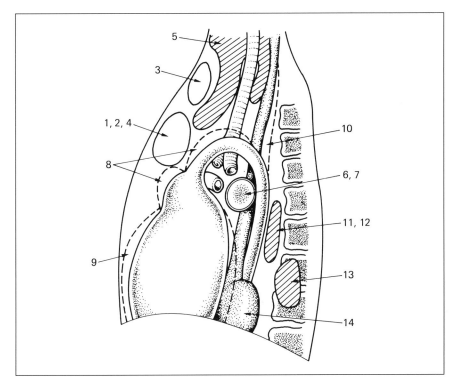

Figure 12.4 Mediastinal masses

Investigations are aimed at the particular part of the mediastinum. They include Tuberculin test, blood count and bone marrow, CT for cysts and tumours, spinal X-rays or MRI for enlarged intervertebral foramina or TB of a vertebral body; barium swallow for oesophageal disorders; thyroid scan for goitre; US for pericardial cyst; urinary catecholamines for neural crest tumours. Bronchoscopy, and thoracotomy may follow.

Wheeze in the first year

Important causes:

1. Acute bronchiolitis.
2. Wheezy baby syndrome.
3. Aspiration syndromes.
4. Bronchopulmonary dysplasia.

  Less commonly:
   Foreign body (above).
   Cystic fibrosis.
   Congenital airway or lung abnormality.

Acute Bronchiolitis

Definition

Coryza for a day is followed by persistent cough, breathlessness, hyperinflation of the chest, and expiratory wheeze in a 1 to 6 (up to 12) month old. Fine crackles and cyanosis correlate with severe disease. Respiratory syncitial virus (RSV) is the usual cause, occasionally parainfluenza.

Epidemiology

1. 1–2% of all infants are admitted to hospital with bronchiolitis. Occurs in winter to early spring.
2. Breast feeding and parental avoidance of smoking, each is protective.
3. Underlying congenital abnormality increases morbidity and mortality (see management (iii) below).

Pathology

1. Inflammation of the bronchioles: secretion of mucus, necrosis of ciliated epithelium, and oedema of the submucosa causing airway obstruction.
2. Hyperinflation and patchy segemental collapse of the lung result, not helped by poorly developed collateral ventilation.

Clinical

1. As in the definition. Severe disease manifest as increasingly rapid respirations and cyanosis in air, inability to feed, head bobbing and unresponsiveness. 1% progress to respiratory failure.
2. Apnoea occasionally, especially in prematures.
3. Cardiac failure is unusual (but often considered due to liver depression secondary to lung hyperinflation), and secondary to underlying cardiac disease.

Investigations

1. RSV identified by immunofluorescence of nasopharyngeal secretions using specific viral antisera.
2. Chest X-ray shows square chest, horizontal ribs, hilar streaking, with subsegmental collapse or consolidation in 35%.
3. Blood gases usually show hypoxia. Hypercapnia common, the level occasionally higher than expected clinically.

Differential diagnosis

1. Wheeze related viral infection (a subdivision of which is the wheezy baby syndrome typically in a plump, less distressed, older at 6–12 months baby, chest X-ray less hyperinflated).

2. Asthma is unusual under 12 months, fine crackles are less prominent. The response to bronchodilators is haphazard.
3. Bronchopneumonia may also be caused by RSV, but the infant is more ill, fever >38°C, no wheeze, fine crackles more localized; chest X-ray differentiates.
4. Cystic fibrosis is similar, but may wheeze for prolonged period.
5. Heart failure: has a very rapid pulse, and liver enlargement which can be differentiated from the downward displacement in bronchiolitis by chest X-ray or ultrasound.

Management

1. Admit to hospital if respiratory or feeding difficulties: minimal handling, suction of secretions if copious, feeding i.v. or via nasogastric tube if indicated.
2. Oxygen for pallor or cyanosis, via tent or head box. Assess severity with transcutaneous haemoglobin oxygen saturation (S_aO_2) by pulse oximetry.
3. Drugs: bronchodilators are of unproven benefit under 6 months, but ipratropium bromide inhalation, in the moderately severe, works in 20 minutes, and may help avoid mechanical ventilation. Ribavirin has some activity against RSV, needs a special nebulizer, and is very costly; reserved for the case with a complication, e.g. bronchopulmonary dysplasia, congenital heart disease, cystic fibrosis, immune deficiency. Antibiotics are not often indicated, nor digoxin or diuretics.
4. Mechanical ventilation. Note that elevated P_aCO_2 is common; blood gases are less important than signs of exhaustion, recurrent prolonged apnoea, or cerebral hypoxia, as indicators of need.

Prognosis

Death is rare, and associated with congenital malformations. Recovery occurs in 7–10 days, occasionally longer. Recurrence of wheeze in 50–75% (wheezy baby syndrome). Abnormal lung function tests may persist for years. A family history of atopy is not more likely, nor a tendency to asthma later.

Wheeze related viral infection (early asthma?)

Definition

Wheeze related viral infection (WRVI) is due to acute viral bronchiolitis, and more likely in the overweight baby, with no increased atopic history.

   Impossible to differentiate from asthma initially, but the latter is likely after repeated recurrences, or seen to be responsive to anti-asthma therapy, especially if eczema is present.

Controversy

WRVI is often a retrospective diagnosis, due to its subsiding by 1–2 years, whereas atopic asthma usually develops after this age.

One view of wheezing children under 3 is that they are all asthmatic, the non-atopic representing a subgroup with age-limited increased bronchial responsiveness to a trigger such as viral infections, as in bronchiolitis and WRVI. Others, with an atopic background, also wheeze to the same triggers but develop airway sensitization to aeroallergens, and become classic asthmatics later.

Management

Ipratropium bromide is effective in 40% of wheezy infants. Prophylactic budesonide via a spacer device with a closely fitting face mask reduces the frequency of recurrence, although there are fears of adrenal supression and growth retardation.

Prognosis

Subsides by 1–3 years old.

Further reading

Leader (1989) Inhaled steroids and recurrent wheeze after bronchiolitis *Lancet*, i, 999–1000
Milner A D (1989) Acute bronchiolitis in infancy: treatment and prognosis. *Thorax*, **44**, 1–5
Wilson N M (1989) Wheezy bronchitis revisited. *Archives of Disease in Childhood*, **64**, 1191–1199

Aspiration pneumonitis

Definition

Inhalation of milk, commonly, causing an acute inflammatory reaction within the bronchi.

Pathophysiology (and relative frequency)

1. Mouth: structural abnormality (uncommon) e.g. cleft palate.
2. Tongue and pharyngeal muscles: weakness or incoordination of sucking and swallowing (frequent), e.g. prematurity, cerebral palsy, CNS depression from drugs, epilepsy.
3. Gastro-oesophageal reflux (fairly frequent) from hiatus hernia or persistent vomiting, e.g. pertussis. Rarely due to a motility disorder like achalasia, or Sandifer's syndrome of torticollis and cerebral palsy.
4. Fistulae of oesophagus (rare), e.g. H-type fistula.

Clinical

Symptoms comprise vomiting or regurgitation, apnoea or cough during feeds, or acute cough and wheeze without URTI.

Recurrent aspiration may lead to interstitial pneumonia, secondary bacterial infection, and eventually even bronchiectasis.

Characteristically the baby is 'propped bottle fed' and has right upper lobe involvement on X-ray.

Diagnosis

1. Observe feeding. Evaluate neurology for cerebral palsy and motor weakness.
2. A chest X-ray typically shows inflammatory changes in the upper lobes.
3. Fat laden macrophages in tracheal aspirate likely.
4. Confirmation of reflux by pH studies or barium swallow.

Main differential is the presence of wheeze and fine crackles of asthma due to viral infections. (Reflux of acid into the oesophagus as a precipitant of asthma has not been convincingly demonstrated). Recurrent cough has many causes.

Management

1. Antibiotics, physiotherapy.
2. Treat the underlying disorder by medication or surgery:

   i   Antireflux: thickener (Gaviscon), motility agents (cisapride, domperidone). Stop drugs exacerbating reflux, e.g. theophylline.
   ii Surgery for medical failures (Nissen's fundoplication) and fistulae.

3. Support, e.g. for prematurity, cerebral palsy.

Further reading

Dinwiddie R (1990) Aspiration syndromes. In *The Diagnosis and Management of Paediatric Respiratory Disease*. Edinburgh:Churchill Livingstone pp. 223–235

ASTHMA

Definition

1. Widespread airway narrowing which reverses spontaneously or with treatment, over short periods of time.
2. Clinical triad: cough, dyspnoea and wheeze.
3. Physiological triad: bronchiolar muscle spasm, mucosal oedema and increased mucus production.

Bronchial hyperresponsiveness can often be detected by challenge tests and reflects increased airway responsiveness to a number of environmental stimuli.

Prevalence

1. Atopy. About 30% of adults are atopic. In children atopy includes infantile or flexural eczema, urticaria, hay fever, and asthma. About 70% of asthmatic children are atopic, and 70% of infants with raised IgE in cord blood develop atopic diseases later. See Allergy.

2. Asthma affects 10–15% of the population. Boys are more often affected than girls, but equilibration between the sexes occurs during adolescence.

Increasing prevalence?

Over a 40 year period, a 3–fold rise in the prevalence of asthma (or wheeze labelled as asthma) in preschool children has been reported. In childhood 80% develop symptoms by 5 years old. Community studies confirm underdiagnosis occurs unless the appropriate questions are asked.

Morbidity and mortality

1% of children with asthma are admitted to hospital annually. Status asthmaticus causes 50 child deaths per year in the UK.

Aetiology

1. Constitutional (i.e. predisposition in that individual).
2. Atopy (inherited autosomal dominant with variable expression) = production of IgE antibody to common environmental allergens, especially those that are inhaled.

Both types have a tendency to bronchial hyperresponsiveness induced by precipitants. The commonest are respiratory infection and atopy or allergy.

Pathophysiology of bronchoconstriction

Can be identified as acute and late phases, and chronic changes, each of which acts to produce or perpetuate wheeze.

1. Acute phase onset in minutes = bronchospasm

Trigger stimulus (i) Of IgE antibody by antigen (type I reaction) → histamine and leukotrienes release (bronchoconstrictors from mast cells)
and/or (ii) Increased airway receptor hyperresponsiveness (vagal reflex) → narrowing and shortening of airways.

2. Late phase

Onset 4–6 h, lasting up to 10 days. Initiated by an allergen challenge, and thought to mimic the changes of chronic asthma (predominantly due to inflammation):

  i Mast cells and alveolar macrophages release leukotrienes, prostaglandins, thromboxanes → bronchoconstriction.
 ii Chemotactic factors attracting neutrophil, eosinophil, and macrophage migration, and platelet activating factor → inflammation and oedema of the airways.

iii Chronic changes: damage to respiratory tract epithelium leads to increased bronchial hyperresponsiveness, maintained by the release of bronchoconstrictor substances, or by local axon reflexes through exposed nerve fibres, lasting for days or weeks.

Most have the acute phase (i), and recover within minutes, or a dual reaction of (i) and (ii), i.e. acute bronchospasm in an allergen challenge, with recovery within minutes, then a second episode 3 to 6 hours later which is relatively resistant to β_2-agonists and probably causes (iii).

Chronic changes = inflammation

Increased smooth muscle bulk and number of submucosal glands produce mucus plugging of the airways, epithelial stripping and a thickened submucosa with cellular infiltrate and many eosinophils.

Wheeze is the result of intraluminal obstruction by oedema and mucus plugging, and, by muscular bronchoconstriction, dynamic airway compression of the intrathoracic extrapleural airways.

Precipitants of asthma attacks

1. Upper respiratory tract infections

Mainly viral: rhino–, respiratory syncytial, parainfluenza.

2. Exercise

Running exacerbates more than cycling, in turn cycling more than swimming. The response depends on inspired air humidity and temperature.

3. Weather changes

Cold air, and humidity, increase fungal spores in the atmosphere.

4. Emotional

Laughing, crying, anger. Acute and chronic anxiety is important in some who subconsciously manipulate their families by illness. Established asthma may be worsened.

5. Aero-allergens

i Seasonal: pollens, e.g. tree in spring, grass in summer, *Cladosporium* and *Alternaria* mould in autumn.
ii Perennial: house dust mite, animals.

6. Food induced

Cola drinks and ice, commonly, and cooking oil rarely, mainly in Asians. Wheeze related to food intolerances are without other symptoms such as urticaria and to be differentiated from those associated with anaphylaxis precipitated by shellfish or cows' milk protein.

7. Irritants

Painting, dust, smoking, paraffin heating.

Onset and course

Intermittent

1. Gradual onset. Cough for one day, progressing to wheeze within another, remitting by day four, and better by the end of the week. In some recurrence is frequent, associated with respiratory infections, commoner in winter than summer and preschool age.
2. May be acute, even explosive, especially if sensitive to a particular allergen. Improves within one to two days.

Chronic

3. Milder symptoms are present much of the time, especially on exercise or at night. Particularly responsive to prophylactic therapy. Occasionally perception of severity is "blunted", a dangerous situation.

Symptoms

Age related. The natural history of atopic children shows a bimodal distribution, with one group who wheeze between 1 and 3 years old, and the other who develop wheeze after that age.

1. Infancy. Persistent/recurrent night cough, repeated wheeze with colds, persistent wheeze with obesity.
2. Toddler. Nocturnal cough is prominent, with recurrent wheeze on exercise, with emotion, and respiratory infection.
3. Children under 5 years old. Cough, may be the only symptom, often worse at night.

Associated symptoms

1. Breathlessness, episodic in nature. Expiratory wheeze. Abdominal pain and vomiting due to forceful coughing.
2. Repeated croup may be due to asthma.

3. Atopic eczema often improves during exacerbations, and vice versa, reason unknown.
4. Severe chronic asthma may stunt growth and delay puberty.

Severity

Mild = less than one attack every 2 months (75% of the total).
Moderate = more than one attack every 2 months (20%).
  Both mild and moderate often have a marked seasonal variation.
Severe:

  i persistent symptoms, exercise limitation and abnormal lung function tests (5%).
  ii Uncommon: very infrequent severe attacks, even life threatening, but asymptomatic with normal respiratory function between episodes.

Poor school attendance

An important reflection of severity/parental anxiety; manipulative school avoidance is unlikely initially, but repeated illness with failure to keep up with class work may cause school failure.
  Up to a third of asthmatic primary and middle school age children miss more than 3 weeks a year. This, with nocturnal wheeze in the early hours ('morning dip'), cyanosis or collapse are each indicative of the need for more effective treatment.

Signs

Mild to moderate attack

- Nasal flaring, prolonged noisy expiratory effort, raised respiratory rate, tracheal tug.
- Hyperinflated chest, plus, if chronic, sulci or grooves at insertions of the diaphragm produce a 'pigeon chest' deformity.
- Auscultation: widespread wheeze with coarse crackles, and often fine crackles in the preschool child.

Severe attack

- Cyanosis in air, grey appearance, progressing to confusion, or coma.
- Use of accessory muscles or difficulty in speaking in sentences are each equivalent to a peak flow <25% of predicted.
- Absent or quiet breath sounds in respiratory failure.
- Pulsus paradoxus >15mm mercury.

Investigations

1. Forced expiration tests of lung function

Effort dependent, highly reproducible in children over 7 years old, and sometimes younger. The normal values are related to height. Accept the best of 3 attempts. The most commonly used and useful tests in diagnosis and monitoring of asthma treatment:

  i The peak expiratory flow rate (PEFR) is the maximal forced expiration, within the first one tenth of a second, through a Wright's peak flow meter or cheap plastic peak flow gauge.
  a. Normal values (Figure 12.5)

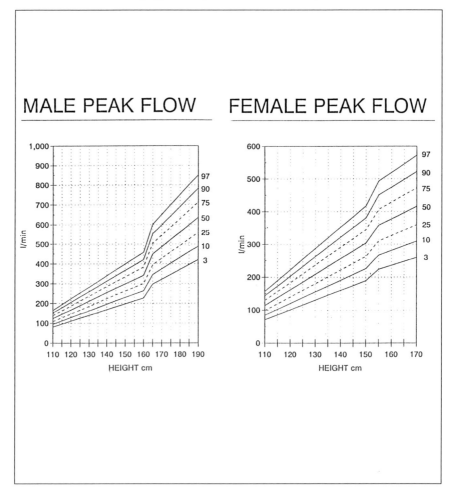

Figure 12.5 Normal values for white children in the UK. Note relationship to height and step increase related to the pubertal growth spurt. (Reproduced by kind permission of the Royal Brompton Hospital)

     b. PEFR below the 5% line *after trying*, requires action.

     c. The response to inhaled bronchodilators can be readily assessed. An increase of 20% or more is diagnostic, but failure to respond does not exclude asthma as bronchoconstriction may need more prolonged treatment.

     d. Variation in airflow obstruction is normal, with lower values of PEFR by 15% being found in the morning. However, low values (20% or more below the evening value) and 'early morning dipping' are important observations for management.

  ii Forced vital capacity (FVC) is the total volume of gas exhaled during forced expiration.

     Reduced in small lungs, stiff lungs, scoliosis, and neuromuscular disorders, e.g. dystrophies, myasthenia.

  iii Forced expiratory volume $(FEV)_1$ is the volume of gas exhaled in the first second. (The $FEV_{0.5}$ is more reliable under 7 years old). Normally 80% of the FVC.

     a. Disproportionally reduced below 80% of FVC in airway obstruction, e.g. asthma, cystic fibrosis.

     b. An increase of 20% in FEV_1 after inhaled β_2-agonists confirms asthma. May fall to <50% of FVC during attacks, and remain low between them.

2. Bronchial challenge tests

These help to clarify or confirm asthma, identify trigger factors (inhalents, foods etc), and the response to treatments.

  i Exercise-induced bronchoconstriction.

     Method: exercise for 6–8 minutes on a bicycle or treadmill to accelerate the heart to more than 170 beats/minute. Then measure PEFR or FEV_1 taken at 0, 5, 10, 15, 20 and 25 minutes from the end of exercise (Figure 12.6).

     A positive response is a fall of 15% or more, usually found at 3–7 minutes.

     Cold air or nebulized distilled water ('fog') are also used in research as challenge tests.

  ii Histamine challenge for bronchial hyper-reactivity, a research tool. Unfortunately, relatively unhelpful in defining the asthma 'grey case'. Method: using doubling concentrations delivered through a nebulizer for 2 minutes at 5 minute intervals until a fall in PEFR or FEV_1 of 20% occurs.

     The response in normal children is usually at far higher concentrations than those with asthma.

     a. This fall, the 'provocative concentration' or PC_{20}, in population studies, correlates with the minimum fall in PEFR for treatment to be required.

     b. Certain foods may increase the responsiveness in susceptible individuals (mainly Asians).

  iii Inhaled allergens. Potentially dangerous, a research procedure.

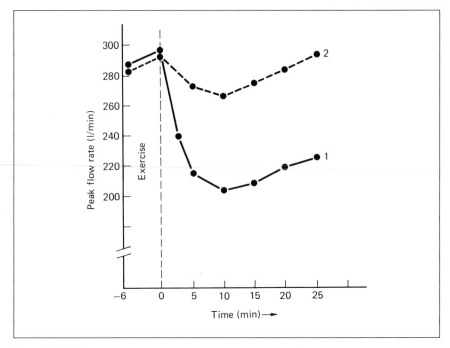

Figure 12.6 Exercise test
1. Positive test, fall of 80 l/min base line = 30%
2. Exercise repeated, with a negative test following pretest inhalation of β_2–agonist.

3. Chest X-ray

Look for hyperinflation and segmental collapse.

Not required in the routine assessment of the wheezy child, but only if symptoms are severe (pneumothorax or pneumonia present?), presence of prominent chest deformity, or a history suggestive of another condition such as cystic fibrosis, foreign body etc (see below).

4. Blood gases in severe asthma

Hypoxia occurs as PEFR or FVC falls.

    i   pH falls: metabolic acidosis from hypoxia and work of breathing.
    ii P_aCO_2 is usually low; if it rises to >5.4 kPa (40 mmHg) it is an indicator of respiratory failure which occurs in about 1% of hospitalized cases.
    iii P_aO_2 may fall significantly when β_2-agonist is given by nebulizer as airways open up in underperfused lung segments. In an acute attack P_aO_2 remains low for days due to ventilation/perfusion imbalance.

5. Other

    i   Eosinophilia (>500/10^9/l) is more common in atopics.

ii Positive skin-prick tests = test substance wheal >4 mm larger than control at 15 minutes, and suggests specific IgE is present. Late reactions at 3–6 hours are also significant (see pathophysiology). Increase in size of reaction and range of allergens with age.

Skin tests (cheap) and blood radioallergosorbent (RAST) antibody tests (expensive) for house dust mite, pollens, animal danders and foods have a 50–80% concordance with symptoms. Positive results do at least support the history. (see Immune disorders).

NB: 30% of the general population have positive reactions but only 25% of these develop asthma and many are free of any allergic symptoms.

Assessment

1. History

i Age at onset, symptoms (may be persistent cough only), their frequency and severity.
ii Other atopic features: eczema, allergic rhinitis, food allergies, irritablity on allergen exposure. Allergens in the house (pets, plants) and bedroom (feather pillow or duvet, pet sleeps on the bed, dust collecting under the bed, in the carpet etc).
iii Seasonal variation and precipitating factors.
iv Other causes of lung abnormality? e.g. neonatal intensive care, pneumonia, repeated aspiration, cystic fibrosis.
v Schooling attainment, time lost from asthma.
vi Exercise related wheeze, interference with sports and games.

2. Examination

In the assessment remember growth, pubertal rating, blood pressure (especially if taking oral steroids, when eyes should also be checked for cataracts).

3. Investigate appropriate to age and findings

Routine respiratory function tests require compliance!

Diagnosis

1. Repeated episodes of cough, dyspnoea and wheeze; +/- presence of infantile eczema and atopic family history.
2. A reduction of 15–20% in PEFR in an exercise test, or increase of >15% in PEFR following β_2-agonist inhalation.
3. Clinical response to a trial of a bronchodilating drug.

4. Characterization of asthma type by respiratory function monitoring (Figure 12.7).

Differential diagnosis

1. Infants

    i Acute bronchiolitis: onset 1–5 days after the start of a 'cold', due to respiratory syncitial virus; fine crackles may be more marked than the expiratory wheeze.

    ii Wheezy baby syndrome/wheezy bronchitis: virally induced wheeze abates by 1–3 years.

2. Any age

    i Cystic fibrosis: failure to thrive, signs of bronchopneumonia, clubbing, abdominal distention etc.

    ii Foreign body. Always suspect this. If a likely object was handled and followed by an episode of paroxysmal coughing +/-cyanosis, investigate even if well on presentation.

    iii Recurrent aspiration: hiatal hernia etc, see Aspiration syndromes.

    iv Rare: bronchiectasis,(+/– immstile cilia syndrome), airways compression from glands, cardiac enlargement, tumour, lobar emphysema, congenital weakness in bronchomalacia, post adenovirus infection in bronchiolitis obliterans, immune deficiency.

Management

General considerations

Co-management, as in many chronic conditions, is a partnership between the patient, the family, and the health professionals.

The cornerstones are (i) understanding the condition, (ii) monitoring of symptoms, peak flow and drug usage, (iii) a prearranged action plan, (iv) written guidlines.

1. Education. Assessment of severity and chest deformity. Frequent checks on inhaler techniques; theophylline levels to optimize treatment; check compliance. The aim is to facilitate a normal life.
2. Sporting performance impaired by exercise–induced bronchoconstriction (EIB) can be helped by pre-activity inhaled β_2-agonist or cromoglycate 5 minutes before. Lasts at least 2 h. Continuous prophylaxis with cromoglycate is equally effective. Nasal breathing reduces EIB. Short burst sports are best, though the child may 'run through' EIB, to a refractory state of reduced bronchial reactivity.
3. Environmental factors:

    i Stop smoking. Avoid allergens, e.g. household pets (better still advise against their introduction into the house in an atopic family). House dust mite numbers may be reduced by impervious mattress covers. Stop smoking.

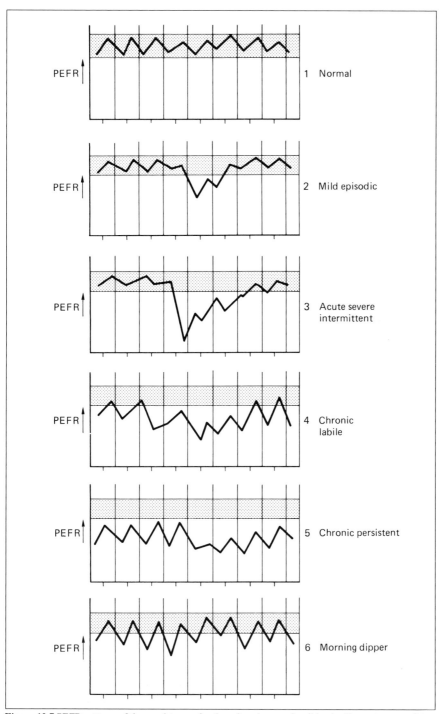

Figure 12.7 PEFR patterns of the usual types of asthma found: normal; mild episodic; acute severe intermittent; chronic labile; chronic persistent; morning dipper.

Humidifiers and ionizers are of unproven value.

ii Hyposensitizing injections may allow a small reduction in medication, at the cost of a long series of injections and danger of anaphylaxis. Worth considering if a very significant reaction occurs to only one or two allergens, in the poorly controlled, severely affected child.

4. Emotional problems within the family may respond to psychotherapy which is not always available. An alternative option is 'parentectomy' by sending the child to boarding school in appropriate severe cases.

Hypnotherapy and acupuncture are of unproven worth in controlled trials.

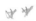 5. Home monitoring: the Daily Record Card. An important monitoring device, listing and grading the severity of symptoms (night cough, wheeze, sleep disruption, daytime cough, wheeze, exercise limitation), and their relation to twice daily PEFRs and treatment.

Insistence on routine monitoring in the well child is unnecessary and psychologically undesirable.

Helping parents interpret the PEFR readings

Predicted PEFR: use the mean value for height if no previous measurements are available when wheeze free (Figure 12.8). At other times, use the best achieved by that individual. The reason is that the normal range is wide, and the maximum for a slim chested, willowy Asian boy is very different from that for a solid Caucasian or Afro-Caribbean of the same height. Take the best of 3 puffs.

   i PEFR below 80% of the predicted is abnormal. Start/intensify treatment.
  ii Below 60% significant airway obstruction. Intensify treatment, as agreed or consult with doctor.
 iii Below 25% is an emergency, requiring urgent medical advice.

NB: The Wright minimeter overestimates by 3% (up to 10% in some hands), and should be borne in mind when interpreting results.

6. Outpatient review. Monitor the response to medication, its side effects, impairment of growth and school progress. The diary and a PEFR in the clinic gives an opportunity to see if the child's or parents' perceptions are exaggerated, accurate or dangerously inadequate.

Nocturnal cough

Troublesome persistent nocturnal cough in an atopic child or with a strong family history is an indication for a trial of β_2-agonist, oral or inhaled, followed by inhaled cromoglycate or steroid, and finally oral theophylline.

Intermittent mild/moderate episodes

1. Mild, the commonest: bronchodilator β_2-agonist, at the time of the attack.

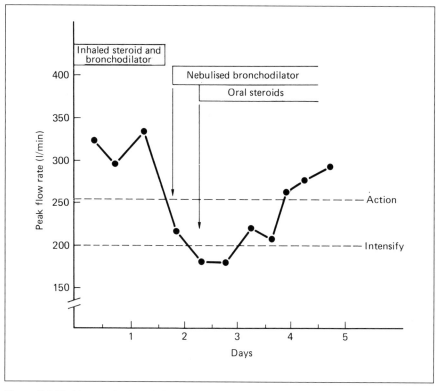

Figure 12.8 Marking a patient's peak flow chart to indicate when previously agreed action should be initiated. In this example, height was 140 cm, mean PEFR = 320 l/min.
Action line (-20%) = 260 l/min,
Intensification line (-40%) = 200 l/min.
Danger (-75%) = 70 l/min

2. Moderate, common pattern in the preschool, occasionally becoming severe:

i Bronchodilator β_2-agonist.
ii If repeated attacks or prolonged for several days then a short course of oral steroids can be administered; they may be given by responsible, competent parents, at home.
iii Antibiotics are rarely indicated yet often prescribed (about 80% of all attacks are viral, less than 5% bacterial).
iv Ipratropium bromide is recommended for those under 18 months, otherwise it is only of limited effect and then only in a mild attack.

Candidates for prophylaxis (drugs: see below)

i Attacks occurring 1–2 per month. May respond even if viral.
ii +/– regular exercise induced wheeze with games.
iii At least one attack severe enough to warrant admission to hospital, unless an isolated (viral) attack or, especially in the older child, an allergic reaction to an animal contact.

Table 12.5 Anti–asthma drugs, action, and important side effects (see status asthmaticus for i.v. drug guide)

Drug		Action	Side effects
β_2–agonist	e.g. Salbutamol: 200 µg 3–4/day inhaled, 0.6 mg/kg/day orally. Turbutaline 250–500 µg/dose 3–4/day inhaled. 75 µg/kg/dose orally, 3–4 daily.	Airway smooth muscle relaxes via cyclic AMP	Tremor, jumpy, tachycardia
	Salmeterol 50 mg twice daily	Not for immediate symptomatic relief	Commoner than with the other β_{-2} agonists
Cromoglycate	Inhaled: spincap 20 mg or metred dose 5 mg, either is given 3–4/day. May reduce to 2/day once symptoms controlled	1 Prevents mediator release from mast cells 2 Reduces reflex vagal stimulation	Nil
Corticosteroids	Inhaled*: e.g. beclomethasone 100–200 µg 2–4/day or budesonide 50–200 µg 2–4/day. Oral: i Prednisolone 2 mg/kg single dose or per day for 4 days ii Alternate day 20 mg/kg	1 Anti-inflammatory 2 β_2 receptors more responsive 3 Phospholipase A2 inhibited, reduces mediator release	Inhaled: oral thrush; hoarse voice; adrenal supression? Oral: adrenal and growth supression if >0.5 mg/kg daily
Ipratropium	Nebulized 100–500 µg Metred 40 µg dose × 2, 2–3 per day	Atropine-like, antivagal	Dries secretions
Theophylline	24 mg/kg/day in 2 doses	1 Airway smooth muscle relaxation by adenosine effect, not by inhibition of phosphodiesterase 2 Improves tired diaphragm contraction 3 Respiratory centre stimulant	GI: Nausea, vomiting CNS: Headache, bad behaviour, school difficulties, fits Enuresis CVS: Arrhythmias, death

* Inhaled steroids: compliance is better if given only twice daily. If the total daily dose excedes 600 µg a spacer should be used to reduce buccal absorption and prevent growth supression.

Frequent episodic or persistent asthma

Symptoms daily, or at least 1–2 days a week, needing continuous therapy for periods of months or years.

1. Prophylaxis

Indications are as in moderate wheeze, and for chest deformity present between exacerbations.

   i Inhaled therapy

   a. Cromoglycate; may take 6–8 weeks to work. Trial of therapy for up to 3 months is recommended.

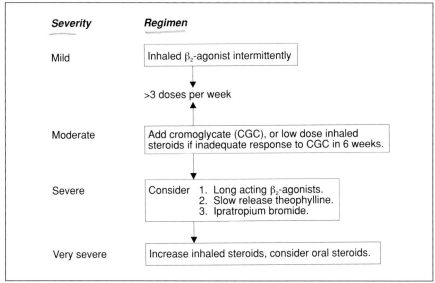

Figure 12.9 Treatment algorithm for asthma

    b. Corticosteroids if cromoglycate is ineffective. Some prefer this from the outset, maintaining their dual action of inhibition of inflammation and reduced bronchial hyper-responsiveness is more efficacious.
    NB An either/or situation. No extra benefit is obtained if both cromoglycate and corticosteroids are given. While receiving systemic steroids i.v., inhaled steroids are not required, but as one progresses to and reduces alternate day oral steroids, inhaled steroids can be added for their independent anti-inflammatory activity.
    c. Salmeterol, a long-acting β-agonist, in older children, especially for overnight wheeze, in whom inhaled steroids are not providing relief.
    NB: *Not* an either/or situation. Continue inhaled steroids and short-acting β-agonist.

ii Oral slow release

    a. Theophylline (Slow-Phyllin) from 1 year old.
    b. Salbutamol from 3 years old (Volmax)–not so effective for cough alone.
       Either a or b is added if high dose inhaled steroids are not controlling symptoms, especially with early morning wheeze, or if night cough is persistent and wakes the child (not just the parent!). For best results using theophylline the drug level must be maintained at 10–20 mg/l and regularly monitored; if the response is satisfactory maintain at a therapeutic dose for 6–12 months, when review is needed.

2. Active treatment

i Bronchodilator β_2-agonist. Ipratropium bromide may be added if excessive side effects occur from the β_2- agonist.

    ii Oral steroids in short courses (2 mg/kg day for 4 days) when PEFR dips more than 20%, and a severe exacerbation could, from experience with past episodes, otherwise ensue.

    iii Continuous alternate day oral steroids (to minimize effects on growth) if persistent severe reduction in lung function, and/or life threatening sudden severe asthma with cyanosis has occurred even *once*.

The drug delivery system

This is determined by age. Choosing an inappropriate method is a common cause of treatement failure and non-compliance.

Delivery systems for asthma treatment by age

1. Under 1 year

Most are unresponsive to β_2-agonists, oral or inhaled, but it is worth trying ipratropium bromide via a tight fitting face mask attached to a low resistance valve spacer (System 22) or nebulizer. Under 18 months inhaled β_2-agonist may cause V/Q mismatch and so lowering P_aO_2; try an oral suspension first.

2. 1–3 years

    i Syrups: salbutamol/terbutaline for a mild/moderate attack. Theophylline syrups need too frequent administration to give stable drug levels for which slow release preparations (SRP) are better. However SRP have more side effects with little increased benefit. Its role is declining in all age groups.

    ii Via nebulizer/compressor (flow rate 8–10 l/min, volume 4 ml): Salbutamol/terbutaline for the moderate/severe attack. Nebulized β_2-sympathomimetics should be driven by oxygen in critically ill infants. The rational is that V/Q imbalance persists for 30 minutes after giving salbutamol, therefore it is unsafe to give nebulized salbutamol at home under 18 months of age. For persistent symptoms: inhaled cromoglycate, nebulized budesonide or beclomethasone. Ipratropium has some effect in mild asthma.

    iii Tight fitting face mask attached to a spacer (see below) to deliver a β_2-agonist, budesonide/beclomethasone,

    iv Coffee cup spacer for those unable to tolerate the close fitting mask.

3. Preschool 3–5 years

    i Metred dose aerosol inhalers can be used by most children, via a spacer, e.g. Nebuhaler/Volumatic 750 ml in size.

    ii Others need a nebulizer (for β_2-agonist, cromoglycate, budesonide, ipratropium) or oral syrup (β_2-agonist), and occasionally a slow release theophylline.

4. Age 5–10 years

 i Powder inhalation devices (β_2-agonists, steroids). A whistle attachment is a useful teaching aid. All require rapid active inspiration.

  a. PEFR of >60 l/min is needed for the rotahaler, spinhaler, and diskhaler, inhaled over 3–4 breaths.
  b. PEFR of as little as 20 l/min will activate the turbohaler, and requires only one inspiration.

 ii Breath-activated inhaler (BAI): minimal inspiratory effort needed is PEFR of 30 l/min, with a long slow inspiration which should be held as long as possible (10 seconds is recommended). Suits 8 year olds and up.
 iii Spacers and nebulizers also have a place; ordinary metred dose aerosol inhaler (MDI) administration is often ineffective due to lack of motivation, or inability to coordinate.

5. Aged >10 years

BAIs and MDIs as well as the above.

Status asthmaticus: indications for hospitalization

- Cyanosis.
- Drowsy/semicomatose.
- Unable to speak.
- PEFR <50% of expected after a β_2-bronchodilator
- Failure to respond to inhaled β_2-bronchodilator and/or as bad within 1 hour of its use.
- Previous severe attack, e.g. collapse/ventilated.

In the Home

1. Oxygen for cyanosis. Give β_2-agonist via a nebulizer driven by oxygen, if available, otherwise give subcutaneous terbutaline or adrenaline.
Start oral steroids, if child is able, as prednisolone 2 mg/kg/24h.
2. Call ambulance, and ensure it has oxygen. (Deaths have occurred as a result of its unavailability during transfer).

In the Hospital (Figure 12.10)

1. History: establish time of last dose of β_2-agonist and theophylline.

2. Monitor colour, pulse, presence of pulsus paradoxus, PEFR, oxygen saturation (maintain saturation at 90–95%). If drowsy, the chest overinflated and silent, blood gases are indicated.

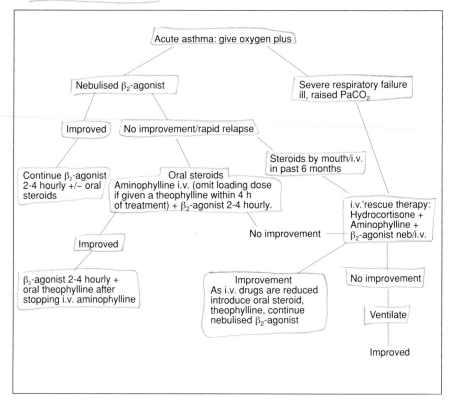

Figure 12.10 Treatment algorithm for hospitalized acute asthmatic attack

Drugs and therapy in status asthmaticus

   i Oxygen driven nebulized salbutamol 2.5–5 mg or terbutaline 2.5–5 mg, frequency 2 hourly at first. Oxygen saturation may fall for a short time due to ventilation/perfusion mismatch. Continuous administration of full strength respirator solutions of salbutamol or terbutaline may be given in hospital.

  ii If in severe failure, in intensive care, and not progressing: i.v. terbutaline 10 μg/kg as a single dose, or iv salbutamol 4–6 μg/kg over 5 minutes, followed by a continuous infusion at 0.6 μg–1 μg/kg/min.

 iii Intravenous aminophylline, loading dose 6 mg/kg (omit if already on oral theophylline) and a continuous infusion of 1 mg/kg/h.

 iv Hydrocortisone 4 mg/kg bolus and 1 mg/kg/ h i.v. Change to oral prednisolone 1–2 mg/kg when i.v. discontinued.

  v Rehydrate. Often insufficient oral intake for many hours, plus increased losses via the respiratory tract. Hyperinflation may stimulate antidiutetic

hormone (ADH) secretion, but overhydration is rarely a problem. Hypokalaemia may develop and need correction.
vi Mechanical ventilation: the indication is progressive respiratory failure with hypoxia and rising P_aCO_2 (>10 kPa or 75 mmHg). Sedate, paralyse and give vigorous physiotherapy to clear mucus plugs. Lavage is not helpful. The ventilator should be volume cycled at slow rates with prolonged expiratory time.

Causes of asthma deaths

1. Crescendo warnings ignored, or not taken seriously. Deterioration in control leading up to the fatal attack. Oral steroids not given or treatment abruptly discontinued.
2. Poor understanding of medication, lack of compliance especially in adolescence.
3. Recent change of family doctor, doctor attending is unfamiliar with the case, or child not attending appointments.
4. Child's perception of severity is blunted as she exerts herself as little as possible and is accustomed to marked physical limitation.
5. During the attack: no oxygen; using a nebulizer not driven by oxygen; over-reliance on the nebuliser causing delay in calling an ambulance; no direct access to ward; away from home and no medication.

Table 12.6 Prognosis

Severity	Children affected (%)	Lung function between attacks	Affected as adults (%)
Mild	75	Normal	15 moderately
Moderate	20	40% have low PEFRs +/- chest deformity	35 moderately 25 severely
Severe*	5	>50% have low PEFRs +/- chest deformity	40 moderately 55 severely

* Girls have the most severe problems as teenagers.
mortality 50 per year in United Kingdom, mainly in 10–14 year olds.

Further reading

Silverman M (1985) *Asthma in childhood.* London: Current Medical Literature
Sporik R, Holgate S T, Cogswell J J (1991) The natural history of asthma in childhood: a birth cohort study. *Archives of Disease in Childhood*, **66**, 1050–1053
Warner J O, Gotz M, Landau L I, *et al* (1989) Management of asthma: a consensus statement. *Archives of Disease in Childhood*, **64**, 1065–1079
Warner J O *et al*. (1992) Asthma: a follow up statement from an International Paediatric Asthma Consensus Group. *Archives of Disease in Childhood*, **647**, 240–248

ACUTE BRONCHITIS

Definition

Acute inflammation of the trachea and bronchi characterized by:

1. Cough, initially dry, becomes loose in 2–3 days, with sputum usually swallowed. Temperature 37–39°C.
2. Later a few coarse crackles and low pitched wheezes are heard.

Aetiology

Common, usually viral, a feature of measles, occasionally due to *Haemophilus influenzae* and pertussis in the young child, often *Mycoplasma pneumoniae* by school age.

Differential diagnosis

High pitched widespread wheeze is likely to be asthma. Persistent cough beyond 2 weeks is suggestive of segmental collapse or secondary bacterial infection.

Management

1. Cough suppressants: may be harmful, so be cautious.
2. Antibiotics: despite growth of bacteria from throat swabs, and purulent sputum, there is little evidence that antibiotics alter the natural history. Amoxycillin, effective against common secondary bacterial pathogens, is permitted if the cough persists for more than 2 weeks. Failure to respond after a week of antibiotic is an indication to consider further investigation (see chronic cough), unless during a mycoplasma outbreak when erythromycin is the drug of first choice, given for 2–3 weeks.

Recurrent bronchitis

Definition

Recurrent episodes (up to 3–4 per annum) of acute bronchitis, affecting as many as 5% of children, mainly in the first 7 years of life.

Viruses are the primary cause, secondary bronchial irritation from cigarette smoking (active and passive), occasionally dust or fumes.

Differential diagnosis includes asthma, sinusitis, foreign body, bronchiectasis, cystic fibrosis, immune disorders, immotile cilia syndrome, tuberculosis.

In community based studies asthma has frequently been misdiagnosed as bronchitis, with a rewarding improvement in symptoms and school attendance after commencing appropriate therapy.

PNEUMONIAS

Overview of causes, symptoms and signs, investigations, management and prognosis

1. Differentiation of bacterial (10%) from viral (90%), or the common from the esoteric is not possible on clinical grounds.
2. Bronchopneumonia is far commoner in the preschool child than a circumscribed lobar pneumonia.
3. Primary, or secondary to prior infection (e.g. measles, pertussis), aspiration or debilitation.

Symptoms and signs

1. Cough. Usually non-specific. If present in a neonate must be taken seriously.
2. Restless, agitated.
3. Signs: grunting, air hunger and tachypnoea. Cyanosis. Head retracted, flaring of alae naesi, sternal, intercostal and subcostal recession.
4. Complications: unusual–pleural effusions occur in pneumococcal, and pneumo-thoraces and empyemas in staphylococcal infection.

Investigations

1. Throat swabs are not diagnostic. Better but barely adequate is a cough swab, or sputum via oropharyngeal suction.
2. Blood cultures are often positive in bacterial pneumonias.
3. Immunofluorescent tests for some viral infections (respiratory syncitial virus, influenza etc) allow rapid diagnosis, otherwise culture delays identification for weeks.
4. Traditional antibody tests with a fourfold rise still have a place, e.g. *Mycoplasma pneumoniae*.
5. Tracheal/bronchial aspirate is indicated if an unusual pathogen (e.g. *Pneumocystis carinii*) is suspected, or response to therapy is slow.
6. Leucopenia: total WBC of <5000/mm^3 has a poor prognosis.
7. Do blood gases if very ill.
8. Chest X-ray (Figure 12.11): may show consolidation before clinical signs are present. Lateral may show unsuspected involvement of the lower lobes. Films should be repeated 3–4 weeks later to ensure resolution.

Management

Observe at home unless toxic, cyanosed, feeding poorly, or parental need for supportive nursing.

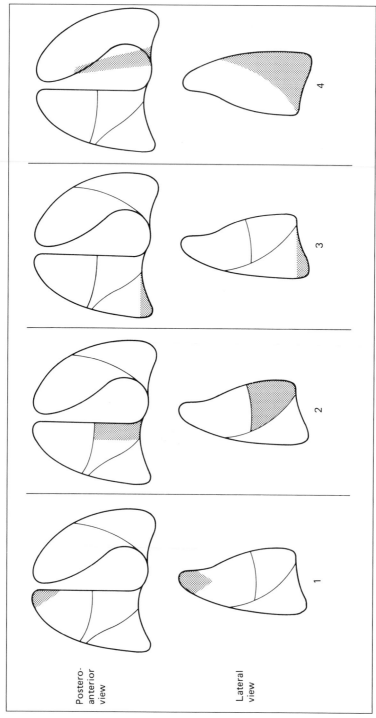

Figure 12.11
Important pneumonic segments not to miss when reviewing postero-anterior X-ray films.
1 = Right upper lobe, upper segment.
2 = Right middle lobe, medial segment.
3 = Right lower lobe, lower segment.
4 = Left lower lobe. Look behind the heart.

If oral fluid administration causes distress, nasogastric or i.v. fluids must be given to avoid dehydration.

1. Oxygen via a tent (max. oxygen concentration possible 30–40%), mask, nasal catheter or prongs according to age and tolerance.
2. Aspiration of nasopharyngeal secretions. Physiotherapy in the recovery phase; use with care, as excessive handling may tip an ill infant into respiratory failure.
3. Medication: antipyretics + antibiotics are administered according to the most likely bacterial pathogens for age, despite most infections being viral.

    i <1 year old: flucloxacillin + gentamicin i.v. covers the common pneumococcus, the not unusual *Escherichia coli*, and rare *staphylococcus aureus*.
    ii >1 year old: penicillin for pneumococcus while ampicillin also covers *Haemophilus influenzae*. If Legionella is suspected, give erythromycin.

4. Drainage of effusion (pneumococcal) or empyema (staphylococcal).

Prognosis

1. Previously well: good. Resolution of pneumococcal pneumonia 7–10 days, viral and mycoplasma 2–3 weeks, staphylococcal 4+ weeks.
2. Underlying abnormality present (congenital heart disease, immune deficiency, cerebral palsy, etc), especially if already in hospital: slower to respond and a higher mortality.

Failure of pneumonia to resolve

1. Inadequate/inappropriate antibiotic therapy.
2. Pleural effusions (aspirate to dryness, may need a drain) or empyema (surgical decortication).
3. Foreign body (non radiopaque) requiring bronchoscopy.
4. Cystic fibrosis and immunodeficiency states.
5. Bronchiectasis.

Pneumococcal pneumonia

Epidemiology

1. The cause of 90% of bacterial pneumonias, commonest in 3–8 year olds. Usually sporadic, but an increased risk exists in schools and nurseries after a preceding viral respiratory infection.
2. Bronchopneumonic pattern in infants, lobar at older ages.

Clinical

1. Respiratory: ill child, herpes febrilis on the lips, fine crackles, consolidation.

2. Abdominal distension and ileus, and, with abdominal pain, may mimic acute appendicitis if the right lower lobe (inflammation of the pleura over the diaphragm) is affected.
3. Febrile convulsion, occasionally meningism (especially with right upper lobe) in the preschool child.
4. Associated focal infection, usually limited to otitis media.

Staphylococcus aureus

Infants are usually the age group affected. Uncommon.

Pathophysiology

May seem an ordinary bronchopneumonia until X-rayed. This shows single or multiple cysts full of pus or air or both developing from areas of consolidation. Ball-valve mechanisms operate, tension cysts (pneumatoceles) develop, (sometimes displacing the mediastinum), which may rupture causing pneumothoraces, empyemas and sudden worsening, all within hours.

Clinical

Preceded by staphylococcal skin sepsis contact, or coryzal for up to a week.

Rapidly become toxic and shocked. Chest involvement is unilateral more than bilateral, right more than left.

Investigations

1. Bacteriology from cough swab, pleural tap, blood culture. (Tracheal aspirate is rarely justified.)
2. Frequent chest X-rays to monitor.
3. Sweat test for cystic fibrosis, screen for immune deficiency.

Differential diagnosis

- Klebsiella pneumonia is similar.
- Foreign body with pulmonary abscess, preceded by an aspiration incident which may have been missed.
- Primary tuberculous pneumonia with cavitation is rarely seen in children in the UK.
- X-ray may be confused with a diaphragmatic hernia.

Management

1. Antistaphylococcal drugs for 4+ weeks.
2. Surgical drainage of empyema.
3. Needling and underwater drainage for gross obstructive distension/pneumothorax.

Prognosis

Prognosis is good if the condition is recognized early. Surprisingly the chest X-ray returns to normal within 2–3 months.

Haemophilus influenzae

Slower onset than pneumococcal, otherwise similar presentation.
   Pyogenic complications are common: septicaemia, cellulitis, septic arthritis, pericarditis, empyema, meningitis.

Mycoplasma pneumoniae

Usually symptomatic in the 5–15 year old age group. Incubation 2–3 weeks, often running in families.

Clinical

Mild respiratory symptoms for days or weeks, not very ill with diffuse signs on X-ray more marked than clinically apparent. Cough productive of mucoid or even blood tinged sputum. Chest pain not uncommon. Occasionally may have a high swinging temperature and be quite toxic. Clinical associations: maculopapular rashes, erythema nodosum, meningitis, myringitis bullosa. McLeod syndrome is a late complication.

Investigation

Cold agglutinins are positive in half of patients. Specific antibody test required for accurate diagnosis.

Management

Erythromycin for 2–3 weeks may be effective.

Adenovirus

Types 3, 7, 21. Especially severe in young children.
   Chronic sequelae, which are rare: hyperinflation, wheeze, recurrent infection and atelectasis due to obliterating bronchiolitis, pulmonary fibrosis, and bronchiectasis.

Chlamydia trachomatis

Uncommon. Acquired during delivery from mother's genital tract, presenting at 4–15 weeks old.
   Pertussis like cough, tachypnoea, fine crackles.

50% have conjunctivitis and/or otitis media.

Interstitial infiltrates and hyperinflation on chest X-ray, mild eosinophilia in the blood. Cultures are needed as antibody tests are unreliable. Erythromycin for 2–3 weeks, to both parents as well as the infant, to prevent recurrence. Chronic cough may persist for weeks.

Pneumocystis carinii

Immune deficiency disorders, primary or secondary, are necessary for infection by this protozoan of low virulence.

Features include dry cough, tachypnoea, cyanosis with variable fever, little on auscultation compared with extensive X-ray changes of infiltrates and a ground glass appearance.

Diagnosis: pneumocystis cysts on lung biopsy or bronchoscopy in small children. Cough induced by hypertonic saline inhalation is productive of cysts in >50% of young adults with AIDS and is less hazardous.

Prognosis

Death if untreated or diagnosis excessively delayed. Give co-trimoxazole (full course, then alternate days for prophylaxis), or pentamidine.

Hydrocarbon aspiration and near drowning.

See Accidents.

ACUTE RESPIRATORY FAILURE

Definition

Elevated PCO_2 during an acute illness (>7 kPa or 49 mmHg, 5.6 kPa or 40 mmHg in asthma). Levels of 8–9 kPa (56–63 mmHg) are consistent with the need for mechanical ventilation.

Low P_aO_2 in air is common.

Pathophysiology

See introduction to the chapter.

Clinical signs are often *more* important than gases: cyanosis/extreme pallor, severe respiratory distress, decreased respiratory effort, 'silent' chest, confused, coma, hypotonia, exhaustion, plus signs from any underlying disease process.

Beware 'healthy' pink vasodilated drowsy child in oxygen rich atmosphere sinking into CO_2 narcosis.

Causes:

1. Previously well

    i Accidents: trauma, burns, drowning, poisoning, foreign body.
   ii Upper airway obstruction: stridor (see causes), tonsillar hypertrophy.
  iii Lower respiratory tract: asthma, bronchiolitis, pneumonia.
   iv CNS abnormality: encephalitis, seizures, polyneuritis.
    v Septicaemia, metabolic disorders.

2. Underlying abnormality

    i Cystic fibrosis.
   ii Scoliosis (severe) with infection, or postoperatively.
  iii Congenital heart disease.
   iv Neuromuscular diseases, e.g. Duchenne muscular dystrophy, myasthenia.

Management

1. Early respiratory failure: treat the underlying condition vigorously. Minimal handling.
2. Established respiratory failure: first consider if an underlying abnormality precludes treatment, e.g. advanced cystic fibrosis, Werdnig-Hoffman disease.

Practical aspects of intubation

1. Bag and mask with 100% oxygen.
2. Endotracheal intubation:

    i Uncuffed tube if under 8 years old.
   ii Tube size not too tight, to avoid pressure necrosis, or too small a diameter with increased airway resistance. Formula = (age/4) +4 = size in mm.
  iii Change to nasoendotracheal intubation, once the airway is controlled, if prolonged support for days is likely.

      Always check:

      a. Air entry lest you are only ventilating the right main bronchus.
      b. Chest X-ray to confirm the tube position (shorten if necessary).

3. Humidification and frequent suction of the tube to prevent blockage.
4. Arm restraints to prevent the child extubating himself. With judicious sedation they may be removed later.
5. Establish an arterial line, repeat blood gases 4–6 hourly, adjust ventilator settings for normalization of gases. Continuous positive airway pressure helps avoid alveolar collapse.
6. As improvement occurs, reduce pressures, oxygen, and rate, in that order.
    Fluids i.v. 0.18% saline + 4.3% dextrose, with added potassium.
    Volume according to weight and condition: e.g. increased in asthma, reduced if a danger of cerebral oedema due to asphyxia or inappropriate antidiuretic hormone release secondary to stress.

CYSTIC FIBROSIS (CF)

Definition

Characterized by malabsorption and failure to thrive due to exocrine pancreatic insufficiency and chronic suppurative lung disease. Inherited in an AR pattern, antenatal diagnosis is possible in informative families.

Incidence

One in 2000 Caucasians, the commonest lethal inherited disorder, carried by 1 in 25 of the population. The incidence is much lower in other races.

Genetic basis for CF and prenatal diagnosis.

The gene on chromosome 7 produces an abnormal CF transport protein 'cystic fibrosis transmembrane conductance regulator' (CFTR) in the cell membrane. Up to 75% of UK children may have the same mutation (delta F_{508}) so their families are informative using DNA probes; 120 affected fetuses could be identified annually.

Chorionic villous biopsy accuracy of prediction is 95% in the first trimester.

Low intestinal alkaline phosphatase in amniotic fluid in the second trimester will correctly predict 90% of fetuses homozygous for CF where the DNA probe pattern proves uninformative.

Pathophysiology

The metabolic defect is CFTR, with reduced ATP binding and defective chloride ion transport.

The mucus gland secretions are more sticky than usual, blocking:

1. Pancreatic ducts, which dilate and become cystic; autodigestion, fibrosis and calcification follow. Digestive enzymes and bicarbonate secretion are severely reduced.
2. Bronchioles; infection results, *Staphylococcus aureus* initially, *Pseudomonas aeruginosa* follows, causing more mucus production, obstruction, fibrosis and bronchiectasis, in a vicious cycle. Progressive respiratory failure leads to cor pulmonale.
3. Liver causing focal biliary cirrhosis; also salivary glands, and vas deferens obstruction resulting in sterile males.

Clinical presentation

Initial presentation:
   Meconium ileus 15%
   Malabsorption 30%
   Chest infection 55%

By age

1. Neonatal: meconium ileus (see Neonatal problems) Some perforate causing peritonitis, and need a temporary ileostomy.
2. Infancy (common)

   i   Recurrent chest infection. Finger clubbing follows later.
   ii Failure to thrive, steatorrhoea.
   iii Developmental delay caused by (i) and (ii).

3. Toddler/child, above plus

   i   Rectal prolapse in 20%.
   ii Heat stroke.

4. Older child, above plus

   i   Asthma in 20%, allergic aspergillosis 10%.
   ii Meconium ileus equivalent in 20% = recurrent colicky abdominal pain, distension, constipation, a mass of impacted faeces in the right iliac fossa. Rarely, complete obstruction from volvulus or intussusception (1%) occurs.
   iii Sinusitis 90%, nasal polyps 10%.

5. Adolescence, above plus

   i   Delayed puberty with short stature is very common.
   ii   Respiratory function deteriorates markedly in females. Haemoptysis, repeated pneumothorax in young adults.
   iii Liver cirrhosis is commonly subclinical–portal hypertension 10%, with bleeding oesophageal varicies 1%. Gallstones in the teens in 10%. Pancreatitis rare.
   iv   Diabetes mellitus in 10–40%, from 10 years of age.
   v   Arthritis: hypertrophic pulmonary osteoarthropathy 10%, intermittent polyarthropathy occasionally.
   vi   Infertility. Males: 97% affected due to atretic vas deferens and epididymus. Females are subfertile due to abnormal cervical mucus.

Consider CF in the following situations

1. Respiratory symptoms

- After a second pneumonia in infancy (or first if staphylococcal).
- Frequent bronchitis (not asthma) with paroxysmal cough.
- Hyperinflated, pigeon chest, intercostal recession and Harrison's sulci are later signs.
- Pseudomonas (mucoid strain) chest infection.
- Staphylococcal pneumonia.

2. Growth and bowel symptoms

- Meconium ileus, meconium plug syndrome.

- Failure to thrive (progressing to gross wasting), voracious appetite, with offensive loose, frequent, small stools which later become bulky, putty coloured, oily.
- Rectal prolapse.

3. Family history and asymptomatic

Diagnosis of cystic fibrosis

1. Sweat test

    i   Sweat sodium of >70 mmol/kg by pilocarpine iontophoresis, weight of sweat >100 mg, on two occasions, is necessary for confirmation of CF. Repeat if >50 mmol/kg.
    ii Osmolality of the sweat obtained >220 mmol/kg, using special collection equipment, has low errors compared with (i), the traditional 'gold standard' test.

2. Screening: serum immunoreactive trypsin (IRT) is raised × 10 normal in the CF newborn. The use of human trypsinogen monoclonal antibody (HTMAB) has improved the accuracy of IRT assay. Guthrie card blood spot is used. Confirm with a sweat test after 1–2 months of age.

3. Genetic studies:

    i   Gene site on chromosome 7 is identifiable in 75% from RFLPs.
    ii Antenatal diagnosis by chorionic biopsy, or estimation of microvillar enzymes in the uninformative families.

Table 12.7 Differential diagnosis of recurrent wheeze

---

1 Reactive airways
Asthma (atopic family history, thriving, though in severe asthma CF must be excluded).
Wheezy baby syndrome often affects chubby (not wasted) infants.
Extrinsic allergic alveolitis will give a history of exposure.
2 Infective
Post pertussis, vomiting prominent.
Loeffler's syndrome, e.g. *Toxocara canis*, drugs.
3 Mechanical
Recurrent aspiration due to hiatal hernia.
Foreign body, compression from glands, tumours, aberrant vessels.
Congenital lung abnormality: bronchogenic cyst, sequestrated lobe, lobar emphysema, cystic adenomatous malformation.
4 Cardiac failure
5 Genetic and acquired impaired respiratory tract defence
Cystic fibrosis
Immune deficiency: unusual organisms may be grown.
Immotile cilia syndrome, including Kartegener's syndrome: (AR, reduced
cilial function due to abnormal cilial structure causes sinusitis, serous otitis, bronchiectasis,
infertility as sperm are immotile, situs inversus in 50%)

Differential diagnosis of causes of failure to thrive

See Growth.

Management

Team of physiotherapists, dieticians, social workers, nurses and doctors. Prognosis for survival may be improved by attending specialist CF treatment centres.

1. Respiratory:

Encourage vigorous daily exercise; use cromoglycate or β-agonists for any exercise induced wheeze.

  i Physiotherapy: passive postural drainage, percussion, forced expiration techniques (huffing), for 10–15 minutes, 2–4 times daily, proportional to sputum production and symptoms. Hypertonic saline (3–5%) inhalation aids coughing. Adolescents often need supervision to keep this up.
  ii Antibiotics for acute infection as sputum culture and sensitivities indicate, for 2–3 weeks.

   a. Early, in infancy: flucloxacillin for *Staphylococcus aureus*.
   b. Later: *Pseudomonas* species appear, and cannot be completely eliminated, but respond to a combination of i.v. aminoglycoside and ureidopenicillin or third generation cephalosporin. Ciprofloxacin has established a place, despite reservations concerning impaired cartilage growth in Beagle pups.
   c. More continuous treatment for increased sputum production and weight loss. Frequent courses inevitably produce resistant strains. *Haemophilus influenzae* causes some exacerbations.
   d. Prevention. Controversy continues concerning its efficacy.
      Infancy: not yet established which is the best policy, whether to give antistaphylococcal drugs either as clinically indicated, continuously for the first 5 years, or for life.
      Late, once colonized by pseudomonas: i.v. antipseudomonal drugs at regular 3 monthly intervals, may be self administered at home via a subcutaneously implanted reservoir.

  iii Inhaled therapy is of proven usefulness in the following situations:

   a. To improve the removal of secretions: hypertonic saline, salbutamol, acetyl cysteine before physiotherapy.
   b. Continued deterioration or frequent hospital admissions, give home nebulized gentamycin + carbenicillin 2 × daily.
   c. Bronchodilatation and reduction of inflammatory oedema: $β_2$-adrenergic bronchodilators, budesonide or betamethasone, or cromoglycate.

  iv Complications of advanced disease: monitored oxygen to avoid CO_2 narcosis; brown sputum is suggestive of *Aspergillus fumigatus*; heart failure occurs due to cor pulmonale.
  v Monitor progress by

   a. Regular (monthly) sputum cultures for organisms and sensitivity patterns.
   b. Chest X-ray (6 monthly). Changes begin in the upper zones.

  c. Assess lung function 6 monthly from 5 years old: FEV_1, FVC, and FEV_1/FVC ratio follow an obstructive airways pattern, influenced by antibiotics, physiotherapy, and diet.

 vi Immunization: pertussis, measles; annual influenza vaccination from 4 years old.

2. Nutrition and growth

Many children are small for age and enter puberty 2 years late. Height and weight must be regularly charted; 90% have pancreatic insufficiency.

 Steatorrhoea occurs when 90% of pancreatic function is lost. Assess by fat balance over 3 days; >10% loss in faeces is abnormal.

 i Caloric requirement is 150% of recommended daily allowance. Maintaining adequate weight is a key factor in long-term survival.

  Full fat diet recommended, for in the past fat avoidance caused unnecessary subnutrition, and possibly contributed to a poorer prognosis.

 ii Cotazyme powder for infants; older ages: enteric coated microspheres of pancreatic enzymes (Creon, Pancrease) up to 4 capsules with meals, 2 for snacks. Excess acidity inactivates these enzyme preparations; add bicarbonate or H_2 receptor antagonist if steatorrhoea, excessive flatus, or abdominal pain persist.

 iii Home intravenous antibiotic/alimentation. Used in the more advanced case, when weight loss predicts serious deterioration. Rationale:

  a. Reduction in hospitalization, its duration and frequency, hence costs and hospital cross infection.

  b. Less disruption and hospital dependency for the family.

  c. Continuity of schooling/employment.

 iv Vitamins: prescribe twice the normal requirements of water (B,C) and fat soluble (A,D,E,K) vitamins as daily Abidec, Ketovite tabs and liquid. Vitamin E and K are given separately.

 v Supplements of protein (skimmed milk powder), fat (medium chain triglycerides) and glucose polymers orally, or via nocturnal nasogastric or gastrostomy tube feeding in malnutrition, or anorexia induced by acute illness.

 vi Sodium supplements in hot weather.

3. Emotional support

This includes the whole family. Guilt feelings in the parents, the demanding daily schedule of treatment and its rejection, delayed puberty and adolescent rebellion, depression, the death of a CF friend, and career guidance, all require some anticipation and an established network of support.

4. Heart-lung transplant

For a selected few is a final treatment option.

Prognosis

Median age of survival is 25 years, 80% reaching adult life in the best treatment centres.

Nutritional factors: stunting leads to a higher mortality. Pubertal females have a high rate of rapid deterioration, cause unknown.

Sedentary/professional occupations are most suitable, and unemployment is little higher than the rest of the population.

Presymptomatic diagnosis of CF by neonatal screening using IRT may further alter the natural history by earlier treatment.

Identification of the CFTR gene sequence makes DNA replacement therapy possible. (See Leader (1990) Cystic fibrosis: prospects for screening and therapy. *Lancet, i*, 79–80.)

Further reading

David T J (1990) Cystic fibrosis. *Archives of Disease in Childhood*, **65**: 152–157

Leader (1988) Survival in cystic fibrosis–How important is nutrition? *Lancet*, ii, 1060–1061

Matthews L W, Drotar D (1984) Cystic fibrosis–a challenging long-term chronic disease. *Pediatric Clinics of North America*, **31**, 133–152

Goodchild M C, Dodge J A (1985) *Cystic fibrosis:Manual of Diagnosis and Management*. 2nd edn. London: Baillere-Tindall

TUBERCULOSIS (TB)

Aetiology

Mycobacterium tuberculosis is transmitted from an adult with caseating disease. Rarely it is spread transplacentally by seeding amniotic fluid. Bovine TB erradicated from the UK.

Malnutrition, measles and immune deficiency increase susceptibility. Dual infection with HIV is an increasing concern worldwide.

Childhood notifications in the UK

Represent 5% of all new TB cases. Almost half are Asian children. The 1983 Medical Research Council survey rate was 5 per 100 000, (2.4 Caucasian, 17 West Indian, 40 Asian) and 25 times higher if born abroad.

Primary lesion in the lung in 75% (higher in Asians), extrapulmonary 25%.

Adult household contact in 80%, with an infection risk of 10% if the adult is sputum positive, 0.5% (non-Asian) to 3% (Asian) if sputum negative.

Pathology

1. Bacilli ingested by macrophages which activate T lymphocytes. Only 1 in 10 of those infected develop disease, the highest risk being in the first 1–2 years after infection.
2. Delayed hypersensitivity reaction (basis of the Mantoux test) after an incubation period of 2–10 weeks, causing massive local tissue reaction = caseation = the body's attempt to seal off the infection.

3. In the brain, bursting of a tuberculoma seeded by miliary spread causes a similar severe inflammatory reaction, then thick gelatinous exudate which gums up the CSF pathways (hydrocephalus), compresses the cranial nerves and obstructs vessels causing infarcts and swelling.
4. Calcification follows over about 6 months.

Timing of presentation after exposure

1. Hypersensitivity phenomena in 2–10 weeks
2. Miliary TB and meningitis within 3 months.
3. Pleural effusion and segmental lesions (see below) 3–12 months.
4. Bronchopneumonia, focal infection of other organs 1–5+ years.
5. Post-primary TB 3+ years.

Clinical

1. Hypersensitivity.
   Asymptomatic or with fever for 2–3 weeks, weight loss, general malaise; occasionally phlyctenular conjunctivitis, erythema nodosum, rarely pleural effusion (usually sterile, may clot on standing, containing lymphocytes, occurs in over 5 year olds).
2. Pulmonary TB (75%)

   i Primary focus with enlargement of hilar lymph glands = primary complex. Heals with calcification.
   ii Mediastinal lymph node involvement with brassy cough (pertussis like), rapid and laboured breathing. Resultant effects:

      a. Gland enlarges, compressing bronchi, causing segmental collapse, or hyperinflation if a 'ball valve' effect occurs.
      b. Contiguous spread of infection into bronchi by erosion and perforation → consolidation + hypersensitivity reaction = 'epituberculosis'. In older children it predominates in the upper lobes; middle and lower lobes in the younger age group.

   iii X-ray changes occur after 3 months (Figure 12.12). Findings on presentation:

Pulmonary shadowing (miliary or pneumonic)	45%
Mediastinal lymphadenopathy	38%
Effusion only	4%
Lymph nodes and effusion	3%
Normal X-ray	10%

3. Extrapulmonary sites (25%):
   'Cold abscess' in the neck (scrofula), overlying skin of red or purplish hue, usually due to bovine TB.
4. Miliary spread and tuberculous meningitis result if a lymph gland erodes into a blood vessel (i.e. post primary TB).
   Commonest age and most at risk are children aged less than 3 years old. Peak onset is 1–6 months after a primary infection.

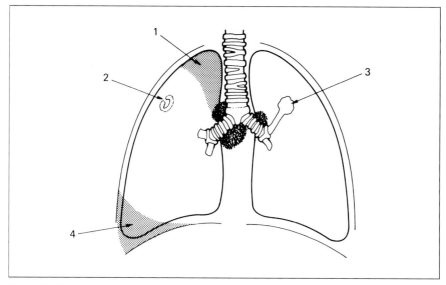

Figure 12.12 Typical changes associated with the primary complex to look for on chest x-ray.
1. RUL collapse due to mediastinal nodes.
2. Nodular lesion of calcified primary complex
3. Cavitation
4. Effusion/empyema

Findings:

    i Fever, anorexia, weight loss.
    ii Respiratory: cough, tachypnoea, pneumonia, with 'snow storm' appearance of generalized mottling on X-ray.
    iii Abdomen: distended by hepatosplenomegaly.
    iv CNS: progressive lethargy, coma, opisthotonus, convulsions; choroidal tubercles in 50%; CSF shows lymphocytosis, low glucose, raised protein, occasional acid fast bacilli.

5. Abdominal TB from bovine source (immigrant from underdeveloped country) or swallowing respiratory tract secretions. Rarely symptomatic, when an ulcerative colitis picture is seen, or tuberculous peritonitis with ascites or matted guts.

Reactivation: adult or chronic TB

Rare in childhood.
Pulmonary caseation and cavitation in adolescents. Kidneys at 3 years, bones and joints (knee, hip, spine) 5 years after primary infection.

Investigation

1. Mantoux, ESR; X-ray of chest, spine or long bone if affected; early morning gastric washings × 3 for acid fast bacilli and culture (takes 6 weeks). Culture

positive 20% in lymph node and pulmonary infection, 50% in meningeal infection. NB: Mantoux may be negative in severe disease, and in up to 40% with TB meningitis.

2. In lymphadenopathy, bone and joint disease: biopsy or aspirate for histology and culture.
3. Bone marrow or liver aspirate is helpful in diagnosing miliary spread.
4. In meningitis obtain CSF, consider CT of the head to identify hydrocephalus and tuberculomas.

 New, experimental diagnostic aids include enzyme linked immunosorbent assay of *M. tuberculosis* antigen and DNA probes of mycobacterial RNA. Rapid confirmation with great accuracy is claimed.

Differential diagnosis includes:

1. Atypical mycobacterial *Mycobacterium avium intracellulare* (MAI): presentation commonly as submandibular and cervical lymphadenitis. HIV associated.
   The Mantoux reaction with PPD is 5–12 mm. Biopsy and culture needed. Standard antituberculous drugs are usually ineffective, but surgical removal is usually curative (see Infectious diseases).
2. Sarcoid: Rare in children, commoner in adolescents. Non-caseating granuloma found in affected lymph gland or on Kveim test (rarely done). Characterized by breathlessness and dry cough. Uveitis and erythema nodosum may be associated. Hilar lymphadenopathy, possibly with widespread infiltrates. Steroids are only indicated for uveitis.

Treatment of TB (Table 12.8)

1.   Active disease (notifiable)

Promptly commence on the basis of a positive Mantoux, or negative but suspicious results in an ill, febrile child from a high risk background.

Table 12.8 First line antituberculous drug regimens and their duration

Initial phase (in months as n/12)	Continuation phase	Months of drugs
1 Active disease any site:* R I P for 2/12	R I for 4/12	Total 6/12
or R I for 2/12	R I for 7/12	Total 9/12
2 Chemoprophylaxis: I for 6/12		Total 6/12
R I for 3/12		Total 3/12

*Treat meningitis for 1 year minimum.
R = rifampicin 10–20 mg/kg/day (colours urine red, warn parents; major side effect hepatitis - substitute with ethambutol).
I = isoniazid 10 mg/kg/day (pyridoxine is unnecessary unless cachectic as peripheral neuritis is not found in children).
P = pyrazinamide 35 mg/kg/day (initial facial flushing, rash, nausea, arthralgia, hepatitis).

Second line drugs for children:

   i Ethambutol 10–15 mg/kg/day usually only until sensitivity of organism is established i.e. the first 2 months (but the risk of optic neuritis, requiring ophthalmic supervision, makes it unsuitable for young children).

  ii Streptomycin for tuberculous meningitis in the first 2–3 months.

 iii Prednisolone lowers raised intracranial pressure, may help in hilar compression, pericarditis, pleural effusion, miliary disease, and is given for 4–8 weeks.

Drug resistance: Caucasians very rare, up to 10% in Asians. To minimize this, 2 or 3 drugs are always given together in active disease.

Compliance must be checked regularly.

Cure is about 95% on the primary course of chemotherapy. Failure, relapse, or toxicity in the remainder will respond to an altered regimen.

Assess progress with serial ESR, X-rays, weight gain, clinical signs.

2. Chemotherapy (does not require notification)

   i Heaf positive, normal ESR and chest X-ray, give if:
No previous BCG and grade 2–4
Previous BCG and grade 3–4

  ii Heaf/Mantoux negative child, recently exposed to known infectious adult.

 iii Previously treated or has become immunosupressed, e.g. from steroids/chemotherapy, AIDS.

 iv Neonate of infected mother: continue breast feeding. Isoniazid for 3 months then check X-ray and Mantoux to determine whether to continue medication. In the UK it is policy to give BCG if negative, not so in the USA.

Contact tracing Delay in diagnosis is a hazard for contacts of the index case, and a large number of children may be infected before action is taken (Figure 12.13).

Prognosis

Excellent with treatment; rarely is there residual lung scarring, or bronchiectasis.

Most deaths occur in infancy and adolescence, which directs preventive strategy at these age groups.

Early diagnosis is critical in TB meningitis to avoid the feared complications (hydrocephalus, blindness, deafness, cerebral palsy, death).

Prevention

1. Screen all new immigrants from India and other developing countries. Identifies those needing treatment, chemoprophylaxis or BCG.
2. Bacille Calmette-Guérin (BCG) is given:

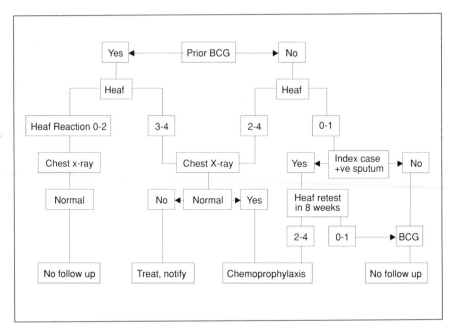

Figure 12.13 Algorithm for TB contact cases

    i At birth: almost 100% protection against TB meningitis and miliary TB in under 2 year olds. Recommended for those of African and Asian origin. Caucasian babies should also be offered it in areas with a high Afro-Asian immigrant mix. Revaccination in adolescence is desirable.

   ii Adolescence: 75% protected for at least 10 years. Routine testing of all children with Tine test or Heaf test at 13 years identifies those at risk. If the incidence of TB continues to fall, and HIV associated TB is contained, routine vaccination may be withdrawn in the mid 1990s.

NB: TB is notifiable to the local Medical Officer of Environmental Health (England and Wales), so that potential contacts are traced and assessed.

Further reading

Leader (1990) Perinatal prophylaxis of tuberculosis. *Lancet, ii,* 1479–1480

Leader (1988) Childhood tuberculosis in Britain. *British Medical Journal,* **297**, 1147–1148

Medical Research Council Tuberculosis and Chest Diseases Unit (1989) *Archives of Disease in Childhood,* **64**, 1004-1012

Snider D E, Rieder H L, Combs D, Bloch A B, Hayden C H, Smith M H D (1988) Tuberculosis in children. *Pediatric Infectious Disease Journal,* **7**, 271–278

Starke J R (1988) Modern approach to the diagnosis and management of tuberculosis in children. *Pediatric Clinics of North America,* **35**, 441–464

IMMUNE RELATED DISORDERS AFFECTING THE LUNGS (ALL RARE)

1. Idiopathic interstitial pneumonitis

Macrophages accumulate in the interstitium. Alveolar epithelial hyperplasia follows, desquamating into the alveoli, blocking them. The result is restrictive lung disease with impaired CO diffusion on testing.

Clinical

Breathless, dry cough, tired, weight loss. Cyanosis, finger clubbing and fine crackles on auscultation.

Investigations

Ground glass lung fields on X-ray. Hypoxia, hypocapnia leading to hypercapnia later.

Management

Steroids or antimetabolites may help, otherwise prognosis is poor.

2. Autoimmune

Complicating rheumatoid arthritis, systemic lupus erythematosus, as part of Goodpasture's syndrome and other connective tissue disorders.

An interstitial pneumonitis with findings similar to the idiopathic variety, but usually more responsive to steroids and antimetabolites.

3. Pulmonary haemosiderosis

Bleeding into the lungs, cause usually idiopathic, occasionally seen in cows' milk protein intolerance and Goodpasture's syndrome.

Clinical

Fever, cough, wheeze and intra-alveolar haemorrhage resulting in anaemia and rusty sputum.

Investigations

Chest X-ray varies from minor areas of consolidation that clear within a week to extensive bilateral mottling. Repeated bleeds cause interstitial opaque nodules.

Gastric aspirate contains haemosiderin laden macrophages.

Management

Transfusion, steroids, iron. Trial of cows' milk avoidance. May respond to anti-metabolites.

Further reading

Textbooks:

Dinwiddie R (1990) *The Diagnosis and Management of Paediatric Respiratory Disease*. Edinburgh:-Churchill Livingstone

Phelan P D, Landau L I, Olinsky A (1990) *Respiratory Illness in Children* 3rd edn. Oxford:Blackwell Scientific

Chapter 13

Cardiorespiratory arrest and hypotension

ABC OF RESUCITATION OF INFANTS AND CHILDREN

Most children present with hypoxia from respiratory failure or in hypovolaemic shock, in contradistinction from adults with cardiac arrest.

1. Place on a firm surface. Summon help.
2. Look for chest movement, listen for breath sounds (cheek close to victim's mouth), feel expired air on your cheek.
3. *Breathing?* Yes → recovery position.

No → Airway

   i Carefully sweep mouth cavity with swab round finger or suction to remove vomit; there is a danger of pushing a foreign body (FB) further down into the airway if FB is not considered.

  ii 'Tilt head backwards, and chin lift' to establish airway, while lifting the tongue off the posterior pharyngeal wall. NB: overextension will kink the soft trachea, excessive pressure under the jaw to the soft tissues of the mouth will force the tongue into the airway.

 iii If still not breathing consider obstruction by:

     a. Epiglottitis.
     b. Foreign body (FB), management:
        Infants: turn upside down and deliver 4 firm blows to the back.
        Children: abdominal compression by upward thrust of fist in the midline above the umbilicus (Heimlich manoeuvre) may move a FB upwards enough to grasp in older children.

Breathing

If still not breathing start mouth to mouth (or mouth and nose), gently breathing into the child until the chest wall rises adequately. Low pressure gives adequate volume avoiding gastric distention.

Best is endotracheal intubation + ventilate by hand, next is oral airway + IPPV via a tight fitting face mask with oxygen. Give 4 breaths initially.

Rate: Infant 24/minute, child 20/minute.

Use an uncuffed tube under 8 years old to avoid pressure necrosis to the trachea.

4. Circulation

Feel for the brachial pulse, alternatively use the carotid or femoral. If inadequate rate or volume, start chest compression. The heart lies under the lower sternum. Surface marking in a child is 2 finger breadths below the line joining the nipples.

Infant: apply pressure with both thumbs on the sternum, fingers encircling the chest.

Toddler: 2 fingers on the sternum, the other hand under the back (suitable for infants too). If a large toddler, use the heel of one hand, compressing 1.5–2.5 cm.

Child: heel of 2 hands, adult style, compressing 2.5–3.5 cm

   i   Smooth compression, not too rapid, enough to produce a pulse.
   ii Rate 100–120/minute.
   iii Release pressure between strokes to allow the sternum to return to its normal position, and time for the ventricles to fill.

Count aloud 1+ 2 + 3 + 4 + 5, then breathe into a small child; 15 compressions to 2 breaths into an older child, or if without an assistant.

5. Drugs (Table 13.1)

Establish i.v., or more rapidly, intraosseous access during resuscitation.

Controversy: hyperosmolar alkali infusions in cardiopulmonary resuscitation may compromise the outcome by reducing coronary perfusion. If the colour remains poor after 5–10 minutes, or frankly cyanosed, sodium bicarbonate 8.4% 1–2 ml/kg and glucose 25% 1–2 ml/kg may be given at the discretion of the resuscitation team leader, preferably after obtaining bloods for pH, glucose, biochemistry, etc.

Further action is rarely required as children usually have healthy myocardia.

6. ECG

Cardiac drugs are given according to the ECG trace. If ECG monitoring is unavailable, it is assumed that asystole is present.

Table 13.1 Drugs useful in cardiorespiratory arrest

Drug	Dose (volume)	Indication
Adrenaline* 1:10,000	10 μg/kg (0.1 ml/kg)	Asystole, severe anaphylaxis
Atropine* (600 μg/ml)	<1 year 0.1 ml, 1–4 years 0.2 ml	Atrial bradycardia/vagal stimu-
	5 years 0.3 ml, 12 years 0.6 ml	lation
Ca gluconate* (10%)	1 ml/year, maximum 10 ml	Cardiac arrest, hyperkalaemia
		Verapamil antidote
Dobutamine	2.5–10 μg/kg/min[+]	Low cardiac output
Dopamine*	2–4 μg/kg/min**	Renal shut down: reduced per-
		fusion
	10–20 μg/kg/min	Cardiogenic shock
Lignocaine 1%	0.5–1 mg/kg (0.05–0.1 ml/kg)	Ventricular tachyarrhythmia
	20–50 μg/kg/min	
Mannitol 20%	2.5–5 ml/kg	Cerebral oedema
Sodium bicarbonate 8.4%	1–5 mmol/kg (1–5 ml/kg)	Severe acidosis

* Inactivated if mixed with sodium bicarbonate
+ Add 2 ml/kg from 250 mg in 20 ml ampoule to 50 ml 5% dextrose. Rate 0.3–1.2 ml/h
** Add 0.5 ml/kg from 200 mg in 5 ml ampoule to 50 ms 5% dextrose. Rate 0.3–0.6 ml/h

  i Asystole: adrenaline is effective if instilled via the ET tube. Avoid the intra-cardiac route, unless in asystole, when adrenaline and calcium chloride are given first.

  ii Bradycardia: atropine *first*, as it may be vagally mediated, then adrenaline/isoprenaline.

iii Ventricular fibrillation/tachycardia: DC shock 1 joule/kg. Double and re-double dose if no response. Consider lignocaine, then bretylium, applying DC shock each time.

     If asystole follows, give adrenaline.

6. *F*ailure of circulation due to shock

If dehydration or pre-existing hypovolaemia is the likely cause of the arrest give albumin/haemaccel/dextrose saline by syringe, 20 ml/kg, as rapidly as possible to a total of 60 ml in the first hour. Follow up with dobutamine or dopamine infusion.

7. Cerebral oedema, renal failure, consumption coagulopathy require to be antici-pated (see relevant sections).

Further reading

Carcillo J A, Davis A L, Zaritsky A (1991) Role of early fluid resuscitation in pediatric septic shock. *Journal of the American Medical Association*, **286**, 1242–1245

Ryder I G, Munro H M, Doull I J M Intraosseous infusion for resuscitation. *Archives of Disease in Child-hood*, **66**, 1442–1443

HYPOTENSION

Causes are hypovolaemia, cardiogenic shock, or peripheral pooling (Table 13.2). All can lead to coma.

Table 13.2 Important causes of shock

Hypovolaemia	Cardiogenic	Peripheral pooling
Haemorrhage	Tension pneumothorax	Septic shock
Gastroenteritis	Pericardial effusion	Anaphylaxis
Diabetes mellitus and insipidus	Arrhythmias	Drugs: e.g. barbiturate
Hypoadrenalism	Congenital heart disease	Toxic shock syndrome
	Cardiomyopathy	

Assessment

1. The history

Vital to determining the cause.

Examples: trauma; access to drugs; infection–contacts or symptoms; sting or medication; increased or reduced voiding of urine; tampon use in an adolescent girl; known heart disease, diabetes, sickle cell, allergies.

2. Clinical

   i Smell: ketones, e.g. diabetes, starvation, hypoglycaemia.
  ii Skin: cyanosis, pallor, dehydration, rashes, trauma.
 iii Neurology: coma, focal signs, meningism, fundi for raised intracranial pressure.
  iv Trunk:
   • Ventilatory effort, added breath sounds.
   • Cardiac arrhythmia or failure, a murmur indicating heart disease.
   • Abdominal distension in necrotizing enterocolitis, surgical or infective problem.
     Organomegaly, e.g. splenic sequestration.
     Mass, e.g. haematoma.
   • Genitalia pigmented or ambiguous in congenital adrenal hyperplasia.

Investigations

1. Blood gases to establish severity of acidosis (usually from hypoperfusion) and hypoventilation.
2. Blood count, blood cultures, coagulation screen.
   WBC count may be raised in infection or stress, or low if overwhelming infection; consumption coagulopathy occurs in septic shock and hypovolaemic shock.

3. Serum electrolytes and urea, liver function and blood glucose. May identify major electrolyte deficits/excess and organ failure (e.g. renal, or liver in Reye's syndrome).
4. Blood and urine for drug screen, organic and amino acids.
·5. Cultures from septic sites, suprapubic urine aspiration, stool, and vagina if toxic shock syndrome is suspected in an adolescent. A lumbar puncture may be delayed if too sick, or raised intracranial pressure likely, as CSF antibodies to common microorganisms can be identified later.
6. Chest X-ray is likely to show pulmonary plethora in cardiogenic shock and peripheral pooling. Widespread or local consolidation in pneumonia. Sometimes little to see in the early stages, especially in staphylococcal pneumonia.
   Heart shape and size may be diagnostic.
7. ECG abnormalities of rhythm, e.g. supraventricular tachycardia, or strain patterns indicative as in endocardial fibroelastosis.

Management

Monitoring: insert a urinary catheter and consider central venous pressure monitoring. Continuous ECG, frequent BP measurement, core-periphery temperature difference (>3°C is significant).

1. Fluids
    i   Blood/plasma expander 20 ml/kg over 20 minutes
    ii In septic shock, give plasma quickly, followed by dextrose-saline to a total of 60 ml in the first hour, and 120 ml/kg within the first 6 h)
    iii Dopamine can be added in hypovolaemic states.

2. Pressor agent, e.g. dobutamine for cardiogenic shock.
3. Diuretic for systemic or pulmonary oedema.
4. Steroids in large dose if:

    i   Septic or toxic shock is likely.
    ii Response to resuscitation is incomplete: adrenal shock is possible, e.g. Waterhouse-Friderichsen syndrome.
    iii Anaphylaxis. First give an antihistamine and adrenaline subcutaneously or i.v.

5. Sodium bicarbonate (see Controversy in resuscitation): may give 1–2 ml/kg or base excess × 0.3 × body weight.
6. Antibiotics if indicated: penicillin and gentamicin or ampicillin and chloramphenicol or ceftazidime and flucloxacillin are standard broad spectrum combinations. Metronidazole may be added if an anaerobic infection is suspected, e.g. an immunocompromised child.

Further reading

Fleisher G R, Ludwig S (1988) *Textbook of Pediatric Emergency Medicine* 2nd edn. Baltimore, MD:Williams & Wilkins
Rogers M C (1987) *Textbook of Pediatric Intensive Care* Baltimore, MD:Williams & Wilkins
Selbst S M, Torrey S B (1988) *Pediatric Emergency Medicine for the House Officer* Baltimore, MD:Williams & Wilkins useful algorithms

Chapter 14

Cardiovascular problems

DEVELOPMENT OF THE HEART AND CONGENITAL HEART DISEASE

The heart begins in the third week of fetal life as a tube and within 4 weeks is a complex 4-chambered and valved organ.

Dextrocardia occurs if the tube bends to the left instead of the right. Defects are common if it is isolated, and uncommon with situs inversus when all the viscera are transposed.

Teratogenic influence

Vulnerable period 15–60 days fetal age.

Causes

Mainly multifactorial.

Others

1. Hereditary, e.g. AD as in Marfan's and Noonan's syndromes, some atrial septal defects, and hypertrophic obstructive cardiomyopathy.
2. Chromosomal, e.g. Down's syndrome, trisomy 13, 18, Turner's syndrome.
3. Maternal disease:

    i Diabetes

      a. Persistent: transposition of the great arteries (TGA), ventricular septal defect (VSD), single ventricle, hypoplastic left heart.
      b. Transient hypertrophic cardiomyopathy resolves by 6 months.

    ii Rubella: patent ductus arteriosus (PDA), pulmonary valve stenosis, branch and central pulmonary artery stenosis, coarctation of the aorta.
    iii Alcohol: VSD, ASD.
      Drugs: lithium and Ebstein anomaly; phenytoin and VSD or ASD.
    iv Phenylketonuria: tetralogy of Fallot, VSD, coarctation of aorta.
    v Systemic lupus erythematosis: complete heart block by Ro antibody.

4. Monozygotic twins.

CONGENITAL HEART DISEASE (CHD)

With renal anomalies, the commonest of persistent congenital abnormalities.

Natural history

25% would die in the neonatal period, 60% in infancy, and only 15% survive to adolescence. Altered by surgical repair and palliation.

Acquired disease is less common in developed countries where rheumatic heart disease and symptomatic infections are rare.

Incidence of congenital heart abnormalities

5–7 per 1000 live births.
Commonest nine overall in the UK (80% of all cases):
Ventriculoseptal defect (VSD) 30%.
2nd equal at 8% each: persistent patent ductus arteriosus (PDA), pulmonary stenosis (PS), atrioseptal defect (ASD).
5th equal: tetralogy of Fallot (TF), coarctation of aorta, aortic stenosis 6% each.
8th equal: transposition of great vessels (TGA), atrioventricular (AV) defect 4% each.
Commonest six in the first year
VSD (15%), TGA (10%), TF (9%), coarctation (8%), hypoplastic left heart (7%), PDA (6%).

Genetic risk and antenatal detection

1. General advice

Other than in Mendelian inherited conditions, the recurrence risk is small, bearing in mind the incidence of a fetal abnormality in any pregnancy is 3%.

  i Siblings 1–3%, and about 10% for left heart obstructive lesions like coarctation and hypoplastic left heart.
  ii Offspring of an affected parent 2–4%, may be higher for some individual lesions.

2. Antenatal diagnosis by US

Optimal US examination, including a four chamber view, e.g. to detect hypoplastic left heart defects, is at 18–24 weeks gestation, with the option of also performing chromosome analysis if appropriate. For example, detection of a complete atrioventricular septal defect may indicate a trisomy 21 which the mother may prefer terminated. If a hypoplastic left heart, termination is likely to be offered as the treatment option has a very high mortality.

Other situations benefiting from US examination:

i   High risk families with existing CHD in a first degree relative.
ii Diabetic mothers, and those taking possibly teratogenic drugs.
iii Other fetal abnormalities: arrhythmias, ascites, non-cardiac abnormalities seen on US.
iv Increasingly as part of the routine US examination in all pregnancies.

Further reading

Allen L D (1989) Diagnosis of fetal cardiac abnormalities. *Archives of Disease in Childhood*, **64**, 964-968

Allan L D, Cook D, Sullivan I, Sharland G K (1991) Hypoplastic left heart syndrome: effects of fetal echocardiography on birth prevalence. *Lancet*, *i*, 959--961

Lin A E, Garver K L (1988) Genetic counseling for congenital heart defects. *Journal of Pediatrics*, **113**, 1105-1109

Some associated syndromes

(Useful 'handles' to identify underlying heart disease.)

1. Asymmetric crying face (septal defects +/– renal, vertebral anomalies, anal atresia).
2. Ellis-van Crefeld syndrome AR: atrioseptal defect, short limbed dwarf, polydactyly, small nails.
3. Kartagener syndrome AR: situs invertus (50%), bronchiectasis, sinusitis, sterility in males due to abnormal dien arms in cilia structure.
4. Noonan syndrome: 1 in 2500; 50% have pulmonary stenosis, atrioseptal defect, or septal hypertrophy.
5. Williams syndrome: supravalvular aortic stenosis, 'elfin face', hypercalcaemia.
6. Associations: VACTERL association: expansion of VATER to include cardiac (VSD, ASD, PDA, Fallot's tetralogy) and limb defects. Incidence 1 in 6000. CHARGE association see Genetics.

EVALUATION OF HEART DISEASE

1. Age at presentation is a useful guide to the underlying lesion (Table 14.1).

Table 14.1 Age at presentation (a rough guide)

Hours or days	Atresia of pulmonary or aortic valve
Days to week	Hypoplastic left heart, complex defect, e.g. TGA, Fallot's tetralogy
One to 3 months	Large left to right shunt, e.g. VSD, PDA
Three months to one year	Fallot's tetralogy, endocardial fibroelastosis, paroxysmal atrial tachycardia, Kawasaki disease
Over one year	Eisenmenger syndrome, systemic hypertension, bacterial endocarditis

2. Symptoms of cardiac decompensation

   i Dyspnoea and slow to complete feeds. In infancy, the effort required is equivalent to an exercise test of cardiorespiratory reserve.

  ii Cyanosis.

 iii Dry cough and wheeze due to pulmonary oedema.

 iv Pallor/shock due to low systemic BP. Sweating, and crying persistently.

  v Excessive, rapid weight gain (>30 g/day) from fluid retention.

3. Precipitating factors

   i Infection, especially respiratory ⎱ Either can cause

  ii Anaemia. ⎰ acute cardiac failure.

4. Specific symptoms

Squatting in tetralogy of Fallot.

Chest pain in aberrant coronary arteries, plus syncope in aortic valve stenosis.

Lassitude, fever, anaemia, and purpura in bacterial endocarditis.

5. Pregnancy: rubella, alcohol, drugs, maternal diabetes.

6. Family history: see genetic aspects.

Examination

1. Observation

   i Abnormal facies/malformations in 10% of infants with CHD.

  ii Mucous membranes for anaemia, cyanosis, digits (fingers and toes) for clubbing.

Cyanosis

Present in the following situations:

   i Newborn with high haematocrit, with otherwise normal oxygen content, if >5 g/dl Hb desaturated.

  ii If >1.5 g/dl reduced Hb, providing the child is not anaemic, when pallor masks the cyanosis.

 iii Central: the tongue is most reliable, as the gums may be darkly pigmented in Asians and Blacks.

 iv Peripheral: hands and feet blue.

Normal in neonates.

Common finding in pyrexial illness as core temperature rises.

Shock.

  v Traumatic: head blue and purpuric from neck compression by umbilical cord/force.

 vi Differential

     a. Coarctation of the aorta with patent ductus → pink upper trunk, cyanosed below.

     b. Transposition of the great arteries with pulmonary hypertension → patent ductus arteriosus → cyanosed upper trunk, pink below.

Causes of central cyanosis

1. Central depression: drugs, immaturity, trauma, asphyxia.
2. Seizures.
3. Respiratory disease

    i V/Q imbalance, e.g. pneumonia, pneumothorax, atelectasis.
   ii Airway obstruction (choanal atresia, laryngeal/tracheal obstruction).

4. Shock: septicaemia, hypoglycaemia, adrenal crisis.
5. Polycythaemia in the newborn.
6. Cardiac disease.
7. Methaemoglobinaemia.

Assessment

1. History, chest X-ray, ECG, right radial (preductal) artery blood gas.
2. *Hyperoxia test*, breathing 100% oxygen for 10 minutes. Positive for CHD = arterial P_aO_2 of less than 20 kPa, in the absence of severe lung disease, or vigorous crying in a normal infant leading to intrapulmonary shunting. Rarely, an infant with significant mixing of systemic and pulmonary blood will appear pink, during the test, due to massive pulmonary blood flow.

Respiration and pulse

A respiration:pulse rate ratio of less than 3:1 is suggestive of a respiratory cause:

	Respiration/minute	Pulse/minute
Infant/toddler:	30 +/– 10	100 +/– 20
Child:	25 +/– 10	90 +/– 10

    i Palpate all 4 limb pulses and carotids.

- Delay or absence of femorals in coarctation may be difficult to evaluate in the infant.
- In a shocked neonate, absent left radial or carotid pulse points to an interrupted aortic arch.
- carotid thrill is found in left ventricular outlet obstruction, e.g. aortic stenosis.

   ii Weak pulse = poor peripheral circulation: e.g. Septic shock, Dehydration, Cardiac:

    a. In the neonate, aortic stenosis, hypoplastic left heart, coarctation with endocardial fibroelastosis, infective cardiomyopathy.
    b. At older ages, cardiac failure from many causes.

  iii Full, 'bounding' pulses: temperature, thyrotoxicosis, arteriovenous fistula, cardiac mixing with rapid pressure 'run off', e.g. patent ductus arteriosus, truncus arteriosus, aortopulmonary window.

3. Auscultation in infants and toddlers, before undressing which is often resented, and can result in crying. Lift vest/shirt or even listen through it!
4. Inspection. Once undressed look for:

   i Neck pulsations: increased in PDA, aortic incompetence, and thyrotoxicosis.
   ii Venous engorgement as a sign of cardiac failure: in <2 year olds it is more reliable to assess liver size.
   iii Precordial bulge = right ventricular hypertrophy. Thoracotomy and sterniotomy scars are indicative of palliative/reparative surgery to the heart and or lungs.
   iv Oedema over sacrum/around the eyes in recumbent infants.

5. Palpation

   i Precordium. Always check for dextrocardia.
      a. Apex beat. Impulse ++ from increased left ventricle stroke volume, e.g. VSD, and prolonged in outlet obstruction, e.g. aortic stenosis, coarctation. Left parasternal heave = right ventricular enlargement.
      b. Thrills are systolic, caused by forcing blood through a small diameter hole, e.g. VSD or narrowed aortic or pulmonary valve.
      c. Palpable pulmonary second sound in second left interspace = pulmonary hypertension.
   ii Liver edge: Normally 1–3 cm below the costal margin in nipple line. Enlargement in cardiac failure. Beware of apparent enlargement from the liver being pushed down by respiratory disease/lobar emphysema/subphrenic abscess.

6. Blood pressure.
   Take the blood pressure once you have gained the child's confidence. The cuff must cover most of the upper arm, with the bladder completely encircling the arm. In infants the Doppler method is commonly used, or the more traditional flush test which measures mean BP.

Normal range:

Age	Median BP	95th centile for systolic BP (mmHg)
Neonate	75	95
2–14 years	95	115

The BP is usually 20 mmHg higher in the legs, so reversal of normal suggests coarctation.
   Diastolic may be indeterminate even in healthy children.

Hypertension

Hypertension = >95th centile. Population screening is not justified. Obesity is the commonest association, and requires diet and sodium restriction.
   Risk factors: Neonatal umbilical artery catheterization. A family history of renal polycystic disease or phaeochromocytoma.
   Select renal disease, diabetes mellitus, neurofibromatosis, and familial hypertension for follow up.

Pathological causes:
  i In the first year renal vascular abnormalities (secondary to umbilical arterial thrombi, renal artery stenosis (RAS), renal vein thrombosis) and coarctation are the commonest causes.
  ii In early childhood mainly renal abnormality (90%):

    a 80%: reflux nephropathy, chronic glomerulonephritis, haemolytic uraemic syndrome, obstructive uropathy, (neurogenic or structural).
    b 10% renal vascular abnormalities (e.g. RAS in von Recklinghausen disease).
       Presentations: failure to thrive, headache, facial palsy.
       Investigate for a and b with US, DMSA, DTPA renal scans and/or micturating cystogram, peripheral and renal vein plasma renin, and angiography of the renal vein.
       Remaining 10%:

    1. Raised intracranial pressure.
    2. Tumours, e.g. neuroblastoma, phaeochromocytoma, Wilm's.
    3. Endocrine: congenital adrenal hyperplasia, Cushing syndrome, primary hyperaldosteronism.

       Characteristic clinical findings with imaging of tumours and urinary amines or steroid excretion.
  iii Older children: obesity and essential hypertension are most likely, and unless secondary hypertension is suspected, examination, family history, normal urinalysis, sterile urine, normal serum electrolytes, bicarbonate and creatinine suffice.

Management of hypertension

1. Surgery for appropriate cases.
2. Mild, and essential hypertension: weight reduction, salt restriction, exercise.
3. Moderate to severe: first try a thaizide diuretic or frusemide, next a β-blocker, finally a vasodilator. Hyper-reninaemia secondary to renal hypertension responds well to the angiotensin converting enzyme (ACE) inhibitor captopril.
4. Hypertensive crisis: the vasodilator sodium nitroprusside, except in acute post infectious glomerulonephritis, when frusemide alone is usually sufficient.

Drug doses
Captopril 0.5–2 mg/kg twice daily.
Chlorthiazide 10 mg/kg twice daily.
Frusemide 1–2 mg/kg two to three times daily.
Hydralazine 0.5 mg/kg three times daily (idiosyncratic hypotension is a danger, so always give a test dose).
Propranolol 0.5–1 mg/kg three times daily, up to 2 mg/kg/dose.
Sodium nitroprusside 0.5–1μg/kg/minute.

Further reading

Report of the Second Task Force on Blood Pressure Control in Children (1987) *Pediatrics*, **79**, 1–25

AUSCULTATION

Order:

1. Heart sounds, concentrating on the second: if single = pathological

Normally the aortic valve closes before the pulmonary valve. The gap widens in inspiration, and its absence requires an explanation. If the younger child cannot regulate breathing, the first few beats on sitting up after lying down will bring out the presence of splitting.

  i   Single and loud in pulmonary hypertension when pulmonary artery pressure approaches systemic, as in a large VSD, where the systolic murmur may disappear as the pressures become equal, i.e. becoming an Eisenmenger's syndrome. Only the quality of the heart sound indicates the severity of the condition.
 ii   Single and soft in aortic stenosis or hypoplastic left heart, and may even be so delayed as to give reversed splitting, i.e. wider in expiration.

Split, fixed and usually wide in ASD, though it may be narrow in infancy, only to be detected in later childhood as the heart rate falls.

Split widely, varying with respiration, with soft second sound in isolated pulmonary stenosis or Fallot's tetralogy (may sound single).

First heart sound: loud in mitral stenosis (rare).

2. Added sounds

Third heart sound during early ventricular filling, is low pitched (best heard with bell):

  i   Physiological and heard in 20% of normal hearts.
 ii   Pathological gallop due to a dilated, poorly contracting, or failing, left ventricle, as in aortic stenosis, or myocarditis.

Ejection click

  i   High frequency, heard in early systole = stenosis with post-stenotic dilatation of aorta or pulmonary artery. Click is absent if the valve is thickened or severely dysplastic.
      Diagnostic confusion occurs when 'aortic clicks' are heard due to truncus arteriosus, dilatation of the aortic root in pulmonary atresia or Fallot's tetralogy, but the infant is more usually cyanosed in these states.
      Site aids identification. Pulmonary valve abnormalities in the pulmonary area (left upper sternal border), aortic at the apex.
 ii   Mid systole = mitral valve prolapse.

3. Murmurs

Listen in systole, then diastole. A murmur may be physiological in systole but never in diastole (*cave* venous hums).

Systolic murmurs

In general, these are due to impeded flow, the intensity proportional to the pressure gradient. Low frequency murmurs are likely to produce a thrill as in VSD or aortic stenosis, but not with high pitched murmurs as in mitral regurgitation.

  i Ejection 'diamond shaped' murmur = high pressure gradient due to obstruction or increased flow:

    a. *Narrow* semilunar valves in:

- aortic stenosis: apical murmur, associated with a carotid thrill, +/- apical click.
- pulmonary stenosis: second left interspace, single second sound or soft pulmonary component. If a pulmonary click is present, the earlier it occurs the more severe the stenosis.

    b. Normal valves with *increased flow*:

- ASD (fixed splitting of the second sound).
- VSD with high pulmonary pressure raising right ventricular pressure, and only the loud second sound is a warning of this potentially irreversible danger.

  ii Pansystolic murmur = low pressure gradient, either through a shunt, or regurgitation through a valve:

    a. *Shunt*: site, radiation and intensity are of help in older infants.

- e.g. VSD, best heard at left sternal border, radiating to the apex and through to the lower back. Loudness is proportional to size, i.e. soft in a small VSD; may be shortened towards the end of systole if due to small muscular defects which close during the contraction.
- PDA, subclavicular, radiating through to the left scapula area. Found in infancy, in which pressures in the aorta and pulmonary artery are equal in diastole at which point no flow occurs across it.

    b. *Regurgitant*: incompetent mitral/tricuspid valve.

- Lower left sternal border (difficult to differentiate from VSD): tricuspid due to persistent pulmonary hypertension in the neonate or obstructed right ventricular outflow as in pulmonary atresia and Ebstein's anomaly.
- Blowing, apical, radiating to the axilla: mitral incompetence. Differentiate from mild mitral valve prolapse, found in up to 5% of normal children and Marfan's syndrome, with its loud mid-systolic click and late systolic murmur using the diaphragm, and not usually heard in infancy.

Diastolic murmurs are always pathological

  i Early diastolic, soft and high pitched: incompetent semilunar aortic or pulmonary valve. Use the diaphragm down the left sternal edge, child sitting forward, holding breath in expiration.

   a. Common after valvotomy for aortic stenosis, valvotomy and repair of Fallot's tetralogy.
   b. To-and-fro murmur. A combination of ejection systolic with early diastolic murmur in the aortic area and lower left sternal edge is indicative of an abnormal and incompetent valve as in:

   • truncus arteriosus (often with an early systolic click), or
   • subvalvular aortic stenosis (no click).
   • Absent pulmonary valve is similar, heard in the pulmonary area.

 ii Middle diastole, tends to be a low pitched rumble. Use the bell:

   a. Usually across normal valves with increased flow due to shunts. Its presence indicates that the ratio of flow through the shunt of pulmonary to systemic circulations is >2:1.

   Tricuspid: lower left sternal edge, increasing on inspiration in ASD, and anomalous pulmonary venous connection.
   Mitral: apical in PDA, VSD.
   b. Stenotic mitral valve in obstructive left heart conditions.

iii Late diastole/presystole: obstructed flow across a 'tight' mitral valve; a VSD's increased flow will accentuate it. Low pitched, rumbling, best heard with the bell.

Continuous murmurs

A pressure difference is present throughout the cardiac cycle.

  i Patent ductus arteriosus in 90% (usually systolic alone in infancy).
 ii Combinations of AS and AI, MI and AI, VSD and AI.
iii Collateral circulation, best heard over the back:

   a. Acyanotic: aortic in coarctation of the aorta, >5 years old.
   b. Cyanosed: bronchial collaterals in pulmonary atresia + VSD.

Venous hum, being continuous, may cause confusion, but it disappears on lying down, applying pressure over the neck veins, or in a Valsava manoeuvre.

Innocent murmurs

Characteristics are:

  i Asymptomatic.
 ii Heart sounds are normal.
iii The murmur is systolic, short ejection. Never diastolic.
 iv Intensity: soft, grade 3/6 or less.

v Localized usually to the left of the sternum. No radiation through to the back.
vi Varies with posture.

Other innocent types heard in childhood

- Venous hum, see above.
- Vibratory: like the buzzing of a bee, becoming softer if sat up and the neck extended.
- Pulmonary systolic murmur (upper left chest → infraclavicular region) with normal splitting in inspiration. Differential is from mild pulmonary stenosis, where a widely split second sound is heard, with ECG and chest X-ray changes.

Investigations

Chest X-ray

Assess cardiac size, presence of pulmonary artery or right–sided aorta, and lung field vascularity. Classic shape, e.g. Fallot's 'coeur en sabot', is absent in 50%.
  Important features to be noted:

1. Cardiomegaly = cardiothoracic ratio of >0.50, due to: congestive cardiac failure, pericardial effusion, myocarditis, cardiomyopathy, complete heart block, Ebstein's malformation.
   Thymus shadow can confuse. The sail/wave signs help to differentiate. Rapid thymic involution in cyanosis/stress.
2. Absent pulmonary artery shadow in pulmonary stenosis/atresia, Fallot's tetralogy, TGA, truncus arteriosus, and tricuspid atresia.
3. A right-sided aortic arch is seen in Fallot's tetralogy (20%), pulmonary atresia with VSD. Less common are TGA and truncus arteriosus.
4. Notched ribs, due to collaterals in coarctation of the aorta, are seen from 5 years old.
5. Lung fields and pulmonary blood flow (PBF)

- Increased vascularity (PBF) in left to right shunts.

   i Acyanotic: PDA, VSD, ASD, atrioventricular canal.
   ii Cyanotic: TGA, truncus arteriosus, single ventricle.

- Venous congestion (hazy lung fields) if back pressure occurs, e.g. heart failure from coarctation, aortic stenosis, hypoplastic left heart, total anomalous pulmonary venous connection (TAPVC).
- Decreased vascularity (PBF)

   i Acyanotic: Pulmonary stenosis. In pulmonary hypertension a 'pruned' appearance with loss of vascular markings towards the periphery of the lung.
   ii Cyanotic: Fallot's tetralogy, atresia of pulmonary/tricuspid valve, Ebstein's malformation.

Electrocardiogram (Figure 14.1 and Table 14.2)

Normal findings:

QRS axis moves anticlockwise with age.

Table 14.2 Selected ECG changes

Type	*Cause*
1 Ventricular hypertrophy: the R wave changes	

i *Right ventricular hypertrophy*
     $V_4R>15$ mm if < 3 months old
     $V_4R>10$ mm if > 3 months old
	1 Acyanotic: pulmonary stenosis
	2 Cyanotic: Fallot's, TGA, pulmonary hyper-
	  tension

ii *Left ventricular hypertrophy*
     V6 > 20 mm if < 3 months old
     V6 > 25 mm if > 3 months old
	Acyanotic: shunts, left heart obstruction and/or
	valve incompetence, cardiomyopathy, endocar-
	dial fibroelastosis

iii *Biventricular hypertrophy* Sum of R+S waves > 70 mm	VSD
2 QRS negative in 1, aVF, + RBBB QRS negative in 1, aVF, no RBBB	Atrioventricular defect Tricuspid atresia
3 RBBB of rsR in V_1, prolonged PR RBBB +/- complete heart block	ASD secundum After surgery for Fallot's, VSD
4 Short PR, broad QRS with δ wave	Wolff Parkinson White syndrome

Echocardiography

Cross-sectional echocardiography shows anatomical detail, pericardial effusions, vegetations. Doppler echocardiography gives information on flow rates and patterns, and gradients of pressure across valves.

Cardiac catheterization

Indications now few, as information is more safely obtained by echocardiography. One such is pulmonary artery pressure in pulmonary hypertension, as operability depends on the severity of pulmonary vascular resistance. However, the velocity of a regurgitant jet from the pulmonary valve, or flow across a PDA, can be measured by Doppler, so catheterization may be unnecessary.

Normal catheterization data

1. Oxygen saturation (%)   right heart 75 +/− 5
                                    left heart 97 +/− 2

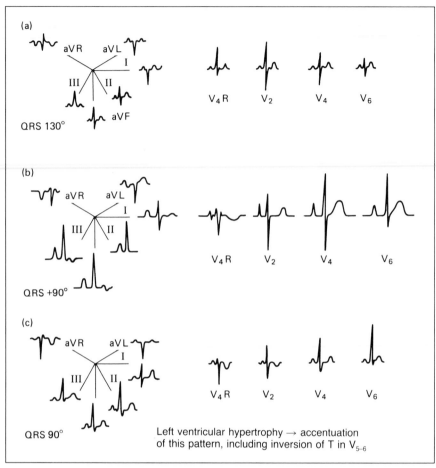

Figure 14.1
a. Newborn normal ECG, with positive QRS complexes in right chest leads, aVR, III and V₄R. At older ages right ventricular hypertrophy has a similar or more accentuated pattern.
b. By contrast, a neonate with pulmonary atresia and intact ventricular septum showing severely reduced right ventricular activity for age, and tall P waves.
c. A child up to 8 years old. Positive complexes in II, aVF, III, and inverted T waves from V₄R to V₃

2. Pressure in mmHg:

right atrium	3–7
left atrium	10–13
right ventricle	25/0
left ventricle	90–120/0
pulmonary artery	25/10
aorta	90–120/50–80
pulmonary arterial wedge	10–13

COMMON PRESENTATION OF CHD IN THE NEWBORN AND INFANT, BASIC MECHANISMS, AND DIFFERENTIATION FROM NON–CARDIAC CAUSES

Presentation is usually with cyanosis, and/or heart failure, and occasionally as an arrhythmia.

Cyanosis

Mechanism: abnormal connection of great vessels, obstruction to flow, or mixing of systemic and pulmonary circulation.

Examples in the newborn

1. Inadequate mixing. Aorta arising from the right ventricle as in transposition of the great arteries (TGA).
2. Obstructive +/– intracardiac defect:

   i Pulmonary valve atresia/critical stenosis +/– ventriculoseptal defect (VSD) or patent ductus arteriosus (PDA).
   ii Pulmonary artery vasoconstriction (dynamic): persistent fetal circulation through a PDA.
   iii Small ventricles: hypoplastic left heart, Ebstein's malformation in which the tricuspid valve is displaced into the right ventricle.

3. Mixing of systemic and pulmonary venous blood as in total anomalous pulmonary venous connection (TAPVC) with obstruction to venous return, and in truncus arteriosus.

Cyanosis, presenting in infancy, caused by mixing of systemic and pulmonary circulations

   i Fallot's tetralogy, tricuspid atresia, Ebstein's, TAPVC, complete atrioventricular defect, or truncus arteriosus.
   ii Acyanotic progressing to cyanotic heart disease:
   Large VSD or ASD with pulmonary hypertension = Eisenmenger syndrome, following the reversal of a L → R shunt in VSD, transposition of the great arteries, and Down's syndrome with VSD or atrioventricular defect. Fortunately rare before 2 years in a simple VSD.

Heart failure

Presentation

Tachypnoea, tachycardia, excessive weight gain, wheeze.
   Pathophysiology due to at least one of the following mechanisms:

1. Obstruction (pressure overload): hypoplastic left heart, coarctation of the aorta, aortic stenosis.
2. Hyperdynamic (volume overload) circulation: PDA, truncus arteriosus. Large arteriovenous fistula in the cranium or liver are rare but warrant auscultation of these organs.
3. Pump failure (myocarditis) is unusual: viral, ischaemia, metabolic.
4. Incomplete diastolic filling (constrictive pericarditis, pericardial effusion, chronic tachycardias) is rare.

   VSD and PDA, the common causes after 3–4 weeks old, are usually asymptomatic before the fall in pulmonary vascular resistance.

   Absence of a heart mumur does not exclude heart disease and is not uncommon in TGA, TAPVC, hypoplastic left heart, and coarctation of the aorta.

   Acyanotic heart disease may present as cyanotic, secondary to cardiac failure and respiratory difficult.

Differential diagnosis

Cyanotic congenital heart disease (CHD) has to be differentiated from:

- respiratory problems
- Persistent pulmonary hypertension
- Myocardial malfunction
- Arrhythmias

Rarely, chocolate coloured blood with the slate blue cyanosis of methaemoglobinaemia is found.

1. Respiratory disorder

Whenever cyanotic CHD is suspected do a hyperoxia/nitrogen wash out test, obtaining blood gases in air and after 10 minutes in 100% oxygen. The P_aO_2 should rise to >20 kPa; if less than 5 kPa, shunting due to pulmonary hypertension or CHD is likely. A raised P_aCO_2 suggests a respiratory cause. This test is not diagnostic, but indicates which line of investigation should be pursued, e.g. echocardiography, Doppler blood flow studies.

2. Persistent pulmonary hypertension (persistent fetal circulation, PFC)

Definition   The shunting of blood away from the lungs via the ductus arteriosus and foramen ovale due to persistently raised pulmonary vascular resistance.

Incidence   1 in 1500 live births.

Aetiology   Usually precipitated by hypoxic delivery, meconium aspiration, hypoglycaemia and maternal diabetes, polycythaemia, or sepsis.

Pathophysiology   Hypoxia → pulmonary artery constriction, mediated by leukotrienes, products of arachidonic acid metabolism. (Prostaglandins are also produced from arachidonic acid, of which E_1 and prostacyclin (PGI_2) can reverse the vasocon-strictive effect).

Presentation Cyanosis, tachypnoea within 24 h of birth, sometimes with very rapid deterioration.

Diagnosis Systolic murmur due to tricuspid incompetence, normal ECG, chest X-ray slightly oligaemic. Echo confirms normal heart.

Treatment
1. Hyperventilate to reduce CO_2 and so peripheral pulmonary arterial resistance, with as high an oxygen concentration as necessary.
   NB: Pulmonary blood flow is reduced by high intrathoracic pressures, so avoid high end-expiratory pressures and an inspiratory to expiratory ratio of greater than 1:1. Pancuronium paralysis is essential.
2. Correct metabolic acidosis with i.v. bicarbonate or THAM.
3. If hypoxaemia persists:

   i   Tolazoline, an α-adrenergic blocker, works best when >7.20 pH. Give i.v., 1–2 mg/kg bolus, then continuous infusion of 0.5–2 mg/kg/h, with dopamine and plasma expanders ready to counteract systemic hypotension.
   ii PGI_2 via pulmonary artery catheter (magnesium sulphate? see PFC in Neonatal problems).
   iii Extracorporeal membrane oxygenation (ECMO) if available.

Prognosis
Mortality 20–40%. Neurological abnormality in up to half of survivors.

3. Myocardial ischaemia

Due to hypoxia or hypoglycaemia causing shock. ECG: T wave inversion, ischaemic/infarct pattern. Chest X-ray: cardiomegaly, pulmonary oedema. Digitalize, diuretics, oxygen.

4. Arrhythmias

i Supraventricular tachycardia
Atrial rate 240–300/minute.
Detected in utero or as attacks of dyspnoea, and/or pallor.

Cause 80% idiopathic; also in ASD, Ebstein's malformation, cardiomyopathy, mitral valve prolapse.

Pathophysiology Usually re-entry of electrical impulse via an aberrant pathway, leading to circular excitation (other less common causes: atrial flutter, ectopic atrial tachycardia). Wolff-Parkinson-White syndrome is the best known. ECG between attacks: short P-R <0.12 s; QRS >0.12 s and abnormal ventricular excitation shows as a slur, i.e. delta wave.

Treatment In utero give mother digoxin.

After birth: ice bag to face is effective in 90% (vagal stimulation), then try i.v. adenosine (short acting, safe) or cardioversion.

Prophylaxis: oral digoxin (50% success), or oral flecainide.

Hazards:

    a. Avoid digoxin in WPW (i.e. delta wave on ECG) which may precipitate ventricular tachycardia.

    b. Verapamil can cause dangerous/fatal hypotension in infancy, or any patient in heart failure.

Prognosis 75% free of recurrence if age <3 months at onset.

ii Ventricular tachycardia
Uncommon in children, usually the result of electrolyte imbalance or structural heart disease. Treatment as in resuscitation section.

iii Complete heart block
Causes: Most are idiopathic congenital. Corrected TGA or maternal lupus erythematosus must be considered in the newborn.

Heart failure and syncope occur if the rate falls below 50/min. If still in utero, deliver early; after birth consider a pacemaker.

5. Other causes of cyanosis and respiratory distress

- Septic shock.
- Seizures, CNS depression by drugs, trauma, asphyxia.
- Reye's syndrome, inborn metabolic error.
- Hypoglycaemia.

Management principles

1. Neonate

Early diagnosis improves prognosis. Ductus arteriosus patency may be necessary for survival, until palliation or repair is achieved. To facilitate this, early referral to a specialist centre in optimal condition is the aim.

    i General: avoid hypoxia as this leads to acidosis, hypoglycaemia, and hypovolaemia. Maintain temperature. Hypothermia is common in cyanosis, acidosis and shock.

Table 14.3 Benefits of establishing/maintaining ductal patency in CHD

Lesion benefiting	Pathophysiological mechanism
Obstructive right heart: pulmonary or tricuspid atresia/stenosis	Pulmonary blood flow maintained until systemic-pulmonary shunt fashioned
Obstructive left heart: preductal coarctation, interrupted aortic arch, severe aortic stenosis, hypoplastic left heart	Renal perfusion is critical, otherwise profound irreversible metabolic acidosis develops
Transposition of the great vessels without a septal defect	Otherwise inadequate mixing of the systemic and pulmonary circulations

ii Prostaglandin E (PGE) i.v./orally to keep ductus arteriosus open

Prostaglandin may induce apnoea (requiring IPPV), raise body temperature, cause seizure, or thrombocytopenia.

Dose: PGE_1 i.v. 0.003–0.005 µg/kg/min or orally PGE_2 25–50 µg/kg hourly, reducing to 2 hourly after a week's treatment.

Supplemental oxygen without PGE can close the ductus arteriosus and worsen hypoxia.

iii Bicarbonate, glucose, calcium as biochemically indicated.

iv Albumin, dobutamine/dopamine to counteract shock and improve cardiac output.

2. Infants and children

i General: Prop up, 30% oxygen, nasogastric feeds in infants. Cool if a large shunt causes a rise in the metabolic rate.

ii Correct biochemical abnormalities: acidosis, hypoglycaemia, hypocalcaemia.

iii Medication:

a. Antibiotic for respiratory infection.

b. Sedation with phenobarbitone if restless. Opiates are avoided as being likely to depress respiration more, especially if already cyanosed.

c. Hypovolaemic shock: colloid and electrolytes (see Hypotension, Gastroenterology problems).

d. Congestive failure:

Diuretics to reduce preload. Potassium supplements are also required if digoxin is administered; alternatively add spironolactone.

Vasodilator: captopril by reducing the after-load is increasingly preferred to inotropic digoxin for a failing heart, especially if due to a high output state, e.g. VSD.

Inotropes: dobutamine +/– dopamine in the acute situation, digoxin for sustained inotropic action.

Digoxin fails to benefit lesions with outflow obstruction, e.g. aortic stenosis, Fallot's tetralogy, and should not be used.

Drug dosages

Captopril: 1 mg/kg 8 hourly, increasing to a maximum of 3 mg/kg/dose.

Digoxin: Digitalization dose: premature 15 μg/kg over 24 h, in older age groups 40 μg/kg over 24 h; 1/2 dose stat, 1/4 at 8 and 16 h. Maintenance 5–15 μg/kg daily. Therapeutic level 1–3 ng/ml.

Diuretics: frusemide 1–3 mg/kg/day, (Potassium chloride 2 mmol/kg/day as supplement unless spironolactone (potassium sparing effect) is used). Hydrochlorthiazide 1–4 mg/kg/day, spironolactone 3 mg/kg/day. Dobutamine/dopamine 5–10 μg/kg/min.

3. Consider surgical options early

Surgical treatment indications

Required by 60% with CHD, 40% of these in the first year of life.

1. Palliative procedures are less favoured than before, as one-stage corrective procedures, e.g. arterial switch in TGA, can now be done from the neonatal period onwards.

   i   Shunts to improve blood supply to the lungs, e.g. pulmonary atresia.
   ii Banding to reduce pulmonary blood supply, e.g. multiple muscular VSD.
   iii Balloon septostomies to improve mixing at atrial level in TGA if the arterial switch is not done (see TGA).

2. Corrective procedures:

   i   Cardiopulmonary bypass. The operative risk is related to the condition, not the procedure.
   ii Balloon dilatation: treatment of choice in pulmonary valve stenosis, aortic valve stenosis, recoarctation of the aorta.
   iii Occlusive devices will increasingly be used, for their low morbidity and avoidance of surgery: double umbrella occluder in PDA >10 kg, clam occluder for ASD, and possibly for VSDs.
   iv Human cadaveric homograft valves for aortic and pulmonary valve replacement are preferred as they do not require anticoagulation and, unlike tissue valved conduits, are not prone to calcific deterioration. Aortic valve homografts may need replacing as children grow.

3. Transplantation: now 50% survival to 3 years.

   i   Cardiac for cardiomyopathies, endocardial fibroelastosis, hypoplastic left heart syndrome.
   ii Cardiopulmonary for Eisenmenger syndrome and pulmonary hypertension, and for cystic fibrosis.

Long-term problems in survivors of operated CHD

1. Bacterial endocarditis.

2. Arrhythmias.
3. Progressive pulmonary vascular disease.
4. Myocardial failure.
5. Replacement of valves and conduits.
6. Advice on employment, genetic risk to offspring, pregnancy.

Further reading

Somerville J (1989) Congenital heart disease in the adolescent. *Archives of Disease in Childhood*, **64**, 771–773

COMMONER AND SELECTED CONGENITAL HEART CONDITIONS

Classify clinically as either *acyanotic* or *cyanotic* and whether *obstructive* or with *increased flow or shunt.*

1. Acyanotic obstructive

Pulmonary stenosis 8%, coarctation of the aorta and aortic stenosis 6% each, and hypoplastic left heart syndrome, which often incorporates the latter two conditions.

Pulmonary stenosis

Definition

Thickened, dome shaped valve with central hole.

Pathophysiology

Right ventricle may hypertrophy and the cavity thus become smaller, further reducing flow to the lungs.

The pressure gradient in mild stenosis commonly does not progress as the child grows, but worsens in severe stenosis.

Clinical

Initially asymptomatic even if the stenosis is severe. Dyspnoea and fatigue appear as severity and decompensation increase.

Cheeks have almost crimson patches, with peripheral cyanosis.

Centrally pink unless a right to left shunt develops through a stretched (from back pressure in the right atrium) foramen ovale.

Low cardiac output is a sign of decompensation, so look for giant 'a' waves in the neck, liver enlargement and presystolic pulsation.

Palpation: right ventricular heave, systolic thrill second interspace, proportional to stenosis.

Heart sounds: the first is followed by a click as the valve opens, and the earlier it is, the tighter the stenosis. The second sound pulmonary component is delayed and may disappear if the stenosis is very severe.

Murmur: harsh loud ejection systolic, maximal second left interspace. The length increases proportional to the stenosis, i.e.:

Mild–ending before the second sound.
Severe–obliterating the second sound due to prolonged right ventricular systole.

Investigations

Chest X-ray: normal size heart, dilated pulmonary artery, diminished blood flow to the lungs.

ECG: right ventricular hypertrophy and peaked P waves develop.

Echo and Doppler show the anatomy and gradient, respectively.

Management

Doppler gradient <30 mmHg–no action; 30–50 mmHg–review; >50 mmHg–proceed to cardiac catheterization and consider balloon valvuloplasty. Right ventricular hypertrophy then subsides.

Coarctation of the aorta

Definition

Narrowing at the isthmus of the aorta due to ductal tissue in its wall. VSD and left heart valve abnormalities are common, and linked with other malformations, e.g. Turner's, congenital rubella.

1. Preductal   Can be detected antenatally as a narrow aortic segment. Supply to the kidneys, liver and lower limbs is through the ductus until it closes. Thereafter circulation is maintained through a very narrow segment. Heart and renal failure, acidosis and hypoglycaemia follow, usually presenting in the first two weeks of life as the ductus closes.

Clinical signs Pallor, shock, poor femoral pulses and blood pressure. Always check using the right radial or brachial artery, as the left subclavian may be post coarctation.

BP normal in arms, low in legs.

Investigations X-ray chest: plethoric lung fields, dilated heart. ECG variable, left ventricular hypertrophy in severe stenosis.

Echo: shows the coarctation. Always look for VSD, and valvular abnormalities. Catheterization is now rarely indicated.

Management

    i Medical emergency. Prompt treatment saves lives. Prostaglandin E$_2$ infusion opens the ductus; also give alkali, glucose, calcium i.v. Combat heart and kidney failure with diuretics and dopamine.

    ii Surgical. Mortality improved by better medical management. The subclavian artery is incorporated into a flap to enlarge the aorta. VSD managed according to size, may need pulmonary artery banding at the same time.

2. Postductal constriction is associated with the development of collaterals across the coarcted segment antenatally. Bicuspid aortic valve may be present.

Clinical signs Presents as weak femoral pulses in infancy or delayed pulses in later childhood once collaterals are well developed. They may be felt and heard round the scapulae.

    BP elevated in the arms. Left ventricular hypertrophy.

Investigations X-ray chest: Penetrated view shows 'figure 3' = aortic bulge, constriction and post-stenotic bulge; reversed on barium swallow. Rib notching from collaterals after 6 years old.

    ECG: Left ventricular hypertrophy.

    Echo: Establishes site of coarctation, and the presence of other lesions. Doppler demonstrates the pressure gradient.

Management Surgery: Mortality <1%. Hypertension may be reactive and settles quickly, or may be more persistent (consider re-coarctation and the need for balloon dilatation) and requires regular follow up for both types of coarctation.

Further reading

Leader (1991) Coarctation repair–the First Forty Years. *Lancet*, ii, 546

Aortic stenosis

Site: valvular, supravalvular (William's syndrome), and subvalvular (diaphragm, hypertrophic obstructive cardiomyopathy) (Figure 14.2).

Aortic valve stenosis

Isolated type Boys>girls. Commoner in Turner's syndrome and coarctation.

Pathology Mild to moderate severity: bicuspid valve is commonest. Severe: unicusp or non-cuspid, like a diaphragm with a hole.

Clinical presentation Infancy: heart failure, sudden death.

    Childhood: asymptomatic murmur or with dyspnoea, central chest pain, and exercise induced faints.

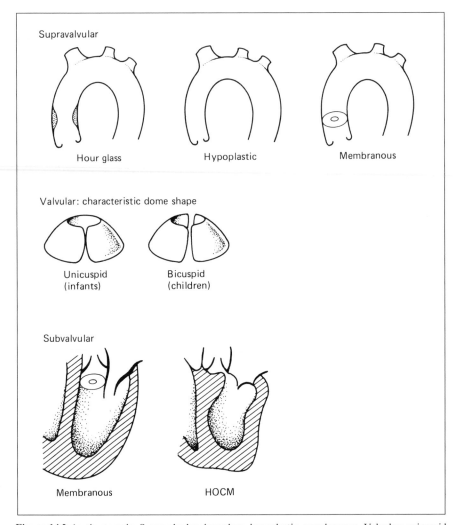

Figure 14.2 Aortic stenosis. Supravalvular: hourglass, hypoplastic, membranous. Valvular: unicuspid (infants), bicuspid (children). Subvalvular: membranous, hypertrophic obstructive cardiomyopathy (HOCM)

Pulse: normal unless severe when it is small volume, 'plateau' type.

Precordium: pulsation seen, systolic thrill felt at suprasternal notch.

Heart sounds: click before first sound, due to mobile aortic valves. Followed by an ejection systolic murmur in the aortic area and up into the neck. The second sound may be normal if mild or moderately stenosed, but single or even reversed with increased splitting on expiration if severe.

Investigations Chest X-ray: post-stenotic dilatation.

ECG: often unhelpful. May show left ventricular hypertrophy.

Echo:

- Cross-sectional: valve cusps may be reduced in number, thickened, and show reduced movement.
- M mode: shows closure of bicuspid valve is eccentric, and size of left ventricle increased.
- Doppler demonstrates gradient. Mild = 20 mmHg, moderate = 50 mmHg, severe = 60–100 mmHg. Catheter studies are now rarely done.

Management

1. Restriction of physical activities in moderate stenosis avoids gross hypertrophy and the dangers of arrhythmias and sudden death. Follow-up is essential to assess the degree of left ventricular hypertrophy.
2. Balloon dilatation is the procedure of choice.
3. Surgical indications for aortic valvotomy.

   i Failure of balloon dilatation of the stenosis.
  ii Neonatal presentation, i.e. severe.
 iii Heart failure or ischaemia detected in moderately severe stenosis.

Valve replacement is rare in childhood, considered for severe aortic regurgitation which may occur after balloon or surgical valvotomy. Complications of prosthetic valves are incompetence and failure to grow with the child.

Further reading

Salley R K (1991) Left ventricular outflow tract obstruction in children. *Cardiology Clinics*, **9**, 381-396

Hypoplastic left heart syndrome

Definition

Underdevelopment that affects the aorta mainly, but also left ventricle and its valves.

Incidence

Accounts for 25% of first week deaths from CHD.

Clinical

Life is sustained by the patency of the ductus arteriosus. Symptoms of dyspnoea, shock, and cyanosis develop at 1–5 days as it closes.
   Differential diagnosis includes septicaemia and inborn errors of metabolism.

Management

Surgery, other than transplantation, has little to offer. Palliation, in which the Norwood procedure couples the right ventricle to the aorta, followed by the Fontan procedure in childhood, is generally not favoured in the UK.

Prognosis

Death within one week, rarely delayed to 2–3 months.

2. Acyanotic shunt from left to right

Ventriculoseptal defect 30%; persistent patent ductus arteriosus (PDA) 8%; atrioseptal defect (ASD) 8%.

Ventricular septal defect (VSD)

The commonest congenital cardiac abnormality (Figure 14.3; Table 14.4); 20% have an associated major malformation/chromosomal abnormality.

Table 14.4 Types of ventricular septal defect (VSD)

Type of defect	Natural history
1 *Muscular*: single hole or, if trabeculated, may be multiple	i Large defects: 75% close spontaneously or become smaller. Only 25% need surgery ii Small defects: All close, most by 2 years. Only risk is bacterial endocarditis
2 *Perimembranous* involving interventricular membrane +/- muscular defect	Spontaneous closure is less common than for muscular VSD as it is mainly a connective tissue defect extending into muscle
	i All are close to the tricuspid valve which is made functionally smaller in 50% by valve tissue sticking to VSD margins = 'pseudoaneurysms' ii Remainder: if many small VSDs they are left, as long as there is no risk of pulmonary vascular disease
3 *Doubly committed subarterial* Muscular defects just below both valves	The VSD is usually large; always needs surgery as the aortic valve prolapses into the defect

Indications for VSD surgery

Dependent on (i) position and size of defect (ii) likelihood of spontaneous closure (iii) pulmonary blood flow and pulmonary vascular resistance.

Clinical situations

1. Asymptomatic small VSD. Most are muscular, so spontaneous closure is likely. Thrill is usually absent, pansystolic murmur best heard at apex, through to the lower back.

2. Moderate to large VSD. Dyspnoea, failure to thrive, recurrent chest infection, heart failure from 2–12 weeks old, as pulmonary vascular resistance falls. Thrill in the third left interspace, harsh pansystolic murmur. Presence of a mid-diastolic murmur indicates a 2:1 pulmonary:systemic shunt.

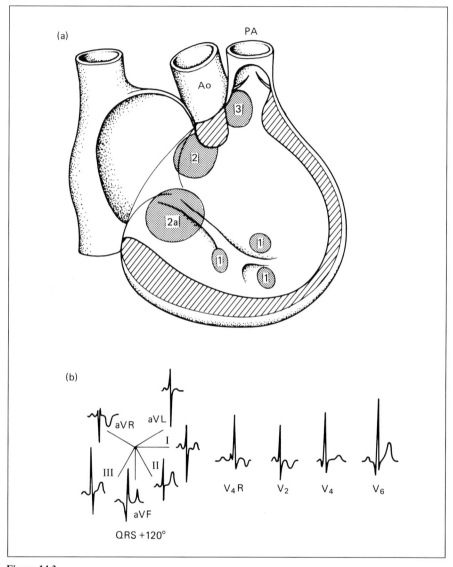

Figure 14.3
(a) Ventricular septal defect, viewed from the right side of the heart. 1 = muscular defect; 2 = perimembranous; 2a = large perimembranous; 3 = doubly committed subarterial. (b) ECG in VSD. Biventricular hypertrophy, R + S wave >70 mm, with right bundle branch block

Investigations   Chest X-ray shows enlarged heart and pulmonary artery, increased vascularity both of hila and at periphery of lung fields.
    ECG: biventricular hypertrophy.
    Echo shows defect, and pseudoaneurysms are well seen. Doppler shows high flow L → R, low pressure gradient between ventricles.

Management Persistent high blood flow may cause pulmonary vascular disease, so:

   i Indications for corrective surgery in a symptomatic infant are:

      a. Failure to thrive.
      b. Persistently raised pulmonary artery pressure.
      c. Calculated shunt ratio of >2:1 pulmonary:systemic circulation.

  ii Pulmonary artery banding is preferred for multiple muscular VSDs, as early corrective surgery may be riskier, and they may close spontaneously anyway.

3. Large VSD with raised pulmonary vascular resistance.

    i Common in Down's syndrome, and late presentation of large VSDs.
   ii Early symptoms of heart failure resolve, so child seems well.
  iii Normal left ventricle, and a hard working right ventricle in which the pressure rises towards systemic, thus no thrill; presence of an ejection systolic murmur, and a loud single second heart sound.
  iv Reversal of the shunt occurs eventually = cyanosis = *Eisenmenger syndrome of irreversible pulmonary hypertension.*

Investigations Chest X-ray: Pulmonary vessel 'pruning' = reduced vascularity at the periphery of the lungs.
  ECG: Right ventricular hypertrophy.
  Echo: Large defect. Left to right shunt.

Management Surgery is contraindicated if the pulmonary vascular resistance is elevated to >8 units, as measured at cardiac catheterization. Heart-lung transplant is the long-term alternative in selected cases.

Further reading

Trowitzsch E, Braun W, Stute M, Pielmeier W (1990) Diagnosis, therapy, and outcome of ventricular septal defects in the 1st year of life: a two-dimensional colour-Doppler echocardiography study. *European Journal of Pediatrics,* **149**, 758–761

Patent ductus arteriosus (PDA)

Normal functional closure occurs within hours of birth. May reopen with hypoxia and excess fluid administration (Table 14.5)

Auscultation

Like the symptoms, dependent on ductal size:

1. Small to medium.
   Thrill in the second left interspace, the classic continuous murmur due to a pressure gradient between the aorta and pulmonary artery throughout the cardiac cycle. The murmur persists on lying down, whereas a venous hum disappears.

The second sound is loud, with both components close together.
2. Large, with raised pulmonary artery pressure due to high flow. Absent thrill, murmur present in systole only, and the characteristic one found in the preterm and term infant. The pressures in the aorta and pulmonary artery in diastole are equal, so no flow can occur then, but a mid-diastolic flow murmur through the mitral valve (increased return to left atrium) may be heard. The second heart sound is loud and single.

Table 14.5 Features of patent ductus arteriosus

	Term infants and older	*Prematures*
Incidence	1 in 2000	Up to 40% in <1500 g
Spontaneous closure	Rare after 2 weeks old	Usually by 3 months old
Clinical 1 Small: asymptomatic. Normal pulses, BP 2 Medium: Tires easily, short stature. Pulse pressure wide, cardiomegaly 3 Large: Failure to thrive, dyspnoea with feeds		Age 3–7 days stiff wet lungs with: i Respiratory distress syndrome, unable to wean off ventilator, or ii Rapid respirations. Both show iii Heart failure with liver enlarged
Complications Heart failure, Eisenmenger syndrome, bacterial endocarditis		Ventricular haemorrhage, bronchopulmonary dysplasia, intractable heart failure

Investigations

Chest X-ray: cardiomegaly and enlarged pulmonary vessels.
ECG: left>right ventricular hypertrophy.
Echo: confirms patency and Doppler shows the direction of flow. In prematures if the left atrial diameter is 1.5 X larger than aorta = large ductus.

Management

Term   Surgical ligation, or umbrella occluder at cardiac catheterization. Leave if pulmonary vascular disease is established, i.e. intervention is too late.

Preterm   Medical if <10 days old, <34 weeks' gestation. Indomethacin (see neonatal problems), fluid restriction + diuretic for heart failure. Delay if sepsis, bleeding, hyperbilirubinaemia, or renal dysfunction. Closure effective in up to 80%.
Surgery if no response or older.

Prognosis

Term Large PDA without surgery 50% dead by middle age.
Operation <1% mortality.
Small PDA: main risk is endocarditis.

Preterm Without treatment 30% die.

Atrioseptal defect (ASD)

Definitions

Defects of the septum may be:

1. Simple, involving the interatrial septum alone = ostium secundum,
2. Complex = atrioventricular septal defect (AVSD) which is either:

> i Partial (ostium primum) if no ventricular component. The mitral valve is usu-
> ally cleft.
> ii Complete if a large central defect due to an ASD and VSD with a single large
> atrioventricular valve. Cyanosis usually supervenes because of pulmonary
> vascular disease. Down's syndrome accounts for 50%, and occurs in 80% of
> Down's with CHD.

Pathophysiology

1. Flow is L → R, secondary to the fall in pulmonary vascular resistance, into the
   low resistance right heart. Further contributions to flow often occur:

> i One or more anomalous pulmonary veins are often present, draining into the
> right atrium (sinus venosus defect).
> ii Primum/AVSD defects: may result in mitral regurgitation producing a pan-
> systolic apical murmur. Complete defects are prone to irreversible pulmo-
> nary hypertension in childhood.

2. Murmurs are due to increased flow across the valves, not the ASD itself.

> i Across pulmonary valve → ejection systolic
> ii Across tricuspid valve → mid-diastolic if >2:1 shunt. The murmur increases
> on inspiration.

3. Fixed splitting of the second heart sound: the increased volume causes prolonged
   contraction time of the right ventricle.

Clinical

Ostium secundum
1 Symptoms rare in childhood. Only in a very large ASD, then like a primum
  defect.
  Adults: heart failure, pulmonary hypertension, atrial fibrilation
2 May be tall, long fingers and toes.
3 Right ventricular heave.

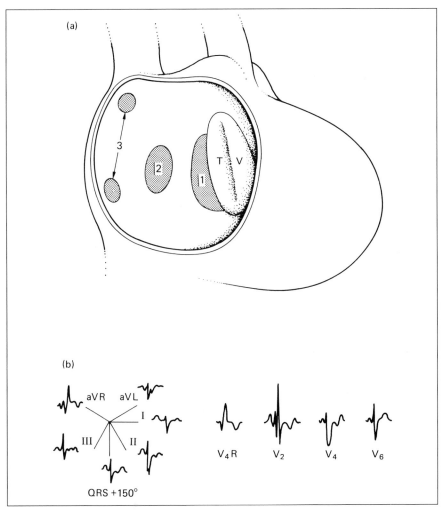

Figure 14.4 Atrial septal defects.
(a) Anatomy: view of the right atrium
    1 = ostium primum
    2 = ostium secundum
    3 = sinus venosus defect
    TV = tricuspid valve
(b) ECG in ostium secundum defect, with peaked P waves in leads II, V_2, right bundle branch block, and right ventricular hypertrophy.
(c) ECG in ostium primum showing biventricular hypertrophy, (unusual unless pulmonary vascular disease is present) right bundle branch block and prolonged P–R interval. (Often shows a superior axis).
(d) Complete atrioventricular septal defect. View from the left side of the heart.
    1 = ASD in the lowest part of the atrial septum.
    2 = common atrioventricular valve in closed position.
    3 = subvalvular VSD.
(e) Surgical repair, of a complete AVSD, with corresponding patches, and reconstruction of the valve into two or replaced by homografts.

Figure continued over the page

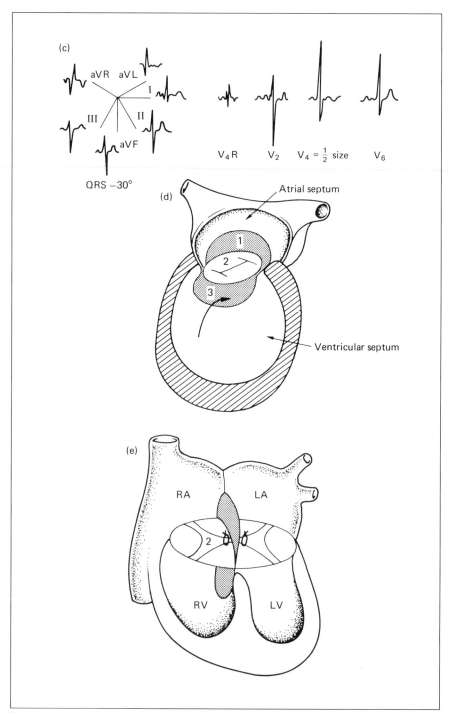

Figure 14.4 *cont'd*

Atrioventricular septal defect

1 Severity of mitral incompetence determines:

   i Symptoms: 50% dyspnoea, tired, frequent chest infections.
   ii Prognosis: Poor without surgery.

2 Often short, Harrison's sulci, bulging precordium.
3 Both ventricles enlarged in complete defects.
4 Heart sounds and murmurs similar for both, plus mitral incompetence murmur in secundum (not loud) type.

   Although a murmur in the pulmonary area may suggest an ASD, a variable splitting of the second heart sound excludes it.

Investigations

Ostium secundum

ECG: Right axis 90–160°, partial right bundle branch block pattern (RBBB).
   Chest X-ray: Prominent pulmonary arteries and vessels to periphery.
   Doppler: Flow shows size of shunt.

Atrioventricular septal defect Left axis superior –60 to –180°, similar RBBB but more right ventricular hypertrophy = rsR in V_4R, V_1 and tall/bifid P waves, PR prolonged.
   Cardiomegaly more likely.
   Shunt, and mitral regurgitation also present.

Surgery

Ostium secundum   Close if shunt >2:1, at 4 years old. Clam occluder is an alternative to surgery. Mortality <0.5%.

Atrioventricular septal defect   Partial atrioventricular septal defect (AVSD) closed before school age. Mortality 1%. Complete AVSD usually needs correction in infancy to avoid pulmonary vascular damage. Mortality 10–20%.

Further reading

Rome J J, Keane J F, Perry S B, Spevak P J, Lock J E (1990) Double-umbrella closure of atrial defects. Initial clinical applications. *Circulation*, **82**, 751–758.

3. Cyanotic obstructive, i.e. *reduced* pulmonary blood flow

Fallot's tetralogy 6%, single ventricle with tricuspid atresia 2%, Ebstein's malformation, pulmonary atresia <1%.

Fallot's tetralogy

Pulmonary stenosis, large VSD, overriding of the aorta and secondary right ventricular hypertrophy (Figure 14.5).

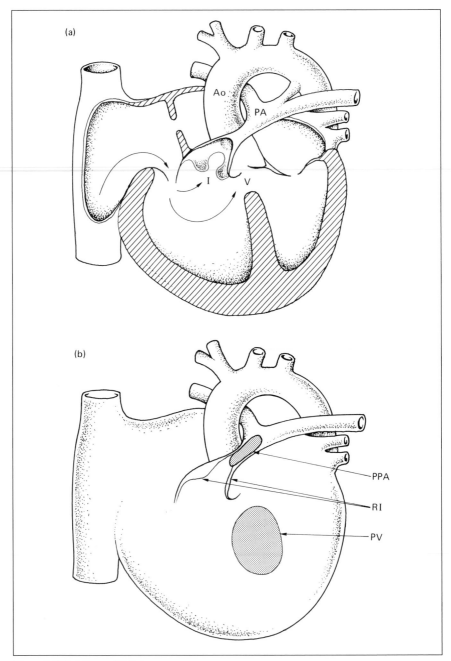

Figure 14.5 Tetralogy of Fallot

(a) Anatomy. I = infundibular narrowing plus pulmonary stenosis. Ao = aorta, PA = pulmonary artery,
     V = VSD

(b) Surgical correction. PPA = patched pulmonary artery +/- homograft valve.
     RI = resected infundibular muscle.
     PV = patched VSD

(c) ECG shows right ventricular hypertrophy and marked right axis deviation.

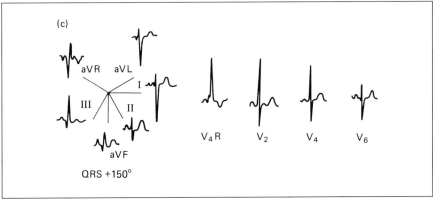

Figure 14.5 *cont'd*

Pathophysiology

The degree of infundibular pulmonary stenosis determines the severity. The right ventricular hypertrophy is secondary to the systemic pressure from continuity with the overriding aorta.

Cyanosis appears:

i From birth if effectively pulmonary atresia, depending on ductus arteriosus and its closure.
ii From 4–6 moths old, 'cyanotic spells' due to infundibular spasm as this portion becomes more narrow as the child grows.
iii After exercise → squatting: reduces blood flow to and from the lower limbs, raises systemic BP and oxygen saturation.

Findings include:

i Poor growth proportional to cyanosis.
ii Clubbing.
iii Cardiac: right ventricular heave, single second heart sound. Murmurs of ventricular defect and pulmonary stenosis may disappear during cyanotic spells due to infundibular spasm, when the pulmonary outlet is obstructed. Heart failure is rare.

Complications

1. Hypoxic attacks can result in brain damage and death.
2. Cerebral thromboses due to high haematocrit, risk increased by dehydration or iron deficiency anaemia (hypochromic RBC's are less deformable).
3. Bacterial endocarditis.
4. Cerebral abscess may be secondary to 2, not 3.

Investigations

See ECG. Chest X-ray:'boot–shaped' heart in only 50%, right-sided aorta 20%. Echo confirms. Cardiac catheterization only if pulmonary artery branch stenoses are suspected.

Management

1. Hypoxic episodes require:

   i   Knee-elbow position
   ii Oxygen
   iii Drugs–morphine + propranolol to ease infundibular spasm, bicarbonate for acidosis. Noradrenaline if unresponsive to propranolol (raises systemic resistance). Digoxin is contraindicated. Early operation is mandated.

2. Surgery.

   i   Early systemic to pulmonary shunt (e.g. Blalock) may be required for severe pulmonary stenosis.
   ii Correction of the outflow tract obstruction, sometimes with a patch through the outflow tract and valve (transannular patch).
   iii Patch the VSD.

Prognosis

Presurgery 30% dead by one year, 75% by 10 years. With surgery 90% survive to adult life, and 90% of them have a normal lifestyle.

Single ventricle with tricuspid atresia

Blood flows from the right atrium through the patent foramen ovale to the left heart, and then through a VSD to the pulmonary artery (Figure 14.6a).

ECG: uncharacteristic left heart predominance in the newborn period.

Surgery: palliative shunt initially, followed by the Fontan procedure where feasible (Figure 14.6b).

Ebstein's anomaly

Definition

'Atrialization' of the right ventricle by posterior and septal leaflets of the tricuspid valve attached to the endocardium below the valve's fibrous ring.

Clinical and investigations

Obstruction to flow to the lungs and dilatation of the right atrium result, seen on chest X-ray and echo. The ECG is characteristic, with tall P waves, right bundle branch pattern. Paroxysmal tachycardia or atrial flutter are typical arrhythmias.

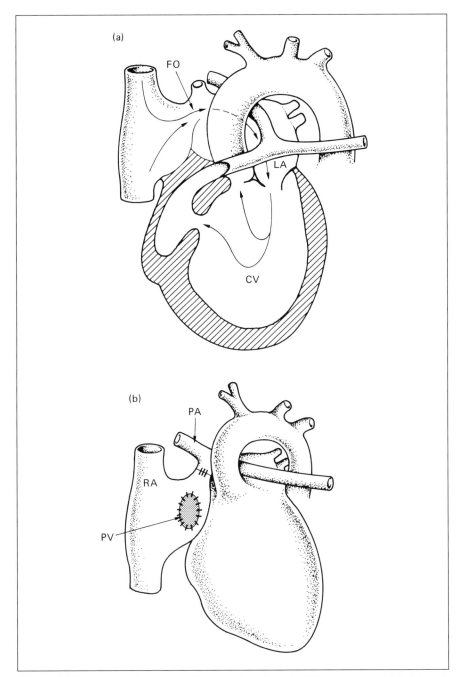

Figure 14.6 (a) Anatomy of a single ventricle with tricuspid atresia. CV = common ventricle, LA = left atrium, FO = foramen ovale
(b) Surgical correction, the Fontan procedure connecting the right atrium to pulmonary artery, disconnecting it from the right ventricle. PA = pulmonary artery, RA = right atrium, PV = patched VSD

Management

Conservative: if pulmonary stenosis is associated consider a shunt. Surgical reconstruction of the tricuspid valve carries a high risk.

Pulmonary atresia

1. With intact interventricular septum–incompatible with life unless the ductus remains patent. The Fontan procedure may be effective.
2. With VSD: similar to Fallot's tetralogy, cyanosis presenting earlier.

The pulmonary circulation is often abnormal, supplied by collaterals which are surgically difficult to correct.

4. Cyanotic with *increased* pulmonary blood flow

Transposition of great vessels, complete atrioventricular (AV) defect (previously called AV canal or endocardial cushion defect) 4% each, and total anomalous pulmonary venous connection.

Transposition of the great vessels (TGA)

Definition

The aorta is attached to the anatomic right ventricle, the pulmonary artery to the anatomic left ventricle (Figure 14.7).

Pathophysiology

Circulations are in parallel instead of in series. If the only connection is through the ductus arteriosus and/or a patent foramen ovale, cyanosis inevitably follows as it closes, unless a VSD is present.

Clinical

Cyanosis within 24 h of birth. No dyspnoea, and a murmur is often absent. Progressive metabolic acidosis.

Investigations

Chest X-ray: 'egg on side' due to a narrow vascular pedicle. May be obscured by the thymus initially, which involutes rapidly due to cyanosis or stress.

ECG: Often normal, later right ventricular hypertrophy.

Echo: Abnormal anatomical relationship of the two great vessels which are in parallel instead of winding round each other. The aorta lies in front of the pulmonary artery, i.e. a reversal of the normal.

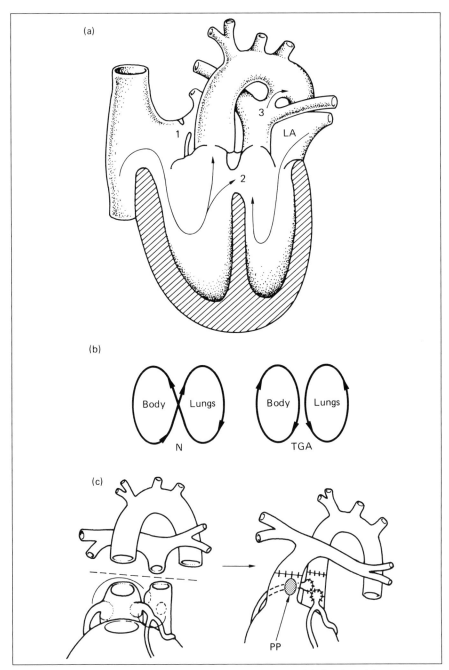

Figure 14.7 Transposition of the great arteries. (a) Anatomy. Potential sites for mixing 1 = foramen ovale, 2 = VSD, 3 = PDA.
(b) Circulation
    N = normal; TGA = transposition.
(c) Surgical arterial 'switch'
    PP = pericardial patch to where coronary arteries have been removed

Management

1. Prostaglandin infusion, support pH with alkali.
      Avoid additional oxygen which may hasten ductal closure, with consequent worsening of hypoxia.
2. Direct arterial 'switch' as the first procedure, of the aorta, with the coronary arteries, to the left ventricle, pulmonary artery to the right ventricle. This correction allows the right ventricle to pump at low pressures and is considered more physiological than the previously preferred balloon septostomy followed by the atrial baffle operation of Mustard or Senning at 6–9 months old. Switch is also the preferred operation if a VSD is present.

Prognosis

Before surgery was available mortality was 80% by 1 year, now 80% survival to adult life is predicted. Operative mortality in the best units is 5%.

Complete atrioventricular defect

See ASD.

Total anomalous pulmonary venous connection (TAPVC)

Definition

The pulmonary veins drain into the right heart not the left atrium. Flow is obstructed or non-obstructed (Figure 14.8).

Pathophysiology

Obligatory right to left shunt → pulmonary congestion with cyanosis:

   i Proportional to the shunt through the stretched foramen ovale.
   ii Most severe in obstructed TAPVC, which is typically infradiaphragmatic.

   In the newborn it may present as respiratory distress syndrome with no improvement despite oxygen administration, or persistent tachypnoea.
   Obstruction due to narrowing of the veins at insertion is invariable in the infradiaphragmatic type, causing pulmonary hypertension.

Non-obstructed drainage

   i Supracardiac via the innominate = 'cottage loaf' X-ray appearance.
   ii Cardiac via the sinus venosus or the coronary sinus. Both present later, in cardiac failure.

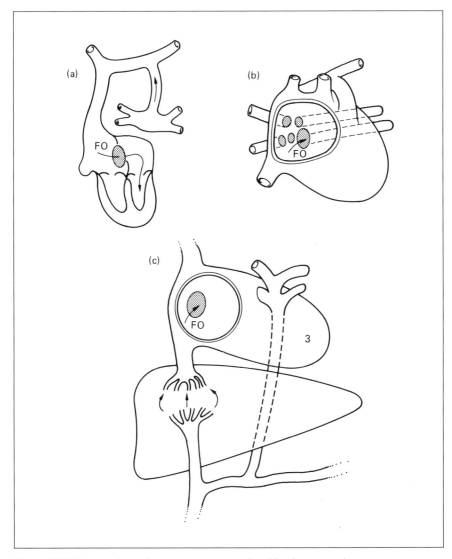

Figure 14.8 Total anomalous pulmonary venous connection. FO = foramen ovale.
(a) Supracardiac via the left innominate vein.
(b) Cardiac. The pulmonary veins drain into the right atrium.
(c) Infradiaphragmatic via the portal vein

Investigation

Difficult to diagnose on echo. An inexperienced echocardiographer may miss the abnormal pulmonary vein connections and misdiagnose as a hypoplastic left heart, or normal if the left ventricle is a good size.

Surgery

Correction is usually urgent.

Mortality 80% without surgery. With surgery 5–30%, depending on age, severity of acidosis, type of obstruction and size of the left ventricle.

INFLAMMATORY HEART DISEASE

Cardiac failure due to bacterial and viral infection, or rheumatic heart disease.

Infective endocarditis

Definition

Bacterial infection occurring at sites of endothelial damage where a jet of blood impinges.

Uncommon in infants, the risk is increased in cyanotic conditions, and after cardiac surgery. *Streptococcus viridans* and *Staphylococcus aureus* are the main pathogens.

Clinical

Fever, pallor, arthralgia, splenomegaly, heart failure, and signs of emboli (haematuria, splinter haemorrhages, hemiplegia, pleurisy).

Prior treatment with antibiotic obscures classic signs, so a high index of suspicion is needed to avoid heart damage, or death (still 25%).

Management

Start treatment as soon as blood cultures have been taken (4 in the first 24 h, 2 in the next 24 h).

Penicillin + aminoglycoside for 6 weeks, adjusted according to microbial culture and sensitivities. High bacteriacidal levels are required.

Prophylaxis

Maintain good oral hygiene and dental care. Fluoride supplements are helpful.
  Antibiotic cover indicated for:

  i   All congenital heart lesions, and always continued for life after cardiac surgical repair (except for a ligated PDA, secundum ASD or spontaneous closure of a VSD).
  ii Acquired: rheumatic heart disease, previous infective endocarditis, acquired valve disease.
  iii Hypertrophic cardiomyopathy, arteriovenous fistulae.

Procedures and recommended antibiotics

1. Dental treatment and operations to the upper respiratory tract: *Streptococcus viridans* is common so give amoxycillin orally/i.m. one hour before treatment 3 g, or 1.5 g if <10 years old.

   For penicillin allergy, erythromycin 1g orally, or 0.5 g if <10 years old, or clindamycin 6 mg/kg.
2. Surgery to gut and renal tract: enterococci common, so give gentamicin 2 mg/kg + ampicillin, 0.5 g under 10 years, 1 g thereafter, both i.m.
3. Prosthetic heart valves best protected by i.m. ampicillin + flucloxacillin, 0.5 g under 10 years, 1 g thereafter, of each, before treatment and at 8 and 16 h after.

Acute myocarditis

Definition

Acute heart failure after a prodromal illness. Usually viral, e.g. Coxsackie, ECHO, influenza, mumps.

Investigations

Echo: dilated heart, reduced ejection fraction.

   ECG: low voltage pattern, arrhythmias, injury as Q waves.

Differential diagnosis

Septicaemia, meningococcal septicaemia, rheumatic fever, Kawasaki disease, anomalous left coronary artery (arising from the pulmonary artery, causes angina and death).

Treatment

Digoxin, diuretics, oxygen.

Prognosis

Recovery 80%, some die, others go on to endocardial fibroelastosis. Neonatal coxsackie B myocarditis has an 80% mortality.

Hypertrophic obstructive cardiomyopathy (HOCM) AD

Definition

Excessive progressive thickening of the left ventricular wall leads to stiffness with poor diastolic filling, and obstruction to outflow.

Clinical

Dyspnoea, chest pain, syncope, sudden death from arrhythmias.

- Double peak to the pulse is pathognomonic, and due to interruption of systolic ejection by septal obstruction.
- Apex beat thrusting, with a double impulse. Mitral regurgitation murmur is heard in some.
  ECG: left ventricular hypertrophy, occasionally with Q waves.
  Echo: thickening of interventricular septum.

Management

Beta blockers or calcium channel antagonists prevent symptoms, and may possibly reverse hypertrophy. Important cause of sudden death in young athletes, so advise against sporting activities.

Endocardial fibroelastosis

Definition

Considered to be the end stage of viral myocarditis or dilated cardiomyopathy.

Pathophysiology

Thickened white endocardium lining a dilated underfunctioning left ventricle, as opposed to the contracted type seen with hypoplastic left heart or secondary obstruction to the left ventricle.

Clinical

Peak age 6 months. May have a regurgitant pansystolic murmur due to gross dilatation of the left heart.

Investigations

Echo: Dilated left ventricle, ejection fraction a third of normal.
   ECG: Left ventricular hypertrophy.
   Chest X-ray: Cardiomegaly.

Treatment and prognosis

As for acute myocarditis. Heart transplant for intractable cases.

Rheumatic fever (RF)

Definition

An autoimmune reaction after a group A β-haemolytic streptococcal pharyngitis, involving skin, joints, the heart and its valves, and the brain.

Incidence

Falling in developed countries to 0.01% compared with up to 1% in Third World urban poverty. Recent upsurge in cases in the USA.

Risk in the UK

1 in 30000 group A β-haemolytic streptococcal infections, a fall from 1 in 300 in 1960; 16 children affected in 1990 (reported to the British Paediatric Surveillance Unit).

Pathophysiology

Cross reaction between a genetically susceptible person's antibodies to streptococcal wall antigen (Lancefield group A) and their own heart, synovial or brain tissues. Family history of RF is common.

Round cells, giant cells and plasma cells, often contained in Aschoff nodules, characterize the inflammatory reaction, except in the brain where the inflammation in chorea is non-specific.

Clinical

Onset: Rare <3 years old, 10–21 days after a streptococcal sore throat/infection. Abdominal pain may precede the following:

1. Arthritis with fever (75%). Large joints are swollen, hot, and painful on movement. Different joints become involved day to day, rarely more than three at a time. Duration 3–4 weeks, resolve completely.

   Mild arthralgia is a commoner presentation, when RF is less easy to diagnose.
2. Carditis. Affects 50%. As part of an arthritis or non-specific illness, with evening fever, weight loss, poor appetite, cough and dyspnoea.

   Pulse: tachycardia, raised sleeping pulse rate. Bradycardia occasionally.

   Cardiomegaly. Heart failure may occur. Pericardial friction rub is rare. Heart sounds become muffled, with tic-tac or gallop rhythm.

   Murmurs:

   Apical
   systolic, high pitched (mitral incompetence, chordae stretched).
   mid-diastolic Carey Coombes (mitral orifice narrowing due to swollen valve leaflets).
   Left sternal edge–early diastolic of aortic incompetence.
3. Rheumatic nodules in 1%, over pressure points. Non tender, containing Aschoff nodules, develop weeks later.
4. Skin rashes. Erythema marginatum, a serpigenous outline which varies over the day, and erythema nodosum, are both found in other conditions.
5. Sydenham's chorea (St Vitus' dance) 15%.

Onset gradual, 5–15 years old. Girls>boys, carditis in 25%. See Involuntary movements in Neurological problems.

Investigations

1. Antistreptolysin O titre raised, streptococci on culture. ESR raised.
2. ECG: prolonged P-R (> 0.2 s), Wenkebach phenomenon.
3. Echo: small pericardial effusion, dilatation and reduced contractility of the left ventricle, stretched chordae of the mitral valve.

Diagnosis

A useful aid to avoid overdiagnosis is Jones' criteria:

1. Major manifestations, a total of 5 (above).
2. Minor manifestations (raised ESR, fever, arthralgia, previous RF or rheumatic heart disease, prolonged P-R).
3. Supportive: recent scarlet fever, rising ASOT, streptococci on culture.

   RF = 2 major or 1 major + 2 minor + preceding streptococcal infection.
   Some cases of RF do not fulfil these criteria, especially if seen early.

Differential diagnosis

1. Arthritis. Conditions commonly confused are:

   i Growing pains: acute pain in leg muscles causes nocturnal waking, often with tears. No fever, normal ESR, joints and heart.
   ii Still's disease: <5 years, fever is diurnal, with maculopapular rash; small joints are often involved, and hepatosplenomegaly and lymphadenopathy, not just liver; pericarditis alone, not pancarditis.
   iii Henoch-Schönlein purpura: any age over 1 year, often no fever, rash is urticarial → purpuric, affects large and small joints. Acute abdominal pain and haematuria are common.

2. Murmurs: characteristics of functional murmurs differ.
3. Chorea: see Involuntary movements, in Neurology.

Management

Penicillin, erythromycin or cephalexin for 10 days.
   Bed rest for painful joints, aspirin 120 mg/kg/day for 14 days, then halved until arthritis and fever have settled.
   Presence of mitral incompetence or ventricular dilatation are an indication for restriction to bed or chair. Steroids are only indicated for heart failure or complete heart block, as rebound on stopping is usual. Limit to bed or chair until ESR <20 mm. Full sporting activities after 6 months.
   Chorea–as for RF. Reduction of movements achieved with haloperidol.

Prevention of recurrence with daily penicillin or erythromycin 250 mg twice daily, probably for life. Follow up is essential to monitor for valvular damage and the taking of antibiotic.

Prognosis

Death from acute and chronic rheumatic heart disease is 2% in childhood.
Chronic rheumatic heart disease occurs in 30% after acute RF.

- Repeated attacks of RF are more likely in these children.
- Severity of valvular damage is related to the number of attacks of RF.
- Mitral and aortic valve damage: mitral stenosis is the commonest sequela.

Further reading

Kavey R W, Kaplan E L (1989) Resurgence of acute rheumatic fever. *Pediatrics*, **84**, 585–586
Gillette P C (ed) (1990) Congenital heart disease. *Pediatric Clinics of North America*, **37**, no.1
Jordan S C, Scott O (1989) *Heart Disease in Paediatrics*. 3rd edn. Butterworths:London
Long W A (1990) *Fetal and Neonatal Cardiology*. Saunders:Philadelphia (for excellent explanations of the physiology and cardiac surgery)

Chapter 15

Gastroenterology problems

PHYSIOLOGICAL EVENTS

1. Fetal ingestion: swallowing 18 weeks, sucking by 24 weeks, gag reflex 34 weeks. The latter is the critical event for avoidance of aspiration. In practice very premature infants are fed earlier, e.g. the 'joey' method (see Nutrition) without harm.
2. Neonatal digestion: fats relatively poorly ('physiological steatorrhoea'), lactose tolerance limited in prematures.
3. Solids chewed from 6 months. Failure to introduce solids by 12–15 months leads to swallowing difficulties.
4. Oesophageal reflux is normal in the newborn (up to 50%), rapidly disappears in the majority, but may persist if the lower sphincter fails to operate normally.
5. Gastric acidity is high at birth, falls rapidly and gradually achieves adult levels in childhood.
6. Intestinal digestive function is adequate for full mixed feeding from 4–6 months. Lactase levels fall after weaning age in some racial groups. The small intestine grows from 2.5 metres in the neonate to 3.5–6.5 metres in the adult, and absorbs 80% of the water ingested. All but 1% is then absorbed by the large intestine.

EXAMINATION

Physical growth, behaviour and responsiveness are necessary aspects of the assessment.

Conventionally the following points are noted.

Head and neck

1. Breath: foetor oris in acute abdomen; ketones in starvation, diabetes mellitus; urine in uraemia; maple syrup etc.
2. The mouth and lips: always look for Koplick's spots, Candida on buccal mucosa, torn frenulum from violence.
3. Tongue and gums

i Underside and edges of tongue should be pink. Gums often have a brown-blue pigmentation in Asians and Africans, who may also have a black line at the gum margin, as in lead poisoning

ii Macroglossia found in normal infants, syndromes (Down's, Beckwith's) and metabolic disease (mucopolysaccharidoses, Pompe's disease)

iii Gingivostomatitis
Important causes

a. Infection especially primary herpes simplex, herpangina, hand foot and mouth disease, streptococci, Vincent's angina, Candida.
b. Aphthous ulcers.
c. Phenytoin.
d. Kawasaki disease or Stevens Johnson syndrome.

4. Teeth

i Eruption of primary teeth occurs from 3 to 20 months, secondary teeth from 6 to 13 years old

ii Bottle caries = brown discoloration with loss of enamel at the base of incisors, due to high sugar feeds from 'dinky feeder' or propped bottle

iii Green/black primary teeth cusps in kernicterus, eroded cusps in neonatal hypocalcaemia/simple dysplasia.

5. Parotid swelling
Above the angle of the jaw: mumps, sialic duct narrowing/stone, AIDS.

Swellings of head and neck

See Respiratory disorders.
   Skin of upper trunk and arms for spider naevi: up to 5 is normal in childhood, if more are present look for jaundice, finger clubbing, ascites.

Abdomen

1. Inspection

Movement with respiration, peristalsis, distension, presence of scars, distended veins on anterior abdominal wall, hernial swellings.
   Umbilical hernias are commoner in prematures, Africans, Down's syndrome, hypothyroidism, mucopolysaccharidoses, and rarely obstruct. Resolve by 2 years, up to 5 years in Africans.

2. Palpation

i Organs, tenderness, guarding. A 'squelch' from the caecum in the right iliac fossa is not found in acute inflammation.
   Avoid retesting for rebound, for if positive, children quickly lose confidence!

ii Inguinal region for hernial orifices and lymph glands.

iii Liver size is measured from the costal margin, in the nipple line: up to 3 cm in infancy, 1 cm by 5 years. Palpation is superior to percussion, though the latter is often used. Remember the liver edge extends beyond the midline.

iv Spleen is frequently palpable in infancy, and commonly enlarges during infection. Smooth in outline, it only becomes notched in late childhood. Palpate from left iliac fossa in infancy, right in older ages. Measure in cm in its long axis.

v Kidneys are easily felt in infants. If hips are flexed, encouraging abdominal muscles to relax, each can be balloted between fingers and thumb.

3. Percussion

i The bladder is an abdominal organ in the preschool child, often palpable/percussable. Obstruction, be it structural or neurogenic, may be detected by persistence of the organ on repeating the examination after voiding.

ii Distension due to fluid or gas is difficult to differentiate by shifting dullness. Fluid is detected by dullness to percussion over the umbilicus when in prone (kneeling child, or held under chest and pelvis in infant)

4. Auscultation

For bowel sounds, vascular bruits (renal artery stenosis, collateral circulation in obstructive liver disease).

5. Anus

For position, inspect for old or fresh fissures, bruising/'tyre' effect, reflex tone and anal dilatation (see Child abuse)

6. Rectal examination (when indicated)

i Digital. Use fifth finger in infants and toddlers. Gripping of total length of finger in Hirschsprung's disease. Pain localized in appendicitis, generally painful in Crohn's, ulcerative colitis.

ii Auroscope: mucosa inflamed and friable in colitis, see extent of fissuring secondary to constipation or trauma.

VOMITING

Fortunately, although half of infants regurgitate food, only 5% have a significant cause.

The majority spit out, vomit through overfeeding, maternal tension, rumination, and later, food refusal as a 1–2 year old.

Cough induced vomiting is common, often occurs at night, and if persistent as in pertussis, may lead to failure to thrive.

Content of the vomit provides clues. If food, is it fresh or partially digested from gastric stasis. Blood streaking is most likely in gastroesophageal reflux if vomiting is chronic, while a large volume of blood welling up suggests bleeding peptic ulcer or oesophageal varicies. Bilious or faeculant vomit is obstructive and surgical until proven otherwise.

Age as a guide

1. Newborn

Onset immediately after birth indicates obstruction, and, in the first few days commonly infection, intracranial injury or bleed, unusually drug withdrawal or peptic ulceration, rarely metabolic inborn error, e.g. congenital adrenal hyperplasia.

2. In older infants

Acute vomiting is most commonly due to infection, gastroenteritis or food poisoning, and accompanied by diarrhoea, both of which usually settle rapidly. Fever suggests it may be a parenteral response, so chest X-ray and urine culture should be taken. Onset of abdominal distention and constipation may however be obstructive, when abdominal pain and bile stained vomitus follow. Pyloric stenosis and gastroesophageal reflux are relatively frequent, often becoming distinguishable from functional disorders through the accompanying weight loss.

3. In childhood

In addition to the common conditions gastroenteritis, upper respiratory infections and onset of exanthema, occasionally urine infection presents in this way. Conditions as diverse as acute hepatitis and diabetes mellitus may mimic appendicitis, but are identified by routine urine testing for bile and glucose. Metabolic disturbance from inborn errors and Reye's syndrome may be precipitated by infection, suggested by profound acidosis and rapidly developing coma.

4. In adolescence

Consider anorexia nervosa and pregnancy.

Chronic vomiting

Almost persistent from birth in gastroesophageal reflux, intermittent in repeated volvulus, migraine or cyclical vomiting (often associated), or peptic ulcer.

Clinically may be only one facet of a systemic illness such as ulcerative colitis or renal failure.

Projectile vomiting

In early infancy it is classically due to pyloric stenosis, but urinary infection, and early, severe gastroesophageal reflux present similarly. A sick infant is likely to be septicaemic or meningitic, or have intracranial haemorrhage. A chronic subdural haemorrhage may fail to thrive. Obstruction due to a duodenal web is usually bilious vomiting and rare, as is a metabolic disorder like congenital adrenal hyperplasia when virilization may be a clue.

In older ages projectile vomiting is unusual, if not rare, e.g. peptic ulcer with epigastric discomfort and nocturnal pain, raised intracranial pressure from hydrocephalus, brain tumour or lead encephalopathy.

Blood stained vomit

Epistaxis is common and needs to be excluded.

Haematemesis is due to bleeding above the ligament of Treitz, and acute or chronic, mild or severe. See below.

History

1. Infectious disease contact, foreign travel or foods likely to be contaminated.
2. A family history of migraine, pyloric stenosis; consanguinity or infant deaths suggest inborn errors.

   Assessment and treatment of the individual conditions follows.

Feeding disorders

- Overfeeding infants is a common cause of regurgitation. Check volume and frequency of feeds offered. Weight gain is satisfactory.
- Tension between mother and baby resulting in refusal, gagging and vomiting. Possible domestic stress and conflict must be explored early.
- Rumination occurs rarely, in infancy, as a self-induced regurgitation which is chewed, pleasurably. May be familial or psychological in origin. Failure to thrive may result.
- Toddler food refusal with deliberate gag and vomit in battles for control. Try allowing the child to feed himself, in quiet suroundings, at the table, instead of spoon thrusts during diversionary games in front of the TV on mother's lap or the settee.
- Anorexia nervosa (see Behavioural problems).

Causes of vomiting

1. Feeding disorders, gastro-oesophageal reflux.
2. Infection especially urinary tract infection, otitis media, gastroenteritis, meningitis.
3. Mechanical causes: gastroesophageal reflux, pyloric stenosis, acute obstruction.
4. Inflammation: acute, e.g. appendicitis, chronic, e.g. ulcerative colitis.
4. Food intolerance, e.g. cows' milk protein intolerance.
5. Metabolic, e.g. diabetic ketoacidosis, adrenogenital syndrome, fructose intolerance.
6. Miscellaneous causes: coughing, e.g. pertussis, asthma, migraine.

Individual conditions associated with vomiting

Gastro-oesophageal reflux

Acid regurgitation into the oesophagus occurs in all infants, but resolves in all but a tiny minority as the neural control of the oesophagus matures.

Pathophysiology

1. The lower oesophageal sphincter shows abnormally prolonged relaxation during a peristaltic wave, or inappropriate periods of relaxation.
2. The segment of oesophagus below the diaphragm is short, preventing abdominal pressure from keeping it closed.

Hiatal hernia

Definition

The herniation of stomach into the chest, where the negative pressure tends to keep the distal oesophageal sphincter open and positive abdominal pressure causes reflux. Sliding hernia is commoner than the paraoesophageal type.

Investigation of gastroesophageal reflux

1. Check Hb.
2. Barium swallow: 30–60% of refluxers identified, but reflux also found in asymptomatic infants.
3. Oesophageal pH monitoring: abnormal if pH falls below 4 for more than 5% of the recording period. Severity proportional to duration, so >20% usually requires surgery.
4. Oesophagoscopy: severity of oesophagitis, any stricture formation assessed.
5. Technetium scan: assessment of volume of reflux and observation of lung aspiration is not commonly done.

Management

Diagnosis may be made on the history and examination alone in mild cases, which respond to thickening feeds, or the introduction of solids if old enough.
   Medical for up to 6 months or until symptom free for 6 weeks.

1. Position: prone at 45° enables stomach bubble to be under oesophageal opening. Alternatively sit upright 60° for an hour after feeds in less severe cases.
2. Thicken feeds with alginate, e.g. Nestargel/Carobel or add cornflour or cereal. Breast fed infants given a few spoons of thick alginate gel prior to a feed.

Clinical

Table 15.1 Comparing hiatal hernia and pyloric stenosis

	Hiatal hernia	*Pyloric stenosis*
Incidence	1 in 500, and frequent in mentally handicapped, and pyloric stenosis	1 in 200, increasing in UK in 1980s Commoner in first born, M:F 4:1
Familial	Recurrence up to 1 in 12 of siblings	Up to 1 in 5 of female index case's sons, 1 in 20 for a daughter
Onset	From birth or first week commonly	At 2–6 weeks, up to 6 months
Vomiting	During and between feeds, copious or regurgitant, partially digested. Oesophagitis → brown streaks, rarely → haematemesis	Projectile, minutes after a feed. Fresh milk, no bile but 'coffee grounds' from oesophagitis seen. Hungry immediately after
Stools	May contain blood	Starvation stools/constipation
Growth	Failure to thrive variable	Recent weight loss, dehydration is usually mild to moderate
Behaviour	Frequently irritable	Appearance: 'Pinched' nose, anxious looking, occasionally jaundiced
Clinical associations	Cyanotic episodes, wheeze, pneumonia. Pallor due to anaemia	Visible peristalsis. Pyloric mass palpable in almost all cases

Drugs

    i Antacid/alginate for mild symptoms, e.g. gaviscon ½ sachet after meals.

   ii H_2 blockers, e.g. cimetidine for oesophagitis 20 mg/kg/day.

  iii Prokinetic drugs which encourage stomach emptying: domperidone 0.6–1.2 mg/kg/day or cisapride 1 mg/kg/day each divided into 3 doses 30 minutes before meals, for 4–8 weeks.

Surgery in the 5–10% non-responders: fundoplication for recurrent aspiration, failure to thrive, haematemesis, low Hb. Dilate strictures.

Prognosis

If simple regurgitation it resolves as the infant sits, becomes mobile and erect, usually by a year old.

Isolated reflux: no stricture develops, surgery not required.

Hiatal hernia (HH): majority well by 18 months, 30% persistent symptoms for more than 4 years, 5% develop strictures. HH radiologically still present in 50% in adult life. Death rare.

Pyloric stenosis

Definition

Anatomical and functional obstruction due to localized muscle hypertrophy.

Aetiology

Partly genetic, with speculation on the role of gastrin and myenteric plexus abnormalities.

Clinical

See Table 15.1.

Diagnosis

- Visible peristalsis like 'golf ball under a blanket'.
- Palpation of olive–shaped mass to right of midline, alternately hard and soft.
- If uncertain, US shows hypertrophied pylorus muscle. If still in doubt, barium meal shows long, narrowed pyloric canal ('string sign'), and 'mushroom' appearance of duodenal cap, with delayed gastric emptying.
- Metabolic alkalosis. May have acid urine if hypokalaemic as kidney conserves $Na^+ > K^+ > H^+$ ion.

Differential diagnosis

- Infection: urine/GI/meningitis/septicaemia.
- Surgical obstruction.
- Food intolerance, e.g. cows' milk, coeliac.
- Raised intracranial pressure.
- Metabolic: renal failure, renal tubular acidosis, adrenogenital syndrome.

Management

1. Prior to surgery rehydrate and correct sodium, chloride and potassium deficits, which allows alkalosis to resolve.
2. Ramstedt's pyloromyotomy. Low risk with <1% mortality. Feeds introduced immediately after are tolerated in most infants.

Cyclical vomiting (periodic syndrome)

Definition

Recurrent nausea and often prolonged, severe vomiting in children may occur spontaneously or be associated with fever or minor infections. Family history of migraine, some are emotionally disturbed. Uncommon.

Clinical

Onset is gradual or sudden, and continued oral fluids exacerbate the vomiting.

Gross dehydration and ketosis result. Must be differentiated from inborn errors of urea cycle and organic acids.

Management

Rehydrate i.v.; severe acidosis may justify alkali i.v. Chlorpromazine reduces vomiting, and if given early may prevent an attack progressing.

Prognosis ultimately good.

ACUTE OBSTRUCTION

Causes

1. Congenital: neonatal presentation common. Duodenal stenosis/atresia, volvulus, malrotation, Hirschsprung's disease, imperforate anus.
2. Acquired: common in the first months of life. Necrotizing enterocolitis, intussusception, strangulated inguinal hernia, testicular torsion.

Clinical

See Table 15.2

Table 15.2 Clinical features of acute obstruction

Signs of obstruction	Differential diagnosis
1 Bile stained or faeculent vomiting	Necrotizing enterocolitis, septicaemia, intracranial bleed, cerebral oedema, meningitis
2 Acute abdominal distension	1 Gastroenteritis, air swallowing, faecal impaction, coeliac, Crohn's meconium ileus equivalent, ulcerative colitis. 2 Ascites. 3 Paralytic ileus: preterm, hypoxia, hypothermia, sepsis.
3 Pain: signs of peritonitis (rigidity, rebound tenderness, guarding)	Common: 1 Gastroenteritis, appendicitis, mesenteric adenitis 2 Cough, pneumonia 3 Urinary tract infection 4 Anaphylactoid purpura (see abdominal pain for complete list)
4 Absent or high pitched bowel sounds	Hypokalaemia, atropine

Investigations

1. Plain X-ray of abdomen pointers to disease process:

   - Loops of distended bowel +/– fluid levels in atresias, meconium ileus, Hirschsprung's disease.
   - Double bubble of duodenal atresia/midgut volvulus with Ladd's bands.
   - Intraluminal gas, dilated 'sentinal' loop in necrotizing enterocolitis.
   - 'Ground glass' due to bubbles of air in the meconium of meconium ileus (not diagnostic).
   - Calcification due to meconium peritonitis.

2. Suspected oesophageal atresia

   - Pass radiopaque feeding tube to determine level of pouch, and X-ray.

3. US for pyloric stenosis, abscesses, duplication cysts
4. Barium enema

   - In meconium ileus, it may be curative. Always do a sweat test, and rectal biopsy.
   - Hirschsprung's disease 'cone' appearance.

5. Electrolytes, acid-base state often deranged and in need of correction. Hb, WBC differential count distinguish, e.g. appendicitis from mesenteric adenitis. Do blood culture.
6. Technetium scan for Meckel's, duplications.

Management principles

Delaying surgery, to resuscitate fully, results in improved morbidity and mortality.

1. Nasogastric tube passed. Free drainage. Aspirate stomach intermittently to assess fluid loss and prevent aspiration pneumonia.
2. Treat shock; i.v. fluids and electrolytes to cover maintenence, deficit and ongoing losses.
3. Bicarbonate for significant metabolic acidosis.
4. Emergency laparotomy–shock, bloody diarrhoea, rigid abdomen = strangulated bowel, perforation likely.
5. Other procedures according to cause, e.g. laparotomy to relieve obstructions due to bands, end to end anastomoses for atresias.
6. i.v. nutrition postoperatively, e.g. extensive resections, necrotizing enterocolitis.

Short gut syndrome after extensive resections; as long as ileocaecal valve is present, 15 cm of small intestine is sufficient for survival, otherwise 40 cm is needed.

Appendicitis

The commonest abdominal emergency. Rare in infancy, when presentation may be atypical and difficult to diagnose so mortality high (Table 15.3).

Table 15.3 Comparing clinical features of appendicitis with mesenteric adenitis

	Appendicitis		*Mesenteric adenitis*
	<5 years	*>5 years*	
Recurrent	No	No	Yes, common
Upper respiratory, tract infection	Maybe	Maybe	Onset within past 24 h, cervical glands
Temperature	39–40°C	38°C	High fever common
Appearance	Ill, becoming toxic early, rapid pulse	Ill, foetor	Flushed
Vomiting	Frequent	Variable	Unusual
Bowel motion	Constipation usual, diarrhoea occasionally		Diarrhoea common
Abdominal examination and pain	Tender +, difficult ++ Pushes examiner's hand away vigorously	Tender ++, to cough or move legs is painful	Vague pain, may vary intermittently, no true rebound
Localization	Poor	RIF/central	RIF/periumbilical
Rectal exam	Pain+/- swelling localized to right		No localized tenderness

RIF = right iliac fossa

Points from the examination

- Ask child to put his hand over the tender area and palpate using his hand to elicit tenderness and guarding, when the examiner's hand is likely to be pushed away vigorously!
- Rebound tenderness should only be elicited once, as it is extremely painful.
- Rectal examination reveals greater tenderness on the right, and perhaps abscess mass if presentation was delayed.

Differential diagnosis

Includes pneumonia (request a chest X-ray to detect a right lower lobe pneumonia), severe gastroenteritis, anaphylactoid (Henoch-Schönlein) purpura, diabetes mellitus, hepatitis. Check urine for infection, glucose, blood and protein.

In appendicitis, the fever and raised WBC with leucocytosis support the clinical findings. X-ray of abdomen may show RIF dilated ileal loops, faecolith or appendix abscess.

Management

1. Observe and review after a few hours if uncertain.
2. Surgery.
3. Peritonitis. Presence suspected if very toxic, or severe ileus. Commoner in small children because their poorly developed omentum often fails to seal off inflammation before perforation occurs.

    Drip and suck, stabilize, broad spectrum antibiotics and metranidazole. Surgery to remove appendix, insert drains.
4. Appendix abscess palpated.

    i Symptoms longer than 48 h: continue with conservative treatment of drip and suck, antibiotics and metranidazole, then interval appendicectomy in 2–3 months.
    ii Unstable, deteriorating, or less than 48 h, treat as peritonitis.

Intussusception

Incidence

1–2 per 1000, 3 months to 2 years, peak 6–9 months.

Pathophysiology

Invagination of proximal into distal bowel segment. Ileocolic commonest, peristalsis causing migration towards rectum where it prolapses. Usually no underlying cause is found, occasionally a Meckel's diverticulum, polyp, or submucosal bleed in Henoch-Schönlein anaphylactoid purpura.

Clinical

1. Sudden onset, repeated at 10–15 minute periods for 1–2 minutes of screaming, drawing up legs, pallor, and vomiting.
2. Stool first, then blood and mucus in 50%, the redcurrant jelly stool.
3. Vomiting becomes bilious, abdomen distended. Temperature and tachycardia from infection and dehydration.
4. Palpation: tender sausage shaped mass in the line of the colon, usually at the hepatic flexure. May be difficult to identify under liver, best examined in prone, legs drawn up under chest. Rectal examination: redcurrant jelly, occasionally the intussusception.

Investigation

Plain X-ray: dilated loops of bowel, absent caecal shadow, and mass with crescent gas shadow to its right.

US: Mass, made of layers of intestine.

Barium enema diagnostic and therapeutic reduction possible if symptoms present for <24 h, i.e. 75% of cases (some now extend this to <72 h).

Management

1. Resuscitate, hydrate.
2. Barium enema reduction as above or surgery.
   Recurrence in 5% after either procedure. Loss of >30 cm terminal ileum leads to vitamin B_{12} deficiency later.

Strangulated inguinal hernia

Common in the first 6 months of life, when 25% will obstruct. Always indirect inguinal hernias in children, M:F 9:1.

Early surgery is indicated for inguinal and the less common femoral hernias to avoid this complication.

Testicular torsion

Table 15.4 Comparison of neonatal and pubertal testicular torsion

	Neonatal	*Pubertal*
Pain	Symptomless	Sudden, recurrent, +/- vomiting
Testis	Hard, enlarged	Swollen, tender, high in scrotum
Scrotum	Bluish	Swollen, erythematous, may be confused with incarcerated inguinal hernia
Salvage rate	Low, detected late	High unless confused with orchitis

Surgery (for both) Untort, fix other testicle to scrotal septum as high rate (50%) of recurrence, due to 'bell clapper' deformity

Dysphagia

Definition

Difficulties in swallowing due to a local abnormality, not an initial lack of motivation, though that may follow. Coughing, choking and aspiration are common symptoms.

Causes

Hydramnios anticipates postnatal dysphagia.

1. First feeds

   i Neuromuscular difficulty in sucking is common, related to prematurity, difficult birth; rarely due to maternal disease such as myasthenia gravis or dystrophia myotonica (shake hands!).

  ii Structural airway difficulties such as macroglossia, Pierre Robin syndrome or choanal atresia, or upper GI atresia of the oesophagus or duodenum are uncommon.

2. Infancy and childhood

Common:

   i Infection causing pain in the mouth or pharynx.

  ii Inflammation due to reflux oesophagitis.

Uncommon:

   i Neurological: isolated pseudobulbar palsy, or as part of cerebral palsy; bulbar palsy, due to polio, Guillaine-Barré syndrome, diphtheria or botulism are rare. Tetanus spasm. Achalasia (absence of oesophageal peristalsis and failure of the lower sphincter to relax) or dermatomyositis affect older children.

  ii Compression by a mediastinal mass, oesophageal duplication.

Assessment

The difference between food refusal and dysphagia is not always evident in the history, and observation of the activity may be diagnostic. Gross obstruction can be eliminated as a cause by passing a nasogastric tube, but a barium swallow and endoscopy will detect stricture, reflux and abnormal motility. Manometry for achalasia is rarely required.

ACUTE ABDOMINAL PAIN

In general, preschool children rarely have a psychological cause, and require careful evaluation whenever they complain of pain.

Types of pain and its localization

Children have a limited vocabulary for pain beyond 'it hurts'. With patience the nature of the pain, its site, radiation, duration and intensity, and factors making it better or worse, will be revealed.

1. Intermittent and colicky = distension or peristalsis of bowel, ureter or bile duct. The appreciation of pain coincides with the embryological dermatome, not the final anatomical site, because visceral and somatic sensory input into the dorsal horn of the spinal cord overlap. Thus pain in the epigastrium comes from the foregut, periumbilical from the midgut, and hypogastrium the hindgut. The diaphragm refers to the shoulder, ureters the flanks.

2. Tender, localized (inflammation of the parietal pleura) becoming generalized in peritonitis, e.g. appendicitis.
3. Dull ache/sharp pain in the suprapubic region comes from the bladder.

Timing of associated symptoms helps in determining the cause. For example, in gastroenteritis, vomiting generally precedes colicky abdominal pain, the reverse in dietary indiscretion (e.g. green apples), and periumbilical pain precedes vomiting in appendicitis. Mesenteric adenitis may be differentiated from the latter by the greater fever, and preceding upper respiratory tract infection.

Extra-abdominal causes to consider: right lower lobe pneumonia, urinary tract infection, diabetic ketoacidosis, spinal nerve compression, shingles.

Causes of acute abdominal pain

1. Medical (90%)

Common

    i Infection: gastroenteritis (Helicobacter, Salmonella, Shigella, Yersinia), mesenteric adenitis, urinary tract infection, hepatitis.
   ii Food poisoning, dietary indiscretion.
  iii Faecal impaction.
  iv Respiratory: cough, pharyngitis.

Uncommon

    i Henoch-Schönlein anaphylactoid purpura.
   ii Sickle cell crises.
  iii Pleurisy, pneumonia, Bornholm disease.

Rare but important

    i Hydronephrosis, renal colic.

2. Surgical (10%)

Common

    i Appendicitis.
   ii Obstruction: strangulated inguinal hernia, volvulus, malrotation, intussusception, testicular torsion.
  iii Trauma: perforation/rupture of intestine, spleen.

Uncommon

Peritonitis, Meckel's diverticulum perforating or causing intussusception.

Rare

Toxic megacolon.

Assessment

In addition to the history of pain, the associated symptoms are all important clues. Urine microscopy and a plain X-ray of the abdomen for fluid levels, large faecal masses, free air, stones or a faecolith; a chest X-ray for pneumonia. A FBC is helpful if appendicitis is a possibility. Other investigations as indicated by clinical findings.

Chronic or repeated episodes of abdominal pain

Common

1. Abnormal gut motility syndromes

   i Infantile colic.
   ii Recurrent abdominal pain, often migraine related, to be distinguished from school phobia, conversion symptom, or depression.

2. Constipation and the gastrocolic reflex.
3. Muscular: strain through exercise or coughing.
4. Food related: lactose intolerance is common in Africans, unusual in Caucasians. Allergy to milk, other proteins.

Uncommon (in the UK).

5. Acid related: gastritis, hiatal hernia, peptic ulceration.
6. Infection: giardiasis, large load of ascariasis.
7. Chronic inflammatory bowel disease, irritable bowel syndrome, TB, subacute obstruction.
8. Others, e.g. cholecystitis, diabetic ketoacidosis, epilepsy: partial complex seizure, hypoglycaemia, acute nephritis, ovarian cyst or tumour, porphyria, pancreatitis, rheumatic fever, splenic infarction in sickle cell disease.

Assessment of recurrent abdominal pain

Every child has a Hb and urine microscopy and culture. In recurrent abdominal pain the functional causes are diagnosed largely by exclusion but have clinical pointers such as the nature of pain being periumbilical, colicky or persistent and dull.

Pointers to an organic cause:

1. The further the site from the umbilicus/radiation away from umbilicus, the more likely it is to be abnormal.
2. Associated signs, e.g. weight loss, anaemia, loss of appetite, fever, diarrhoea, blood in stools, growth failure.
3. Preschool or >10 years old.

The organic reasons have distinctive histories if the correct questions are asked.

Frequency of bowel movement, the onset after an episode of dehydration or anal fissure, and confirmation of constipation on rectal examination rarely require further investigation.

Pain near the points of insertion of the rectus and oblique muscles which is elicited by pressing there and persists on straining is musculoskeletal.

A detailed dietary history, with improvement on removing the offending item, is practical. Confirmation is by challenge on 2 or 3 occasions, some weeks apart.

Stool examination for ova and cysts, as well as bacteria, especially if the family has travelled abroad, may identify pathogens. In infants and young children urine microscopy and culture are often diagnostic.

If in some doubt, arrange a consultation at the time of the pain to identify precipitant, take viral/bacterial cultures of throat, urine, stool, blood for ESR, glucose, (amylase, porphyrins if indicated) and an erect plain X-ray of the abdomen, if it is distended, for obstructive causes.

Specific indications for further tests

US of abdomen where pain is localized to back/loin (renal), upper abdomen (right–gall bladder, left–spleen), lower abdomen (ovarian).

Endoscopy for epigastric tenderness of peptic ulceration, or colonoscopy, barium follow through for inflammatory bowel disease symptoms–pain intermittent with lethargy, anaemia, fever, raised ESR.

Hydrogen breath test or stool fluid Clinitest for suspected lactose intolerance.

Management is discussed in the individual conditions.

Infantile colic

Definition

Paroxysmal abdominal pain, persistent severe crying, abdominal distension by gas and a wish to suck often, occurring in the first 3 months of life. Most frequent in the evenings.

Incidence

10–20%.

Cause

Unknown in the majority. Some have cows' milk protein (CMP) or lactose intolerance.

Differential diagnosis

Includes acute otitis media, strangulated hernia, intussusception, urinary tract infection, anal fissure.

Management

Some improve on casein protein hydrolysate milks or maternal CMP avoidance. A 2-week trial is warranted, and continued, if beneficial, until 3 months old. Sedatives are of dubious benefit, and antispasmodics are associated with a risk of cot death.

Recurrent abdominal pain (RAP)

See Behavioural problems for discussion and management.

Constipation

Definitions

Constipation is the passing of a hard stool, to be differentiated from straining at stool, common among babies, and the infrequent passage of a normal stool. 'Normal average' is 4 stools daily in newborn, 1–2 by a year.

Soiling is the involuntary passage of a semisolid or liquid stool, often with a retained rectal faecal mass.

Encopresis is often used interchangeably, for soiling, and the voluntary deposition of normal stool anywhere but the proper place.

Causes to consider

1. Physiological:

   i   constitutional and familial
   ii starvation, dehydration

2. Voluntary: encopresis, anal fissure
3. Obstruction, paralytic ileus
4. Neurological: mental retardation, hypotonia, cerebral palsy, spina bifida/spinal injury.
5. Metabolic: rickets, hypothyroidism, hypercalcaemia, lead poisoning, renal tubular acidosis, diabetes insipidus.

Differential diagnosis of major organic causes

In infancy

1. Passage of meconium delayed beyond 24 h old, recurrent diarrhoea, abdominal pain and distension is an indication for investigation for Hirschsprung's disease and cystic fibrosis.
2. Anal stenosis → ribbon or toothpaste like faeces.
3. Abdominal distension, vomiting and constipation due to partial intestinal obstructions from malrotations, strictures and diaphragms, paralytic ileus.
4. Hypothyroidism may give a history of prolonged jaundice and slowed growth, rickets is suspected clinically, hypercalcaemia has a characteristic elfin face, renal tubular acidosis and diabetes insipidus excessive thirst, and all may be failing to thrive.
5. Anal tone, saddle area sensation and intrinsic muscles of the feet are assessed, the spine examined for abnormal neurology. A developmental history identifies the mentally handicapped.

6. Excessive cows' milk feed, without roughage, or dietary changes, to solids or from breast to cows' milk, or a period of illness, with fever, or witholding food, contribute to constipation.

In the toddler or older child

Voluntary control is the commonest cause of soiling, through holding back defaecation or lack of training. It must be differentiated from the failure to have ever achieved reliable faecal continence due to abnormal neurology. Hirschsprung's disease, especially if of the ultra short segment variety, may not be identified early, but has a history from birth. Hypothyroidism occurs at any age. Occasionally, an anteriorly placed anus, with a posterior rectal shelf, is found to be obstructive.

Simple constipation

Constipation is familial in 50%, frequency every 2–5 days. Soiling affects boys> girls, 1–2% of children over 4 years old; 30% are also enuretic.

Character

1. Hard motions, small or large.
2. Secondary leakage of liquid faeces ('spurious diarrhoea') around large impacted masses of faeces is common. Inappropriate prescribing of antidiarrhoeal remedies worsens the situation.

Pathophysiology

Precipitating event: constipation →pain → fear → retention → pain.

Examples

1. Infant negativism, exacerbated by punitive parental attitude.
2. Anal fissure or hard stool during acute illness with reduced fluid intake. A constipating medication may have been prescribed, e.g. iron, antacids, diuretic.
3. Emotional trauma of new sibling, or school.
4. Environmentally unpleasant to pass stool, so retained, e.g. toilets at school smelly, lacking in privacy.

Resulting physiological abnormalities

   i Failure of relaxation of internal anal sphincter despite rectal dilatation.
  ii Reduced rectal sensitivity and increased rectal compliance reducing the urge to defaecate.

Clinical

Presentation: 18 months old upwards, symptoms usually for many months before seeking medical help, i.e. behavioural pattern often well established. Important factors include dietary fibre intake, previous medications, and parental response to soiling. Blood streaking of the stool is common, and parents may have noted an anal fissure. Examination may reveal a midline faecal mass rising out of the pelvis is craggy, indentable, and painless.

Assess neurology of perineum and lower limbs for paresis, or sensory loss.

Anus may be obscured by faecal liquid if overflow is present. Buttocks may be tensed, anus dilated. Clean it up and look for fissures, skin tags, reflex anal dilation (common?), and signs of abuse.

Rectal examination: the anal canal is shortened, seek the tight grip of Hirschsprung's and beware the associated gush of faeces and air, resistance to dilatation of anal stenosis, and the posterior shelf of an anteriorly placed anus.

Table 15.5 Differentiation of constipation from Hirschsprung's disease

	Simple constipation	*Hirschsprung's**
Failure to thrive	Absent	Usually present by late infancy
Abdominal pain	Common	Absent unless obstructed
Stool size	Normal/bulky	Narrow, ribbon like
Stool on PR	Present, anus often smeared	Empty rectum
'Tight' anus	Extreme, but voluntary	Even when relaxed

* Additional symptoms: delay in passing meconium, constipation from birth, diarrhoea and constipation, vomiting, severe abdominal distension.

Other causes

See above.

Investigations

A Hb check in excessive intake of milk for related iron deficiency, and a plain X-ray of the abdomen are justified, whereas a barium enema for idiopathic megacolon is not.

Management

Graduated according to severity.

1. Carefully explain to the parents and, appropriate to age, the child, the pathophysiology of megacolon, the reduced rectal sensation in faecal soiling, and the need for a behavioural approach. Consider psychological support.

   Check fluid intake and dietary fibre is adequate; soluble fibre in fruit is not as valuable as the insoluble bran and cellulose fibre found in cereals.
2. Establish effective evacuation of retained faeces. Stepwise approach. Mild 5–10 ml senna once, followed by 2 weeks docusate. If moderate, picosulphate, which may be repeated in 6 h. Severe justifies a microenema or phosphate enema, with

full cooperation or under appropriate sedation, or a manual evacuation (some also give an anal stretch) under anaesthesia.

3. Maintain an empty rectum with stool softener and laxative, increasing the dose stepwise to achieve at least one motion daily, while avoiding abdominal cramps and diarrhoea as these lead to treatment failure.

   i   Stool softeners: docusate sodium 12.5–25 mg 2 times daily, lactulose 5–15 ml 3 times daily, methylcellulose 5 ml after meals.

   ii Laxatives: Senna 2.5–20 ml at night. A weekly picosulphate or microenema is reasonable for a few weeks, in the severe case, to aid involution of the megacolon.

Continue for several months, then gradually reduce.

4. Regular toileting 5–10 minutes within 30 minutes of each meal is strictly enforced.

   Optimal conditions for success include: making time to avoid hurry, sitting comfortably, feeling physically and emotionally secure. Reinforce success with praise and star chart, and appropriate rewards.

5. Biofeedback by rectal manometry claims success in improved awareness and cleanness.

Prognosis

Ultimately good, but relapse is common, especially in the socially deprived.

Further reading

Clayden G S (1990) Constipation. In *Recent Advances in Paediatrics*, (T J David ed) Edinburgh:Church-ill Livingstone pp. 41–59

Loening-Bauke V (1989) Factors determining outcome in children with chronic constipation and faecal soiling. *Gut*, **30**, 999–1006

Loening-Bauke V (1990) Modulation of abnormal defecation dynamics by biofeedback treatment in chronially constipated children with encopresis. *Journal of Pediatrics*, **116**, 214–222

DIARRHOEA

Acute diarrhoea

Definition

An increase in stool water; an often subjective increase in stool frequency and looseness, i.e. no satisfactory definition.

Annual incidence world wide

100 million attacks in the 300 million under 5s, 4 million deaths (late 1980s).

Epidemiology

Highest risk groups

1. < 6 months in developed world.
2. From weaning into the second year in developing countries. The principal cause of malnutrition in children (anorexia, catabolism from infection, practice of starvation 'therapy').

Pathogens

Rotavirus commonest single agent in infants, *Helicobacter jejuni* commonest invasive pathogen.

Environmental factors

i Poverty = overcrowding, no clean drinking water supply, reduced hand washing, sewage not dealt with.
ii Malnutrition from recurrent diarrhoea, lack of appropriate food → reduced stomach acidity = reduced barrier to infection.
iii Bottle feeding.
iv Antibiotics alter bacterial flora: pseudomembranous colitis.

Pathophysiology

1. Normal water and electrolyte transport

Water shifts passively, accompanying solute. Glucose and salt transport are coupled, i.e. each is enhanced by the presence of the other. It is an active transport process across mucosal cell membranes, at a shared receptor site.

2. Mechanisms inflicting damage by microorganisms

i Direct attack by microorganism, producing mucosal damage.
ii Toxin produced after ingestion, e.g. enterotoxigenic *Escherichia coli*, cholera.
iii Toxin produced before ingestion, e.g. staphylococcal food poisoning, always the result of poor hygiene and hand washing. Onset hours after ingestion, lasting 1–2 days. *Bacillus cereus* toxin from cooked rice contamination, *Clostridium perfringens* from contaminated meat.

Pathophysiology of the diarrhoea

1. Secretory diarrhoea

Membrane transport is deranged → decreased absorption of sodium and chloride through increased activation of cyclic adenosine monophosphate (AMP) by toxins (e.g. cholera, enterotoxigenic *E. coli*), and Ca^+ calmodulin (e.g. *Clostridium difficile*), through cell damage by cytotoxic enterotoxins (e.g. Shigella, *Bacillus cereus*), and sodium-potassium ATPase inhibition from bile acids deconjugated by anaerobic bacteria in a small intestine contaminated by bacteria.

2. Decreased absorption

  i   Mucosal damage by microorganisms or small intestine surgical resection. In cryptosporidiosis and acute viral gastroenteritis (e.g. rotavirus) damaged villi cells are replaced by immature crypt cells → impaired absorption of water, electrolytes and sugars.
  ii Osmotic diarrhoea due to unabsorbed intraluminal sugars as in primary disaccharidase deficiency or from mucosal damage.
  iii Increased gut motility reducing transit time.

Classification linking clinical picture to causal organism by mechanism of injury

1. Watery diarrhoea = non inflammatory, due to toxins (food poison toxins, cholera and toxigenic *E. coli*), and damage to the brush border (enteropathic *E. coli*, e.g. 055, 0111, 0119, cryptosporidiosis, *Giardia lamblia*).
2. Dysentery = mucosal invasion (fever often present)

  i   Localized: Shigella, enteroinvasive *E. coli.*
  ii Mucosal invasion and spread to local lymph glands:
      Helicobacter, Yersinia, non-typhoid salmonella.
  iii Mucosal damage, marked rectal bleeding:
      enterohaemorrhagic *E. coli* 0157

3. Variable, intestinal symptoms may be absent, e.g. mucosal invasion and septicaemic spread in *Salmonella typhi*.

Table 15.6 Organisms commonly causing acute gastroenteritis in UK

Viral	Bacterial
1 Rotavirus 50%	1 Helicobacter 6%
2 Norwalk virus 10%	2 Cryptosporidiosis 4%
3 Adenovirus 5%	3 Salmonella 2%
4 Shigella 1%	

Rotavirus Winter peak, most severe under 2 years old, though usually mild in neonates (maternal antibody?). Droplet and faecal–oral spread.
   Incubation 1–3 days, lasts 7 days. Respiratory illness in 50% +/- fever, precedes watery diarrhoea and vomiting. Transient glucose malabsorption common.

Helicobacter jejuni, Gram negative rod, commonest cause of dysentery with severe abdominal pain, bloody diarrhoea due to invasion of mucosa. Source: contaminated milk, chicken, water. Incubation 3–5 days. Lasts 10–14 days. Erythromycin if prostrated or prolonged.

Cryptosporidiosis. Mainly 1–4 year olds. Several outbreaks in day nurseries, from animals on farm visits by schoolchildren, or contaminated water supply. Peaks in spring and autumn. Incubation 7 days, watery diarrhoea × 6–9 daily, abdominal cramps, prolonged in 20%, worse in immune deficiency, e.g. HIV. No specific treatment.

Salmonella enteritidis P4 Increased reports to Communicable Disease Centre from contaminated poultry-egg production.

Clinical pointers

- Preceding upper respiratory tract infection: rotavirus.
- In contact with diarrhoea, or to a common food source in a communal outbreak.
- Foreign travel: Asia: cholera, amoebic dysentery; giardiasis, dysentery; Northern Europe/Russia: giardiasis, cryptosporidiosis.
- Dysentery = abdominal pain, blood and mucus = invasive organism likely (see mucosal invasion).
- Reduced immunity: persistent rotavirus excretion, more than one virus, cryptosporidium, yeasts.
- Rarely, arthritis, iritis, erythema nodosum follows: *Yersinia enterocolitica.*

Clinical

General: fever, anorexia, vomiting, abdominal pain, diarrhoea.

- Stool may be so fluid as to be mistaken for urine.
- 'Diarrhoea' may be starvation stools: mucousy, watery, green.
- Febrile convulsions particularly associated with Shigella.

Assessment of dehydration

1. 5%: dry mucous membranes, decreased skin turgor, slightly sunken eyes, fontanelle.
2. 10%: obvious skin laxity, sunken eyes and fontanelle. Rapid pulse and respiration. Restless/lethargy. Oliguria.
3. 10–15%: shock, coma, anuria.
   Obesity may mask skin signs.

Hyponatraemic dehydration

Serum sodium <130 mmol/l in 5–10%, signs of circulatory collapse occur earlier as water shifts from hypotonic extracellular fluid into normotonic cells. More common among malnourished breast-fed infants in developing countries.

Hypernatraemic dehydration

Serum sodium >150 mmol/l, in 1–2% (historically in 1960s up to 20% in temperate regions). Water shifts out of cells into the circulation, which is maintained longer, so the degree of dehydration is greater when symptoms show. Irritability and lethargy greater than expected for degree of dehydration. Skin 'doughy'. Osmolality of serum higher than expected from sum of electrolytes, due to presence of 'idiogenic osmols'.

Brain damage in 10–20%, exacerbated by too rapid rehydration causing cerebral oedema.

Commoner in the 1960–70s due to the then permitted higher sodium and protein content in infant formula milks. Also due to insufficient water or giving salt as emetic/abuse/Munchausen by proxy.

Differential diagnosis of acute vomiting and diarrhoea

Common

1. Gastroenteritis.
2. Food poisoning.
3. Parenteral response to infection elsewhere, e.g. septicaemia, urinary infection, meningitis.
4. Surgical: appendicitis, intussusception, Hirschsprung's disease.
5. Bowel reaction, e.g. food intolerance, coeliac disease, chronic inflammatory bowel disease.

Uncommon

Congenital adrenal hyperplasia, diabtetes mellitus, haemolytic–uraemic syndrome.

Investigations

Pursued according to severity of illness.

Stool culture: microscopy for pus cells and red cells in dysentery, *Giardia lamblia*, *Helicobacter jejuni*, 'hot stool' to identify amoeba, culture; electron microscopy and tissue culture for viruses.

Blood count: leucopenia classically associated with *Salmonella typhi.*

Serum biochemistry reveals sodium level; potassium may be normal or high initially in the presence of the usual metabolic acidosis due to loss of bicarbonate in stools; urea is often raised.

Blood glucose may be raised in hypernatraemia, and may cause initial confusion with diabetes mellitus, but returns to normal as rehydration continues. Measure blood pH and base deficit if clinically acidotic or shocked.

Urine microscopy and culture are essential. Blood culture +/- CSF if septicaemia or meningitis is likely.

X-ray the abdomen if it is distended or tender. Fluid levels in both the ileus of gastroenteritis (may be due to hypokalaemia) and surgical obstruction or peritonitis mandate a rectal examination, and may need a surgical opinion.

Management

1. Weigh on admission and regularly thereafter for realistic monitoring of progress.

2. Oral rehydration therapy (ORT) saves millions of lives in developing countries. 'Greatest medical advance this century' claim in 1983 *Lancet* editorial.

Based on preservation of sodium–glucose coupled transluminal transport mechanism even in severe secretory diarrhoeas, e.g. cholera.

WHO oral rehydration solution (ORS): sodium 90 mmol/l, potassium 20 mmol/l, chloride 80 mmol/l, bicarbonate 30 mmol/l, glucose 110 mmol/l, (sucrose a suitable alternative). Used successfully in 90–95% of cases in developing countries where hyponatraemia is common.

Solution with sodium 35–50 mmol/l, carbohydrate up to 200 mmol/l (e.g. Dioralyte) recommended for use in developed countries to avoid hypernatraemia.

Amino acids, e.g. glycine, alanine, act additively to transport of sodium and glucose, confirming the benefit of 'folk remedy' rice water (which is now available commercially as Ricelyte, containing sodium 50 mmol/l, rice-syrup solids 30g/l).

3. Fluid replacement = RMO

   i *R*ehydration: 50 ml/kg if mild, 100 ml/kg moderate, over first 6 h unless hypernatraemic, where 24–48 h is safer.
   ii *M*aintenance: 100 ml/kg/24 h up to 10 kg, plus 50 ml/kg for the next 10 kg, then 25 ml/kg thereafter.
   iii *O*ngoing losses from vomiting and diarrhoea.

Method

Little and often = 5–10ml every 5–10 minutes by spoon or nasogastric tube. If tolerated for 30 minutes at 15 ml/kg/h, increase to 30 ml/kg/h.

   a. Replacement in 6 h, offering extra (10 ml/kg) after each large vomit/fluid stool. Ratio of 2 volumes ORS to 1 of water. Breast feeding should recommence after 4 h.
   b. If still mildly dehydrated give 50 ml/kg ORS over next 6 h.
   c. At 12 h start maintenance 100 ml/kg/24 h.
   d. Regrading: begin after 24 h, cows' milk (whole or powdered), half strength for first 24 h, and starches reintroduced over 1–3 days. Under 3 months old, hydrolysed milk may be preferred for a few days to avoid postenteritis lactose and cows' milk protein intolerance. Both are usually transient.

In developing countries
   a. Local fluid alternatives to ORS: rice water, coconut water, clear soups (electrolyte and carbohydrate content are suboptimal).
      Fruit used for potassium replacement, e.g. banana.
   b. Early refeeding the cornerstone in preventing the cycle of diarrhoea and malnutrition using full strength milk from the beginning. Failures no worse than with graduated regrading.

4. Intravenous therapy
   Indications: shock, coma, ileus.

   Often given in developed countries in less severe dehydration, as more convenient, less labour intensive (but the pumps used still need to be monitored), and fear of hypernatraemia (now rare).

Shock: plasma/plasma substitute/albumin 20 ml/kg immediately over 20–30 minutes.

Half strength Dextrose/saline initially 60 ml/kg over 4 h.

Sodium bicarbonate added if base deficit greater than 10 mmol/l, according to the formula: 0.3 × weight × base deficit.

Complete rehydration using 0.18% saline plus 4% dextrose over 24 h as calculated for Replacement, Maintenance + Ongoing losses above.

Add potassium to infusion once urine flow is established unless: Renal failure should be suspected when urine output <0.5ml/kg/h. Differentiated from prerenal by (i) urine:plasma urea ratio >4, or osmolality ratio >1.3, and urinary sodium <10mmol/l. These findings, after adequate rehydration, are an indication for frusemide and reducing intake to 80 ml/kg/24 h.

In hypernatraemic dehydration total fluid is restricted to 150 ml/kg/24 h, and rehydration spread over 2–3 days if necessary.

Medication

1. Antibiotics

  i Specific indications and first choice until sensitivities known:

Cholera:	tetracycline
Severe shigella:	co-trimoxazole
Helicobacter persistent and severe:	erythromycin
Giardiasis, amoebiasis:	metronidazole
Yersinia:	co-trimoxazole
Salmonella < 2 years old or septicaemic:	chloramphenicol, co-trimoxazole

  ii Suspected septicaemia

Antibiotics are otherwise contraindicated as:

  i Bacteria develop resistance.
  ii May prolong carriage, e.g. *E. coli*, salmonella.
  iii Cause pseudomembranous colitis (treat with vancomycin).

Antidiarrhoeals

Use accepted in older children and adults, rarely in infants. Loperamide is effective and safe. Diphenoxylate (Lomotil) may cause respiratory depression in young children; Kaolin etc have no place.

Further reading

Leader (1983) Oral hydration in context. *Lancet,* ii, 118

Regrading failure

Regrading failure (20%) and the postenteritis syndrome = failure to tolerate cows' milk.

1. First regrade failure: clear fluids for a day is usually sufficient to return to normal.

2. Second regrade failure: consider lactose or cows' milk protein intolerance and introduce hydrolysed or soy and lactose free milk.
3. Third regrade failure: comminuted chicken, glucose polymer and medium chain triglyceride oil feed.

Prognosis

Mortality <1% hospital cases in UK. Secondary food intolerance 5%. Prolonged malnutrition in established postenteritis syndrome.

Further reading

Wharton BA, Pugh R E, Taitz L S, Walker-Smith J A, Booth I W (1988) Dietary management of gastro-enteritis in Britain. *British Medical Journal*, **296**, 450–452

Chronic diarrhoea

The implication of stool frequency and consistency is best considered in its impact on growth.
1. Normal growth, loose or semiformed stools

   i Toddler diarrhoea.
   ii Constipation with overflow.
   iii Laxative abuse (Munchausen by proxy, bulimia nervosa).

2. Failure to gain weight or actual weight loss with persistent loose watery stools for 2 weeks or more.

Common causes

   i Persistent enteric infection (amoeba, salmonella, schistisoma, shigella, TB, yersinia); associated with immune deficiency.
   ii Post enteritis lactose or cows' milk protein intolerance. Intractable diarrhoea and where relevant, tropical sprue (cause unknown in either but often linked to prior infection).
   iii Food allergy.

Uncommon

   i Inflammatory bowel disease: food allergy, Crohn's disease, ulcerative colitis (beware misdiagnosing enterocolitis actually due to Hirschsprung's disease).
   ii Malabsorption: coeliac disease, cystic fibrosis, Shwachman syndrome (rare).

Iatrogenic

Antibiotic induced, chemotherapy induced.

Assessment

1. The nature of the stool may give a clue:

   - A fluid stool should be tested for reducing sugars.
   - An offensive greasy stool suggests malabsorption.
   - Offensive with mucus +/- blood may be infective or chronic inflammatory bowel disease.
   - Partially digested vegetables in a healthy 6–36 month old is indicative of toddler's diarrhoea.

2. Age at onset

   i   From birth. Apart from infection, and post necrotizing enterocolitis, a primary lactase or even rarer glucose–galactosse monosaccharidase deficiency, or chloridorrhoea may be present. Hirschprung's disease may be missed unless the intermittent nature of the diarrhoea is appreciated.

   ii Persistent neonatal jaundice, and onset of greasy pale stools may be biliary atresia or neonatal hepatitis.

   iii In the first few months of life cows' milk and soy protein intolerance, cystic fibrosis as well as a postenteritis malabsorption need to be considered. Dietary manipulation can be therapeutic. Rare causes include intestinal lymphangiectasia, and inborn errors of absorption, e.g. chloridorrhoea (HCO_3^- :Cl^- exchange), acrodermatitis enteropathica (Zn deficiency).

   iv After 4–6 months, coeliac disease and various food allergies/intolerance join the list, with the introduction of weanings as the clue.

   v   In the first year, ulcerative colitis (UC), exacerbated by cows' milk, is commoner then than at any subsequent age. Immune deficiency syndromes usually present within the year, SCID and yeast opsinization defect early, immunoglobulins later.

   vi After the first year HIV infection assumes importance. UC remains unusual, but increasing in childhood is Crohn's disease. Gut hormone secreting tumours and neuroblastoma occur at any age.

Clinical pointers

Normal height for age and weight for height implies no serious organic disturbance, the converse if growth is failing. Previous recordings of weight are therefore extremely useful.

Diet, any changes in it, and the management of previous diarrhoeal episodes, or the use of antibiotics in the last 6 weeks for any reason, may be implicated. Dilution of feeds with inadequate caloric intake resulting in weight loss is common.

Infectious disease contact, foreign travel, previous acute diarrhoeal episodes suggest an infective aetiology.

Intermittent vomiting may be a feature of food intolerance, Hirschsprung's disease, intermittent volvulus with post-iscaemia malabsorption.

A history of laxative abuse may be withheld, and requires careful observation in hospital.

Clinical

Alertness: apathetic and irritable in coeliac disease. Pallor, rickets, in malabsorption; joint swelling, iritis, erythema nodosum in chronic inflammatory bowel disease.

Merasmus or marasmic kwashiorkor in profound protein–calorie deficiency. The additional findings of rectal prolapse or chest infection suggest cystic fibrosis.

Eczema with infection suggest immune deficiency, or HIV infection.

Abdominal distension may be coeliac, meconium equivalent in cystic fibrosis, or hepatomegaly from biliary atresia which should prompt looking at the superficial abdominal veins for a caput medusae.

Investigations in context

Commonly, specific signs are rarely found, so often as much relies on the dietary assessment and response to feeding as to laboratory investigation.

Stool cultures, preferably hot to identify protozoa, stool water for sugars (and if positive, a lactose load and hydrogen breath test), a FBC, a sweat test and, if symptoms are suggestive, barium contrast X-ray, followed by jejunal biopsy for coeliac disease or colonoscopy for inflammatory bowel disease.

Second pass investigations look for the less common conditions.

Further reading

Walker-Smith J A, McNeish A S (1986) *Diarrhoea and Malnutrition in Childhood.* London:Butterworths

INDIVIDUAL CONDITIONS CAUSING CHRONIC DIARRHOEA

Toddlers diarrhoea (irritable bowel syndrome of infancy)

A functional bowel disorder of frequent passage of loose, offensive stools. Similarly affected family members are common.

Pathophysiology postulate

Prostaglandin E increased in plasma, may reflect increased secretion, and rapid small bowel transit delivers bile salts to the colon stimulating a secretory diarrhoea.

Clinical

Onset 6 months to 2 years, sometimes following gastroenteritis, remits by 5 years. Boys: girls = 2:1

Stools may alternate between constipation and loose mucuosy and undigested ('peas and carrots syndrome'), exacerbated by roughage. Frequency 1–10 per day.

Very active behaviour is common.

Normal growth velocity in height and weight.

Investigations

Stool culture, stool water for reducing substances.

Management

Explanation of natural history, avoidance of fibre, reduction of sucrose, possible addition of fat to the diet to slow motility.

Loperamide 0.1 mg/kg/24 hours for 7 day courses if the diet is unsuccessful.

Persistent gastrointestinal infections

1. Yersinia enterocolitica

Gram negative rod, producing acute abdominal pain, watery diarrhoea, for 1–3 weeks.

2. Parasitic infections

i Causing prolonged diarrhoea in temperate climates (also found world wide).

Giardia lamblia
Life cycle: cyst ingested → trophozoite in small intestine → cysts spread by contaminated water or food.
Clinical: incubation 1–3 weeks followed by severe diarrhoea and abdominal pain for a week. Chronic diarrhoea +/– malabsorption and failure to thrive may follow. Common in malnutrition, immune deficiency.
Investigation: Examine fresh stool and/or duodenal aspirate.
Treatment: Metronidazole 3 days or single dose of tinidazole.

Amoebiasis (Entamoeba histolytica)
Life cycle: cysts → trophozoites in small intestine → cysts, colonization of colon.
Clinical: Incubation 2 weeks–months. Blood and mucus in intermittent diarrhoea. Invasion of mucosa commoner in tropics, with spread to liver, occasionally lung, brain, forming abscesses.
Investigation: Hot stool for cysts and amoebae, serum antibodies raised.
Treatment: Metronidazole 5 days.

ii Causing protracted diarrhoea in the Tropics

Examine stool for eggs/larvae

Whipworm (Trichuriasis) Estimated 500 million cases. Common. Usually asymptomatic, may have abdominal pain, diarrhoea, rectal prolapse.
Treatment: Mebendazole.

Roundworm (Ascaris lumbricoides) Estimated 1000 million cases.
Life cycle: eggs ingested → larvae hatch in small intestine→ lungs via blood stream → trachea → swallowed → gut to become adults 15–35 cm long → egg production. Migration takes 1–2 weeks, egg production 2 months → soil.
Clinical: Often asymptomatic or abdominal discomfort, occasionally obstruction or wheeze due to pulmonary infiltrates and eosinophilia.
Treatment: Mebendazole. Piperazine in <2 years old or for obstruction.

Hookworm Estimated 900 million cases.
Life cycle: After penetration of intact skin (e.g. bare feet) by larvae, itchy vesicular eruption at the site, otherwise similar to roundworm. Attach to gut mucosa.
Clinical: Occasionally malabsorption, hypoproteinaemia, anaemia; usually asymptomatic.
Treatment: Bephenium hydroxynaphthoate, or mebendazole in >2 year old.

Strongyloides Similar to hookworm, with larva skin eruptions around anus from reinfection as the worm is voided. Treatment with thiabendazole.

Schistosomiasis 200 million children and teenagers swimming/paddling in infected pools.
Life cycle: Like hook worm, with snail as intermediate host. *S. mansoni* in Africa and South America, *S. haematobium* Egypt, *S. japonica* in China, eastern Asia.
Clinical: Incubation 1–2 months → fever, urticaria, diarrhoea/dysentery. Hepatoplenomegaly, cirrhosis → oesophageal varices in mansoni, japonica; haematuria and dysuria in haematobium; cerebral migration → epilepsy in japonica.
Diagnosis: Stool, midday urine for eggs.
Treatment: Praziquantel.

iii Ubiquitous, nuisance only

Threadworm (Enterobius vermicularis)
Life cycle: eggs ingested → larvae hatch, sexually reproduce in caecum → females containing eggs pass out of bowel at night → shed eggs on perianal skin which cause itching → scratching → reinfection.
Clinical: Pruritus ani, mainly at night, 1–2 cm white 'threads' on stool. Whole family may be infected.
Treatment: Trim fingernails, apply mittens to prevent scratching. Mebendazole single dose, or piperazine in <2 years old. Treat the whole family.

Cows' milk protein intolerance (CMPI)

Definition

Temporary intolerance to lactalbumin and lactoglobulin, which may be primary immune, usually with an atopic family history, or secondary to damage to gut wall from gastroenteritis and subsequent immune reaction to milk, the foreign protein. Appears in the first months of life, resolves by 1–2 years.

Incidence

1 in 200 (range an extraordinary 0.3–7%).

Clinical presentations

1. Diarrhoea:

    i Acute onset with vomiting leads to rapid withdrawal of cows' milk.
    ii Persistent diarrhoea and vomiting with failure to thrive, +/- blood and mucus.

2. Oedema, generalized, due to protein losing enteropathy, and anaemia.
3. Allergic: nasal discharge, wheeze, eczema. Anaphylaxis and angioneurotic oedema are rare.

Investigation and diagnosis

1. Empirically by elimination of cows' milk or other suspect protein (e.g. soy). Confirm diagnosis with at least one positive challenge, performed at the end of the first month. Three challenges have been suggested (Goldman criteria) but rarely complied with, as the risk of anaphylaxis in young infants is real, and parents are often reluctant once they see a thriving infant.
    Breast fed babies' mothers should have a trial of cows' milk elimination diet.
2. Raised IgE, food antibodies, skin tests, eosinophilia may be present, but are not essential for diagnosis.
3. Jejunal biopsy is only required if uncertainty as to coeliac or post-enteritis. Findings are similar to coeliac disease, but usually not so severe.
4. Peripheral eosinophilia, with blood and mucus in the stool: consider CMPI related eosinophilic colitis in which colonoscopy reveals erythematous patches of colitis containing eosinophils and plasma cells in the lamina propria. An otoscope may show inflammatory changes in the rectum.

Management

1. Which milk?

    i Soy milk, containing a glucose polymer as carbohydrate source as many also have lactose intolerance.
    ii However, soy protein intolerance is also present in 30%, so persistent symptoms indicate need for cows' milk protein hydrolysate, e.g. Pregestimil, Nutramigen, or goats' milk.

2. Reintroduce CMP milk at 2 years old, in hospital if necessary if initial presentation was severe, or anaphylactic.
    Method: 1 ml fresh cows' milk, doubling hourly to 32 ml at 5 h, monitoring stools and vital signs. Discharge after 24 h, to increase intake gradually at home.

Prognosis

If mild, weeks to months, the more severe may take up to 6 years. Adverse reactions to other foods is frequent. Stopping CMP does not prevent atopic disease (asthma, eczema and allergic rhinitis).

Further reading

Bishop J M, Hill, D J, Hosking C S (1990) Natural history of cow milk allergy: clinical outcome. *Journal of Pediatrics*, **116**, 862–867

Soy milk intolerance

Similar to CMPI. Less common at present, but incidence is likely to increase, due to inappropriate advice or parental hopes that by cows' milk allergen avoidance eczema may be prevented. At present the evidence for the latter is conflicting.

Carbohydrate, especially lactase, deficiency

Absence of brush border enzymes which metabolize dietary sugars. (Absence of maltase and isomaltase is clinically unlikely.)

1. Lactase: Lactose $\rightarrow$ glucose + galactose
2. Sucrase: Sucrose $\rightarrow$ glucose + fructose

Causes: congenital and secondary to mucosal insult. Lactase is particularly vulnerable.

Clinical

- Stools watery, frothy ('fermented'), acid causing perianal excoriation
- Failure to thrive

Lactose intolerance

Reduced or absent lactase activity in small bowel.

Table 15.7 Lactose intolerance

Primary	Secondary
1 Non-Caucasian AR adults world wide. Onset may be in early childhood, leading to recurrent abdominal pain. Residual activity allows small amounts of lactose to be tolerated.	1 Post gastroenteritis
	2 Protein-energy malnutrition
	3 Cows' milk protein intolerance
	4 Coeliac disease in relapse
2 Congenital AR, onset in newborn due to almost complete absence of lactase, rare	5 Post gastrointestinal surgery
	6 Neonatal: prematurity, hypoxia, necrotizing enterocolitis
Pathology: Normal histology	Often subtotal villous atrophy

Diagnosis

Reducing substances >0.5% in stool water:water mix of 1:2 tested using Clinitest. Stool pH <5.5, not reliably present.

Breath hydrogen test. Hydrogen, released by bacterial breakdown of any unabsorbed sugars passed into the large intestine, is carried by the circulation and excreted via the lungs, i.e. not specific for lactose. >20 p.p.m. above base line is a positive result.

Jejunal biopsy for enzyme assay is not justified in clearcut secondary disaccharidase deficiency.

Management

Lactose free diet. Remember lactose is often used as a filler in pill medicines.

In secondary intolerance CMPI may coexist, so soy milk is often used. Recovery follows within days to weeks unless merasmic, so cows' milk challenge permitted after a fortnight and usually allows return to a normal diet.

Monosaccharide malabsorption

Congenital glucose–galactose malabsoption AR is rare, due to a transport defect in the brush border. Severe diarrhoea, with normal disaccharidase activity. Only fructose is tolerated, i.e. sucrose, lactose and glucose free diet.

Secondary glucose malabsorption

   i A transient state in acute gastroenteritis, for 2–3 days.
  ii Rarely, in under 3 months old, may persist for weeks as intractable diarrhoea, postenteritis, or rarely, as a familial condition (consider immune deficiency, inborn errors of absorption), needing total parenteral nutrition for a period. Trimethoptim and metronidazole are added. Cholestyramine, cromoglycate, steroids and loperamide may help, though effect is often transient.

Inflammatory bowel disease: Crohn's, ulcerative colitis

Definition

Chronic inflammatory diseases of unknown aetiology affecting any part of the gastrointestinal tract (Crohn's) or limited mainly to the colon and premalignant (ulcerative colitis) (Table 15.8).

Table 15.8 Comparison of Crohn's disease and ulcerative colitis

Crohn's disease	Ulcerative colitis (UC)
Site: Ileum (mainly terminal ileum) and anus 80%, colon 50%. Anywhere from mouth to anus	Colon and rectum always involved Small intestine only 10%
Distribution: Skip lesions, normal bowel between them	Continuous
Pathology: Transmural chronic inflammation (100%), fissuring (25%), submucosal ulceration, granulomata 50%	Mucosal ulceration, goblet cell mucus depletion. Abscess formation begins in the crypts

Crohn's and ulcerative colitis, a comparison

Incidence

1 each per 20000 population. Crohn's increasing in children and more frequent than UC. Commoner among first degree relatives and Jews.Onset
Less than 20 years of age in 30 - 40% of adult cases.

Clinical

1. Growth failure:

   - Crohn's>UC, may be a late sign in the latter.
   - Precedes gastrointestinal symptoms by 1 or more years in some.
   - 'Nutritional dwarves' due to (i) anorexia with reduced intake (to avoid symptoms of diarrhoea and abdominal pain?) (ii) increased need for calories (iii) malabsorption: > subsequently delayed puberty.

2. Gastrointestinal symptoms

   i Diarrhoea:
      Blood and mucus, tenesmus and faecal incontinence are characteristic of UC. Diarrhoea and rectal bleeding may be minor in Crohn's.
   ii Abdominal pain:
      Often more severe and left sided in UC.
         In Crohn's more intermittent, +/– abdominal mass in right iliac fossa consisting of either matted loops of bowel, obstruction from stricture or abscess.
   iii Abdominal distension in UC = toxic megacolon, an emergency. Severe diarrhoea, abdominal pain, tender on palpation, peritonitis, weight loss, increased pulse and respirations.
   iv Perianal fissures, fistulae and tags common in Crohn's, but rare in UC.

3. Fever, fatigue.
4. Extra-intestinal disease common to both:

   i Common: clubbing, arthritis, mouth ulcers.
   ii Uncommon: uveitis, erythema nodosum, pyoderma gangrenosum.

iii Liver involvement: UC>>Crohn's, especially adults, consisting of chronic active hepatitis, biliary cirrhosis.

Investigations

1. Stool culture.
2. Blood for ESR, an indicator of activity. Albumin low in 50%, iron deficiency common in both; thrombocytopenia in UC.
3. Serology for amoeba, salmonella, yersinia.
4. Multiple biopsies from affected areas to distinguish Crohn's from UC.
5. X-ray:
   Crohn's–skip lesions, ulcers, strictures.
   UC–distal changes, continuous, shortening of bowel, reduced motility and haustral pattern.

Differential diagnosis

1. Mis-labelled recurrent abdominal pain, anorexia nervosa, school refusal due to listlessness. Weight loss, fever and bowel symptoms help to distinguish.
2. Other causes of growth failure and delayed puberty.
3. Infection: stool for amoeba, organisms. *Clostridium dificile* toxin present and colonoscopy in post antibiotic pseudomembranous colitis.
4. Food intolerance, especially cows' milk protein and soy. Response to dietary elimination, and characteristic biopsy if in doubt.
5. Pyrexia of unknown origin.
6. Local disease: ulcerative proctitis carries a good prognosis, recovery within 6–12 months.

Medical management

1. High calorie diet. Elemental diet in Crohn's is effective. Parenteral nutrition may be necessary in toxic megacolon.
2. Steroids. Topical enemas for ulcerative proctitis and distal disease. Systemic prednisolone 1–2 mg/kg/day for 4–6 weeks if extensive disease or toxic, then weaning off.
3. Aminosalicylates: Sulphasalazine. Particularly effective in UC. Helps steroids obtain remission, and maintain it. Up to 3–4 g/day is usual. Olsalazine may be preferred in UC.
4. Others: Cromoglycate in UC may be beneficial, metronidazole in Crohn's with abcesses or fistulae.

Support for child and family through the difficulties with school attendance, acceptance of surgery, ileostomy/colostomy, delayed puberty.

Surgery

Crohn's disease

85% come to operation within 15 years from diagnosis for removal of toxic segments of bowel.

Ulcerative colitis
Indications 1 toxic megacolon; 2 unresponsive to steroids; 3 perforation; 4 bad bleeding. After 10 years: collectomy and removal of rectal mucosa or 6 monthly endoscopy and biopsy of suspicious lesions.

Prognosis

Crohn's: relapse 30% within 2 years. Mortality up to 10% in children. UC: cancer risk 3% first 10 years, then 2% per year.

MALABSORPTION

When food is not properly absorbed or transported across the intestinal mucosa, malabsorption is present, and usually presents as failure to thrive.

Failure to thrive due to gastrointestinal disorders

Definition of failure to thrive

Weight below the third centile for age, or earlier presentation as persistently downwards crossing of centile lines. (A comprehensive approach appears in Growth problems.)

Common in the UK

1. Emotional deprivation with impaired utilization of food.
2. Enteritis: acute bacterial or viral, post enteritis syndrome (mainly lactase deficiency).
3. Food intolerance: cows' milk protein, soy protein, and others, e.g. egg, chicken, fish, goats' milk.

Common world wide

1. Protein energy malnutrition-enteritis cycle.
2. Tropical sprue.
3. Giardiasis.

Uncommon

1. Coeliac disease.
2. Cystic fibrosis.

Rare

1. Chronic inflammatory disease: Crohn's disease, ulcerative colitis.
2. Biliary atresia.

3. Immune deficiency and Shwachman syndrome.
4. Inborn errors of absorption, e.g. abetalipoproteinaemia, transcobalamin II deficiency, primary lactase deficiency, glucose-galactose malabsorption.
5. Blind loop syndrome.
6. Hirschsprung's disease.

Clinical

Common

Diarrhoea, often as steatorrhoea. Abdominal distension, wasting of muscles and subcutaneous fat → wrinkled skin around thighs, buttocks, upper arms. Hypotonia and weakness are related. Irritability and lethargy may be striking, and mislabelling as spoilt or difficult is likely.

Longer term: growth failure, delayed puberty in the chronic causes.

Uncommon

Oedema (hypoproteinaemia), bleeding (vitamin K deficiency), hypocalcaemic tetany.

Clinical pointers to individual conditions

1. Respiratory infections: cystic fibrosis, immune disorders.
2. Skin abnormalities:

   a. Eczema, lymphopenia/neutropenia, repeated infections: HIV, Shwachman syndrome.
   b. Herpes like lesions on back and buttocks, in mid childhood: dermatitis herpetiformis:
   c. Eczema around the mouth: acrodermatitis enteropathica.

3. Anaemia (megaloblastic): transcobalamin II deficiency.
4. Hepatomegaly, diarrhoea (+/– ascites and oedema, bruising from hypoprothrombinaemia): biliary atresia, chronic hepatitis.
5. Finger clubbing: cystic fibrosis, chronic hepatitis, Crohn's, ulcerative colitis (joint swelling may precede).
6. Asymmetric limb lymphoedema in intestinal lymphangiectasia with protein loosing enteropathy.
7. Ataxia, peripheral neuropathy, retinopathy and cirrhosis: abetalipoproteinaemia.

Investigation of suspected malabsorption

1. Check that caloric intake is for the average weight at that age. This should result in weight gain within days, or up to a month in the severely emotionally deprived.
   Occasionally nasojejunal feeding is justified to demonstrate that weight can be gained, after investigations have been initiated.
2. Check dietary intake with care. First step is either a supervised trial of feeding in hospital, or at home of parent–child interaction, mealtime behaviour, and feeding

practice, unless symptoms and signs suggest an organic cause when investigation should not be delayed.

Persistent failure to gain weight during the trial or the infant/child is clearly mal-absorbing

i First line

Stool for culture, parasites, fat droplets and blood, and reducing substances in stool water.

Urinalysis and culture.

FBC, serum ferritin, and if megaloblastic, or an older child, B_{12} and folate levels.

Biochemistry for electrolytes, urea, rickets, liver function, albumin.

A chest X-ray and a sweat test if respiratory symptoms, voracious appetite, meconium ileus.

Breath hydrogen if carbohydrate intolerance is likely.

ii Second wave

Barium meal and follow through for Crohn's, enema for ulcerative colitis.

Duodenal aspirate for giardiasis.

Jejunal biopsy if coeliac or severe post enteritis: it may also detect abetalipopro-teinaemia fat laden villi.

Shilling test for terminal ileum Crohn's disease.

iii Less commonly tested, only when specifically indicated

Immune function tests if infection chronic or repeated or multiple.

Low Zn in acrodermatitis enteropathica.

Low cholesterol and β-lipoprotein, presence of RBC acanthocytes in abetalipro-teinaemia.

Protein electrophoresis for transcobalamin II deficiency.

Lymphopenia and uniformly severely lowered plasma proteins is a clue to pro-tein losing enteropathy, detected by Cr^{51} labelled albumin excretion test.

Management

See the individual disorders.

Coeliac disease

Definition

Lifelong gluten induced enteropathy of the proximal small bowel resulting in mal-absorption, which remits completely on gluten withdrawal.

Pathophysiology

Intolerance caused by a toxic, immunologically mediated response to the alpha glia-din fraction of gluten, a cereal protein found in wheat and rye (oats and barley too, but less toxic). The turnover rate of small bowel epithelial cells is increased.

IgA antibodies (gliadin, antireticulin, antiendomysium) present at diagnosis, rise and fall with gluten challenge and its withdrawal.

Histology shows flat mucosa, crypt hypertrophy, cuboid epithelium, increased intraepithelial lymphocytes and plasma cell infiltration of lamina propria.

Damaged brush border causes low lactase activity, secondary lactose intolerance.

Inheritance

Familial in 10%. Associated with HLA types DR4 in all, HLA-DR3 or DR7 in over 90%.

Incidence

1 in 2000 UK and USA, as high as 1 in 300 in Galway, Ireland.

Falling incidence in last decade attributed to more breast feeding, later weaning and introduction of gluten.

Clinical presentations

1. Failure to thrive after weaning, onset usually by 2 years, with diarrhoea, some-times vomiting.
   General: wasted, hypotonic, pale, irritable and anorexic.
   GI signs: Abdomen distended. Faeces soft, pale, sticky, frequent. May be loose secondary to lactose intolerance.
   Oedema due to protein losing enteropathy is rare.
2. Short stature, pubertal delay.

Investigations

- Iron deficient anaemia (folate deficient rare).
- Rickets (uncommon).
- Hypoprothrombinaemia (vitamin K malabsorption–always check prothrombin time before doing a jejunal biopsy).
- Hypoalbuminaemia.
- D-xylose 5 g in 50 ml water with blood at one hour <20 mg/100ml supports the diagnosis.
- Jejunal biopsy by capsule is still preferred to a smaller sample obtained at endos-copy.
- Duodenal aspirate and faeces for giardia.
- Immunoglobulins for deficiencies, and IgA antibodies.

- Salivary IgA antibody is more specific and sensitive.
- Note fat balance studies are now rarely done.

Differential diagnosis

1. Causes of subtotal or total villous atrophy:

    i Coeliac disease, transient gluten intolerance
    ii Gastroenteritis, postenteritis syndrome
    iii Cows' milk protein intolerance, soy intolerance
    iv Giardiasis, immune deficiency, e.g. HIV, IgA deficiency.

2. Causes of malabsorption and failure to thrive:
    Cystic fibrosis, distinguished by failure to thrive and oily very offensive stools from birth, voracious appetite, recurrent chest infections, lively personality.
    Schwachman syndrome AR Pancreatic insufficiency with normal sweat test. Bony changes with short stature, leucopenia which may be cyclical, and thrombocytopenia common. Continuous pancreatic replacement, vitamins and courses of antibiotic as indicated. Lymphoma relatively common. Chromosomal breaks on culture.
3. Toddler diarrhoea/irritable bowel syndrome – often intermittent, no evidence of failure to thrive, or abdominal distension.
4. Emotional deprivation with abnormal feeding behaviour, and subsequent accelerated growth on social work/psychiatric interview, or if that fails, removal from home.

Diagnosis

1. Classical criteria: 3 biopsies (European Society of Paediatric Gastroenterology criteria)
    First: at diagnosis.
    Second: demonstrating return to normal on gluten free (GF) diet.
    Third: relapse on challenge with gluten of 15g/day for 3 months.
2. Alternative criteria, all 3 required for diagnosis.

    i One characteristic biopsy, not repeated if response to GF diet is full and unequivocal.
    ii IgA gliadin, antireticulin, antiendomysium antibodies (though note 3% of coeliacs are IgA deficient), which disappear on GF diet.
    iii Cows' milk protein intolerance, post-enteritis syndrome and giardiasis excluded, which they cannot be with confidence if diagnosis is made in the first year of life.

    Any doubt about the diagnosis or response to GF diet is an indication for a control biopsy on treatment followed by gluten challenge.
3. Transient gluten enteropathy is found in some under 2 years at diagnosis. Challenge after 2 years of GF diet, preferably after 6 years old. Rarely, may take 5–7 years on gluten to relapse, so follow up is essential.
    Conditions associated with coeliac disease include dermatitis herpetiformis, which, with skin manifestations, may respond to gluten free diet, and diabetes mellitus.

Management

Gluten free diet for life, unless lactose or cows' milk intolerance suspected as the true cause, when challenges to each may be necessary after 3–6 months, time for the mucosa to recover.

Advise dietetic supervision and membership of the Coeliac Society.

Occasionally needs lactose free diet initially, or steroids if in coeliac crisis (biopsy deferred if very ill).

Gluten challenge after 2–4 years to allow 'catch up' growth (takes up to a year) preferably before school age. Thus if no longer affected the child can have school meals.

Prognosis

Adolescence a time of spontaneous 'remission', despite indiscretions, only to worsen in adult life with general malaise, anaemia, infertility, osteomalacia.

Gluten free diet may be protective against lymphoma and GI malignancy.

Further reading

Guandalini S, Ventura A, Ansaldi N, *et al*, (1989) Diagnosis of coeliac disease: time for a change? *Archives of Disease in Childhood*, **64**, 1320-1325

Holmes G K T, Proir P, Lane M R, Pope D, Allan R N (1989) Malignancy in coeliac disease – effect of a gluten free diet. *Gut*, **30**, 333–338

Report of the Working Group of European Society of Paediatric Gastroenterology and Nutrition (1990) Revised criteria for diagnosis of coeliac disease. *Archives of Disease in Childhood*, **65**, 909–911

Dietary treatments

1. Hyperactivity and the Feingold diet

This postulates that 30–50% of 'hyperactive' children benefit from exclusion of additives, colourings and salicylates. Some children do benefit in the short term.

2. Atopic eczema and elimination diets

Skin tests and food antibody tests are unhelpful.

Diets are probably only worthwhile in extensive eczema. Dietician support is essential.

Guidelines

   i Parents enthusiastic, child likely to cooperate by age (<1 year) or by inclination (disfigured body image).

  ii Staged approach, according to severity and dietary clues

Stage 1: Eliminate those 'trigger' foods implicated by observation.

Stage 2: 'triggers' plus cows' milk protein and egg.

Stage 3: includes food additives, wheat, fish, legumes, tomatoes, citrus, berries, currants, nuts.

iii Few food diet (stage 4): strict exclusion except for turkey/lamb, potato, rice, carrot and leafy vegetable, pear, bottle water.

iv Continue stage 1–4 for 4–6 weeks. If successful, gradually re-introduce a new item of food every 5 days.

Prognosis

10% of children benefit from cows' milk elimination, and up to 25% of those severe enough to try using the few food diet.

3. Migraine

Elimination of the 4 Cs: cheese, chocolate, citrus fruits, caffeine. On the few foods diet other triggers are also improved.

4. Few food diet (oligoantigenic) diet

Indications range though intractable seizures, migraine, hyperactivity, eczema, vaginal discharge, abdominal pain.

Further reading

David T J (1989) Dietary treatment of atopic eczema. *Archives of Disease in Childhood*, **64**, 1506–1509

Egger J, Carter C M, Wilson J, Turne M W, Soothill J F (1983) Is migraine food allergy? *Lancet*, ii, 865–869

HAEMORRHAGE

Although common, gastrointestinal haemorrhage is not usually life threatening.

Factors to consider in bleeding from the gastrointestinal (GI) tract:

1. Site: upper or lower GI tract.
2. Acute or chronic

   Acute e.g. 'red currant jelly' stool of intussusception, bleeding from varicies, Meckel's diverticulum, peptic ulcer.

   Chronic loss is usually blood streaking as in constipation, proctitis, hiatus hernia, or mixed with faeces in inflammatory conditions (cows' milk intolerance, infective, Crohn's).
3. Severity. Assessed by volume of vomitus or aspirate, or stool content. Shock in acute large bleeds contrasts with relative cardiovascular stability in all but the severest chronic blood loss.
4. Age.

   i The neonate swallows maternal blood (Apt's test distinguishes), and is prone to bleeding disorders (check vitamin K administered).

   If stressed or shocked, then haemorrhagic gastritis, erosions or ulcers, and with bilious vomiting and abdominal distension, necrotizing enterocolitis, must be considered. The latter may be indistinguishable from midgut volvulus unless abdominal X-rays are regularly taken.

Minor bleeds from anal fissures (and rectal thermometers) or feeding tubes are readily identified.

ii Throughout infancy, anal fissuring from constipation is very common.

Blood mixed with stool is commonly enterocolitis from bacterial infection (cultures helpful), occasionally cow or soy milk colitis, when their exclusion is diagnostic.

Occult loss may be significant in gastroesophageal reflux.

Intussusception and congenital malformations (Meckel's, volvulus, duplications, vascular) are individually uncommon but can cause severe acute bleeding.

iii The 1–5 year old, like the infant, is prone to constipation and infection. The latter may precede the haemolytic uraemic syndrome if a verotoxin is produced.

In the upper GI tract swallowed blood from epistaxis and oesophageal tear through vomiting becomes common, but is rarely due to varices, from portal hypertension.

Abdominal pain is acute in intussusception, and may precede the rash of Henoch-Schönlein anaphylactoid purpura.

Intermittent painless rectal bleeding may be profuse with malaena in Meckel's diverticulum, and rarely, haemangiomas, or less severe from polyps (which may be familial).

iv The older child also experiences epistaxis, vomiting and infection, but is now more prone to peptic ulceration and bleeding from localized proctitis, and be systemically unwell if due to Crohn's disease or ulcerative colitis. Haemorrhoids are uncommon and may be due to portal hypertension.

At any age accidental or non-accidental trauma (duodenal injury) and sexual abuse are primary considerations; bleeding disorders, ulceration due to aspirin and stress, and tumour, are less common.

Causes of bleeding from the upper gastrointestinal tract

1. Swallowed blood: maternal, at birth or cracked nipple, and nasopharyngeal inflammation.
2. Oesophagus: hiatus hernia, oesophageal varices, foreign body.
3. Stomach and duodenum: haemorrhagic gastritis, peptic ulceration, acute gastric erosions, pyloric stenosis.
4. Drugs: aspirin, iron poisoning.
5. Bleeding disorders, e.g. haemorrhagic disease, thrombocytopenia, von Willibrand's disease.
6 Munchausen by proxy.

Causes of blood in stool or bleeding from rectum

1. Local: constipation causing anal fissure, sexual abuse.
2. Swallowed maternal blood in the newborn.
3. Infection: dysentery.

4. Upper GI bleeding: hiatus hernia, peptic ulceration.
5. Lower GI bleeding: intussusception, peptic ulceration in Meckel's diverticulum and duplications, polyps.
6. Inflammatory bowel disease: cows' milk colitis, ulcerative colitis, Crohn's, proctitis.
7. Bleeding disorders.
8. Portal hypertension.
9. Munchausen by proxy.

Assessment

1. Distinguish blood in vomit or stool from food colours or beetroot, or black stool containing iron, by guaic or ortho-toluidine.
2. Haematemesis is occasionally described as being blood 'coughed up', but a careful history will clarify. Swallowing blood from a nose bleed may have preceded the event. 'Coffee grounds' = gastric acid action on blood.
3. Establish whether the haematemesis or malaena is due to bleeding proximal to the ligament of Treitz, by a positive test for blood in gastric aspirate. Unfortunately, an aspirate negative for blood does not exclude it, as bleeding may have stopped, or, if the pyloris remains closed, failed to reflux back into the stomach.
4. Origin of blood passed rectally (generalization):

   i Malaena = bleeding proximal to the caecum, e.g. peptic ulcer, Meckel's diverticulum. Occasionally, brisk duodenal bleeding results in rapid transit and the passing of a bloody stool.
   ii Red currant jelly = ileocolic intussusception or midgut volvulus.
   iii Bright red blood = colonic bleed from ulcerative colitis, arteriovenous malformation, haemangioma, telangiectasia.
   iv Dark red, jelly = colonic inflammation, e.g. shigella, yersinia, salmonella, enterohaemorrhagic *E. coli*, amoebae. Rarely due to *Clostridium difficile* toxin in pseudomembranous colitis.
   v Stool mixed with red blood = polyp, ulcerative colitis, proctitis.
   vi Stool with blood smeared on the outside = anal fissure.

5. History: elicit presence and duration of pain and its character, diarrhoea, fever, weight loss, growth retardation, joint swellings. History of foreign travel, family history of bleeding, polyposis or inflammatory bowel disease, indicate the direction of investigations. An excessively calm parent presenting grossly blood stained clothing may have had previous 'cot death', and be a Munchausen by proxy.
6. Clinical points:

   i Physical growth may be reduced in chronic abuse, or inflammatory bowel disease.
   ii a. Lips and mucous membranes: pigmented spots of Peutz-Jegher's (AD familial intestinal hamartomas)
   b. Nose bleed
   c. Skin for purpura or signs of violence.

iii Pulse, blood pressure, pallor.
iv Abdomen

    a. Enlarged liver and/or spleen (cirrhotic bleeding disorders, varices).

    b. Discrete mass under the liver from intussusception, right iliac fossa in Crohn's disease, anywhere for duplication.

    c. Tenderness and guarding may be severe in acute abdominal emergencies (intussusception, volvulus, strangulated bowel), localized in peptic ulceration to the hypochondrium, or left side of the abdomen in ulcerative colitis. Although usually painless, occasionally a Meckel's mimics appendicitis.

  v Anus and rectum for fissure, evidence of abuse, digital examination for constipation, local pain from ulcerative colitis, auriscope for low polyps, visualisation of friable mucosa from infection, pseudomembranous colitis, or food intolerance.

Investigation

1. Blood count, ESR, coagulation studies, stool culture. Liver function tests if splenomegaly is present.
2. X-ray

  i Plain film of abdomen for signs of necrotizing enterocolitis, or distended bowel proximal to obstruction, e.g. intussusception

  ii Barium enema to confirm intussusception, chronic inflammatory bowel disease, polyps. Rare findings are Hirschsprung's disease or colonic duplication.

    Barium swallow is rarely helpful in an acute bleed, but detects some hiatus herniae and peptic ulcers.
3. Technetium scan for Meckel's/duplications may be helpful if persistent/recurrent or in a single severe bleed before colonoscopy.
4. Endoscopy performed early is often the most helpful investigation:

  i Upper GI endoscopy diagnostic in most cases of upper GI bleeds, enables biopsies to be taken for Crohn's, and oesophageal varices to be injected with sclerosant.

  ii Lower GI: auriscope to see anal tear and extension. Proctoscopy enables view of ulcerative colitis, milk colitis, most juvenile polyps, though colonoscopy may be needed to assess the extent of these, Crohn's disease, vascular abnormalities, and bleeding from lymphonodular hyperplasia seen after infections.

Management

See individual conditions for details. General approach:

1. Resuscitate, give blood if necessary.
2. Laboratory tests of coagulation, plasma urea, ESR, liver function tests. X-ray abdomen looking for mass, fluid levels, free air.

3. Locate site of upper GI bleeding:

   i If nasal, may need packing.

   ii Pass a nasogastric tube, if blood is aspirated bleeding is above ligament of Trietz (but see above). Iced saline gastric lavage until bloody aspirate is almost clear seems to help.

   iii Endoscopy will usually determine whether due to ulceration requiring antacids and an H_2 blocker, or varices needing i.v. vasopressin or sclerosant.

   iv Angiography if severe bleeding continues and accurate localization needed to identify varices or severe bleeding ulcer, give i.v. vasopressin and embolize by intra-arterial injection with a gelatin preparation.

4. Lower GI bleeding:

   i Malaena may require urgent transfusion, and endoscopy. A small bowel barium may be unhelpful, and a pertechnetate 99[Tc] scan to identify the gastric mucosa of a Meckel's diverticulum or duplication should be ordered.

   ii Acutely ill with redcurrant jelly stool should have a barium enema, which reduces 75% of intussusceptions if up to 72 h old.

   iii Colonoscopy is preferred in colitis, when toxic megacolon may be precipitated by a barium enema, and for minor recurrent bleeds.

   iv Barium enema, in which double contrast is reserved for identifying polyps and ulceration of inflammatory bowel disease.

Peptic ulceration and gastritis

Definition

A peptic ulcer occurs where mucosa is exposed to acid and pepsin.

Pathophysiology

1. Peptic ulceration = imbalance between acid secretion and mucosal defence. Acid output tends to be increased in children with chronic duodenal ulcer.
2. Proof that gastritis in children is caused by *Helicobacter pylori* is as yet inconclusive.
3. Psychological associations with bereavement and separation.

Epidemiology

Usually secondary to stress and drugs in infancy and childhood. Primary in adolescence, boys twice as often as girls, and are 4 times more likely to have a duodenal ulcer than girls. Antral gastric ulcer is often transient and commoner than duodenal ulcer which tends to be chronic. A family history of duodenal ulcers in up to 50%.

Clinical presentation

Unlike adults, pain is often periumbilical, not associated with mealtimes, and periodic.

Night pain prominent in a third of children. Dyspepsia and vomiting are common.

Haematemesis or malaena occurs in a third, sometimes without prior pain.
Epigastric tenderness on palpation.

Diagnosis

Confirm site and extent by endoscopy which is twice as likely to detect ulceration as a barium meal, which does show distortion of the duodenal cap.

Managment

1. Drugs for active ulceration:

    i   Antacids 1h (and 3 h if actively bleeding) after meals.
    ii Cimetidine once or twice daily, 20–30 mg/kg/day or ranitidine up to 150 mg twice daily, for 4–8 weeks.
    iii Sucralfate if not responding.

2. Prophylaxis: H_2 antagonist for 12 months reduces relapse rate in that time of over 50% in adolescents to 10–25%.
3. Surgery: selective vagotomy and pyloroplasty for failed medical therapy.

Repeated ulceration requires gastrin levels to detect Zollinger-Ellison syndrome of acid hypersecretion due to islet cell tumour.

Further reading

Murphy M S, Eastham E J, Jimenez M, Nelson R, Jackson R H (1987) Duodenal ulceration: review of 110 cases. *Archives of Disease in Childhood*, **62**, 554–558

Nord K S (1988) Peptic ulcer disease in the pediatric population. *Pediatric Clinics of North America*, **35**, 117–140

Abdominal masses

A high index of suspicion that an abdominal mass is malignant is required. The exceptions may seem obvious, but are so by history and associated findings. If in doubt, full investigation is necessary.

1. Retroperitoneal:

    i   Renal: hydronephrosis, Wilm's tumour, multicystic and polycystic kidneys.
    ii Neuroblastoma.

2. Gastrointestinal, and differential diagnosis in that area:

    i   Right iliac fossa: appendix abscess, Crohn's matted loops of bowel, TB, ectopic kidney, ovarian tumour.
    ii Right hypochondrium: intussusception (may migrate to left hypochondrium), pyloric stenosis, choledochal cyst.
    iii Left iliac fossa: faeces, intussusception, ulcerative colitis, ovarian tumour.

    iv Duplication, lymphoma anywhere.

    v Suprapubic: bladder, faeces.

3. Hepatosplenomegaly: see liver disorders.

Investigations

1. Hb, WBC, ESR, Mantoux, early morning gastric aspirates.
2. Urinalysis and culture.
3. US + history most likely to identify which organ, whether a solid or fluid containing lesion, or pyloric stenosis, and whether or which further test is required.
4. Barium meal for chronic inflammatory bowel disease, duplications.
5. Radioisotope scans for renal function, duplication, bone metastases.

Management

1. Treatment of infection (urinary tract, TB).
2. Surgery for tumours, pyloric stenosis, intussusception, appendix abscess.
3. Radiotherapy for large tumours; may precede surgery in Wilms'.
4. Chemotherapy according to type of tumour.

Abdominal tumours

See Oncology.

Further reading standard references:

Anderson C M, Burke V, Gracey M (1987) *Paediatric Gastroenterology* 2nd edn. Oxford:Blackwell

Milla P J, Muller D P R (1988) *Harries' Paediatric Gastroenterology*. Edinburgh:Churchill Livingstone

Tripp J H, Candy D C A (1985) *Manual of Paediatric Gastroenterology*. Edinburgh:Churchill Livingstone Useful for revision.

Chapter 16

Hepatobiliary disease and jaundice

HEPATOMEGALY

Causes

1. Infection

    i   Bacterial: septicaemia, brucella, leptospirosis.
    ii Viral: hepatitis A, B, the transfusion-associated non-A non-B, C (now 90% of such cases) and D; infectious mononucleosis, cytomegalovirus, HIV.
    iii Protozoal: malaria, toxoplasmosis, amoebiasis.
    iv Parasitic: hydatid, ascariasis, schistosomiasis.

2. Haemolytic: sickle cell, thalassaemia.
3. Congestive cardiac failure.
4. Malignancy: hepatic tumours, leukaemias, Letterer-Siwe disease, secondaries from Wilm's tumour, neuroblastoma.
5. Cystic fibrosis.
6. Metabolic:

    • Reye's syndrome.
    • Storage disorders: glycogenoses, mucopolysaccharidoses, lipidoses, e.g. Gaucher's.
    • Galactosaemia, fructose intolerance, Wilson's disease, α-1 antitrypsin deficiency.
    • Poisons, drugs.

7. Chronic diseases: Still's, Crohn's, ulcerative colitis, chronic hepatitis.
8. Portal hypertension (see below).

    History and clinical findings will usually indicate the direction of investigation. First exclude downward displacement of the liver by hyperinflation.

1. Skin manifestations: spider naevi, palmar erythema in chronic liver disease. Jaundice: see below.

2. Tender liver with soft edge suggests infectious hepatitis, infectious mononucleosis, leptospirosis, abscess, cardiac failure.
3. Huge enlargement, firm edge, in storage disorders, malignancies, established congestive cardiac failure.
4. Absence of splenomegaly in metabolic disorders, except storage disorders.
5. Developmental delay is associated with storage disorders.
6. Hard irregular liver edge favours tumour, polycystic disease, hydatid disease.

Serology for alphafetoprotein and chorioembryonic antigen, antibodies to amoeba (+ stool) and hydatid.

Abdominal, chest X-ray and skeletal X-rays, early US, CT, technetium scintiscan, for primary and secondary deposits, hydatid cysts.

VMA urinary excretion, bone marrow for neuroblastoma.

JAUNDICE

Jaundice after the newborn period

Acute onset

1. Prehepatic: haemolytic.
2. Hepatic: infection, drugs, poisons.
3. Post hepatic: obstruction.

Chronic persistent jaundice

1. Hepatic

   i Chronic hepatitis: chronic persistent hepatitis, chronic active hepatitis.
   ii Inborn errors: Gilbert's syndrome, Wilson's disease etc (see neonatal jaundice).

2. Post hepatic: biliary atresia, choledochal cyst.

Assessment of jaundice and hepatitis: points relevant to childhood

Relative frequency

Hepatitis A is common in children and young adults, but only 1% of all UK hepatitis B notifications are of under 15 year olds, most being due to contact within the family. Reye's syndrome occurs 1 in 2000 influenza B, 1 in 4000 chickenpox cases.

History

1. Contact with hepatitis:

   i Foreign travel in hepatitis A virus (HAV) within the past 6 weeks
   ii Parenteral (including blood products) or sexual transmission (abuse) in hepatitis B virus (HBV) or non-A non-B hepatitis, in the last 6 months.

2. Institution for the mentally handicapped (HBV).
3. Mother affected by HBV: vertical transmission to infant.
4. Recent viral infection and aspirin taking in Reye's syndrome.
5. Drugs: valproate risk in under 24 months old, mentally handicapped, taking multiple anticonvulsants.

    Ingestion of paracetamol rarely produces serious liver damage in young children.
6. Swimming in canals or rivers may lead to leptospirosis.
7. Family history in Wilson's disease.
8. Pre-icteric phase: fever and abdominal pain may suggest an infectious fever or appendicitis. Difficult to diagnose if the child remains anicteric.

Clinical

1. Fever, anorexia, nausea. Abdominal discomfort in the right upper quadrant, worse on exercise is common in older children. Diarrhoea in half the children with HAV.
2. Begins to feel better with the onset of jaundice in HAV, not usually with HBV. Enlarged tender liver, with splenomegaly in 30%. Dark urine and pale stools if significant cholestasis is present.
3. Illness lasts 2–4 weeks in acute hepatitis A or B.
4. HBV associated disease:

    i Acute: urticaria, arthritis, rarely Henoch-Schönlein purpura, Guillain-Barré syndrome, renal failure due to endotoxin.
    ii Chronic: papular acrodermatitis (non itchy, papular rash over face and limbs for 2–4 weeks), membranous glomerulonephritis.

    Chronic signs to look for: clubbing, spider naevi, caput medusae, Kayser-Fleischer ring.

Worsening of behaviour, unconsciousness and biochemical indices in established hepatitis signal the onset of encephalopathy.

Persistent jaundice (rarely, no jaundice), the onset of bleeding, the development of ascites and liver shrinking are ominous signs of fulminant or subacute hepatic necrosis.

Investigations

1. Urine for bilirubin confirms obstructive element.
2. Serum bilirubin up to 250–300 mmol/l.
3. Liver transaminase enzymes raised 10–20 × upper limit of normal.
4. Alkaline phosphatase usually no more than 1.5 × upper limit. Higher values, with prolonged prothrombin time, indicate chronic or fulminating hepatic failure.
5. Antibody tests for HAV, HBV, Paul Bunnel, TORCH, leptospirosis. Tropical parasitic diseases sought in appropriate cases.
6. Atypical cases:
    Consider a paracetamol level.

US for choledochal cyst, liver architecture.

Raised reticulocyte count in haemolytic diseases, e.g. glucose 6–phosphate dehydrogenase, or Wilson's disease.

7. Persistently raised enzymes/bilirubin for 4–8 weeks: caeruloplasmin (for Wilson's disease), autoantibodies, e.g. antinuclear antibody and anti-double stranded DNA present in 50% with chronic active hepatitis.

Liver biopsy is necessary to diagnose chronic active hepatitis, chronic persistent hepatitis and Wilson's disease, providing the prothrombin time is satisfactory.

8. Encephalopathy: arrange investigations 1 to 7 *plus* blood for raised ammonia (best indicator), low glucose, sodium and potassium, albumin, blood urea, and abnormal gases, low prothrombin and disseminated intravascular coagulation, autoantibodies. EEG shows generalized slowing.

Management

1. Establish whether acute or chronic or acute on chronic. Based on the clinical and laboratory findings.
2. Acute hepatitis. Supportive. Bed rest as required, not mandatory. Fats may help resolution, although often worsens nausea.
3. Chronic active hepatitis. Steroids are indicated providing it is non-HBV–they may be started even if low prothrombin prevents biopsy.
4. Fulminant hepatitis

   i Prevent worsening of encephalopathy by reducing the protein intake and ammonia production from bacteria in the bowel by neomycin and lactulose.
   ii Established encephalopathy: counter cerebral oedema (with mannitol), bleeding, renal failure, secondary infection, and consider exchange transfusion to reduce the ammonia level. See Reye's syndrome.

Prognosis

1. HAV: 90% anicteric, a mild disease common in young children. No carrier state, does not progress to chronic liver disease.
2. HBV

   i Infants infected at birth/breast feeding: usually asymptomatic,but 70–90% develop the carrier state, with a high risk of hepatoma as an adult.
   ii Older children: the majority recover completely, 1–20% become chronic carriers, (especially the preschool Chinese where the figure is 25%).
   Of these, 10% develop chronic persistent and chronic active hepatitis, 3% cirrhosis; hepatoma as an adult is much less common than for transmission at birth.
3. Chronic persistent hepatitis: good, no treatment.
4. Chronic active hepatitis: HBV see 1 and 2 above. The autoimmune type has a poor prognosis without steroids +/– azothiaprine, but after treatment 70% are normal at 5 years. The remaining 30% progress to cirrhosis and liver failure.
5. Acute liver failure: 30% mortality, proportional to the severity of coma.

Prophylaxis and prevention

1. Hepatitis A. Gamma globulin 0.04 ml/kg i.m. in the incubation period.
2. Hepatitis B in mother's HB surface antigen (HBsAg) positive, or e antigen (HBeAg) positive.

    Maternal carrier status is 0.5% in Caucasians in Europe and USA, and 10–20% in Asians and Africans.

    Risk of transmission:

    Maternal acute hepatitis in the third trimester = 50%.

    At/after delivery, if mother is HBeAg+ve, 85% infants become carriers, and even if HBe antibodies are present 25%, but if HBsAg+ve alone = 10–20%.

    Prognosis: chronic active hepatitis, cirrhosis, and/or carcinoma in up to 25%.

    Vaccination is offered to all newborn of mothers HBsAg+ve regardless of HBeAg status.

    i Within 24 h of birth, repeated at one month and 6 months.
    ii Additional specific antihepatitis B immunoglobulin 0.5 ml, if mother is HBeAg+ve, at birth.

3. Hepatitis B after sexual abuse

    Specific antihepatitis B immunoglobulin 0.06 ml/kg as soon as possible after exposure.

    Other risk groups: include the immunosuppressed, Down's syndrome, receiving chronic haemodialysis.

Further reading

Balistreri W F (1988) Viral hepatitis. *Pediatric Clinics of North America*, **35**, 637–669

CHILDHOOD HEPATITIS SYNDROMES

Chronic active hepatitis

Causes

1. Viral hepatitis (mainly HBV–HBsAg, HBeAg persist).
2. Autoimmune.
3. Others: Wilson's disease, drugs, chronic inflammatory bowel disease, α-1 antitrypsin deficiency.

Autoimmune

A chronic aggressive hepatitis, often with cirrhosis, raised serum immunoglobulin IgG and autoantibodies. Sporadic, girls 3:1, rare before 6 years old. HLA antigen B8 DR3 found in 80%.

Clinical

Insidious onset is usual, less often acute with amenorrhoea, anorexia, fever, spider naevi, jaundice (unusual), hepatosplenomegaly, bleeding, +/- weight loss, arthralgia, and erythema nodosum.

Diagnosis

Liver biopsy shows inflammatory cell infiltrate, 'piecemeal' hepatocellular necrosis, whereas in chronic persistent hepatitis there is only an inflammatory cell infiltrate.

Treatment

Immunosuppressive doses of steroids, with azothiaprine if unresponsive or serious steroid side effects, until well for a year/histology has returned to normal.

Wilson's disease

AR, gene on chromosome 13. (Indian childhood cirrhosis is related.)

Definition

An abnormality of copper metabolism, with impaired excretion causing symptoms and signs to appear, in order:

1. Haemolytic anaemia (due to copper uptake by RBCs) +/– liver failure with jaundice in <3 years old.
2. Deposits in the eyes (Kayser-Fleischer brown or grey-green rings).
3. Kidney (Fanconi syndrome) >5 years old.
4. Brain (choreathetosis, school failure. Unusual in childhood).

Diagnosis

Slit lamp, low serum caeruloplasmin, raised urinary copper, increased copper in liver biopsy.

Management

Penicillamine or trientine for life prevents irreversible damage. Prognosis is therefore dependent on early diagnosis, for without treatment it is fatal.

Alpha-1 antitrypsin deficiency

Definition

AR, the affected are homozygous for Pi (protease inhibitor) ZZ. The gene is on chromosome 14.

Pathophysiology

Absence of the proteolytic enzyme inhibitor α-1 antitrypsin may allow damage to liver and lungs by proteases released by the tissues.

Incidence

1 in 5000.

Clinical

85% asymptomatic, 10% develop neonatal cholestasis, 5% minor liver dysfunction.
Presentation at 3–12 weeks with cholestatic jaundice, resolving over 6 months.
Chronic bronchitis and emphysema in older child.

Prognosis

Liver disease in infancy slowly progresses to cirrhosis in >50%. Risk of hepatic carcinoma is substantial.

Cirrhosis

Hepatocellular failure + portal hypertension. The end result of hepatitis, biliary
atresia, cystic fibrosis, chronic active hepatitis, alpha-1-antitrypsin deficiency,
Wilson's disease etc.

Clinical

1. Hepatocellular: failure to thrive, oedema, ascites, spider naevi, liver palms,
   bleeding tendency.
2. Portal hypertension: see below.
3. Obstruction: jaundice, pruritus, xanthelasma.

Investigation

Liver function tests, tests for cause of cirrhosis from history.

Management

Fat soluble vitamins A, D, K by i.m. injection, high carbohydrate diet.

Prognosis

Poor, consider liver transplant depending on aetiology.

Liver transplantation indications

1. Biliary cirrhosis.
2. Metabolic: chronic parenchymal disease, decompensating (ascites resistant to
   diuretics, prolonged prothrombin, low albumin, failure to thrive, bacterial peritonitis) e.g. Wilson's disease, α-1-antitrypsin deficiency, glycogen storage diseases; also tyrosinaemia.
3. Cholestatic disorders and congenital biliary atresia.

4. Acute fulminant hepatitis.
5. Liver tumours without metastases.

Survival after transplant: for a year 80%, for 5 years 64%, not so good under one year of age. Dividing a donated liver allows several children to benefit.

Controversy: will transplant supercede the Kasai procedure? Certainly consider if over 120 days old, with a large hard liver.

Causes of portal hypertension in childhood

1. Intrahepatic: cirrhosis
2. Extrahepatic venous obstruction:

   i Portal vein thrombosis:
     idiopathic.
     umbilical vein sepsis, catheterization.
   ii Hepatic vein thrombosis: Budd Chiari syndrome.
   iii Vena caval back pressure: congestive cardiac failure, cor pulmonale, constrictive cardiac failure.

Presentations

Acute bleeds (varices), hypersplenism (pancytopenia); haemorrhoids (a portocaval anastomotic site) are rare in childhood.

Clinical

1. Ascites, splenomegaly.
2. Portal-systemic venous anastomoses (oesophageal varicies, caput medusae, haemorrhoids, upper abdomen venous hum).
3. Jugular venous pressure (JVP) is raised if vena caval pressure is raised, but if the cause is heptic vein obstruction the JVP fails to rise on pressure on the liver.

Investigations

1. Differentiation between cirrhosis and extrahepatic venous obstruction:

   i Normal liver function = extrahepatic obstruction.
   ii Technetium scan: normal liver scan = extrahepatic obstruction.
   iii To identify the site of extrahepatic venous obstruction, use US, and abdominal CT.

2. Identify bleeding/state of varices by endoscopy.

Management

1. Bleeding varicies:

   i As a single bleed is common, and a tendency to improve with age, adopt an expectant policy.

ii If severe and acute, i.v. pitressin helps reduce portal venous pressure, and is followed by sclerosing injection therapy. A portovenous anastomosis may eventually be needed.

2. Cirrhosis: fat soluble vitamins A, D, K, by i.m. injection and a high carbohydrate diet.

SPLENOMEGALY

Palpability: normally palpable in 30% of term infants, <10% by the end of infancy. Thereafter, enlarges 2 to 3 times normal to become palpable.

Causes

1. Infection.
2. Blood disorder: anaemia, haemolysis (+ splenic sequestration in sickle cell disease), extramedullary haemopoiesis as in thalassaemia major.
3. Infiltration:

    i Malignant: leukaemia, lymphoma, Langerhan's cell histiocytosis.
    ii Storage disorders: Gaucher's disease, Niemann-Pick disease.

4. Congestion: cardiac failure, portal hypertension which is either:

    i Extrahepatic: umbilical vein catheterization, sepsis, or
    ii Intrahepatic: cirrhosis due to hepatitis, cystic fibrosis, metabolic errors, e.g. Wilson's disease, galactosaemia, α-1 antitrypsin deficiency. Shistosomiasis and malaria in endemic areas.

5. Connective tissue disease: Still's disease, systemic lupus erythematosus.

Clues from the history

Pyrexia +/- foreign travel: infection, especially infectious mononucleosis, bacterial endocarditis, malaria.
  Neonatal umbilical catheterization or sepsis causing portal vein thrombosis.
  Jaundice: haemolytic diseases, e.g. spherocytosis, sickle cell disease (+ race).
  Purpura, bleeding from infiltration or hypersplenism.

Clinical pointers and appropriate investigations

1. Spleen tender if acute, firm if congested or infiltrated. A FBC for anaemia, spherocytes or sickling. Target cells indicate a need for Hb electrophoresis; thick film for malaria if travel abroad. Virology for infectious mononucleosis, cytomegalovirus, HIV; blood culture for bacterial endocarditis; serology for Widal, brucella, leptospirosis.
2. Inability to get one's fingers above it, that it moves with respiration, along the line of the 9th and 10th ribs is spleen. Nevertheless, an US should be done to ensure it is not a splenic cyst or Wilm's tumour or other renal enlargement.

3. Hepatomegaly and lymph node enlargement accompanying indicated malignancy, Still's disease, Langerhan's cell histiocytosis. A bone marrow aspiration distinguishes malignant infiltration from infiltration due to Gaucher's disease or Neimann-Pick disease.
4. Splinter haemorrhages, fundal haemorrhages in subacute bacterial endocarditis (+ cardiac murmur) or liver disease.
5. A reduction in one of the three blood elements (anaemia, leucopenia, thrombocytopenia) indicates hypersplenism. Haemorrhoids, caput medusae, or haematemesis is an indication for liver function tests for cirrhosis, and endoscopy, barium swallow for varices, and a splenic puncture for portal vein pressure.
6. Joint swelling and transient rashes in connective tissue disorders require serology.

Further reading

Mowat A P (1987) *Liver Disorders in Pediatrics* 2nd edn. London:Butterworths
Tanner S (1989) *Paediatric Hepatology.* Edinburgh:Churchill Livingstone

Chapter 17

Haematology

DEVELOPMENT OF THE HAEMATOPOIETIC SYSTEM

Of mesenchymal origin, the stem cells of the blood islands in the yolk sac migrate to the liver, the main organ of haematopoiesis in the first two trimesters of fetal life, with support from spleen, lymph glands and thymus.

The bone marrow (BM) takes over in the third trimester. At birth all bones are active; during childhood BM activity regresses progressively from the long bones.

CHANGES IN HAEMOGLOBIN PRODUCTION AND NORMAL VALUES

Fetal haemoglobin (HbF) 50–80% at birth, 5% at 6 months, <2% at a year.

Adult HbA at birth 15–40% → over 90% by 6 months.

Mean corpuscular volume (MCV) is high in the neonatal period and declines to a steady state in childhood, rising to adult values in adolescence.

Table 17.1 Normal values of haemoglobin

Age	Hb (g/dl)	Packed cell volume	MCV (fl)
Birth	19	60	110
2 months	11	35	100
1–10 years	12	40	80
Adolescence	14	40	90

WHITE BLOOD CELL COUNTS, TOTAL AND DIFFERENTIAL

Total: At birth $9–30 \times 10^9/l$
           One year $6–8 \times 10^9/l$
           Childhood $5–15 \times 10^9/l$

Neutrophils predominate in the early neonatal period, superceded by relative lymphocytosis from 3 weeks to 9 years.

IMPORTANT CAUSES OF CHANGE IN WBC COUNTS

Neutropenia

Definition

Less than $1.5 \times 10^9/l$. Presentation: usually signs of sepsis, or oral ulceration.

Pathophysiology

1. Both decreased production and increased destruction:

    i Infection
    ii Drugs.

2. Decreased production: congenital, malignant infiltration, folate or B_{12} deficiency.
3. Increased destruction: neonatal isoimmune, juvenile rheumatoid arthritis.

Mode of onset and aetiology

1. Acute, previously well:

    i Infection: e.g. overwhelming sepsis, typhoid, brucella, TB, viruses, malaria.
    ii Drug ingestion:

        a. Suppression, e.g. antimetabolites, chlorpromazine, chloramphenicol, indomethacin, antithyroids, gold.
        b. Immune, e.g. penicillins, sulphonamides, anticonvulsants.

    iii Infiltration: leukaemia, malignancy.

2. In the neonatal period:

    i Isoimmune from maternal antibodies, recovers slowly over 4–8 weeks.
    ii Bone marrow neutrophil maturation arrest (Kostmann disease, AR), bone marrow transplant needed.

3. Recurrent from infancy:

    i   Hypogammaglobulinaemias, cyclical neutropenia.
    ii Associated 'handles': Shwachman syndrome AR (malabsorption, short stature), Chediak-Higashi AR (partial albinism).
    iii Chronic benign neutropenia: mild skin and oral infections. Some are immune mediated lasting a year, others of unknown cause improve in adolescence.
    iv With failure to thrive: a sign of various forms of immunodeficiency as well as malabsorption.

Assessment

1. History: of drug administration (improvement on stopping is diagnostic), exposure to X-rays, similarly affected family members or consanguinity.
2. Clinical: lymphadenopathy, hepatosplenomegaly suggest infective cause. Do culture and serology.
3. Investigations: weekly FBC for cyclical neutropenias, and bone marrow examination if infiltration is likley.
   Autoantibodies in connective tissue disease, and antineutrophil antibodies if suspected to be immune mediated.

Treatment

1. Antibiotics: prophylaxis is not indicated. Broad spectrum cover for suspected sepsis.
2. Steroids controversial in immunoneutropenias.
3. Granulocyte colony-stimulating factor: initial results promising in congenital agranulocytosis, chemotherapy-induced and cyclical neutropenias.
4. Granulocyte transfusions now rarely used.

Further reading

Quesenberry P (1989) Treatment of a marrow stem-cell disorder with granulocyte colony-stimulating factor. *New England Journal of Medicine*, **320**, 1343–1345

Lymphocytosis

Physiological: relative lymphocytosis from 3 weeks old to 9 years .

Table 17.2 Commoner causes of lymphocytosis

Clinical	Cause and appropriate investigation
Infection Acute	1 Marked lymphocytosis: infectious mononucleosis, cytomegalovirus, acute infectious lymphocytosis, toxoplasmosis, pertussis 2 Moderate lymphocytosis: common exanthema, roseola infantum brucella, typhoid, infectious hepatitis Investigations: culture, paired serology.
Chronic	TB. Do ESR, Mantoux, chest X-ray, gastric washing
Leukaemia	Acute lymphoblastic leukaemia: Bone marrow
Systemic juvenile chronic arthritis	Raised ESR, fever with rash, +/- joint swelling, eye signs, lymphadenopathy, i.e. clinical diagnosis, as serology is rarely helpful

Eosinophilia

Definition

Greater than $0.5 \times 10^9/l$, e.g. in atopy; up to $2 \times 10^9/l$ in worm infestations.

Table 17.3 Causes of eosinophilia

Cause	Appropriate investigation
Prematurity	Rarely may be seen in sepsis, otherwise a normal finding in thriving small for dates infants
Atopy	History, IgE, skin prick tests
Infestation	1 Antibody tests, e.g. toxocara, stool examination, e.g. ascaris 2 Complement fixation tests (CFT): hydatid 3 Tropical: stool for trichinosis, hookworm, strongyloides, blood film for filaria, malaria, CFT for schistosomiasis
Infection	Mantoux, Epstein-Barr virus and aspergillus antibodies
Drug reaction	History. Antibodies available for some, e.g. penicillin
Connective tissue or vasculitis	Autoantibodies, DNA antibodies
Malignancy	Lymphoma likely, do lymph node biopsy and bone marrow aspiration + trephine

Anaemia

Definition

A reduction in haemoglobin concentration.
Normal value varies with age, and later, sex.

Causes

Impaired RBC production, blood loss or haemolysis.

History and useful pointers

1. Age at onset

    i First 3 months

       a. Preterm infants
          1–2 months: infection, iatrogenic, acute bleed.

2–3 months: dilutional anaemia, folic acid and vitamin E haemolytic anaemia.

b. Newborn, regardless of gestation.

Acute and chronic blood loss.

Haemolysis due to isoimmunization, glucose 6–phosphate dehydrogenase deficiency, congenital and acquired infection, spherocytosis etc. (see Haemolysis).

c. 'Physiological' anaemia.

ii 3–6 months

Hereditary haemoglobinopathies, e.g. HbS, thalassaemia.

iii Over 6 months.

Nutritional, especially prematures and Asians.

2. Family history, e.g. jaundice or gall bladder removal with spherocytosis.
3. Sex linked disorders, e.g. glucose-6-phosphate dehydrogenase deficiency (G6PD) among Asians, Greeks, Kurds.
4. Race: HbS in Blacks, β-thalassaemia among Whites, Asians, α-thalassaemia in Black and Yellow races.
5. Geographical and ethnic: β-thalassamia in the Mediterranean area.
6. Diet: reduced intake of nutrients, e.g. iron, vitamins B_{12}, C, E, folic acid.
7. Exposure

   i Lead, toxins.
   ii Drugs: haemolysis (redox/immune mediated), aplastic anaemia (chloramphenicol), megaloblastic (phenytoin).

8. Infections: haemolytic uraemic syndrome (HUS), in spherocytosis, parvovirus in haemoglobinopathies.
9. Diarrhoea: malabsorption, inflammatory bowel disease, HUS.

Clinical clues

1. Skin

   i Petechiae/purpura = thrombocytopenia.
   Causes

      a. Consumption, e.g. disseminated intravascular coagulation.
      b. Trapping and destruction, e.g. immune idiopathic thrombocytopenia, or large cavernous haemangiomata in the Kasabach-Merritt syndrome.
      c. Reduced production, e.g. aplastic anaemia.

   ii Echymoses/soft tissue/joint swelling: coagulation factor deficiency, e.g. haemophilia.
   iii Jaundice: haemolytic causes (see Newborn).
   iv Hyperpigmentation: Fanconi's anaemia, also sallow in uraemia.
   v Leg ulcers in adolescence: HbS, HbC.

2. Mouth

   i Ulceration: aplastic anaemia, leukaemia, chronic inflammatory bowel disease.
   ii Glossitis and angular stomatitis in iron deficiency anaemia.

iii Sore red tongue: B_{12}, folic acid deficiency.

3. Skull enlarged +/– 'mongoloid' features in haemoglobinopathies. HbS, β-thalassaemia.
4. Eyes
    i Cataracts: glucose-6-phosphate dehydrogenase, galactosaemia.
    ii Tortuous, proliferative retinal blood vessels in HbS, HbC.
5. Limbs: triphalangeal thumbs in RBC aplasia; radial aplasia in Fanconi's anaemia and thrombocytopenia.
6. Splenomegaly: haemolytic anaemia, leukaemia, malignancy, infection, portal hypertension.
7. Lymphadenopathy
    i Localized, e.g. infection, Hodgkin's lymphoma.
    ii Generalized in infection, leukaemia, eczema.

Investigation of anaemia

FBC, reticulocyte count and a blood film.

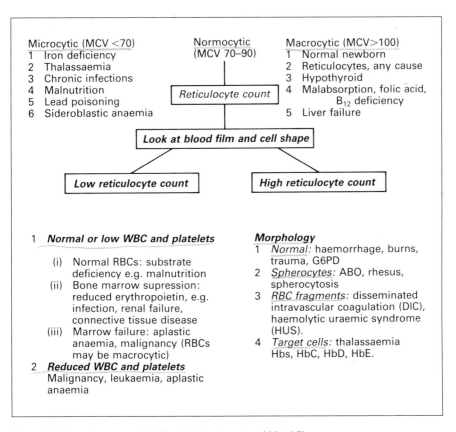

Figure 17.1 Algorithm using the FBC, reticulocyte count and blood film.

Hypochromic microcytic anaemia and differentiation of its causes

1. Iron deficiency by finding a low serum ferritin.

   i Worldwide, nutritional deficiency is the primary cause, plus hookworm infestation in developing countries.
   ii Menstruation from adolescence onwards.

2. Thalassaemia trait by finding a normal RBC count and haemoglobin electrophoresis if a genetic likelihood (Asian or Mediterranean parents).
3. Blood film for basophilic stippling and lead level if exposure is likely.
4. Serum copper level if premature and prolonged intravenous feeding.
5. If still unexplained, look for autoantibodies, do a bone marrow and stain for sideroblasts (ring of dark iron granules around the nucleus of the RBC). Sideroblastic anaemias are rare, inherited or idiopathic, or secondary to lead or drug exposure.

Normocytic anaemias and differentiation of causes

1. Raised reticulocyte count identifies high turnover states. Infection is often a trigger, especially in glucose-6-phosphate dehydrogenase deficiency (G6PD), sickle cell disease (HbS), spherocytosis, disseminated intravascular coagulation (DIC), and haemolytic uraemic syndrome (HUS), and must be screened for.
2. If the RBC morphology is normal

   i Look for acute or chronic blood loss by testing for occult blood loss.
   ii By sex and race give appropriate priority to:

      a. G6PD and pyruvate kinase enzyme levels (remember that levels may be normal in the presence of a high reticulocyte count, as young cells have relatively more enzyme activity).
      b. Sickle cell screening test, Hb electrophoresis for HbF and HbA_2.

   iii Coombs' test for autoimmune haemolytic anaemia, serum complement for low levels of C3, C4, CH_{50} and DNA autoantibodies in systemic lupus erythematosus.

3. If blood film identifies morphological abnormalities

   i Spherocytes require osmotic fragility test, and the parents' blood if positive.
   ii Fragmented RBCs are associated with consumption of coagulation factors in DIC and HUS. In HUS raised serum creatinine and urea are also found.

4. Low reticulocyte count may be secondary to

   i Reduced erythropoietin

      a. Chronic infection: normal red cell distribution width, look for systemic signs, do cultures.
      b. Renal failure: raised serum urea, creatinine.
      c. Rheumatoid arthritis: clinical findings, serology.

ii Marrow failure

    a. Pure red cell aplasia, congenital/acquired (drugs, infection).

    b. Pancytopenia: infection, or with congenital abnormalities, e.g. Fanconi's anaemia.

    c. Infiltration by disseminated malignancy or leukaemia.

If in doubt, always obtain a bone marrow. ⚹

Macrocytic anaemia and differentiation of its causes

1. History of drugs, e.g. phenytoin.
2. Look for malabsorption states, folate or B_{12} deficiency: bone marrow is megaloblastic, absent in other causes of macrocytosis.
3. Endocrine causes: identified clinically, e.g. hypothyroid, hypopituitarism, hypoadrenalism, and biochemically by free T4, TSH levels, cortisol, ACTH.
4. Other: aplastic anaemias and malignancy need bone marrow trephine and aspiration to identify them.

SPECIFIC ANAEMIC CONDITIONS

1. Bone marrow failure

i Aplastic anaemia

Definition

Diagnosed by reduction in two of the following three blood cell lines: neutrophils $<0.5 \times 10^9/l$, platelets $<20 \times 10^9/l$, and reticulocytes $<1\%$. The bone marrow shows markedly reduced cellularity. Rare in childhood other than due to immunosuppression.

Causes

1. Genetic: e.g. Fanconi's anaemia (AR, growth retarded, abnormalities of forearm bones, heart, kidneys, a defect in DNA repair increasing the risk of malignancy; 2-year survival without treatment), Shwachmann's syndrome (pancytopenia in 25%).
2. Viruses (e.g. hepatitis), drugs (e.g. immunosuppressives, sulphonamides, chloramphenicol, phenylbutazone), toxins, e.g. DDT, benzene.
3. Idiopathic.

Presentation

Purpura and haemorrhage, oral ulceration, bacterial infection, and finally anaemia due to the long life span of the RBC.

Age at diagnosis of marrow involvement in genetic forms is variable, e.g. in Fanconi's 80% are between 2 and 13 years old.

Management

1. Transfuse when Hb falls to 6 g/dl. Limit their frequency if bone marrow transplant is likely, e.g. for Fanconi's, to prevent the development of WBC antibodies, and always use CMV negative blood products (see management of leukaemia).
2. If HLA match is available: bone marrow transplant, including for Fanconi's in which previous results were poor, outcome improved with pretreatment 'conditioning' by immunosuppressives to reduce graft versus host disease.
3. Granulocyte-macrophage colony-stimulating factor (GM-CSF) infusion. Otherwise: Antilymphocytic globulin +/− androgens, and immunosuppressives.

Prognosis

With supportive care 20% to 1 year, increases to 80% 5-year survival after bone marrow transplant.

Further reading

Webb D K H (1990) Aplastic anaemia: continued cause for concern. *Archives of Disease in Childhood*, **65**, 1105–1106

ii Pure red cell aplasia

  a. Congenital: Diamond-Blackfan syndrome, usually sporadic, pale at birth, 90% diagnosed by 1 year. HbF increased. Steroid responsive in 75%. Maintain with blood transfusions when Hb falls to 6 g/dl.
  b. Parvovirus infection → aplastic crisis in haemolytic anaemias, e.g. HbSS, spherocytosis, β-thalassaemia. Supportive care for 1–2 weeks until the marrow recovers.
  c. As for aplastic anaemia: drugs, toxins.

2. Iron deficiency anaemia

Commonest cause of anaemia.

Prevalence

5–10%, mainly up to 2 years old and in adolescence. Increased in the inner city and Asian population.

Mild anaemia may contribute to reduced concentration and preschool learning.

Causes

1. Diminished intake:

    i Doorstop cows' milk. Excessive intake, >1 litre daily after the optimal time of weaning. Formula milk is fortified with 6 mg iron/l. Although breast and cows' milk each contain 1 mg/l, the bioavailability is 50% and 10% respectively.

    ii Malabsorption. A relatively uncommon cause.

2. Blood loss

    i Acute: perinatal, postnatal, e.g. peptic ulcer, Meckel's diverticulum.
    ii Chronic

        a. Gastrointestinal: cows' milk protein intolerance, peptic ulcer, duplication, chronic inflammatory bowel disease, telangiectasia.
        b. Parasites, e.g. hookworm is the commonest cause in the developing world.
        c. Menstrual loss in adolescence.
        d. Aspirin taken in chronic rheumatic disease.

3. Rapid growth, e.g. increased demand in prematures, catch-up in small for dates, after malnutrition, and in adolescence.

Clinical symptoms

1. Gastrointestinal: anorexia, pica.
2. Behavioural: listless, irritable, impaired concentration, retardation of development and school progress.
3. Poor exercise tolerance and of sustained physical work.
4. Infections: upper respiratory infections commoner, bacterial infections reduced (inhibition due to lack of available iron, all being bound to transferrin).

Clinical signs

Pallor, spoon nails, angular cheilosis and glossitis, tachycardia, progressing to cardiac failure.

Diagnosis

1. Anaemia = Hb < 10g/dl after 6 months in a term infant, with low mean corpuscular haemoglobin (MCH), mean corpuscular volume (MVC), serum ferritin, and increased red cell distribution width (RDW).
2. Borderline anaemia = <11, >10 g/dl. Indices may be otherwise normal. Treat for a month, iron 3 mg/kg/day. If the Hb rises by 1 g/dl iron deficiency is confirmed; continue treatment for 2 months to replenish stores.

Differential diagnosis

1. Acute infection. A transient fall in Hb is common.

2. Persistently low Hb in repeated infection or chronic disease, e.g. renal failure, juvenile chronic arthritis. Serum ferritin may be 'normal' at >15 mg/l, but if <50 mg/l may still benefit from treatment as iron stores are not mobilized and food iron is not so well absorbed in these conditions.
3. β-thalassaemia trait. A very low MCV, around 55–60, with relatively high/normal RBC count, and normal RDW is very suggestive. A low serum ferritin is an indication for treatment. Repeat the FBC on its completion and then do Hb electrophoresis if parameters remain relatively unchanged.
4. Protein-calorie malnutrition. Clinically distinct.

Management

1. Ferrous sulphate 3 mg/kg: single daily dose in infancy, twice daily thereafter.
    Response: reticulocytes appear in 1–2 weeks, Hb two thirds corrected by a month. Maximum rise of Hb 0.25–0.4 g/dl/day.
2. Blood transfusion. Only contemplate if ill. Danger of cardiac failure if transfused at Hb 4–5 g/dl.
    If due to bone marrow infiltration, e.g. by leukaemic cells, and a reaction to blood occurs, hydrocortisone may be given. This will lyse abnormal cells and obscure the diagnosis. If in doubt, check the blood film, and a bone marrow if at all suspicious.
3. Iron dextran by i.v. or i.m. route is rarely indicated. Danger of anaphylactic reaction which may be fatal.

Prevention

1. Daily recommended requirements:

    i   Term infants 1 mg/kg/day to maximum of 15 mg daily.
    ii Preterm 2 mg/kg/day (up to 4 mg in <1 kg birthweight) from a month old, to a maximum of 15 mg daily.
    iii Childhood 10 mg/day.
    iv Adolescence 18 mg/day.

2. Cyanotic congenital heart disease and sickle cell disease. Anaemic RBCs are more rigid, hence thrombotic complications are more likely. Give iron.

Screening

A case has been made for routine screening:
    Prematures at 4 months
    Term infants at 8 months
    All children at 18 months, 5 years and adolescence, especially the Asian and inner city high risk groups.

Further reading

Marder E, Nicoll A, Polnay L, *et al*, (1990) Discovering anaemia at child health clinics. *Archives of Disease in Childhood*, **65**, 892–894

Folate and B_{12} deficiency

Deficiency results in a macrocytic, megaloblastic anaemia. May rarely be caused by hereditary orotic aciduria.

Table 17.4 Folate and B_{12} deficiency

	Folate	B_{12}
Cause		
1 Inadequate intake	Boiled milk, goats' milk	Mother a breast feeding vegan
2 Absorption impaired	Small intestine injury: Crohn's, coeliac, surgical resection	1 Lack of intrinsic factor in stomach 2 Transcobalamin II transport protein absent from blood 3 Terminal ileum: Crohn's or surgical resection
3 Increased requirement	1 High cell turnover, e.g. premature or chronic haemolysis 2 Metabolic effects of phenytoin, phenobarbitone	
Clinical	Anaemia +/- related signs of malabsorption/haemolysis/ epilepsy	Weight loss, diarrhoea, subacute combined spinal cord degeneration
Diagnosis	Folate level	B_{12} level, Schilling test
Treatment	Folic acid 5–10 mg/day	B_{12} 1000μg i.m. then 3 monthly

HAEMOLYSIS

Disruption of the RBC may be from within (intracellular, membrane) and without (intravascular).

1. Intracellular abnormality: Hb molecule in the haemoglobinopathies, and enzymes, e.g. glucose-6-phosphate dehydrogenase deficiency, pyruvate kinase deficiency.
2. RBC membrane abnormality: spherocytosis, elliptocytosis, stomatocytosis.
3. Plasma: antibodies, autoantibodies and endotoxins (e.g. in septicaemia) to RBCs.
4. Hypersplenism.
5. Capillary: haemolytic uraemic syndrome, disseminated.
6. Vascular: giant haemangiomas, artificial heart valves.
7. External agents: injury due to trauma or burns.

Assessment

History and examination will indicate the likely cause, aided by a reticulocyte count, a film (i) showing red cell fragments, and abnormal coagulation tests in 2 and 3 and (ii) abnormal morphology in spherocytosis, and the haemoglobinopathies.

A FBC showing reduction in WBCs and platelets as well as Hb implicates hyperplenism if it is palpable. RBC antibodies and autoantibodies may be detected in plasma, or a Gram negative septicaemia isolated. Specific enzyme tests for G-6-PD and pyruvate kinase, and the sickle test and Hb electrophoresis determine which haemoglobinopathy.

Haemoglobinopathies

Definition

Characterized by abnormal production and structure of the Hb molecule, and an advantage for carriers against falciparum malaria.
  Molecular basis: amino acid substitutions in the β-chain of adult Hb.
  Inheritance: autosomal recessive.

Table 17.5 Some haemoglobinopathies' distinguishing characteristics

	Normal	Iron* deficient	β-thalassaemia trait	β-thalassaemia+	HbAS	HbS	HbSC	HbSβ-thalassaemia
Film	Normal (N)	MH	MH	MH	N	Target cell Sickle++	Target Sickle+	MH, target Sickle +
HbF%	<1	<1	1–5	50–95	<1	2–20	5	2–30
HbA$_2$%	3	3	4–7	4–7	3	4+	3	4+
HbA%	95	95	90	1–50	35	0	0	0–15
HbS%	0	0	0	0	60	80–90	90	50–85
Spleen	–	+	–	+++	–	++ → –	++	++
MCV(fl)	80–100	60–70	60–70					
MCH(pg)	27–37	17–25	17–25					

* Treat with iron and repeat tests to exclude iron deficiency unless serum ferritin is normal.
+ Check for HbH by looking for 'H' bodies in RBC's and Hb Barts on electrophoresis.
MH = microcytic hypochromic.

Sickle cell disease

This term includes homozygous sickle cell anaemia (SS), sickle cell trait (AS), and the double heterozygotes HBS + HbC = SC disease, and HbS + Hb β- thalassaemia trait = Sβ-thalassaemia, which may be slightly milder than SS, but are treated similarly.

Pathophysiology

Deoxygenated HbS molecules polymerize → sickling. Sickled RBCs intertwine, occluding small blood vessels and causing infarction.
  Precipitants of sickling: hypoxia, dehydration, fever, acidosis. Sickled RBC life span is reduced from an average120 days to 20 days. No drug prevents sickling, clinically.

Despite anaemia (Hb 8 g/dl), no discomfort except during crises, as HbS gives up oxygen more readily than HbA.

1. Sickle cell (SS): valine for glutamic acid at position 6. Distribution 30 million sufferers world–wide.

   i Blacks from central Africa have a carrier rate of 20%. Taken to the Americas, Caribbean, Europe.
   ii Non-blacks. A milder disease, among Asians, Arabs, Greeks.

2. Homozygous HbC (West Africa), HbD (Pakistan, north India), and in South-East Asia some 30 million have HbE. If any anaemia, it is usually mild, +/– splenomegaly.
3. HbSC and HbSβ-thalassaemia: chronic haemolytic anaemias more severe than with either trait alone. Mild to moderately severe, occasionally with fatal crises. Unlike SS no painful infarctive crises, as mean red-cell Hb concentration is lower and sickling is less likely. Splenomegaly persists.

Clinical manifestations of sickle cell anaemia

1. Age and presentation

Early at 3–6 months

1. Infection, e.g. meningococcal meningitis → disseminated intravascular coagulation.
2. Pallor and anaemia. Hepatosplenomegaly +/– jaundice.
3. Infarction → pain +/– swelling:

   i Hand-foot syndrome.
   ii Bones, joints, liver, spleen.

Later, still under 2 years old
Untreated cases have a 20% mortality.

1. Infection, e.g. pneumonia, malaria.
2. Acute splenic sequestration, recurs and may be rapidly fatal.
3. Stroke, may recur.

Over 2 years old

1. Infarction crises

   i Acute chest syndrome masquerading as 'pneumonia' may be due to infection or infarcted bone marrow emboli. Fever, tachycardia, tachypnoea, chest pain. Chest X-ray shows basal infiltration, consolidation or collapse.
   ii 'Acute abdomen' due to infarcted liver (may abscess), spleen (autosplenectomy), and lymph glands.
   Simulates surgical emergency, but recurrent and without rebound tenderness.
   iii Retinal emboli → neovascularization → haemorrhages → blindness.
   iv Bone and joint pain. Aseptic necrosis of femoral or humeral head.

2. Haematological crises

   i Aplastic crisis: sudden fall in RBC production. Susceptible due to high marrow turnover. Occurs in parvovirus infection, a 'flu like illness, and lasts up to 14 days.

  ii Hyperhaemolysis precipitated by infection. Glucose-6-phosphate dehydrogenase deficiency may contribute.

3. Splenic involvement

   i Hypersplenism: Hb falls to <6 g/dl, reticulocytes >15%, platelets reduced.

  ii Hyposplenism: repeated sickle infarcts →autosplenectomy→ increased susceptibility to infection especially Salmonella, pneumococcus, *Haemophilus influenzae*.

4. Renal manifestations

   i Painless haematuria: papillary necrosis.

  ii Polyuria and enuresis: impaired concentrating ability.

5. Growth problems: failure to gain weight, delayed puberty.
6. Adult: priapism, leg ulcers.

Diagnosis

In an emergency, screen all who are likely to be susceptible with an illness attributable to HbS.

1. FBC. In HbS the Hb averages 5–10 g/dl, with sickled cells, reticulocytes 10–30%.

   In health the HbS carrier has a normal blood film and indices.
2. Sickling test or solubility test: diagnostic for HbS and carrier state, but fails to distinguish between them.
3. Hb electrophoresis: HbF 5% (similar in HbS, carrier and HbSβ-thalassaemia).

   Further investigation: search for cause of crisis, e.g. infection, dehydration.

Management

1. Prophylaxis: may be initiated in asymptomatic individuals detected by neonatal screening. Applicable in HbSC and HbSβ-thalassaemia.

   i Vaccination: pneumococcus, *H. influenzae*.

  ii Folic acid, penicillin V daily from 6 months old.

 iii Avoid stress: cold, dehydration, excessive exertion.

 iv Transfusion

     a. Preoperatively.
     b. To prevent recurrence:

       After femoral head necrosis for 6–24 months.
       After hemiplegia for 2 years or until adulthood!

v Travel in a pressurized aircraft (commercial airline cabin pressure is satisfactory, set to 3,000 feet).

2. Acute crises

i Search for infection, meanwhile prescibe broad spectrum antibiotic. A raised WBC is unhelpful as often raised in crises.
ii Oxygen, only if pulmonary signs are present.
iii Hydration adequacy: if in doubt, establish an i.v. infusion, rate 3 l/m²/24 h.
iv Analgesia must be effective: codeine, DF118, pethidine.
v Tranfuse: if anaemic or in crisis. Consider exchange if slow to respond.

3. Life style at school and in employment.

i Understanding of absences through illness, and the need for frequent urination.
ii Light physical activity in sports and employment.

4. Genetic counselling, antenatal screening and diagnosis (see thalassaemia). The NHS Haemoglobinopathy card given to the parents identifies the type of Hb abnormality, vital for subsequent medical contacts. Family counselling by specialist nurses and support from the Sickle Cell Society are available in areas with large Afro-Caribbean populations.

Thalassaemia

Definition

Anaemia due to underproduction of one or more of the globin chains, commonly alpha or beta, which make up the Hb molecule.

Pathophysiology

The reduction in production of one globin chain results in relative overproduction of another. Within RBCs it accumulates as an unstable aggregate which precipitates, causing premature destruction of the RBCs, mainly in bone marrow and spleen.

Beta thalassaemia major AR

Pathophysiology

β-Thalassaemia results from a change in β-globin chain gene DNA structure. B^0 = no production, B^+ = reduced production.

A compensatory increase occurs in those haemoglobins not containing β chains, i.e. HbF (α and γ chains) and HbA_2 (α and δ chains).

Distribution: Blacks B^+ (less severe), Mediterranean B^0 (severe) and B^+.
Onset from 3 months old, as δ chain and HbF production falls.

Clinical

1. Anaemia.
2. Failure to thrive, diarrhoea and vomiting: hypoxia causes growth failure and increased susceptibility to infection.
3. Hepatomegaly +/– splenomegaly +/– jaundice due to high breakdown rate of haem pigment, later causing gall stones.
4. Increased bone marrow activity results in 'mongoloid' facial appearance, large skull (hair on end appearance on skull X-ray).
5. Puberty delayed or absent, leg ulcers in adults.

Investigations

1. FBC: Hb 3–7 g/dl, increased RBC count. Leucocytosis is common.

   i Film: severe hypochromia, microcytosis, target cells, moderate reticulocytosis, with basophilic stippling, inclusions (Heinz bodies), and abnormally shaped red cells.
   ii Red cell distribution width within normal limits, as against iron deficiency when width is increased.

2. Hb electrophoresis: HbF >50% in B⁺ thalassaemia, up to 95% in B⁰.
3. Serum ferritin raised: due to increased absorption from increased marrow activity, iron in blood transfusion (1 mg/ml in packed cells), and inability to excrete excess.

Management

1. Transfusion. A high transfusion programme, at 2–4 week intervals, to maintain Hb at 12 g/dl, permits growth, and inhibits the ineffective erythropoieses and hypersplenism.
2. Iron chelation therapy to prevent iron overload complications (failure of puberty, cardiac siderosis, cirrhosis, hepatoma, pancreatitis, infertility, infection with *Yersinia enterocolitica*, skin pigmentation). Commence when serum ferritin >1000 µg/l, by continuous subcutaneous desferrioxamine 35–60 mg/kg/night. Predictably, compliance is low in adolescence.
3. Splenectomy only after 5 years old, (the annual blood requirement is >1.5 times that of splenectomized), or for hypersplenism.
4. Future potential therapies: bone marrow transplant (used for selected patients at present); gene therapy using modified retrovirus vectors.
5. Genetic counselling

   i Antenatal screening of maternal blood for carrier status. If found, check partner's. This allows informed choice to interrupt pregnancy, following chorionic villous biopsy for DNA studies, or fetal blood, to identify affected homozygotes. The result has been a return to the normal family size for those communities using this approach. Previously, it would have been limited to that at the birth of the first affected child. See Genetic Counselling.
   ii Population screening and premarital counselling to enable carriers to avoid each other.

Beta thalassaemia trait, and differentiation from iron deficiency anaemia

β-Thalassaemia trait is asymptomatic. Carriers are usually picked up by their pallor.

A mild anaemia with a blood picture similar to iron deficiency of low mean corpuscular volume.

The normal RBC count and narrow red cell distribution width of β-thalassaemia discriminates from iron deficiency.

If the serum ferritin is low, treat with oral iron for 2 months and repeat FBC and ferritin. Hb electrophoresis is required if it is still suggestive of β-thalassaemia trait (HbA$_2$ 4–7%, HbF >1%).

Further reading

Rebulla P, Modell B (1991) Transfusion requirements and effects in patients with thalassaemia major. *Lancet*, i, 277–280

Alpha thalassaemia

Alpha thalassaemia is due to loss of α gene(s). Distribution: Blacks 20%, widespread in the Mediterranean, Middle and Far East.

A normal individual has 2 α genes per chromosome, i.e. a total of 4.

Clinical

Manifestations are proportional to the number deleted.

Loss of 1 or 2 alpha genes is asymptomatic.

Haemoglobin H disease

Loss of 3 α genes: as α chains are present in normal HbA ($\alpha_2\beta_2$), HbF ($\alpha_2\gamma_2$) and HbA$_2$ ($\alpha_2\delta_2$), anaemia, with HbH (4 β-chains) on electrophoresis.

Clinical

Anaemia, marked splenomegaly, aplastic and haemolytic crises.

Investigations

  i Hb 6–10 g/dl, reticulocytes 5–10%, low mean corpuscular haemoglobin and mean corpuscular volume.

  ii Blood film: 'H' bodies present = Hb precipitants.

 iii Hb electrophoresis: HbH (4 β-chains) 4–5%, some Hb Barts (4 γ chains).

Haemoglobin Barts = No alpha genes, 4 γ chains.

Hydrops fetalis or neonatal death. Commoner than rhesus hydrops in Asians.
 Hb electrophoresis: Hb Barts 85%.

Further reading

Huntsman R G (1987) *Sickle Cell Anaemia and Thalassaemia: A Primer for Health Care Professionals.*
 Canadian Sickle Cell Society

OTHER HAEMOLYTIC CONDITIONS

Spherocytosis

Definition

Deficiency of spectrin, a major structural protein in the RBC membrane, causes it to
take up a spherical shape. This is more readily trapped in the sinusoids of the spleen
and removed.

Autosomal dominant, one third are new mutations with no family history. Rarely
AR.

Presentation and assessment

1. Neonatal: Jaundice day 1 may be severe enough to require exchange transfusion.
   Related to perinatal hypoxia or stress. Differential diagnosis of spherocytosis:
   ABO incompatibility and infection. The red cell fragility test may be inconclusive, so repeat in 3–6 months.
2. Early childhood: acute anaemia with jaundice secondary to haemolytic crises
   precipitated by infection. Occasionally aplastic crisis due to parvovirus infection.
   Spleen moderately enlarged, firm and tender. Between episodes mild anaemia,
   and icteric conjunctivae.
3. Late childhood: presents as chronic anaemia, or as an asymptomatic family
   member after detection in another. In the adult, symptoms of gall bladder stones,
   leg ulcers, and corneal opacities.

Investigations

1. Haematology: haemoglobin 5–8 g/dl, varies with haemolysis. Reticulocytes
   about 10%. Coombs' test negative.
2. Red cell osmotic fragility test: more easily lysed than normal RBCs, effect
   enhanced by incubation at 37°C for 24 h.
3. Biochemistry: Raised serum bilirubin, urinary urobilinogen.

Glucose-6-phosphate dehydrogenase

See Inborn errors.

Vitamin E deficiency

An unusual cause of haemolytic anaemia, found in:

1. Prematures at 2–3 months.
2. Cystic fibrosis.

Clinical

Peripheral oedema.

Blood film

Acanthocytes, increased platelets.

Treatment and prevention

See Neonatal problems.

BLEEDING CHILDREN

Bleeding is the result of loss of haemostasis. The character of the bleeding may give an indication of which of the three main mechanisms (there may be more than one) is involved: (i) vascular (ii) platelet or (iii) coagulation abnormality.

History

Recurrent epistaxes are common, and reliably stopping within minutes is unlikely to require further investigation. Easy bruising too is non-specific. Be specific, e.g.:

1. Intercurrent illness

    i Acute, e.g. diarrhoea (haemolytic uraemic syndrome), septicaemia, meningo-coccaemia (disseminated intravascular coagulation). Rickettsial spotted fevers.
    ii Recent viral: idiopathic thrombocytopenic purpura.
    iii Insidious: bacterial endocarditis.

Table 17.6 Haemostasis and clinical characteristics of bleeds from vascular or platelet defect and coagulation defect

Haemostasis factors	Examples of disorders	Clinical
1 Vascular integrity	Henoch–Schönlein purpura, scurvy, infections, Ehlers–Danlos, hereditary haemorrhagic telangiectasia	1 Petechiae, purpura, echymosis
2 Platelets	i Quantitative: idiopathic thrombocytopenia	2 Epistaxis, GI bleeds, menorrhagia
	ii Qualitative: von Willebrand, asprin	3 Bleeds stop on local pressure
3 Coagulation	i Alone: haemophilia	1 Cut → *delayed* onset of bleed
	ii Combined: disseminated intravascular coagulation (+platelets consumed)	2 *Deep* bleeds, single site e.g. joint, muscle. Haematuria.
		3 Local pressure fails to stop bleeding

2. Incidents recalled, e.g. bleeding after circumcision (factor VIII), cord separation (factor XIII), immunization. Bruising after minor falls.
3. Response to trauma, e.g. factor VIII suggestive if persistent bleed occurs after a torn frenulum, or loss of deciduous teeth. Healing by large scars as in Ehlers-Danlos syndrome.
4. Previous surgery: satisfactory haemostasis makes a serious coagulopathy unlikely.
5. Family history:

    i Sex linked: haemophilia, platelets + eczema + infection in the Wiskott-Aldrich syndrome.
    ii Autosomal dominant: von Willebrand disease.
    iii Autosomal recessive: Bernard-Soulier giant platelets syndrome.
    iv Other: autoimmune disease (thyroid, lupus) associated with idiopathic thrombocytopenia.

6. Drugs: e.g. platelet function (aspirin) and platelet count (quinine, penicillin, cotrimoxazole, valproate).
7. Factitious: self induced (arms/wrists) or Munchausen by proxy.

Examination

1. Is the child sick or well?
2. Character of the bleeding (see Table 17.6).
3. Associated congenital malformations, e.g. thrombocytopenia, absent radii syndrome (TAR), giant haemangiomata.
4. Specific features

    i Hepatosplenomegaly + jaundice in disseminated intravascular coagulation (DIC).

ii Splenomegaly

  a. Large in some malignancies, hypersplenism from portal hypertension.

  b. Moderate in haemolytic uraemic syndrome, DIC, infection, Gaucher's disease.

  c. Small or impalpable spleen in idiopathic thrombocytopenic purpura.

iii Eczema + infection in Wiskott-Aldrich syndrome.

iv Telangiectatic vessels: inspect the lips, mucous membranes, mouth, and nose in the presence of epistaxis and GI bleeding.

Tests of coagulation

Comprise platelet count and tests of haemostatic function.

Table 17.7 Normal coagulation values

	Partial thromboplastin time (PTT) (seconds) INT	Prothrombin time (seconds) EXT	Bleeding time (minutes)
Normal values			
Child/term infant	45–55	13–17	3–5
Premature	up to 1.5 × normal (90)	up to 1.5 × normal (20)	Same as child
Factors involved	XII, XI, X, IX, VIII, V, II, or fibrinogen	X, VII, V, II or fibrinogen	Platelets and capillaries

Platelet disorders: general principles

1. Quantitative: thrombocytopenia due to decreased production or reduced survival. Thrombocytopenia = <100 × 10^9/l.
2. Qualitative: bleeding with normal platelet numbers, but abnormal function. Congenital (e.g. giant platelets of Bernard-Soulier syndrome) or acquired (e.g. aspirin)

Investigations

1. Blood film, platelets, coagulation tests. Bone marrow aspiration and trephine if infiltration or aplasia likely.
2. Guided by clinical state:

  i In the sick child: bacterial, viral cultures and serology, plasma electrolytes and urea, liver function tests.

  ii Well child: platelet antibodies, viral acute and convalescent serum.

Table 17.8 Clinical categorization of thrombocytopenia: sick or well?

Sick	Well
Coagulation tests are usually abnormal, with excess consumption of platelets, and RBC fragments (or acanthocytes in liver failure).	Coagulation normal, generally not acutely ill. Bone marrow examination helps further categorization:
1 Usually acutely ill	1 Increased megakaryocytes, i.e. increased destruction
i Disseminated intravascular coagulation (DIC)	
ii Haemolytic uraemic syndrome (HUS)	i Idiopathic thrombocytopenic purpura (ITP)
iii Liver damage	ii Drug induced e.g. co-trimoxazole, valproate
	iii Autoimmune (rare)
2 Relatively well, may become sick: increased removal/sequestration, e.g. Giant haemangioma (hypersplenism has similar mechanism, but coagulation is normal, and bleeding is unusual)	2 Reduced megakaryocytes, i.e. diminished destruction
	i Congenital: isolated or associated with rubella, radial aplasia (TAR), Fanconi's anaemia, Wiskott-Aldrich syndrome
	ii With abnormal bone marrow Leukaemia or malignant infiltration Aplastic anaemia Storage disorder

Management principles

1. Sick: treat primary cause, support with platelet transfusion if the count is <30 × 10^9/l, and coagulation factors as indicated. Giant haemangioma: shrink with steroids.
2. Well: if drug related, stop it. Idiopathic thrombocytopenia treatment is controversial.
3. Congenital or acquired aplasia/Fanconi's anaemia/Wiscott Aldrich syndrome: reconstitution by bone marrow transplant.
4. Infiltration: chemotherapy.

Disseminated intravascular coagulation

Definition

Intravascular consumption of platelets and clotting factors with fibrin formation which is deposited throughout the body.

Pathophysiology

Fragmentation of RBCs and microangiopathic anaemia result from mechanical injury and immune mechanisms.

Result

1. Fragmented RBCs → anaemia.
2. Coagulation cascade - plasminogen - lysis mechanism initiated:

    i Reduction in fibrinogen, factors V and VIII → prolonged thromboplastin time (TT), prothrombin time (PT), partial thromboplastin time (PTT).

    ii Fibrin degradation products (FDPs) rise as the clots are lysed by plasmin, and further derange coagulation.

3. Thrombocytopenia.

Causes

1. Tissue injury, e.g. trauma, burns, haemorrhagic shock, dead twin fetus, necrotizing enterocolitis (NEC).
2. Endothelial injury, e.g. infection, hypoxia, e.g. respiratory distress syndrome, malignancy, liver failure.
3. Platelet or RBC injury, e.g. incompatible blood transfusion, haemolytic uraemic syndrome, anaphylactic shock.

Clinical

Purpura, bleeding from mucous membranes, from venepuncture sites, gastrointestinal and urinary tract. Progresses to hypotension, acidosis, anuria, seizures.

Management

1. Treat the primary cause to halt the condition, e.g. antibiotics, oxygen/assisted ventilation.
2. Counter shock (blood/fresh frozen plasma), acidosis, electrolyte disturbances.
3. Replacement:

    i Platelet concentrate 1 unit/10 kg.

    ii Cryoprecipitate if fibrinogen <0.5 g/l.

    iii Fresh frozen plasma (multiple clotting factors) 10 -15 ml/kg.

Controversy

Heparinization only in fulminant meningococcal septicaemia if thromboses are affecting the brain (multifocal neurology) and kidneys (acute renal failure).

Idiopathic thrombocytopenic purpura (ITP)

Definition

Platelets <100 × 10⁹/l, shortened platelet survival, with increased megakaryocytes in the bone marrow. It becomes chronic in 10%, i.e. persists for >6 months.

Incidence

1 in 25000 children annually.

Pathophysiology

Immune mediated, usually secondary to a viral infection (occasionally rubella, infectious mononucleosis) in the preceding weeks. IgG platelet antibody in 75%. Increased production and turnover of platelets, which, being young, are slightly larger than normal. Destruction occurs mainly in the spleen.

Clinical

Table 17.9 Clinical features of ITP

	Acute ITP	*Chronic ITP*
Proportion	90%	10%
Age (years)	Usually <10	>10 More common
Sex ratio	M:F = 1	M:F = 1:3
Onset	Acute	Insidious

In acute ITP 70% have purpura or bruising only, in an otherwise well child, as bleeding is only likely if the platelet count falls below 20×10^9/l. The 30% with active bleeding have epistaxis, malaena, and haematuria.

Complication: intracranial haemorrhage occurs in 1%, independent of duration of the disease, and may be fatal.

Diagnosis and management

1. Platelet count and full blood count help identify possible aplastic anaemia, or infiltration due to leukaemia.
2. Splenomegaly points to acute lymphatic leukaemia, or hypersplenism. Bone marrow essential.
3. Bone marrow, and consider viral studies and DNA binding antibodies. Do a Coombs' test if Hb is also low, as it may be Evans anaemia, with antibodies also against red cells.

Controversy

1. Is bone marrow (BM) aspiration and biopsy necessary in all cases? If the clinical picture and peripheral blood picture are characteristic of acute ITP only regular platelet count monitoring is required. BM must be done if steroids are to be given, which may temporarily eliminate atypical/leukaemic cells and precipitate a tumour lysis crisis as inadequately prepared and hydrated for this complication.
2. Are steroids necessary in acute ITP? Platelet count may rise before steroids could have worked, but a European study found most children did respond to steroids, with a more rapid rise in count to protective levels.
   Indications: bleeding and platelet count $<30 \times 10^9$/l.

Dose and duration: prednisolone 2 mg/kg 2–3 weeks, and repeated for relapses. (Corticosteroids act by rapidly stabilizing capillary membranes against leaking platelets and reducing destruction of sensitized platelets.)

3. High dose i.v. IgG (HD IgG)? In acute ITP 80% respond only transiently to HDIgG. Chronic ITP is not prevented, and although effective, HD IgG is required every 3–4 weeks, but does reduce the need for splenectomy.

   Dose: 0.4–2 g/kg for 5 days. (i.v. IgG blocks Fc receptors of reticuloendothelial system).

4. Splenectomy, indications:

   i Duration for 2 or more years and unresponsive to steroids, high dose IgG, or immunosuppressives.

   ii With dangerous bleeds.

Prognosis

Recovery in 90% of acute ITP by 4 months, and 90% of chronic ITP in time.

Further reading

Lilleyman J S (1984) Idiopathic thrombocytopenic purpura–where do we stand? *Archives of Disease in Childhood*, **59**, 701

COAGULATION DISORDERS OF IMPORTANCE

Haemorrhagic disease of the newborn

See Neonatal problems.

Haemophilia

Descriptive title for deficiency of factor VIII (haemophilia A) and factor IX (haemophilia B or Christmas disease), both XL.

Incidence

1 in 10000 boys, 8 out of 10 due to haemophilia A, remainder are Christmas disease; 30% have no family history, being new mutations.

Pathophysiology of haemophilia and von Willebrand disease

Absence of either factor prolongs the partial thromboplastin time and prevents clot formation.

1. Factor VIII molecule abnormalities

   i In haemophilia A: factor VIII procoagulant activity (FVIII:C) site is absent or defective. Thus thrombin (acts on fibrinogen →fibrin) formation from prothrombin is reduced.
   ii In von Willebrand: reduced Factor VIII-related von Willebrand factor FVIIIR:WF). It acts as a carrier protein for FVIII:C, which is thereby lowered as in haemophilia A. FVIIIR:WF is also necessary for normal platelet adhesion to endothelial surfaces, i.e. impaired plugging of blood vessels also occurs.

2. Factor IX

Activates factor X in the presence of factor VIII, calcium and platelets. Without it a fibrin clot cannot form.

Clinical

Severity proportional to the level of factor.
Manifestations by age tend to accord with severity.
1. The severely affected have <1% activity = 50% of sufferers.

   i Neonate after circumcision.
   ii Under 1 year: bruising from falls as he learns to walk.
   iii Toddler: deep muscle bleeds and haemarthroses by 3 years, oral and gum bleeds from minor lacerations and shedding teeth.
   iv Older children's joints gradually destroyed and ankylosed.

   Deaths due to cerebral, retroperitoneal and gastrointestinal bleeds were common prior to prophylaxis, especially in adults.
2. Moderate = 1–5%, bleeds after mild to moderate trauma, seldom spontaneous.
3. Mild = 5–25%, bleeding after moderate to severe trauma, or surgery.
   Complications of treatment: viral hepatitis, HIV, analgesic addiction.

Diagnosis

1. Family history.
2. Prolonged PTT.
3. Individual factor VIII or factor IX level reduced.

   Carrier detection: measured coagulant activity is less than the level of factor VIII-related antigen (FVIIIR:Ag).
   DNA studies allow antenatal diagnosis.

Management

1. Replacement: monoclonal or heat–treated factor VIII concentrate has eliminated the risk of HIV. In the severely affected, prophylactic i.v. administration by the parents at home has revolutionized life style and prognosis.

2. Antibodies to factor VIII develop in 10% and may need prothrombin complex concentrate.
3. Desamino D-arginine vasopressin (DDAVP) is useful in boosting factor VIII levels in the mild to moderate group.
4. Pain relief must be effective, and may require opiates.
5. Genetic counselling; carrier identification will establish whether a familial problem.

Prognosis

Those with severe disease not HIV positive can look forward to a near normal life span.

Von Willebrand disease

Inheritance

Usually autosomal dominant, prevalence half that of haemophilia.

Pathophysiology

(See haemophilia.)
1. Abnormal platelet function.
2. Prolonged bleeding time (BT) and partial thromboplastin time (PTT) due to an abnormal or reduced factor VIII, the von Willebrand factor FVIIIR:WF.

Clinical

Picture is similar to haemophilia but mild unless factor VIII activity is very low. Tendency to bleeding episodes improves with age.

Diagnosis

Prolonged BT, PTT. Assay the individual factors. The ristocetin-induced platelet agglutination is reduced.

Management

Mild disease: DDAVP increases levels of FVIII:C and FVIIIR:WF.
   Major bleed: cryoprecipitate. Factor VIII concentrates lack FVIIIR:WF, so are ineffective.

Prognosis

Death from haemorrhage is rare, and life span usually normal.

Further reading

Standard texts

Hann I M, Gibson B (1991) *Paediatric Haematology*. London:Ballière Tindall
Nathan D G, Oski F A (1987) *Hematology of Infancy and Childhood*. Philadelphia:Saunders

Chapter 18

Oncological problems

CHILDHOOD MALIGNANCIES

Incidence

1/10000 annually or a risk of 1/600 in childhood. Overall 60% survival. Third commonest cause of death in childhood.

Relative frequencies

Acute lymphoblastic leukaemia 30%.
Brain tumours 20% (see Neurology).
Lymphoma (Hodgkin and non-Hodgkin) 15%.
Soft tissue sarcoma = mainly rhabdomyosarcoma 10%.
Neuroblastoma 7%.
Retinoblastoma, Wilm's and Ewing's tumours each 5%.

Aetiology

1. Genetic:
    i Mendelian, e.g. neurofibromatosis (AD) may give rise to sarcomas, Wilm's tumour, neuroblastoma.
    ii Familial clustering of leukaemias and lymphomas: risk at least doubled if one sibling is affected.
    iii Point deletion on chromosomes, e.g. in Wilms' tumour on chromosome 11, retinoblastoma on chromosome 13. Mechanism is probably through loss of regulation of oncogenes, allowing tumours to form: e.g. in retinoblastoma the *N-myc* oncogene is amplified.
    iv Immunodeficiencies: Wiscott-Aldrich syndrome and lymphoma.
    v Fragile chromosome syndromes with defective DNA repair: e.g. ataxia-telangiectasia and lymphoma, Bloom syndrome and cancers, Fanconi anaemia and leukaemia.
2. Therapeutic X-rays and chemotherapy for a previous malignancy is a substantial risk, and up to 3% develop 'secondary' cancers.
3. Viruses: Epstein-Barr is associated with Burkitt's lymphoma (which shows a chromosomal translocation of the *c-myc* oncogene), the human immunodeficiency virus with lymphoma and lymphosarcoma. Postulate: New Town children

exposed at a critical age to infection predisposes them to malignancy. Verdict: unproven.
4. Vitamin K i.m. at birth may double the risk of malignancy?

Peak age at presentation

1. Infancy: neuroblastoma.
2. 2–4 years: Wilm's kidney tumour, rhabdomyosarcoma.
3. 4–7 years: acute lymphoblastic leukaemia (ALL), non-Hodgkin's lymphoma.
4. >10 years: acute myeloid leukaemia, Ewing's sarcoma.

Table 18.1 Trends in 5 year survival rates (%) (from the Manchester Children's Tumour Registry, 1954–83, and National Cancer Registry 1989)

	1954–63	1964–73	1974–83	1989
Overall survival	21	34	49	60
Acute lymphatic leukaemia	2		60	65
Retinoblastoma	84	85	87	86
Wilms' tumours	31	59	85	75
Brain tumours				50
Ewing's tumour	9	14	41	33

Improved prognosis

Incidence of cancers has remained constant, whereas survival and quality of life continues to improve.

Factors

1. Presymptomatic screening in familial and syndromic cases.
2. Better understanding of disease processes.
3. Improved drugs and radiotherapy, and surgery coordinated with these therapies.
4. Prevention of secondary spread, e.g. CNS prophylaxis.
5. Improved management of treatment induced complications with platelets, blood products (including WBCs), and immunoglobulins.

Treatment centres and agreed protocols have contributed significantly to these advances, improving survival by 15–25% compared with care at non-specialist centres not in trials.

Shared care between the centre and referring hospital is increasingly practised: part of the treatment is done locally, convenient for the family, more local support, better use of the centre's resources.

General considerations

Differential diagnosis of leukaemia or malignancies from among the following presentations:

- Lymphadenopathy
- Purpura

- Anaemia
- Bone pain +/– swelling
- Stomatitis

Lymphadenopathy +/– hepatosplenomegaly

1. Infections:

    i Infectious mononucleosis with Paul Bunnel or monospot test, pertussis lymphocytosis by the history and cough swab, cat scratch disease by a primary lesion at the scratch site and localized lymphadenopathy.

    ii Serology for rubella, Echo, coxsackie virus, toxoplasmosis, brucellosis, leptospirosis.

    iii Mantoux for tuberculosis, atypical TB.

    iv Eczema, sometimes exacerbated by low grade infection.

2. Malignancies: leukaemias, lymphomas, metastatic disease. Rapidly progressive enlargement of glands over 2–3 weeks are an indication for FBC, Mantoux, biopsy. Cannot be easily clinically differentiated from simple infective lymphadenopathy.

3. Still's disease with high intermittent fever, lymphadenopathy, rash, lymphocytosis, joint swelling. FBC, ESR. Usually seronegative.

4. Drug reaction producing serum sickness: history of exposure.

5. Kawasaki disease: tender lymphadenopathy with fever, red lips and tongue, peeling finger tips, myocarditis.

6. Storage disorders, e.g. Gaucher's: do biopsy, enzyme estimation.

Purpura

1. Vascular: Henoch-Schönlein (anaphylactoid) pupura, meningococcaemia, bacterial endocarditis.

    History, distribution of lesions and severity of illness is usually diagnostic; swabs, blood culture, FBC and echocardiography clarify.

2. Thrombocytopenia: idiopathic, consumption, or malignancy.

    FBC, and coagulation if unsure. Bone marrow is diagnostic.

Anaemia +/- splenomegaly

Sickle cell, thalassaemia, haemolytic anaemias: require FBC, electrophoresis, fragility testing, glucose-6-phosphate dehydrogenase assay, Coombs' test.

Rare aplasias and infiltrations detected by bone marrow aspiration.

Bone pain +/- swelling

1. Infection.

2. Inflammatory conditions, e.g. Still's disease.

3. Neuroblastoma, leukaemia, eosinophilic granuloma.

    Signs of infection are usually obvious, but osteogenic sarcoma may present similarly. FBC, ESR, skeletal survey and bone scan are helpful. Bone trephine may clarify.

Radiological features to look for:

Vertebral collapse from metastatic deposits, but intervertebral disc space preserved. In pyogenic infection both are affected.

Metaphyseal lytic lesions in neuroblastoma, leukaemia, as well as infections. Malignant tumour has poorly defined edges, shows periosteal reaction, destruction of structure. It is often painful with overlying soft tissue swelling. Benign tumour or cyst has a well defined border, bone swelling, no bone destruction or periosteal reaction, and is usually pain free.

Stomatitis

1. Primary infection, e.g. herpes simplex, Vincent's angina.
2. Secondary to agranulocytosis, immune deficiency.
   Swabs, FBC, immunoglobulins and serology are informative. Consider HIV.

Other presenting signs

Abdominal masses: see Gastroenterology problems.
Soft tissue swellings: see Orthopaedic problems.

PHARMACOLOGY OF DRUG TREATMENT

1. Cytotoxic drug action is related to the effect on the cell growth cycle, though it is largely ignored in therapeutic shedules!

   i Phase specific: only a certain number of cells are likely to be vulnerable at any one time, i.e. prolonged exposure may be beneficial, but not increasing the dose e.g. cytosine arabinoside, vincristine, etoposide.

   ii Cycle specific: act at any stage of the cell cycle, i.e. dose related e.g. cyclophosphamide, cisplatin.

2. Antiemetics have significantly improved, and encouraged increased patient acceptability of even the most toxic cocktail. Metoclopramide and stemetil, sometimes dexamethasone, are standard drugs. For particularly emitogenic protocols which include cisplatin, high dose cyclophosphamide or ifosphamide, Ondanestron, a serotonin receptor antagonist, is usually the first choice. In children the dopamine antagonists are more likely to induce extra-pyramidal reactions, particularly metoclopramide, domperidone less so.

TREATMENT PRINCIPLES FOR THE LEUKAEMIAS

1 Isolation

No need to isolate against infection; almost all episodes of febrile neutropenia arise from endogenous gastrointestinal organisms. Providing the neutrophil counts >100 × 10^6/l they may mix with their peers at school and play.

2 Multiple chemotheraphy

Nationally agreed protocols for the UK for treatment of the leukaemias and solid tumours are prepared by the Medical Research Council (e.g. the 1990 acute lymphoblastic leukaemia (ALL) trial protocol is UK ALL XI), and the UK Children's Cancer Study Group.

The reader is advised to study the latest protocol available.

Treatment is determined by the prognosis for that child. In ALL high risk is related to high WBC total, age <2 or >12, presence of CNS or testicular disease at diagnosis, and cell type. Such children are assigned even more intensive treatment.

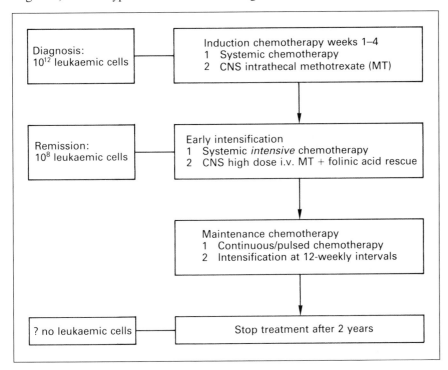

Figure 18.1 Outline of chemotherapy for acute lymphoblastic leukaemia

Acute lymphoblastic leukaemia

The treatment is divided into blocks of chemotherapy over 2 years (Figure 18.1), with continuous co-trimoxazole prophylaxis against pneumocystis infection.

   i Induce remission
      Induction weeks 1 to 4: prednisolone, vincristine and duanorubicin, L-asparaginase,
  ii Early and late intensification weeks 5 and 23.
      A week's intensification to reduce the relapse rate, give 3 additional drugs: cytosine, arabinoside, etoposide or teniposide.

iii Treating 'sanctuary' sites where leukaemic cells may be present at diagnosis and can persist:

CNS directed therapy is now intrathecal (methotrexate, hydrocortisone, cytarabine). Prophylactic cranial irradiation has been discontinued in low risk children, but may be given at a year in high risk cases. Rationale: high dose methotrexate eliminates the need for irradiation and hence may avoid the fall in IQ found after it.

Testicular disease at presentation must be confirmed by biopsy in ALL. Presence of leukaemic cells at diagnosis or subsequently is an indication for irradiation despite the inevitable sterility.

iv Maintenance in ALL: daily 6-mercaptopurine, weekly methotrexate. Evaluation of pulsed steroids, vincristine, methotrexate with leucovorin rescue, and other drug combinations continue in an effort to further improve prognosis.

Acute myeloid leukaemia

Current approach: myelosuppression followed by autologous bone marrow transplantation, or further chemotheraphy in the 70% of children without an HLA-identical sibling. Extremely myelosuppressive, using powerful drugs (cytosine arabinoside, daunorubicin, VP16) which produce prolonged periods of marrow aplasia requiring antibiotics and blood products.

3. Support

i Give blood and platelets whenever required. Indications: Hb <8 g/dl; platelets <20 × 10⁹/l, or <40 × 10⁹/l with fever.

All blood products must be CMV negative in case bone marrow transplant (BMT) is needed. CMV complicates about 20% of allogenic BMT.

ii Anticipate the acute' tumour lysis syndrome' in the first 24 h treatment. Most at risk are those with a high WBC count ALL, and bulky non-Hodgkin's lymphoma → hyperuricaemia, metabolic acidosis, hyperkalaemia. Adequate fluids (4 l/m²/day) and allopurinol are routinely given. Occasionally hyperkalaemia requires i.v. frusemide or even peritoneal dialysis.

4. Suspected infection

If neutropenic (<1000 × 10⁹/l neutrophils) and a pyrexia of 38°C, even a single spike, do not wait to see if it persists:

i After taking cultures give the locally agreed antibiotic cocktail (often ceftazidine/ureidopenicillin + gentamicin). If already on prophylaxis (see below), continue the oral antifungal and co-trimoxazole.

ii Continuation of therapy depends on the results of culture, and WBC.

a. Culture negative and afebrile after:
2 days, stop antibiotics after 5 days, regardless of WBC.
5 days, continue antibiotics for further 3–5 days.

b. Positive cultures: continue antibiotics for 10 days.

iii Persistent temperature + neutropenia needs repeat cultures. Consider adding amphotericin after 96 h even if culture negative. Change therapy on the basis of results or deterioration. Acyclovir for lesions of herpes simplex/zoster.

5. Prophylaxis

i Antifungal orally during induction and consolidation phases.
ii Co-trimoxazole against *Pneumocystis carinii* throughout treatment, on alternate days.
iii Hyperimmune zoster immunoglobulin after chickenpox contact. Parents must be warned of this need.
iv Live vaccines are avoided. Inactivated polio vaccine, and DPT are safe, with best response between courses.

6. Allogeneic bone marrow transplant

Indications: relapse, older child with ALL, B cell ALL or acute myelogenous leukaemia (AML). 5-year survival 60% when done in second remission ALL, 60% in first remission in AML.

Contentious, inconclusive: autologous (own) bone marrow transplant, purged of leukaemic cells, in older children with ALL, and in AML at any age.

STAGING OF SOLID TUMOURS

1. Staging is a guide to the intensity of treatment required, and is related to the prognosis at the time of diagnosis.
   The definitions for staging vary with the nature of the tumour and the treatment currently appropriate.
   Cannot be applied to leukaemia which is a disseminated disease.
2. Generally:
   Stage I = Localized to organ of origin.
   Stage II = Local spread; if surgically treated some tumour may remain.
   Stage III = Extends horizontally across the vertical midline or to both sides of the diaphragm.
   Stage IV = Disseminated disease.
3. Further subdivision indicating systemic involvement:
   A = Asymptomatic.
   B = >10% weight loss, pyrexia >38°C, night sweats.

SOLID TUMOUR TREATMENT PROCEDURES

Philosophy is 'contain or cure with least cost' to avoid mutilation and unacceptable side effects, by weighing up the likely outcome, then planning intervention using modalities 1–5 in the most appropriate way.

1. Removal by surgery, or shrink tumour mass first with chemotherapy.
2. Postoperative radiation therapy.

3. Chemotherapy: cytotoxic agent.
   Example: all three modalities are used in Wilm's kidney tumour: surgery + radiotherapy + chemotheraphy (actinomycin D).
   Antiemetics are an important adjunct.

Variations

4. Megatherapy: chemotherapy with autologous bone marrow rescue is under investigation for management of solid tumours with poor prognosis.
5. Reconstructive surgery, e.g. in Ewing's and osteogenic sarcoma: endoprosthetic replacement of diseased bone + aggressive chemotherapy. Mutilation is avoided, so more acceptable to the patient, without significant reduction in prognosis.
6. Bone marrow transplant, in disseminated disease after total body irradiation. Used in neuroblastoma, with an autologous marrow transplant, made possible by purging it of tumour cells using isotope tagged monoclonal antibodies.

GENERAL SUPPORTIVE MEASURES

Family support

Maintain schooling. Parent support groups.

Palliative care

400 children die of cancer annually in the UK. Increasingly, specialist support nurses, symptom care teams, and hospices provide support.

Further reading

Goldman A, Beardsmore S, Hunt J (1990) Palliative care for children with cancer–home, hospital, or hospice? *Archives of Disease in Childhood*, **65**, 641–643

HAZARDS OF THERAPY

1. Irradiation

i Cranial

- Short term: drowsiness.
- Long term: reduced IQ, learning problems, difficulty in social relationships.
- Reduced growth hormone production at puberty, short stature. May induce premature puberty. Other forms of hypopituitarism are less common.

ii Spinal

If half of the spine is irradiated → scoliosis due to asymmetry of spinal growth, e.g. as part of an abdominal field in Wilm's tumour. When vertebral bodies are equally irradiated → short trunk which becomes manifest at puberty.

iii Gonads

- Ovaries: failure after Wilms' tumour is proportional to dose. Increase in miscarriages, no increase in congenital malformations. Premature menopause due to loss of germ cells.
- Testes: for ALL → severe oligospermia, but normal testosterone production.

iv Eyes

Cataracts from total body irradiation for bone marrow transplant and rescue therapy.

v Secondary tumours

From within the irradiated field.

2. Chemotherapy

i Organ damage

- e.g. Bleomycin → lungs fibrosis.
- Cisplatin → kidney damage, high tone hearing loss.
- Doxorubicin (adriamycin) → myocardial weakness, cardiac failure.

ii Immunosuppression

Measles is the major cause of death in children receiving treatment, for unlike the other potentially fatal viral infections a specific antiviral agent is not available. Chickenpox fatalities are reduced by hyperimmune globulin and acyclovir. Pneumocystis infection is reduced by trimethoprim prophylaxis.

iii Sterility

In Hodgkin's disease treatment with mustine and procarbazine.

3. Bone marrow transplantation

   i Opportunistic infection up to 3–12 months after grafting.
   ii Graft versus host disease (GVHD) in allogeneic transplants. Occurs despite histocompatibility matching by human leukocyte antigen (HLA). The attack is mounted by donor T cells against the recipient's skin, liver and gastrointestinal tract. Termed acute GVHD in the first 100 days, chronic thereafter.

Management

T cell depletion of donated marrow before engrafting, and/or cyclosporin may reduce its occurrence.

Steroids, antithymocyte globulin, azothiprine, or cyclosporin A are used in established GVHD.

4. A second malignancy

Unrelated to the first, but due to the therapy, occurs in 3% by 15 years from diagnosis.

Further reading

Poplack D G (ed) (1988) The leukaemias. *Pediatric Clinics of North America*, **35**

Morris-Jones P H, Craft A W (1990) Childhood cancer: cure at what cost? *Archives of Disease in Childhood*, **65**, 638–640

Rivera G K *et al* (1991) Improved outcome in childhood acute lymphoblastic leukaemia with reinforced early treatment and rotational combination chemotherapy. *Lancet*, i, 61–66

SPECIFIC CONDITIONS

Acute lymphoblastic leukaemia (ALL)

Definition

The uncontrolled proliferation of a clone of immature lymphoid cells from a single abnormal cell. 85% of childhood leukaemias are ALL, the remainder of acute non–lymphoblastic leukaemias (ANLL) are mainly acute myeloblastic. ALL>ANLL association with Down's syndrome and defects of DNA repair (see introduction).

Tumour marker

95% of all ALL have an enzyme not found in ANLL – terminal deoxynucleotidyl transferase (Tdt).

Prognosis

Linked to morphology and immune cell type, less so to chromosomal abnormality (Table 18.2).

1. Morphology

85% of childhood ALL have small round lymphoblasts (L1 lymphoblasts in the French–American–British classification), with higher remission and long–term survival than the other cell types in ALL (L2 = larger, kidney shaped nuclei 12%, L3 = large, basophilic, one or more nucleoli <3%).

2. Immunophenotypes

Most ALL lymphoblasts are in the B cell line, but the more the monoclonal antibodies react the worse the prognosis. 80% of ALL have non-T, non-B cell lymphoblasts (common ALL antigen, 60% from an early pre-B cell, 20% a pre-B cell line), and have a better prognosis. 20% are T-cell type and have a poor prognosis, and the 1% with B-cell type a very poor prognosis.

3. Chromosomal studies

These show that leukaemic cells usually have more than 46 chromosomes. The higher the number (>50) the better the prognosis. Translocation of genetic material from one chromosome to another may worsen the prognosis.

Overall 50–70% have a 5-year disease free survival.

After the first relapse 30% still have a good prognosis if given a compatible bone marrow transplant.

Clinical

Duration of symptoms is usually weeks, rarely a month or more. Peak age 4–7 years old. Lethargy, anorexia, bone pain, bleeding and fever are common.

Pallor, purpura, lymphadenopathy, and hepatosplenomegaly are usual.

Investigations

1. Bone marrow aspirate is diagnostic if >25% lymphoblasts present.
2. Chest X-ray for mediastinal mass.
3. CSF for ALL cells.
   2 and 3 present in 5% at diagnosis and associated with a poorer prognosis (usually T cell).

Differential diagnosis and treatment

See above.

Table 18.2 Clinical and laboratory features influencing prognosis of ALL

Feature	Good prognosis	Poor prognosis
WBC (most predictive)	<10000 × 10^9/l	Very high
Age	1–10 years	<1 or >11 years
Race	Caucasian	Black
Sex	Girl	Boy
Haemoglobin	Low	Normal
Platelets	Plentiful	Low
Lymphadenopathy	Little	Diffuse + mediastinal glands
Bone marrow (BM) cell type	pre-B cell	B cell
Morphology (FAB classification)	L1	L2 or L3
BM response to treatment	Normal in 14 days	Incomplete
CSF	Clear	Contains ALL cells
Chromosomes of ALL cells	Normal	Translocation, in 80% = t(8;14)

Acute non-lymphoblastic leukaemia (ANLL)

Definition

A monoclonal disease like ALL, it comprises 15% of childhood leukaemias.

Presentation

As for ALL.

Diagnosis

Bone marrow aspirate containing >30% myeloblasts.

Morphology (FAB classification) and cytochemistry classify ANLL into 6 subtypes, e.g. acute myeloblastic (AML) is FAB M1 or M2, and myeloperoxidase positive. Monoclonal antibodies reacting with myeloid blasts (but also react to normal myeloid precursors), chromosomes (e.g. AML has an 8:21 translocation), and Tdt enzyme estimation (absent in 95% of ANLL) are guides to prognosis and cell type, though not as clear cut as ALL.

Treatment

More intensive than ALL as remission is more difficult to obtain and maintain. Early allogeneic bone marrow transplant may offer the best chance. See above.

Prognosis

30% survival to 3 years.

Poorer prognosis: WBC >100000, <2 years old, acute monoblastic leukaemia, particularly with chromosomal translocations.

INDIVIDUAL SOLID TUMOURS

Lymphomas

Incidence

1 in 100000 annually, non-Hodgkin's commoner than Hodgkin's, present in late childhood/adolescence, M>F.

Hodgkin's disease

Definition

A malignant lymphoma characterized by the Reed-Sternberg multinucleated giant cell, and T-cell dysfunction increasing susceptibility to infection.

Clinical

Initial presentation is progressive lymph gland enlargement in the neck. Night sweats, fever and weight loss appear in advanced disease.

Management

1. Biopsy and staging.
2. Radiation for local disease.
3. Combined chemotherapy and extended field radiation if the disease is more extensive.

Prognosis

Excellent 95% cure if localized, down to 50% in stage IV with symptoms of advanced disease at diagnosis.

Non-Hodgkin lymphomas

Definition

A malignant lymphoma of the B-cell or T-cell lymphocyte, non-Hodgkin lymphoma (NHL) is the most rapidly growing of all human tumours.

Epidemiology

Most cases are sporadic, but the incidence is increased in primary and acquired immunodeficiencies.

1. African. Endemic. After immunosuppression by malaria, measles etc, the Epstein-Barr (EB) virus may induce Burkitt's lymphoma in extranodal sites, e.g. jaw, organs, spinal cord, by unchecked B-cell proliferation.

2. Sporadic. In contradistinction to the endemic type, the EB viral genome is rarely found, and the usual site is a lymph node.

Prognosis, presentation and sites

Related to histology and stage at diagnosis. Best is 90% 5-year survival if localized, falling to 20% for CNS involvement.

1. Favourable and localized, stage I and II. Relatively unusual. Cough, sore throat with enlarged neck glands or tonsils, or in the ileo-caecal region presenting as intussusception.
2. Unfavourable, the majority. Obstructive symptoms. Rapidly enlarging:

   i Mediastinal tumour T cell: respiratory or superior vena cava obstruction.
   ii Infiltrative, large retroperitoneal B-cell tumour: vomiting and pain in the abdomen.

iii Dissemination (stage IV) is likely, presenting as an acute lymphoblastic leukaemia with masses.

Diagnosis

Biopsy and bone marrow. Staging does not require routine laparotomy.

Management

- T-cell NHL: chemotherapy and CNS prophylaxis as for ALL. Improved prognosis in T-cell stage III with UKALL X protocol giving a 90% 4-year survivial.
- B-cell NHL: Aggressive pulsed chemotherapy regimen for stage IV disease using alkylating agents and methotrexate, is improving survival. Tumour lysis syndrome is particularly likely.
- Surgery is only indicated for emergency tumour obstruction of airway, bowel or bladder.

Reference

Wheeler K, Chessells J M (1990) An effective treatment for stage III mediastinal non-Hodgkin's lymphoma. *Archives of Disease in Childhood*, **65**, 252–254

Rhabdomyosarcoma

Definition

Embryonal small round and spindle–shaped cell tumour, arising from muscle mesenchyme, is found in 80% of cases, and has the most favourable histology.
 Peak age 2–5 years and second peak in adolescence.

Sites and clinical associations

Metastases present in 20% at diagnosis, and may be responsible for the mode of presentation.
 A third each occur in:

1. Head and trunk: proptosis, chronic otitis, pressure effects.
2. Bladder: urinary retention, frequency, haematuria, straining–mass often palpable on bimanual palpation or rectally. Includes botryoides (grape like) tumour of the vagina.
3. Muscle of the limbs, usually in adolescence.

Treatment

After diagnosis by biopsy and imaging for metastases.

1. Surgery to remove or debulk but not mutilate.
2. Drugs (e.g. ifosfamide, vincristine, and actinomycin D as cyclical therapy), plus local radiotherapy, according to locally agreed protocols.

Prognosis

Poor for limbs, retroperitoneal sites, and metastatic disease. Histologically, alveolar has a poorer prognosis than embryonal. 80% 5-year survival if localized completely resectable (stage I) disease, 20% for stage IV disease.

Wilms' tumour and Neuroblastoma

Embryonal tumours. Inherited in 20%, sporadic in 80%.

Wilms' associations: chromosome 11 point deletion, aniridia, hemihypertrophy, genitourinary anomalies, Beckwith's syndrome.

Neuroblastomas have a variety of presentations, few due to catecholamines, mainly compression (spinal cord, Horner's), or size, and metastases. Site in 75% is abdominal, 25% in the posterior mediastinum or neck.

Incidence

1 in 10000 for each during childhood.

Controversy: presymptomatic diagnosis of neuroblastoma

Neuroblastoma in situ (NIS) found in 1/260 infant autopsies, thus many regress. Japanese studies screening babies' urine aimed at demonstrating that early diagnosis and treatment can prevent deaths have failed to convince.

Further reading

Murphy S B, Cohn S L, Craft A W, *et al* (1991) Do children benefit from mass screening for neuroblastoma? *Lancet,* i, 334–345

Osteogenic sarcoma, Ewing's sarcoma

Tumours of adolescence, commoner in males, ratio 5:1 Osteogenic sarcoma twice as common as Ewing's sarcoma.

The spindle–shaped cell of osteogenic sarcoma is distinct from the round cell tumour type of Ewing's also found in neuroblastoma, rhabdomyosarcoma and non-Hodgkin lymphoma.

Clinical

Pain and local swelling. Ends of long bones are the usual sites. Ewing's is also found in the pelvis, ribs and scapulae, occasionally involving the soft tissues.

Fever and weight loss with metastatic disease in Ewing's.

Metastases to the lungs are common in both.

Table 18.3 Differentiating features of Wilms' tumour and abdominal neuroblastoma

	Wilms' tumour	*Neuroblastoma*
Embryonal origin	Metanephros	Neural crest
Peak age	2–3 years, 75% <5 years old	<2 years, 30% <1 year old
Clinical	Well, swollen abdomen, abdominal pain occasionally. Hypertension 25%	Presentation with stage 4 disease common: ill, pale, weight loss, fever, bone pain, abdominal pain. Hypertension in 10%. Proptosis, Haematuria, usually microscopic. Ataxia, diarrhoea due to vasoactive intestinal peptide
Abdominal mass	Lobulated, firm	Irregular edge, 'craggy' hard
Crosses midline	Rarely	Commonly
Bilateral	Common if hereditary	
US	Grossly distorted renal echo	Mass above kidney pushing it down. Fine calcification may be seen. Collecting system not distorted
Metastases at diagnosis	Occasional (15%)	Common (66%), diffuse, to bone, lungs, classically to orbits, skin, liver
Diagnostic tests	US of both kidneys and liver, plus X-ray chest AP + lateral for staging. Bone trephine. CT may be indicated if brain secondaries clinically likely	24–h urine for VMA amd HVA. ^{99}Tc and ^{123}I MIBG bone scan. Leucoerythroblastic blood count. Serum ferritin >150 ng/ml has a poor prognosis
Staging	Stage V = bilateral renal disease (5%)	Stage IVS = stage I or II + liver, skin or bone marrow involvement, usually confined to infants
Differential diagnosis	Hydronephrosis	'Growing pains', early rheumatoid, cerebellar ataxia
Order of treatment	1 Surgical removal of whole affected kidney 2 Chemotherapy: 1, 2, or 3 drugs for stage I, II, or III respectively 3 3 drug chemo +/– irradiation for stage IV, i.e. lung metastases	As disseminated disease at presentation is usual: 1 Chemotherapy = cyclical doxorubicin, cisplatin, VM26, and cyclophosphamide → remission in 50% 2 Chemo + resection of residual post-chemo neuroblastoma tissue precedes autologous bone marrow transplant with high dose melphalan 3 Surgery for localized stage I or II disease 4 Surgery + chemo for stage III

Prognosis for 5–year survival	1 90% in the 85% with well differentiated tumours
	
	2 50% in poorly differentiated, anaplastic types
		1 Under 1 year old good stage I, II, IVS. Spontaneous remission is common, and 90% long–term survival
		2 >1 year old, stage IV: poor, 20% survive. Tumour markers for poor prognosis:
		  i High serum ferritin
		  ii High number of *n-myc* oncogene copies

Diagnosis

1. X ray:
   - i Osteogenic sarcoma 'sunburst' sign = extension through the periostium.
   - ii Ewing's 'onion skin' caused by layers of new bone.
2. CT of lung
3. Bone scan.
4. Marrow aspirate and trephine biopsy.
5 MRI of tumour.

Treatment

Limb conservation surgery with endoprostheses and chemotherapy. Local radio-therapy for Ewing's improves survival.

Prognosis

50% 5-year survival.

Ewing's: poor in proximal femoral site; proportional to the volume of the tumour, and as pelvic tumours are large they have a particularly poor prognosis.

Both: poor for metastatic disease.

Retinoblastoma

Definition

Intraocular malignancy arising from one, or several, sites in the retina.

Incidence

1:20 000 live births

Aetiology and presentation

1. Genetic: 40% of neuroblastomas, AD with variable penetrance. Presentation before 12 months old, usually multifocal with bilateral disease and a tendency to other tumours too. A quarter of them have a family history of retinoblastoma.
2. Sporadic: 60% due to 'two hit' mutation (see Genetics). Usually older, 1–2 years of age, unilateral, with only a small risk of retinoblastoma in offspring.

Clinical

White 'cat's eye' pupil, absent red reflex. Occasional strabismus. Metastasizes late, along the optic nerve to meninges and via blood to bone.

Treatment

As disease is usually limited to the globe of the eye, surgical enucleation alone suf-fices for large unilateral tumours. Small tumours receive laser or cryotherapy. Chemotherapy is of limited benefit even in bilateral or disseminated disease.

Prognosis

Excellent unless disseminated.

Prevention

Regular ophthalmic examination in siblings in affected families and their offspring up to age 2 years.

DNA markers identify individuals at risk within carrier families.

Germ cell tumours

Contain all three embryonic germ cell layers. Two thirds are extra gonadal. Rare (3% of all childhood cancers), commoner in females.

1. Sacrococcygeal tumour is the commonest solid tumour in the newborn. Arises between the buttocks, very variable in size. Usually benign but has malignant potential if not surgically removed.
2. Testicular tumour presents under the age of 2 years.

Investigations

Elevated serum alpha fetoprotein (AFP) and occasionally human chorionic gonado-trophin (HCG), are markers of malignancy. Continued elevation of AFP or failure to fall is an indication for further therapy.

Langerhans cell histiocytosis (Histiocytosis X)

Definition

A group of rare conditions due to proliferation of phagocytic histiocytes or Langer-hans cells.

Cause

Reactive, not malignant but often treated as such because of historically poor prognosis in multisystem involvement with organ dysfunction.

Systems involved

1. Skin

- Purpura, generalized eczema, trunk nodules, scalp seborrhoea like crusts and punched out ulcers.
- Eczematous otitis externa.
- Chronic otitis media from mastoid involvement, unresponsive to antibiotics.

2. Organs

- Lymphoreticular: generalized lymphadenopathy.
- Hepatosplenomegaly with hypoproteinaemia, hyperbilirubinaemia.
- Lungs: involvement ranges from asymptomatic 'honeycomb' infiltrates to cough, tachypnoea, cyanosis, and spontaneous pneumothorax.
- Bone marrow: infiltration with anaemia, neutropenia, thrombocytopenia.

3. Skeleton

Lytic lesions, eventually may show new bone formation and heal spontaneously.

Investigation and evaluation

1 Biopsy of suspicious skin lesion, lymph node, bone marrow.
2 X-ray skeletal survey, pituitary fossa.
3 Lung function for restrictive lung involvement.
4 Blood: anaemia, biochemical liver involvement.
5 Urine: test for diabetes insipidus.

Definitive diagnosis

Depends on finding Birbeck granules in lesional cells on electron microscopy, and T-6 antigenic determinants on their surfaces in biopsy material.

Characteristic clinical presentations, treatment and prognosis

1. Multisystem disease

Letterer-Siwe disease occurs in infants, involving skin, lymphoreticular system, lungs and bone marrow. Failure to thrive is common.

- Diagnosis by skin or lymph node biopsy.
- Treatment is chemotherapy: prednisolone and second line drugs vincristine, cyclophosphamide or etoposide
- Prognosis: good if skin involvement only. Poor if under 2 years, multisystem soft tissue disease and showing a vital organ dysfunction.

2. Bone and skin

Hands-Schuller-Christian disease is uncommon in infants, tends to chronicity, usually involves skeleton and skin, and has a better prognosis.

- Classical triad of proptosis, lytic skull lesions, and diabetes insipidus due to granuloma around the pituitary stalk, occurs in 10%.
- Treatment: radiation to orbits, and mastoid if involved; chemotherapy as for Letterer-Siwe if disease is extensive.

3. Bone

Eosinophilic granuloma is rare in infants.

- Lytic bone lesions, sites of local swelling and pain, pathological fracture.
- Diagnostic curettage of a solitary lesion may be curative.
- Excellent prognosis if limited to bone.

Further reading

McLelland J, Broadbent V, Yeomans E, Malone M, Pritchard, J (1990) Langerhans cell histiocytosis: the case for conservative treatment. *Archives of Disease in Childhood*, **65**, 301–303

General reading

Ekert H (19) *Childhood Cancer, Understanding and Coping* Boston:Gordon & Breach
Horowitz M E, Pizzo P A (eds) (1991) Solid tumors in children. *Pediatric Clinics of North America*, **38**, no 2
Plowman, Pinkerton (eds) (1991) *Pediatric Oncology, Clinical Practice and Controversies*. New York:-Chapman & Hall

Chapter 19

Immunological problems

THE IMMUNE SYSTEM

The immune response comprises two complementary systems, the non-specific and specific, which must interact for effective protection of the body.

Recognition of failure of the defences is the first step in identifying immunodeficiency.

Non-specific host defences

Exposure to viruses, bacteria or toxins activate the cellular and non-cellular mediators (cytokines and plasma factors) of the inflammatory response.

1. Cells: neutrophils, monocytes, macrophages, platelets, natural killer cells.
2. Cytokines (locally acting hormones) released by macrophages:

    i   Interferons. Active against viral infections, they enhance major histocompatibility (MHC) antigen expression of cells infected by virus and hence their destruction by cytotoxic killing.
    ii Colony stimulating factors and platelet activating factor cause neutrophils and other cells to multiply.
    iii Tumour necrosis factor contributes to shock as part of the inflammatory response.
    iv Interleukins induce T cell proliferation, B lymphocyte differentiation, and acute phase reactants.

3. Plasma factors: complement activation by the classical or alternative pathways. By opsonization, it coats antigen or microorganisms and enhances ingestion and killing.

Specific host defences

These comprise antibody production, antigen recognition and the inflammatory response, culminating in killing.

1. Active response to antigen/microorganism depends on:

    i Memory of previous exposure.

    ii Prediction, despite no previous exposure, by the process of random genera-tion of DNA sequences during lymphocyte production. Ensures survival against changing microorganisms.

2. Immunity is humoral or cellular. Stem lymphocytes differentiate into humoral B (bone marrow) cells, or cellular T (thymus) cells.
3. Antigen recognition occurs at T-cell receptors and B cell immunoglobulin secre-tory sites → cellular proliferation, the differentiating T and B cells acting together, the T cells as enhancers (helper cells, mainly CD4) or suppressors (mainly CD8) of the response.

   CD4 is selectively destroyed by HIV, CD8 spared.
4. Cytokines are released to aid or multiply the inflammatory process.
5. Leucocyte adhesion is enhanced by glycoproteins as a prelude to lysis. Absence results in leucocytosis, recurrent bacterial and fungal infection from birth, with delayed cord separation.
6. Lysis occurs by one of three possible mechanisms:

    i Release of perforins by T cells and natural killer cells.

    ii Complement cascade with B cells.

    { target cell membrane's per-meability increases allow-ing influx of fluid and then its rupture.

    iii Antibody dependent cellular cytotoxicity: coating of target cell with anti-body, allows neutrophils or macrophages to attach to the antibody's Fc receptor and release perforin to lyse it. This oxidative 'respiratory burst' is measured by the nitroblue tetrazolium test and chemiluminescence.

Immunodeficiency is a breakdown in any part of this process.

RECURRENT INFECTION

Infection is commonplace and necessary in the developing child to develop resist-ance to the common environmental pathogens.

    Normal frequency is increased in a poor socio-economic environment, bottle feeding (hygiene), and parental smoking. Upper respiratory tract infections nor-mally recur about 6 per annum.

    An increase in frequency of infections occurs in preschool care facilities, and when the first-born goes to school and brings them home to his younger siblings.

    Underlying disorders may predispose, e.g. cystic fibrosis to bronchiectasis, cleft palate to otitis media.

Warning signs

Abnormal response, persistent or unusual infections, or failure to thrive, should alert to possible immunodeficiency.

    Secondary causes far outnumber primary, and are mainly due to malnutrition or after exanthema such as measles, chickenpox, (common) or other increasingly important and frequent causes such as HIV.

In addition, reinfection with the same organism, arthritis, vasculitis, progressive neurological deterioration and malignancy are associated with primary immunodeficiencies.

SECONDARY IMMUNODEFICIENCIES

As a group, relatively common even in developed countries, and diagnosis is rapidly arrived at by the history of a primary disorder, except in the case of suspected HIV (counselling must precede testing).

1. Malnutrition and post exanthema.
2. Infection, e.g. HIV.
3. Protein losing, e.g. nephrotic syndrome, protein losing enteropathies.
4. Drugs, e.g. steroids, immunosuppressives.
5. Splenectomy.
6. Infiltration, e.g. disseminated malignancy.

PRIMARY IMMUNODEFICIENCY DISORDERS

Rare.

Incidence

1 in 10000
Types of deficiency:
  antibody alone 50%
  combined cellular and antibody 20%
  phagocytic 18%, cellular 10%, complement 2%.

Pointers to diagnosis

1. Family History

  i Consanguinity: autosomal recessive examples

  a. In severe combined immune deficiency (SCID) 20% have the enzyme deficiency adenosine deaminase (ADA).
  b. Schwachmann's syndrome, includes neutropenia.

  ii Male relatives suffering early death, or recurrent infection: ratio of boys:girls affected by primary immunodeficiency = 4:1 as many diseases are X linked (XL) e.g. all Wiskott Aldrich syndrome and XL hypogammaglobulinaemia, most SCID and chronic granulomatous disease.
  iii Connective tissue and lupus-like syndromes: complement deficiency.
  iv Autoimmune disease, pernicious anaemia, thyroid disease: hypogammaglobulinaemia.

2. Pattern of infection unusual

   i   Unusual organism, e.g. *Pneumocystis*, or persistent, e.g. *Giardia*.
   ii Two or more anatomical sites.
  iii Unpredictable course, poor response to antibiotics, periodic, e.g. 3-weekly in cyclical neutropenia.
  iv Increased frequency of infection, examples:

     a. Two or more episodes of pneumonia in a preschool child, or
     b. Six or more episodes of otitis media, tonsilitis or bronchitis in a year often points to a humoral or phagocytic disorder.
     c. Repeated meningococcal infection in complement deficiency.

   v Type of organism may be a clue to the underlying deficiency, e.g.

     a. Cell mediated if viral (especially if multiple infection), fungal, *Pneumocystis* or BCG-osis.
     b. Humoral – common pathogenic bacterial, *Giardia*, all enteroviruses.
     c. Phagocytic – staphylococci or *Candida*.
     d. Complement – *Meningococcus, Pneumococcus, Haemophilus*.

3. Dysmorphic features in the presence of recurrent infection

i Neonatal:

a. Di George syndrome of midline facial cleft, absent thymus and parathyroids, with hypocalcaemic tetany in the first week, and severe congenital heart disease (usually an interrupted aortic arch).
b. Oculocutaneous albinism: Chediak-Higashi abnormal neutrophils.

ii Short stature plus:

a. Malabsorption +/-eczema: Schwachmann's neutropenia with exocrine pancreatic dysfunction.
b. Fine hair: cartilage-hair hypoplasia with T cell dysfunction, prone to severe chickenpox.

iii Coarse features, recurrent superficial and deep Staphylococcus aureus infection, chronic dermatitis

Hyperimmune IgE syndrome (AD), due to T and B cell dysfunction.

iv Eczema with bleeding

a. Wiskott Aldrich syndrome (XL), T cell dysfunction, small platelets rapidly destroyed by the spleen.
b. With short stature and neutropenia in 'lazy leucocyte' syndrome.

v Progressive 'cerebral palsy' and lymphomas

a. Ataxia telangiectasia: progressive ataxia and choreoathetosis, telangiectasia on bulbar conjunctivae and antecubital fossae in mid-childhood, chronic pulmonary infection, death from lymphoproliferative disease due to defective DNA repair. 95% have raised alpha fetoprotein, chromosome 14 abnormality, abnormal T and B cell function, low IgA, and IgG.
b. Lymphoproliferative syndrome (XL): after Epstein-Barr virus infection an uncontrolled monoclonal B cell proliferation occurs.

4. Age at onset

Generally, the more severe, the earlier the onset, and the worse the prognosis.

i Less than 6 months

Cellular immunodeficiency (T +/- B cell) is the most common form. Examples: SCID, Di George's syndrome. Antibody production is often reduced as well, as T cells are important modulators of B cell activity.

Clinically a lack of lymphoid tissue, and a small/atrophic thymus is seen on X-ray.

a. Chronic infections: e.g. diarrhoea (rotavirus, cryptosporidiosis, *Giardia lamblia*), lung infection (respiratory syncytial virus, cytomegalovirus, adenovirus, parainfluenza), candida.
b. Life-threatening infection by organisms of low pathogenicity, e.g. *Pneumocystis carinii*, BCG-osis, as well as by Herpes simplex or zoster.
c. Failure to thrive from a few months old.
d. Erythroderma within days to weeks of birth: graft versus host disease from maternal lymphocytes or other transfusion.
e. Delayed separation of the cord for 3 weeks or more in leukocyte adhesion defect.
f. Eczema with bleeding from thrombocytopenia in the Wiskott Aldrich syndrome (WAS).
g. Neurodegeneration: spastic cerebral palsy, in adenosine deaminase deficiency (ADA) is found in 20% of SCID patients.

Prognosis Complete deficiency causes death in weeks, others within 1–2 years without treatment. Reconstitution with thymus (Di George) or bone marrow (SCID, WAS) is effective in some.

ii Over 6 months

Antibody deficiency emerges as maternal transplacental IgG wanes. Organisms are usually extracellular.

a. Recurrent or persistent sepsis (bronchiectasis, meningitis, arthritis, furunculosis) with common bacterial pathogens.
b. Chronic diarrhoea, malabsorption, with cryptosporidiosis, *Giardia lamblia*, campylobacter.

c. Risk of vaccine poliomyelitis and persistent enterovirus infection.
d. Arthritis, aseptic in 75%, affecting one or more large joints.
e. Malignancy develops eventually in 10%.

Conditions causing hypogammaglobulinaemia (IgG <2g/l, low IgA, IgM) may be:

Persistent:

i Inherited XL with little lymphoid tissue (also called Bruton's disease).
ii Sporadic 'common variable' hypogammaglobulinaemia with normal or large
glands +/– splenomegaly, otherwise indistinguishable from the XL form. Onset
at any age.

- Secondary to EB virus in XL lymphoproliferative syndrome.
- Transient due to delayed switching on of immunoglobulin production. Recovery
by 5 years.

Selective hypogammaglobulinaemia A low IgA alone is usually healthy, but IgA
with IgG_2 deficiency is associated with pneumococcal infections.

Phagocytosis defects Present below a year old with superficial and deep *Staphylococcus aureus* infection slow to respond to antibiotics: chronic granulomatous disease, hyperimmune IgE syndrome.

Prognosis Severe deficiency may be fatal in early childhood, but immunoglobulin
replacement allows survival to adulthood; so too for most phagocyte defects. Partial
(IgA, IgG_2) deficiency is compatible with a normal life span.

iii Over 5 years old

Still mainly antibody deficiencies, but also complement and phagocytosis defects.
   Delay in diagnosis is increasingly common as age increases, with a lack of its
recognition as the cause of chronic suppurative otitis, sinusistis, bronchiectasis, or
diarrhoea +/– malabsorption, arthritis, or neurodegeneration.

a. Hypogammaglobulinaemia: chronic ECHO encephalitis.
b. Complement deficiency → increased pneumococcus, haemophilus, meningococcus: lupus-like syndrome with fever, arthralgia, vasculitis, glomerulonephritis.
c. Phagocyte dysfunction: see above.
d. Neurodegenerations: see above.

Management Principles

1. General

i Early diagnosis and decision on treatment improves survival, and reduces
long-term complications, e.g. bronchiectasis.
ii All blood transfusions must be irradiated to prevent graft versus host disease.
iii Avoid live vaccines, except measles vaccine in HIV.

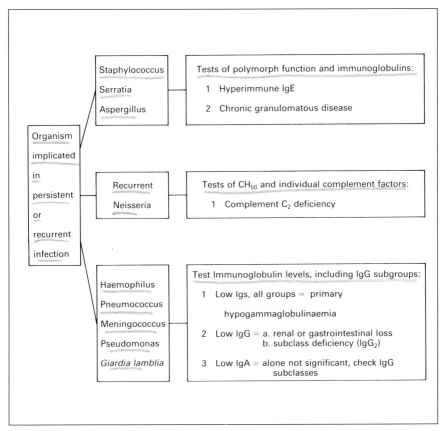

Figure 19.1 Algorithm for recurrent bacterial infection

2. Reconstitution by bone marrow transplant e.g. SCID, ADA deficiency, WAS, and some chronic granulomatous disease. In haplotype transplants (usually a parent) depletion of mature T cells before engraftment reduces graft versus host disease (GVHD). Radiation ablation of the marrow is unnecessary in SCID.

3. Replacement of IgG in hypogammaglobulinaemia, and selected cases of IgA associated with IgG_2 deficiency.

4. Cytokines: colony stimulating factor in neutropenia, aplastic anaemia; gamma interferon in chronic granulomatous disease.

5. Prophylactic antibiotics

   i Co-trimoxazole against *Pneumocystis carinii* in combined immunodeficiencies; in chronic granulomatous disease; cyclical neutropenia; IgG subclass deficiency.

  ii Penicillin against meningococcus, pneumococcus in complement deficiency.

6. Antenatal diagnosis is increasingly possible: by T cell function, gene probes and enzyme estimations on fetal blood, as well as female carrier detection in informative families by restriction fragment length polymorphism.

Table 19.1 Investigation, diagnosis, and treatment of specific immunodeficiencies

Dysfunction	Condition and relevant investigation	Treatment

T cell	SCID: 1.Lymphocytes: count <1 × 10^9/l
	  i T cells <25% of total (variable)
	  ii Reduced lymphocyte transformation response to stimulation e.g. to PHA
	2. Chest X-ray: small/absent thymus
		Early bone marrow transplant, if HLA identical 90% success, reduced to 50% if HLA non-identical

	ADA deficiency: adenosine deaminase detoxifies its substrate, an inhibitor of DNA synthesis	BMT is less sucessful, 50% and 25% for HLA and non-HLA identical
	'Bare lymphocyte' syndrome: lack of major histocompatability antigens on the T cells reduces antigen responses and antibody production	Antibiotic prophylaxis only, no specific treatment available
	Di George: T cells low in number and function, normal B cell function, Ig's, antibodies	Fetal thymus graft. Cardiac surgery (danger of GVHD if non-irradiated blood products are used at by-pass)
	WAS: small platelets, thrombocytopenia. Progressive lymphopenia in mid-childhood	BMT 80% success. Splenectomy helps (risk of infection increased)
	Ataxia telangiectasia: low IgG, IgE, absent IgA. Raised alpha fetoprotein, chromosomal breaks increased by irradiation	In selected cases i.v. Ig. No benefit from fetal thymus graft

B cell	Hypogammaglobulinaemia:
	1 Low serum immunoglobulin levels, must be repeated and related to age
	2 Lack of blood group antigens (IgM)
	3 No antibodies to *E. Coli*, vaccination
	
	  X linked — B cell function absent — T cell function normal
	  Common variable — B cell function low/normal — T cell function low in some
		i.v. IgG, 200–400 mg/kg every 2–3 weeks, aiming for serum IgG level of 5 g/l. Preferred to i.m. as easy to administer at home and severe anaphylactic reactions are rare

	Subclass deficiency: low IgG$_2$ in recurrent Pneumococcus, Haemophilus infections	Prophylactic antibiotic, selective i.v. IgG
Phagocytosis	Neutropenia: <1500 × 10^9/l, bone marrow. Isoantibodies to neutrophils present (like Rhesus)	Identify cause
	Cyclical neutropenia: repeated counts to identify periodicity	Surgical incision and drainage, prophylactic antibiotics
	Leukocyte adherence: target lysis by T cells reduced	BMT if prophylactic antibiotics fail
	Chronic granulomatous disease: reduced NBT, chemoluminescence, killing	Prophylactic co-trimoxazole. High dose antibiotics for infections. Incision and drainage of abscesses. Gamma interferon transfusion, BMT
	Hyperimmune IgE syndrome: IgE >4800 µg/l neutrophil movement impaired	H$_2$ antagonists
Complement	C1–C9, properdin. Screen for low or absent: 1 Classical pathway haemolytic activity (CH$_{50}$) 2 Alternative pathway haemolytic activity (AP$_{50}$) 3 Individual factors if 1 or 2 is low.	Penicillin prophylaxis

Further reading

Graham Watson J, Graham Bird A (1990) *Handbook of Immunological Investigations in Children.* London:Wright

Heaney M, (1990) The detection and management of primary immunodeficiency. In *Recent Advances in Paediatrics* vol. 9 T J David (ed). Edinburgh:Churchill Livingstone pp 21–39

Hong R (1990) Update on the immunodeficiency diseases. *American Journal of Diseases in Children,* **144**, 983–991

Pelham A, Kinnon C, Levinsky R J (1991) Prenatal diagnosis and carrier detection of inherited immunodeficiency disorders. *Pediatric Allergy and Immunology,* **1**, 51–59

Windebank K P (1990) The cytokines are coming. *Archives of Disease in Childhood,* **65**, 1283–1285

ALLERGY

Definition

A change in the immune response after exposure to an allergenic substance, be it environmental, drugs or constituent of one's own body.

Allergic disorders

Atopy

A term coined by Coka and Cooke for IgE mediated asthma, hay fever, and atopic eczema. Often familial, it clearly does not include all cases of asthma or atopic eczema, where other mechanisms may operate.

Prevalence 20% of the population, 12% asthma, 5% each hay fever and atopic eczema.

Incidence and severity increased over the past 20 years. Postulated causes: air pollution and ozone production by car exhaust gases.

More than one condition may coexist, e.g. 50% of atopic eczema have asthma, 80% of asthmatics have hay fever.

A family history of atopy is found in 70% of asthmatics.

Factors influencing the development of allergy in the predisposed infant include: the month of birth and aeroallergens in the environment, maternal diet during breast feeding, parental smoking, and an infant feeding regimen coupled with environmental allergen avoidance.

Identification of allergens

History, skin testing, serum radio-allergosorbent test (RAST) are often used. Less frequent are nasal instillation, and more hazardous, inhalation of allergens.

Skin testing, and correlation of results with other tests

Select antigens from the history. Skin test interpretation: see Table 19.2.

1. Skin tests in asthma and hay fever: house dust mite, *Aspergillus fumigatus*, animal dander of the house pet, mixed grass pollens and feathers will identify 90% of those who are reactive.

Table 19.2 Classification of hypersensitivity reactions (after Gell and Coombs)

Type, antibody, clinical onset	Reaction	Clinial examples in childhood	Investigations
Type I: IgE Onset immediate	Anaphylaxis Reagin (IgE) dependent: IgE binds to mast cells and eosinophils. They then release histamine and prostaglandin activators on contact with antigen	1 Anaphylaxis 2 Hay fever, asthma 3 Uticaria 4 Food allergy 5 Drug allergy, e.g. penicillin	IgE, Radio-aller-gosorbent test (RAST). Skin prick tests: weal of 3 mm or flare 10 mm larger than saline control is positive. For drugs use RAST, e.g. penicillin RAST
Type II: IgG/IgM Onset minutes to hours	Cytotoxic: IgG reacts with antigen bound to cell membrane $\rightarrow$ damage/lysis by complement activation.	1 Rhesus, ABO iso-immunization 2 Drug induced	Specific antibodies to Rhesus, A, B. Leucopenia, haemolytic. anaemia, thrombocytopenia
Type III: IgG, IgM Onset: hours to days	Circulating soluble immune complexes of antigen + antibody combine in the presence of complement to form microprecipitates damaging small blood vessels (Arthus phenomenon)	1 Post-streptococcal glomerulonephritis 2 Systemic lupus erythematosus 3 Erythema multiforme e.g. to sulphonamide 4 Serum sickness e.g. penicillin	Antibodies e.g. to streptococci, DNA. Low complement levels, low CH_{50}, and C3 or C4, whichever pathway is activated
Type IV: T cell Onset: days	Cell mediated or delayed hypersensitivity. Sensitized lymphocytes react with antigen fixed at a local site	1 Mantoux skin test 2 Rejection of transplant or graft 3 Drug: e.g. phenytoin lupus like reaction	Prior exposure to TB Lymphocyte HLA antigens. Biopsy of lymph gland

Table 19.3

Onset	Regression
1 Atopic eczema (after 3 months)	80% in the first year, 90% by 5 years, 90% of the remainder by adulthood
2 Asthma 50% by 3 years old	80% by adolescence. Hay fever tends to persist

Eosinophilia of $>0.5 \times 10^9/l$ and raised serum IgE found in most (70%) cases.

False positives are common, false negatives unusual. Correlation between skin tests and RAST is 80%.

Bronchial hyper-reactivity to the same allergen is only 50%.

2. In atopic dermatitis, prevalence of food allergy is at least 10–15%. Most common allergens are cows milk protein, eggs, wheat, fish, and nuts. False positive

skin tests are often found, RAST also. Oral challenge, if neccessary by 'single blind challenge', is the most reliable. Consistent response to three separate challenges is taken as proof positive. The danger of anaphylaxis during repeated challenge is small but real.

Principles of management

1. Allergen avoidance. This empiric approach is based on history and diary records, with some support from skin testing. Best results are obtained if there are only one or two allergens, usually identified from the history alone.

2. Hyposensitization. A procedure with significant morbidity and mortality, to be considered if a significant systemic reaction to an allergen has occurred e.g. bee sting, but not for hay fever.

3. Modification of trigger factors. Emotion can be a potent factor needing psychotherapy; smoking in the home should be avoided.

4. Medication Mast cell stabilizers, e.g. cromoglycate to conjunctivae, nose, or inhaled; antihistamines e.g. terfenadine for hay fever, and bronchodilators +/- steroids for asthma.

Individual conditions

Anaphylaxis

An IgE mediated type I hypersensitivity reaction.

Common causes

Antibiotics (e.g. penicillin, cephalosporins), food allergens (see above), X-ray contrast media, bee or wasp sting.

1. Immediate, within minutes.
    - Skin: itch, urticaria and angioedema.
    - Respiratory: bronchospasm, laryngeal oedema.
    - Cardiovascular: tachycardia, hypotension.
    - Gastrointestinal: vomiting, diarrhoea, abdominal pain.
2. Delayed phenomenon, 2–48 h after the immediate reaction. → Generalised anaphylaxis, as above.

Management

1. Adrenaline subcutaneously, 10 µg/kg of 1 in 1000 = 0.01 ml/kg, maximum dose 0.4 ml, may repeat every 15 minutes.
2. Oxygen, nebulized salbutamol 2.5 mg, i.v. aminophylline 4 mg/kg for bronchospasm, consider IPPV.
3. Maintain blood pressure by i.v. plasma expander, and dopamine 2.5–5.0 µg/kg/minute.

4. Antihistamine: chlorpheniramine maleate 0.2 mg/kg i.m./i.v./orally 4–6 hourly for up to 2 days to minimize the delayed phenomenon.
   Note how steroids play no part.

Hay fever

Definition

Congestion of nasal mucosa, conjunctiva, venous congestion under the eyes, transverse nasal crease secondary to repeatedly rubbing the nose (allergic salute). Nasal turbinates pale and oedematous, best seen with an ear speculum.

Seasonal (grasses, trees) intermittent (periods of high humidity and warmth increase fungal spores; exposure e.g. to cats) or perennial (house dust mite).

Asthma

See Respiratory problems.

Atopic eczema

See Dermatological problems.

Food and drink reactions: allergy, intolerance or aversion?

1. Allergy: immunologically mediated, immediate anaphylactoid or delayed >1 h. Commonly to milk, egg, wheat, nuts, fish, soy.
2. Intolerance: chemical (e.g. histamine release from cheese), enzymatic (e.g. lactase deficiency).
3. Aversion: psychological base in the child, or parent as a form of Munchausen by proxy.

Examples

1. Cows' milk protein (CMP) intolerance

Incidence

1–3%.

Clinical

Primary, within a week of starting CMP feeds, or secondary to infective diarrhoea.

Symptoms vary from acute anaphylaxis (IgE mediated) through failure to thrive (malabsorption, colitis, protein losing enteropathy), gastrointestinal bleeding, to rhinitis and skin rashes. Atopy often present.

Controversial cause of colicky infants: one study found up to 25% may show improvement on CMP exclusion diet, including mother's diet if breast fed.

No proven link with serous otitis media, and rarely the sole cause of wheeze. No proven benefit from CMP exclusion in these conditions.

Investigations

Eosinophilia, positive skin prick test in 25%. Lacking in sensitivity or specificity are IgE milk antibodies and RAST.

Diagnosis

Rests on milk challenge, conducted in hospital if anaphylaxis thought likely.

Day 1: 10, 20, 30, and 60 ml cows' milk fed at 30–minute intervals.
Day 2: 120 ml and day 3, 240 ml as a single morning dose. Normal intake thereafter if no immediate response, but waiting for a delayed response for up to a week.
Rechallenge every 6–12 months to see if it is outgrown.

Differential diagnosis

Gastrointestinal, respiratory or urinary tract infection, coeliac disease, cystic fibrosis, lactose intolerance, immunodeficiency.

Prognosis

30% tolerate milk within 2 years, but 20% may take 6 or more years. Prone to atopic disease, even if they become milk tolerant.

2. Atopic eczema

At least 10% of eczema sufferers benefit from allergen avoidance. Infection and heat play a part in exacerbations. Skin or RAST tests are *unhelpful* in constructing exclusion diets.

Stage 1: colouring and preservatives: exclude colourings (azo-dyes) and preservatives (benzoates), cows' milk, egg, wheat, fish for an initial period of 4 weeks. If successful, continue, reintroducing potential allergens one each week. May take up to 2 years to achieve tolerance.
Stage 2: few food diet: in more severe cases may only respond to extreme exclusion by special 'hypoallergic' diet comprising lamb, rice, cauliflower, pears and bottled water. Claims are made that this treatment plan is successful in food intolerance, rhinitis, migraine, seizures, hyperactive behaviour; any benefit is generally short lived.

Prophylaxis

Breast feeding is no longer considered reliably protective against atopic eczema, though it may benefit babies with an elevated cord IgE.

3. Urticaria

Most episodes are acute, occasionally chronic, and recurrent. No cause is found in up to 80%. Antihistamines and systemic steroids are indicated according to severity, and allergen avoidance if the cause is identifiable:

  i   IgE mediated: bee/wasp stings, drugs (e.g. penicillin), foods (e.g. shellfish, milk, eggs) some viral and bacterial infections.
  ii Leukotrienes by activation of the arachidonic acid pathway: foods, food colourings, and salicylates.
  iii Histamine release from mast cells and basophils:

  • by morphine, bacterial toxins.
  • by physical agents cold, sun, pressure, sweat etc.

  iv Complement mediated: recurrent angioedema due to C1 esterase inhibitor deficiency is AD, and shows as a low C4 serum complement. Triggered by injury and infection, the swelling involves deep tissues, and may affect the airway. Confirm the diagnosis by enzyme assay. Tranexamic acid and danazol are helpful.

4. Asthma

Food triggers include not only allergens (e.g. egg, chocolate, peanuts), but also intolerance to chemicals (e.g. tartrazine) and physical agents (e.g. ice, acid colas or orange squash). Commoner in Asian children. (See Respiratory problems.)

Drug Allergy

Antibiotics

May occur in first apparent exposure, but must have been previously sensitized e.g. through antibiotics in milk or vaccines.

Overdiagnosed, alternative possibilities include:

1. Rash: underlying infection (e.g. measles, rubella), colouring agent (tartrazine) or preservative (benzoic acid).
2. Loose stools: viral infection, altered flora especially *Clostridium difficile* overgrowth in pseudomembranous colitis.
3. Other medication or antibiotic (parents often report 'penicillin prescribed').

Ampicillin associated non-allergic maculopapular rash may appear a week after starting treatment.

Adverse reactions

Hazardous to repeat dose if:

1. Immediate and accelerated reaction occurs within 1–72 h comprising laryngeal oedema, urticaria, wheeze, anaphylaxis.

2. Late reaction >72 h later, includes a maculopapular rash, urticaria, serum sickness, erythema multiforme, haemolytic anaemia, thrombocytopenia, neutropenia.

Action

1. Treat anaphylaxis.
2. Assess which medication is the most likely cause.
3. Readministration?

   - antibody tests unhelpful clinically.
   - avoid cross-reaction e.g. penicillins-cephalosporins.
   - if essential (e.g. penicillin in endocarditis) give orally before i.v., in progressive doses; risk of anaphylaxis is ever present.

Non-steroidal anti-inflammatory drugs (NSAID)

Aspirin and other NSAID cause angioedema, asthma.

Further reading

Hill D J, Hosking C S (1990) Cow's milk allergy. *Recent Advances in Paediatrics* vol 9 (T J David, ed.) Edinburgh:Churchill Livingstone pp 187–206

Leader (1989) Penicillin allergy in childhood. *Lancet*, i, 420

Warner J O (1985) Allergies in childhood. *Progress in Child Health* vol 2. (J A Macfarlane ed.) Edinburgh:Churchill Livingstone pp 63–76.

Chapter 20

Infectious disease problems

The downward trend in deaths from infectious disease continues for the present. Increasing numbers of immunocompromised children from HIV and chemotherapy may reverse this. Doubtless, many deaths and much morbidity remains preventable. Delay in diagnosis for lack of specific signs, and sudden overwhelming of the body systems in infancy remain the greatest obstacle.

PATHOPHYSIOLOGY

The competence of the immune system is essential to survival (see Immunology). It has become increasingly evident that once the process of defence has been initiated, the symptoms, signs and complications of many disease states are more often the result of the body's reactions to these mechanisms than the infection which triggered it.

Taking septic shock as an example: bacterial infection results in triggering of inflammation. The production of exotoxins, endotoxins, and activation of the specific and non-specific defences result in a triad of adversity: increased vascular permeability, vasoconstriction/vasodilatation, and microthrombosis.

Table 20.1 Mortality from infectious disease UK 1987 (source: OPCS)

	Under 1 year	1–4 years	5–9 years	Total
1 Respiratory infection: pneumonia, acute bronchitis/bronchiolitis	210	51	14	275
2 Meningococcal infection	53	40	9	102
3 Meningitis	40	33	4	77
4 Viral, including CNS	32	23	12	67
5 Septicaemia	25	5	6	36
6 Diarrhoea	14	3	1	18

Others, at no particular age band: Chickenpox 7, measles, viral hepatitis 5, pertussis 4, herpes simplex 3, tuberculosis 1

Clinical trials

1. Dexamethasone in haemophilus meningitis given 20 minutes prior to antibiotics has shown a reduction in tumour necrosis factor α and interleukin-1β, and in the relative risk of deafness and neurological sequalae by a factor of four.
   Controversy: similar benefits may occur in cerebral malaria (see below).
2. Monoclonal antibodies to endotoxins (to prevent activation of the non-specific defences), and tumour necrosis factor, show promise.

Further reading

Levin M (1990) The inflammatory response to infections. In *Infection in the Newborn*. (J de Louvois and D Harvey, eds.) Bristol:John Wiley. A comprehensive review of the mechanisms involved.
Odio C M, Faingezicht I, Paris M, *et al*, (1991) The beneficial effects of early dexamethasone administration in infants and children with bacterial meningitis. *New England Journal of Medicine*, **324**, 1525–1231
Ziegler E J, Fisher C J, Sprung C L, *et al*, (1991) Treatment of Gram-negative bacteraemia and septic shock with HA-1A human monoclonal antibody against endotoxin. *New England Journal of Medicine*, **324**, 429–436

Table 20.2

Pathophysiological response	*Postulated mechanisms*
1 Increased vascular permeability → reduced blood volume, venous return and so cardiac output	A strong negative charge normally present on the endothelial lining is neutralized by strong cations released by inflammation
2 Changed vasomotor tone	
i Vasoconstriction increases resistance to perfusion of both systemic and pulmonary circulations	Prostaglandins and leukotrienes are powerful vasoconstrictors and dilators
ii Vasodilatation leads to peripheral pooling, reduced perfusion and venous return. Cardiac output fails	Vasodilatation is an effect of prostacyclin
3 Microvascular obstruction of organs from deposition of fibrin and platelets. If widespread becomes disseminated intravascular coagulation	Thromboxane encourages platelet aggregation. Prostacyclin is an effective vasodilator, and is being used in severe sepsis to reduce the consequences of this deposition

MANAGEMENT OF INFANTS SUSPECTED OF INFECTION

1. In the community

  i Most infections are minor, coryzal, and require advice on temperature reduction and an antipyretic. If a source of infection is identified, e.g. pharyngitis, otitis media, an antibiotic may be appropriate.
  ii Early recognition of the acutely ill infant in the community by parents and family practitioners is an essential first step to bringing the individual for paediatric assessment and reducing morbidity and mortality.

    a. Advise regular observation and temperature taking 4 hourly. Stress that in the neonate a subnormal temperature is of greater significance than fever.

    b. Draw parents' attention to 'sinister' signs being an indication for urgent medical attention: e.g. continuous inconsolable crying for >2 h, rapid breathing when at rest, seizure, excessive drowsiness, purpuric rash. Low accuracy limit their usefulness.

    c. A more comprehensive approach is the Baby Check 19 point scoring system, with claims of a high sensitivity and specificity, for use by parents and family practitioners.

    d. If referral to hospital is likely, avoid antibiotics except in the case of suspected meningococcaemia, when penicillin should be given i.m. immediately.

2. In the Accident and Emergency Department

    i Sick. Evaluation for focus of infection. If no focus is found, blood culture and urine (clean catch or suprapubic) should be obtained for culture, and in an ill infant an LP must be considered. Admit.

    ii Pyrexial, no focus clinically, but well enough to go home. Consideration has to be given to prescribing a broad spectrum antibiotic. Given 'blind' i.e. before the results of culture could be available, results in lowering the septicaemia rate, without masking possible urinary tract infection and the need for further investigation.

Further reading

Hewson P H, Humphries S M, Roberton D M, McNamara J M, Robinson M J (1990) Markers of serious illness in infants under 6 months old presenting to a children's hospital. *Archives of Disease in Childhood*, **65**, 750–756

Morley C J, Thornton A J, Cole T J, Hewson P H, Fowler M A (1991) Baby check: a scoring system to grade the severity of acute sytemic illness in babies under 6 months old. *Archives of Disease in Childhood*, **66** (a series of articles, pp 100–120)

DIFFERENTIAL DIAGNOSIS OF RASH, USUALLY WITH FEVER

The three main categories are purpuric, maculopapular and papulovesicular. The acute exanthemata of childhood comprise the majority, but an awareness of other important causes is essential.

1. Purpura with fever

Generalized distribution

First thought must be meningococcaemia!

  i Common–Septicaemia: meningococcaemia, *Haemophilus influenzae*, Group A β-haemolytic streptococcus, pneumococcus.

  ii Relatively unusual and mild – Viral: rubella, measles, varicella, ECHO 9 and coxsackie A9, respiratory syncytial virus.

  iii Unusual–Haematological: idiopathic thrombocytopenia, leukaemia.

Localized or circumscribed distribution

  i Child abuse: distribution over the limbs, face, buttocks; the presence of grip marks, linear bruises.

  ii Anaphylactoid (Henoch-Schönlein) purpura: erythema and purpura over extensor surfaces, joint swelling, abdominal pain, haematuria.

  iii Venous congestion → purpura on head and neck: e.g. cough caused by pertussis.

  iv From the appropriate geographical area, typhus (trunk) and Rickettsial spotted fever, (palms and soles). Both are maculopapular and purpuric.

Management

Generalized purpura: cefotaxime is now the first line antibiotic in hospital. Delay may be fatal. Both meningococcal and Haemophilus infection present similarly, and penicillin resistance to the former is now appearing.

Leucocytosis and/or increased band forms and C reactive protein are supportive. Bacterial and viral studies may eventually determine the pathogen.

2. Maculopapular rash with fever

  i Viral

    a. Measles and rubella, less frequent through MMR vaccination, coxsackie and ECHO becoming relatively more common.

    b. Mild fever, slapped cheek sign with parvovirus B19 (previously called 5th disease).

    c. The rash of roseola appears as the fever abates.

    d. Pityriasis rosea (rotavirus?): no fever, but if intercurrent temperature occurs it could cause confusion. Herald patch is followed by more generalized itchy papules. Lasts 2–12 months.

  ii Bacterial

    a. Meningococcaemia before the onset of purpura.

    b. Scarlet fever's circumoral pallor is distinctive.

  iii Kawasaki disease: strict criteria for diagnosis.

  iv Drug rash, e.g. ampicillin (especially with infectious mononucleosis).

  v Erythema multiforme: rash, may develop target lesions; Stevens Johnson syndrome also includes stomatitis, conjunctivitis, urethritis. Secondary to herpes simplex, *Mycoplasma pneumoniae*, enteroviruses, as well as drugs.

Assessment

  i Contact history, medication taken.
  ii Prodromal history useful:

    a. High fever: roseola 2–5 days, Kawasaki disease 5 days.
    b. Coryzal: measles.
    c. Sore throat, vomiting: scarlet fever, toxic shock, Kawasaki, rickettsia.
    d. Influenza-like: meningococcaemia, rickettsia.
    e. None: usually in rubella, 5th disease, enteroviruses, (drug rash or toxic erythema may simulate any of the above, but are generally afebrile).

  iii Rash: spread and distribution are helpful.

    a. From head downwards: measles, rubella.
    b. Flexor surfaces becoming generalized: scarlet fever also desquamates 1–2 weeks later.
    c. Central (trunk)
    spread to limbs and face in roseola.
    swollen hands and feet early, peeling after 1–3 weeks, in Kawasaki disease.
    oedema of face and limbs and peeling in staphylococcal scalded skin, toxic shock.

    (If from abroad, consider rickettsial spotted fever even though a tick bite may not be evident.)
  iv Characteristic signs e.g. Koplik's spots in measles, slapped cheek in 5th disease, tonsillitis, lymphadenopathy and splenomegaly in infectious mononucleosis, strawberry tongue in scarlet fever.

Investigations

Depending on severity of illness and likely cause, throat swab and viral antibody titres, blood culture +/– CSF if appropriate.

3. Vesicular eruptions

Differentiation between small vesicles and larger blisters (bullae) is helpful.

Table 20.3 Differentiation between vesicles and bullae

Vesicular	*Bullous (>1 cm diameter)*
1. Acute viral: herpes simplex, zoster/ chickenpox, hand foot and mouth	1. Bacterial, e.g. bullous impetigo, Gram negative septicaemia, scalded skin syndrome
2. Insect bite: papular urticaria, scabies	2. Chemical: plants, medication e.g. barbiturate
3. Chronic viral: molluscum contagiosum	3. Burns: accidental and non-accidental, sun.
	4. Skin disorders, e.g. erythema multiforme (due to herpes simplex, *Mycoplasma pneumoniae*), and chronic bullous diseases of childhood.

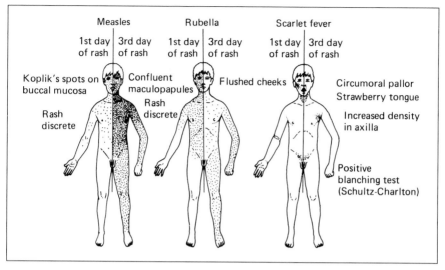

Figure 20.1 Difference in appearance, distribution and progression of rashes of measles, rubella, scarlet fever. (From *Infectious Diseases of Children* (eds Krugman S, Katz S L, Gershon A A, Wilfert C) (1985) 8th edition Mosby: St Louis p 457)

PERSISTENT FEVER

A distinction must be made between one episode, (albeit with 1–2 days of normal temperature), from discrete episodes perceived by the family as continuous, or so called 'pseudo fever of unknown origin', a stable mate of unexplained lethargy/myalgic encephalopathy.

Pyrexia of unknown origin

Definition

A fever of 38.5°C for 2 weeks, (or a week documented in hospital and reportedly at home), in which a careful initial assessment fails to find a cause. The pattern of fever is generally unreliable.

Causes

Common conditions occur commonly!

1. Infection 50%:

   i 'Viral' 40% including infectious mononucleosis, hepatitis.
  ii Bacteraemia: in order of frequency,
      Common   Urinary tract infection.
                  Pneumonia (especially mycoplasma).
                  Upper respiratory: sinusitis, chronic pharyngitis.

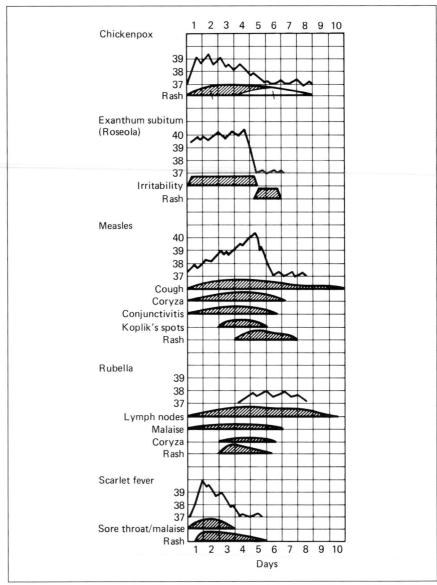

Figure 20.2 Diagnostic clinical features of 5 commoner infections causing a rash. From *Manual on Infections and Immunisations in Children* (Rudd P, Nicoll A, eds) (1991) 2nd edn Oxford University Press:Oxford p 14

Uncommon TB.
              Septic arthritis.
              Typhoid fever.
              Lyme disease.
              Endocarditis.
Rare   Brucellosis, listeriosis.

  iii Foreign travel: typhoid, malaria, TB, Lyme disease, typhus, brucellosis (see below).

2. Connective tissue disorders (15%): juvenile chronic arthritis, rheumatic fever, systemic lupus erythematosus.
3. Malignancy (7%): leukaemia, lymphoma, neuroblastoma, sarcoma.
4. Inflammatory bowel disease (4%): Crohn's, ulcerative colitis.
5. Undiagnosed 12%: many resolving by the time of presentation.
6. Uncommon important: Munchausen by proxy (factitious fever), drugs, Kawasaki disease.

Clinical pointers

Importance of history, (infectious contacts, foreign travel, medication) and examination: together suggest/indicate diagnosis in 60% prior to any test.

Investigations

1. Initially: urine microscopy and culture, chest X-ray and Mantoux, blood cultures, FBC, blood film, and thick film if from a malarial zone. ESR. First serum for viral antibodies, Paul Bunnell.
2. Fever persists: repeat WBC, differential, blood culture, ESR; typhoid, paratyphoid, brucella agglutinations, second viral serum 10 days after the first. Bone marrow for malignancy + culture for TB.
3. Negative results after this may indicate: bone scan, lymph node biopsy for malignancy, serology for connective tissue disease. Consider factitious fever.

Progress

Fever pattern and response to antipyretics are unreliable indicators of cause or severity of the disease. Repeated review and time reveal (almost) all!

Further reading

Pizzo P A, Lovejoy F H, Smith D H (1975) Prolonged fever in children: review of 100 cases. *Pediatrics*, **55**, 468–473
McCarthy P L, Lembo R M, Baron M A *et al* (1985) Predictive value of abnormal physical examination findings in ill-appearing and well-appearing febrile children. *Pediatrics*, **74**, 167–171

SUSPECTED INFECTION AFTER FOREIGN TRAVEL BY A CHILD, OR A FOREIGN VISITOR IN CONTACT WITH A CHILD

The first step is knowledge of the countries visited and duration there, or arrival of a visitor from abroad capable of passing on an illness.

Tropical infections often come in twos, so finding one should not necessarily halt further investigation, especially if symptoms persist.

Infections range from common in UK e.g. rotavirus, Campylobacter, through unusual, e.g. TB, to rare, e.g. polio, diphtheria, or only from abroad e.g. rabies, malaria.

1. Fever: from Asia or Africa consider:

    i Malaria no matter how long ago the travel and despite taking prophylaxis.
    ii Typhoid, hepatitis A (or B if injected, or transfused while abroad), meningo-coccus. A rash may be present (also consider Dengue haemorrhagic fever virus).
    iii TB.

2. Diarrhoea.

    i Acute onset: viral, commonly Campylobacter, *E. coli*, dysenteric organisms.
    ii Persistent diarrhoea with abdominal pain is suggestive of *Giardia lamblia*, with mucus +/- blood in amoebiasis.
    iii Worm infestation is often asymptomatic.

3. Fever + neurological symptoms: polio, falciparum malaria, typhoid, rabies.
4. Fever + sore throat: common infection likely but diphtheria must be remembered.
5. Fever + jaundice: viral hepatitis; with pallor in malaria; varies from 'flu-like symptoms to a shocked state in yellow fever.

The variability in symptoms must be born in mind when considering the infection control consequences.

Chronic fatigue syndrome with preceding febrile illness

A not uncommon condition in late childhood or early adolescence, of unknown cause, after an influenza-like illness. Girls>boys. Duration for 6 months before hospital referral is common.

Hypotheses as to pathophysiology

Viral infection. Serology/culture positive for Epstein-Barr virus (EBV), Coxsackie B, herpes virus type 6, VPI antigen, among others.

Postulates: chronic as a result of persistence, or reactivation, of infection, or exaggerated/abnormal immunological response.

Psychiatric illness, even in those with positive EBV serology, found in at least one study. Secondary gains may be useful to the sufferer.

Clinical

Previously well, the child becomes lethargic, unable to sustain concentration or effort. Headaches, dizziness and muscle weakness are precipitated by exertion. Sore throat, slight fever, mild lymphadenopathy, and arthralgia are common. Often tired on waking despite long sleep. Symptoms persist for days or weeks at a time, and a cycle of relapse and recovery is established.

Diagnosis

Prominent diagnostic features: reduced activity for 6 months, prolonged school absence, normal weight gain and laboratory investigations. Occasionally related to change of schools, other stress or a family history of similarly affected siblings.

Differential diagnosis

Infection (bacterial, HIV, toxoplasmosis etc); psychiatric illness; chronic inflammatory disease of bowel, joints, connective tissue; malignancy; endocrine disorders; drug dependency.

Management

After careful history and complete examination, check ESR, FBC, tests for infectious mononucleosis, Mantoux, urinalysis and urine culture if not already done.

Reassurances of normality (the parents have doubtless already had them) must be accompanied by discussion of underlying concerns and followed by a graduated programme of activities and schooling. If too rapid, relapse may follow. So much time may have been lost that extra help in the classroom may be required. Physiotherapy is valuable. Antidepressants are rarely required.

Prognosis

Many months and often more than one medical opinion before resolution.

Further reading

Kleiman M B (1982) The complaint of persistent fever. Recognition and management of pseudo fever of unknown origin. *Pediatric Clinics of North America*, **29**, 201–219
Smith M S, Mitchell J, Corey L, *et al* (1991) Chronic fatigue in adolescents. *Pediatrics*, **88**, 195–202

Infection in the immunocompromised

E.g. Primary, secondary to HIV, immunosuppressives, malnutrition.

Organisms

1. Naturally occurring viruses: measles, chickenpox (VZ), herpes simplex (HS) and cytomegalovirus (CMV).

2. Vaccine related: live polio and BCG.
3. Grafted organ/blood contaminated by cytomegalovirus. (Also spread naturally and by sexual contact). Clinically 6–12 weeks after transplant/transfusion: fever, hepatitis, retinitis, pneumonia, diarrhoea, leucopenia.
4. Bacteria: Gram negative organisms, e.g. pseudomonas, coliforms, *Staphylococcus aureus*, *Staphylococcus epidermidis* (especially with indwelling catheters), TB, atypical mycobacteria.
5. Fungi: candida or aspergillus infection of the mouth and/or anus, pneumonia, meningitis.
6. Protozoa

    i *Pneumocystis carinii* pneumonia (PCP).
    ii Cryptosporidiosis. Protracted diarrhoea.

Commoner presentations

1. Fever: in some, the only sign of potentially overwhelming bacterial or viral sepsis, and always requires careful evaluation. A single flick of temperature in the neutropenic is usually sufficient indication for treatment (see below).
2. Pneumonia: usual signs, but rapidly progressive. Chest X-ray: widespread infiltrates spreading from the hilar region, progressing to consolidation. PCP, CMV, TB, candida.
3. Gastrointestinal

    i Dysphagia/sore mouth: Candida.
    ii Vomiting, severe diarrhoea: cryptosporidiosis, *Giardia lamblia*, Campylobacter, *Clostridium difficile*.

4. Arthritis affecting one or more large joints.
5. Meningitis.
6. Skin: furunculosis, candida of the nails.

Investigation

Cultures: blood cultures from all lines and peripherally × 2, urine, skin lesions, faeces, CSF if clinically indicated. Viral swabs, blood for virology baseline sample, vesicular fluid for HS, HZ. Fungal cultures. Consider lung biopsy or bronchial lavage for PCP. Chest X-ray and FBC are helpful.

Management

1. Avoid contact with exanthema, cold sores.
2. Prophylaxis

    i Co-trimoxazole during chemotherapy, in HIV positive infants and AIDS.
    ii Immunoglobulin therapy.

        a. In hypogammaglobulinaemias and, recently, in HIV.
        b. After contact: measles – gamma globulin 0.5–1.5 ml/kg; VZ – hyperimmune zoster immunoglobulin.

3. Vigorous antimicrobial treatment to cover likely pathogens:

   i   3rd generation cephalosporin/piperacillin + gentamycin +metranidazole.
   ii Antifungal if Candida in nose, mouth, or antigens present in the blood.
   iii Co-trimoxazole against pneumocystis if pneumonic and not already on it.
   iv Acyclovir (herpes group: VZ, HS, CMV) for lesions of HS, VZ, with septi-
       caemia, pneumonia, aseptic meningitis, or chickenpox despite zoster immu-
       noglobulin.
   v   Antibiotic for infections normally allowed to run their course, e.g. in persist-
       ent cryptosporidiosis, use spiramycin.

Duration, and change of treatment depends on results and response, re-assessed
at 3 days, and is rarely less than 2 weeks. Amphotericin may be added empirically
after fever >5 days on treatment without positive cultures, and checking for Candida.
4. 'Rescue' granulocyte infusions in neutropenics with resistant septicaemia and
   deep tissue infection not responding to antibiotics.

MENINGITIS

Definition

Inflammation of the meninges due to infection; rarely, chemical, cytotoxic drugs,
sympathetic response to local inflammation or malignancy.

Bacterial meningitis

Epidemiology in the UK

Incidence

Neonatal 1 in 500, progressive decline throughout childhood. Commoner in winter.

Organisms

1. Neonatal: Group B β-haemolytic streptococcus, coliforms, *Listeria monocytogenes*.
2. 4–12 weeks old: neonatal or those found in older ages, i.e. overlap.
3. Post neonatal:

   i   *Haemophilus influenzae* type B (Hib), commonest up to 2 years rarely after 5
       years.
   ii *Neisseria meningitidis* next most common, from one month to 5 years, and
       commonest in late childhood and adolescence.
   iii *Streptococcus pneumoniae* is third, most common in adolescents and adults

Table 20.4 CSF findings in intracranial infection

	WBC (mm³)	Protein (g/l)	CSF glucose
1 Normal:			
i Neonatal	<30	0.2–1.7 (3.0 in prems)	>50% blood glucose (BG)
ii Older ages	<5	0.2–0.4	>66% (BG)
2 Cells: polymorphonuclears predominate			
Acute bacterial	>100, often 1000s	0.5–5.0	<66% BG, often <2 mmol/l
3 Cells: either polymorphonuclears or lymphocytes predominate			
i Partially treated bacterial	Variable, Any number	>0.2	Normal or low
ii Brain abscess	10–200	0.3–5.0	Normal
4 Cells: polymorphonuclears predominate very early on, later lymphocytes predominate			
i Viral	25–1000	0.5–2.0	Normal, low in 20% of mumps
ii TB meningitis*	10–500 >If CSF block	0.1–2.5	<2 mmol/l
iii Fungal	25–500	0.25–2.0	Normal

* CSF Spider web clot occasionally, bacilli rarely found on ZN stain.
  CSF glucose also low in medulloblastoma, CNS leukaemia

Pathophysiology

Entry due to bacteraemia, occasionally locally via sinuses or fracture, or site of infection elsewhere, e.g. pneumonia, abscess. Direct extension from otitis media is probably rare.

Exudate over the brain, and ventriculitis, may cause obstructive hydrocephalus in addition to damage from cortical thromboses, hypoxaemia, bacterial toxins and bacterial invasion. Atrophy follows.

See pathophysiology of septicaemia.

At special risk

1. Sickle cell: *S. pneumoniae*, salmonella.
2. i.v. lines.
3. Neurosurgical procedures, shunts: coagulase negative Staphylococcus.
4. Burns, cachectic.
5. Immunocompromised.

Age at infection, likely pathogen and clinical course

1. Neonatal

Organisms: Group B streptococcus (GBS) 25%, *Escherichia coli* with K1 antigen, 17% other Gram–negative organisms, *Listeria monocytogenes* 5%.

Factors: low birthweight, maternal colonization by GBS.

Clinical

1. Early onset (<7days old): as part of a septicaemia, with shock, respiratory illness, jaundice.
2. Late onset (>7 days old): feeding poorly, shrill cry, apnoea, seizures.

   Non-specific but useful sign in the neonatal period is temperature instability. Infrequent signs (in delayed diagnosis?): bulging fontanelle, neck stiffness.

Investigation

1. LP mandated, but may be delayed if very sick. Even neonates can cone! CSF
   i Gram stain: 50% positive. ii Culture. iii Latex agglutination for GBS.
2. Blood culture, urine culture, swabs for microbiology, FBC, platelets, coagulation, blood and urine osmolality and electrolytes.
3. Monitor for hypoglycaemia and hyponatraemia (common), hypocalcaemia.
4. Head circumference at diagnosis, daily during admission. Rapid growth requires head US for early hydrocephalus.

Management
CSF penetration: Good, with inflammation, for ampicillin and third generation cephalosporins, poor for aminoglycosides.
   Initial antibiotic, either combination suitable:

1. Cefotaxime for *E.coli*, GBS (or ceftazidime where Pseudomonas suspected) + ampicillin for Listeria.
2. Ampicillin + gentamicin: if Listeria (the two antibiotics may act synergistically), GBS, Gram negative organisms suspected.

   LP is repeated after 48–72 h to check on CSF sterility; do drug levels and consider a change of antibiotic if not clearing.
   Administration i.v. for 2 weeks for GBS and other Gram positives, 3 weeks for Gram negatives after CSF cultures become sterile, changing to the most effective drug according to bacterial sensitivity tests.
   Hazards to be avoided:

   i Chloramphenicol, despite good CSF penetration: potentially toxic in the neonate (grey baby syndrome) and erratic levels if phenobarbitone is also administered.
   ii Intrathecal adminstration of gentamicin, to overcome poor CSF pentration: death and neurological complications commoner than if only given systemically.

Prognosis
Mortality:
   Early onset 20–50% (GBS, *E. coli*)
   Late onset 10–20% (GBS, *E. coli*, Staphylococcus, Pseudomonas, Klebsiella).
   Morbidity 50%, severe in 30% of survivors, related to rate of clearance of infection as reflected in CSF. Comprises mental handicap, seizures, hydrocephalus, cerebral palsy, deafness, blindness.

2. >3months

In the UK the meningoccocus (B:15 commonest, then A and C) now second to *H. influenzae* type B (Hib), while *S. pneumoniae* is isolated in only 15%.

Clinical Fever, irritability, headache, lethargy, vomiting, photophobia.
  Meningism unreliably present under 18 months.
  Seizures.
  Purpura: meningococcus, ECHO, Hib.
  Meningitis present in 50% of those with a meningococcal rash.
  Coma from cerebral oedema may lead to death from transtentorial herniation of the brainstem. Shock due to the latter, or endotoxic shock.

Investigation Early diagnosis alters prognosis. LP every first fit with fever under 18 months, unless very sure you are dealing with a simple febrile convulsion.
  CSF Gram stain positive in 90%, blood culture in 50%. Blood and urine as for <3 month old group.
  Coma, decerebration or papilloedema (a late sign) a contraindication to LP. Best start treatment and do latex particle agglutination for Hib, GBS, and meningococcus on CSF obtained at LP after the child's condition has stabilized. CT scan helpful if available.
  LP hazardous in meningococcaemia. One may assume seeding of meninges has occurred as this is the case in 50%.

Management Antibiotic for 10 days.

1. Traditional. Ampicillin + chloramphenicol cover the 3 major organisms. 20% of *H. influenzae* strains resistant to ampicillin, rarely to chloramphenicol. Change to the most effective single antibiotic once sensitivities are known.
2. Single agent. Cefotaxime is the preferred third generation cephalosporin at present. (Ceftriaxone, requiring only a once daily dose, may become available in the UK). Effective against *N. meningitidis*, *H. influenzae* (including β-lactamase producing strains), *S. pneumoniae*, *E. coli*, proteus, klebsiella: good levels in CSF, safe, non-toxic, no resistance yet reported. Especially useful in partially treated meningitis when the organism is usually not identifiable on Gram stain.
   After *H. influenzae*, eliminate possible persistent carriage with rifampicin as for chemoprophylaxis.

Controversy Dexamethasone administration. To date shown to reduce the duration of fever, and frequency of neurological complications including severe deafness (from 14% to 1% in Hib). Even greater effect if commencement precedes the antibiotic. Dose 0.15 mg/kg every 6 hours for 4 days.

Management applicable to meningitis at all ages

1. Shock and disseminated intravascular consumption in 10%.
   Monitor peripheral perfusion, BP, and central venous pressure if shocked. Immediately set up i.v. line, give albumin and fresh frozen plasma. Volume required in septic shock may be up to 60 ml/kg in the first hour, 120 ml/kg in the first 6 hours.
2. Cerebral oedema.
   i After correcting hypovolaemia, fluid restrict to 60% of normal requirements to avoid hyponatraemia (due to inappropriate ADH secretion, so maintain osmolality 280–300 mOsm/kg water).

ii Consider mannitol, and mechanical hyperventilation to lower P_aCO_2. Intra-cranial pressure monitoring is increasingly used, especially in older children.

3. Seizures occur in 20–30%. Diazepam immediately, and to prevent recurrence, phenytoin (10 mg/kg via nasogastric tube or i.v. (not im)) or phenobarbitone, loading dose 20 mg/kg followed by 5 mg/day 24 h later.
4. Monitor for and treat:
   Hypoxia from apnoea, hypoventilation.
   Hyperpyrexia.
   Subdural effusions (especially in *Haemophilus influenzae*).
5. Partially treated meningitis: previous exposure to antibiotic alters the CSF total WBC and culture, though not the differential count, glucose and protein. Treat as for full blown meningitis.
6. Investigate fever persisting beyond 10 days, which occurs in 10%.
   Causes, in order of frequency:

   i Intercurrent viral infection.
   ii Thrombophlebitis.
   iii Immune complex disease.
   iv Drug fever.
   v Abscess, subdural effusion.

7. Indications for a repeat LP. (CT before LP if a mass lesion is suspected):

   i Failure to improve.
   ii After improving, the development of a seizure or focal neurological signs.
   iii Fever for 10 days.
   iv Less than 3 months old.

Prognosis outside the neonatal period

Mortality 5–10%.

Deafness 10%. Always arrange hearing test for one month after discharge from hospital.

Other neurological sequelae in 10–20%: epilepsy, school problems, mental handicap, blindness, cerebral palsy.

Partially treated meningitis has a similar prognosis, after diagnosis and appropriate treatment.

Chemoprophylaxis

1. Meningococcal infection. Offered to all household contacts, classmates, kissing or mouth to mouth resuscitation contact. Rifampicin 10 mg/kg twice daily for 2 days.
2. *Haemophilus influenzae* B (Hib):
   All household members.
   Playgroup contacts under 4 years old where two cases of invasive Hib disease occur within 120 days.
   Rifampicin 20 mg/kg once daily for 4 days, to a maximum of 600mg.
   Exceptions: pregnant and nursing mothers, or hepatic impairment.

3. Remember administration to index case to prevent persistent carriage.

Vaccination has a limited role at present.

1. Only effective against A and C meningococcal strains, whereas 60% of cases are due to B.
2. Conjugated Hib vaccine introduction 1992/3 (see Community). Administration at times of DPT vaccination.

Tuberculous meningitis

Due to haematogenous spread from other site, e.g. chest, gland, miliary (see end of Respiratory problems).

Viral meningitis/encephalitis

Causes

1. Epidemics associated with exanthema e.g. measles 1/1000, influenza, mumps.
2. Local outbreaks of polio, coxsackie, ECHO.
3. Sporadic: individual response to primary infection (80%) or recurrence of herpes simplex 1 (labial) or 2 (genital, principal cause of neonatal h. simplex encephalitis).
4. Altered immunity: congenital infection – rubella, CMV; congenital or acquired – HIV.

Presentation

Preceded by respiratory or gastrointestinal infection in 20%.

Meningitis: Sudden onset of headache, fever, meningism, vomiting.

Encephalitis: Behaviour altered, may progress to coma. Seizures, hemiparesis, cranial nerve palsies.
   Absence of vesicles in H. simplex is not uncommon, and may present as encephalitis, jaundice, or necrotizing enterocolitis. Macular rash suggests ECHO virus.

Exanthema: Chickenpox, measles, glandular fever, herpangina (coxsackie 16, 22).

Investigations

1. CSF (may be normal in herpes simplex viral encephalitis).

   i WBCs: lymphocytosis 20–200/mm^3, occasionally 1000's.
      Polymorphs may predominate in early phase.
   ii RBCs present may be due to herpes simplex encephalitis (up to 500/mm^3)

Interpretation of traumatic tap

Ratio of RBCs:WBCs in peripheral blood is usually 500:1. A relative excess of WBCs in CSF is suggestive of meningeal inflammation.

   iii Protein 0.5-1g/l, glucose normal.

2. Viral studies: swabs, paired sera.
   For suspected herpes simplex:

    i CSF: antigen detection and polymerase chain reaction for viral DNA has high specificity.
   ii EEG often shows periodic lateralizing epileptiform discharges, or temporal lobe abnormalities.
  iii MRI is more sensitive than CT in showing early disease.
   iv Brain biopsy is diagnostic, but rarely done.

Differential diagnosis

1. Other infections e.g. partially treated pyogenic meningitis, brain abcess, TB (skin test, ZN stain, primary lesion on chest X-ray), leptospirosis (immersion in canal/infected river, serology), Lyme disease (skin lesion around the bite, arthritis, serology), brucella (goats' milk ingestion, serology). Fungi (prematures, immunodeficient).
2. Parainfectious illness, e.g. Guillain-Barré (high protein, otherwise normal CSF).
3. Post immunization encephalopthy.
4. Leukaemia, rarely amoeba, toxoplasmosis, sarcoid or Behcet's syndrome.
5. Causes of coma, e.g. drugs, hypoglycaemia, Reye's syndrome.

Management

1. Supportive, reduce cerebral oedema, fluid restrict to 60% of normal intake to reduce danger of inappropriate ADH secretion.
2. Acyclovir for h. simplex if suspected clinically.
3. If in doubt, e.g. partially treated meningitis possible, either wait and repeat the LP after 8–12 h, or start antibiotic until results of latex agglutination and culture become available.

Prognosis

Viral meningitis: 95% complete recovery.

Encephalitis

1. Herpes simplex: untreated = 60% mortality in neonates, 30% older ages, 50% of survivors handicapped. Improved by early acyclovir treatment.
2. Measles: 15% mortality, 25% neurological sequelae.

Further reading

Addy D P (1987) When not to do a lumbar puncture. *Archives of Disease in Childhood*, **62**, 873–875
Bell W E, McCormick W F (1981) *Neurologic Infections in Children* 2nd edn. Philadelphia:Saunders

Klein J O, Feigin R D, McCracken G H Jr (1986) Report of the task force on diagnosis and management of meningitis. *Pediatrics*, **78**, 959–982

Lebel M H *et al* (1988) Dexamethasone therapy for bacterial meningitis. *New England Journal of Medicine*, **319**, 964–971

Levin M, Heyderman R S (1991) Bacterial meningitis. *Recent Advances in Paediatrics*, (David T J, ed) Edinburgh:Churchill Livingstone pp 1–19

de Louvois J, Blackbourn J, Hurley R, Harvey D (1991) Infantile meningitis in England and Wales: a two year study. *Archives of Diseases in Childhood*, **66**, 603–607

Table 20.5 Sudden onset of paralytic weakness due to infection

Condition	Distribution	Related clinical and laboratory findings
1. Polio like	Asymmetric	Fever, meningism, CSF lymphocytosis Coxsackie and polio titres requested
2. Ascending	Symmetrical Legs → arms → bulbar.	CSF: 'dissociation cytoalbuminic' of Guillain-Barré.
3. Descending	Urine retention Cranial nerves	i Facial nerve: central/peripheral in Lyme disease. Bell's palsy in viral infections ii Ptosis, diplopia → swallowing difficulties; + progressive weakness, respiratory failure, sudden cardiac arrhythmia in botulism
4. Paraplegia	Definable level	Associated with exanthema, e.g. chickenpox i.e. transverse myelitis. Rarely due to a spinal epidural abscess. Urgent CT to identify a treatable cause
5. Acute hemiplegia	Flaccid → spastic	Hyperpyrexia and seizures with infection in acute infantile hemiplegia. CT with enhancement to exclude A-V malformation. Mantoux, as TB meningitis may present similarly.

SELECTED INFECTIONS WITH CONCERNS SPECIFIC TO CHILDREN

Viral

Herpes viruses

Herpes simplex virus (HSV)

Incubation 2–12 days. Type 1 = oral, and type 2 = genital characterize the usual, but not exclusive, sites. In the neonatal period HSV type 2, of maternal genital origin, predominates, thereafter type 1.

Primary infection   In addition to herpes of the lip. It takes many forms:

1. Neonatal (see Neonatal problems)
    i   Oral ulcers, vesicles on the skin, eyes.
    ii Encephalitis/meningitis.
    iii Jaundice/disseminated/necrotizing enterocolitis +/- rash.

2. Infancy: infected nappy rash.
3. 1–3 year olds:

   i Herpetic stomatitis is a common presentation at this age and lasts 5–14 days. Febrile and anorectic, with a painful mouth and non-tender cervical lymphadenopathy. The mouth ulcers are towards the front, while herpangina is over fauces and pharynx.
   ii Vulvovaginitis (consider sexual abuse, although it may be transmitted on carer's hands).
   iii Ophthalmic infection.

4. Kaposi varicelliform eruption: infected atopic eczema.
5. Aseptic meningitis/encephalitis: primary (uncommon) or reactivation. Commonest identifiable cause of non-epidemic encephalitis.

Reactivation of latent infection

1. Miscellaneous: labial HSV lesion associations: in acute fevers (eg bacterial pneumonia, meningitis), herpetic whitlow from finger sucking, sunlight.
2. Serious infection:

   i Meningoencephalitis.
   ii Local tissue necrosis or disseminated HSV in the immunosupressed.

Investigations   In emergency: rapid diagnosis by direct immunofluorescence. Routinely: viral culture, 4–fold rise in antibody titre.

Treatment

1. Stomatitis: mouth care, paracetamol, and acyclovir orally/i.v. if i.v. hydration is necessary.
2. Local HSV: acyclovir cream for labial herpes in pre-eruptive, 'tingling' phase or as a 3% solution in HSV eye involvement.
3. Systemic infection: acyclovir i.v. 10–15 mg/kg (neonate) or 750–1500 mg/m^2 (older ages) 3 × daily for 10–14 days is used in severe HSV infection, otherwise orally 200 mg 5 × daily if able to swallow. Monitor renal function.
4. Maternal genital HSV infection: management of the newborn.

   i Primary: Prophylactic Caesarian delivery if active genital herpes and membrane ruptured <4 h. Swab baby's eye, throat, ear and umbilicus for viral culture.
   Prophylactic acyclovir i.v. is controversial.
   ii Recurrent: risk of infection is 2%. Observe for the first 10 days of life, treat if symptomatic.

Chickenpox/zoster

Incubation 13–17 (up to 21) days.

Communicability From 2 days before to 7 days after start of the rash, and vesicles crusted (dry).

Clinical

1. Skin: vesicles begin on the face, spread to the trunk and proximal parts of the limbs.
   Complications: pneumonia, ataxia, Reye's syndrome.
   Progressive chickenpox in the immunosuppressed is often severe with significant mortality unless treated.
2. Shingles: unusual. Also seen in the immunosuppressed previously infected in early childhood. Rash lasts up to 4 weeks, and persistent pain for many more weeks.
3. Neonatal: severe if mother develops rash within the 7 days before or after delivery.
4. Intrauterine: rare, skin scarring, limb damage, malformed brain and eye.

Management

1. Symptomatic, with fever, give antipyretic but not aspirin (associated with Reye's syndrome in this exanthema); antibiotic for secondary bacterial infection.
2. Prophylactic zoster immune gammaglobulin, best within 4 days, may give up to 7 days after exposure to:

   i Immunosuppressed/cystic fibrosis.
   ii Mother in late pregnancy.
   iii Newborn at risk, and to a contact born before 28 weeks.

3. Acyclovir (see HSV) for:

   i The severely infected.
   ii Immunosuppressed showing early signs—give i.v.
   iii To mother and infant prophylactically if she develops spots immediately before delivery, both via i.v. route.

4. Avoid hospitalization to protect other immunosuppressed patients, or isolate.

Glandular fever—Infectious mononucleosis

The Epstein-Barr virus is a herpesvirus.

Incubation 4–6 weeks.

Communicability Several months, via saliva.

Clinical

1. Anginose: fever, headache, sore throat.
2. Lymphoreticular: generalized lymphadenopathy, tender slightly enlarged spleen, less commonly hepatomegaly and jaundice. Subclinical hepatitis is common (abnormal liver function tests in 50%).
3. Neurological: aseptic meningitis, polyneuritis, rarely transverse myelitis.
4. Pneumonia rare, except in the immunosuppressed or AIDS.

Complications:

   i Common is inappropriate ampicillin administration → maculopapular rash (almost diagnostic!).

  ii Uncommon: upper airway obstruction.

 iii Rare: spontaneous splenic rupture.

Diagnosis

1. Triad of sore throat, lymphadenopathy and splenomegaly is characteristic, but cytomegalovirus and toxoplasmosis may only be distinguishable serologically. A FBC helps exclude acute leukaemia, and usually has 'atypical' lymphocytes.
2. Presence of one or two components of the triad are also found in streptococcal throat, diphtheria, rubella, and viral hepatitis.
3. Monospot is positive in 35% of EBV in children under 4 years, 80% aged 4–11 years. Worth repeating as it may develop over 3–4 weeks.

Management   Supportive. Exceptionally, needs intubation + steroids for airway obstruction by massive tonsillar enlargement.

Hand foot and mouth disease

Coxsackie A virus.

Incubation

3–5 days.

Communicability

Virus excreted in faeces for several weeks.

Clinical

Mainly 1–5 year olds. Papular–vesicular rash on palms and soles, oral ulceration.

Hepatitis A

Incubation

30 days

Communicability

For 14 days before to 7 days after the onset of jaundice.

Clinical

Anicteric, itchy, anorexic → jaundice, pale stools, dark urine. Liver tenderness and abdominal pain simulate appendicitis.

Diagnosis

Aminotransferase (ALT) peaks in symptomatic phase, anti-HAV IgG appears later.

Management

Supportive. Human normal immunoglobulin for vulnerable close contacts.

Human immunodeficiency virus (HIV)

Worldwide one million children HIV infected, of whom half have the acquired immune deficiency syndrome or AIDS (WHO estimate 1990).

Mode of transmission and prognosis

1. Vertical by materno-fetal spread (75% of total childhood HIV at present. Predominantly from heterosexual spread, some i.v. drug users). In 1991 inner London HIV +ve test found in 1 in 500 pregnancies, 1 in 16000 in another region. Prenatal transmission far commoner than by breast milk (seven cases reported in the literature).

    i   Incidence probably 100–200 annually in UK in 1990.
    ii 13% of infants born to infected mothers in Europe become HIV +ve. Of these, AIDS develops in a quarter by a year (of whom the majority die of HIV related disease within that time), four fifths by 4 years.
    iii Over 80% of those infected have clinical or laboratory (see below) evidence of HIV infection within 6 months of birth.

2. Horizontal by infected blood or blood products (200 haemophiliac children in UK from contaminated factor VIII, no new cases since 1986).
   Differences from vertical transmission

    i   Incubation period longer: 20% of the HIV +ve developed AIDS within 2 years, but of these 95% have died within 5 years.
    ii Infection and lymphocytic interstitial pneumonitis (LIP) less common. Exposure at a later age probably permitted some immunological development, denied those infected vertically.

Presentation

1. Infections, becoming recurrent:

    i   Bacterial pneumonia, meningitis, recurrent otitis media, sinusitis.
    ii Oral candidiasis, persistent and recurrent, and herpes stomatitis.
    iii Acute interstitial pneumonitis = cough and dyspnoea, extensive infiltrates on X-ray. It should promote a search for Pneumocystis pneumonia (PCP), which occurs in 75%. Mortality at first presentation and from AIDS over the ensuing 5 years is high. Other infections include TB, CMV, opportunistic infections.
    iv Chronic lymphocytic interstitial pneumonitis (LIP), mean onset 14 months. Restrictive disease on respiratory function testing, proceeds to respiratory

distress and hypoxia. Chest X-ray: hilar glands, lung infiltrates. Hypergammaglobulinaemia (>30 g/L).

iv *Mycobacterium avium intracellulare* ('atypical'). High mortality.

Table 20.6 Presentation of HIV infection

AIDS indicator diseases	Other HIV manifestations
Opportunistic infections	Persistent/recurrent oral candidiasis, parotitis
Severe recurrent bacterial infections	Persistent diarrhoea
LIP	Persistent hepatosplenomegaly, lymphadenopathy
Severe failure to thrive	Severe/recurrent varicella
HIV encephalopathy	Thrombocytopenia, nephropathy, cardiomyopathy
Malignancy	

2. Failure to thrive, malabsorption. Poor appetite aggravated by the pain associated with oropharyngeal candidiasis.
3. Non-specific. Lymphadenopathy, hepatosplenomegaly, eczematous skin rash, monilial nappy rash, persistent diarrhoea (75% initially present in this way).
4. Parotid gland swelling.
5. Encephalopathy (50%). Developmental delay or regression, pyramidal signs, ataxia, cortical atrophy. Differentiate from other CNS infection, deprivation, hospitalization, and constitutional causes.
6. Malignancies. Unusual in children: Kaposi's sarcoma, lymphoma.

Diagnosis

HIV antibody in first 18 months may be passively acquired from the mother. If still present later the child is HIV infected. If the child develops signs or symptoms of disease before this time, the diagnosis can be made earlier.

Indicative of infection Polyclonal hypergammaglobulinaemia, and low CD4 (cluster determinant) lymphocyte counts. Reversal of CD4:CD8 ratio occurs. Normal values for CD4 vary with age, are higher than adults' especially in infancy. (To give some idea of normal counts, CD4 $1-6 \times 10^9/l$, CD8 $0.5-3 \times 10^9/l$, CD4 > CD8). In contrast to adults, although the CD4 falls, the WBC differential remains normal, and the polymerase chain reaction (PCR) to detect HIV proviral DNA fails to detect infants earlier. LP is usually unhelpful.

Gold standard Viral culture, p24 core antigen in <15 months old, PCR thereafter.

Differential diagnosis Primary immune disorders, cystic fibrosis, CNS degenerative disease.

Classification

1. Centres for Disease Control Classification for Paediatric HIV infection

   P-0 Indeterminate infection.

P-1 Asymptomatic infection: immune function A = normal, B = abnormal, C = not studied.

P-2 Symptomatic infection: A = non-specific signs and symptoms, B = progressive neurological disease, C = lymphocytic interstitial pneumonitis, D = secondary infectious diseases, E = secondary cancers, F = other possible diseases due to HIV.

2. In those parts of the world where sophisticated diagnostic methods are unavailable, a clinical case definition (WHO), divided into major and minor, is used.

   i Major: weight loss or failure to thrive; persistent diarrhoea, recurrent unexplained fever.

  ii Minor: generalized lymphadenopathy, oropharyngeal candidiasis, repeated common infections, persistent cough, generalized dermatitis, confirmed maternal HIV infection.

Management

1. Perinatal.

   i Resuscitation with gown over plastic apron, surgical gloves and eye protection. Mechanical suction only. Wash to remove blood from baby's skin to avoid HIV transmission.

  ii Breast feeding avoided by at risk/HIV infected mothers in UK, but encouraged in developing countries where the risk of death from malnutrition and diarrhoea is greater.

2. Confidentiality and HIV testing.
Parental consent should be obtained, but a child can be tested without if it is essential to that child's care (British Medical Association advice). The family should be informed of the importance of the knowledge of testing/diagnosis to the family doctor. Other agencies informed at the family's discretion.

3. Potentially HIV positive: test at birth and follow carefully for signs and symptoms of disease. Repeat test at 18 months.

4. Asymptomatic HIV positive. Avoid segregation as there is no evidence for transmission from child to child. Blood rituals and biting to be avoided! Schools are already advised to treat all blood/excreta from any child as if potentially infective.

Zidovudine (AZT) may prevent or delay the onset of AIDS, trials in progress.

5. Symptomatic HIV (AIDS)

   i Vigorously treat infections. Atypical TB responds poorly to conventional antituberculous therapy. Pneumocystis pneumonia (PCP) may respond to co-trimoxazole, pentamidine by inhalation/i.v., and steroids in severe PCP but despite therapy mortality remains high.

  ii Prophylaxis: co-trimoxazole on alternate days, dose based on 5 mg/kg of the trimethoprim component, as prophylaxis against pneumocystis. Its introduction is related to the CD4 count at a given age.

 iii Zidovudine (AZT) administration increases weight gain, improves cognitive function, and prolongs survival.

iv Immunoglobulin infusions, 3 weekly, if suffering recurrent bacterial infections, but mortality not significantly reduced.

6. Immunisation whether symptomatic or not

   i Check mother's hepatitis B status, vaccinate if appropriate.

   ii Routine immunizations: diphtheria, tetanus, pertussis + live measles, mumps, rubella. Inactivated polio vaccine.

   iii Pneumovax after 2 years old, and 5 yearly.

   iv Influenza vaccine at the appropriate season.

   v No BCG after the neonatal period.

7. Supportive care: nutritional supplements, nasogastric feeding, handicap team for the encephalopathy.

8. Community aspects:

   i Mother may be single, unsupported, drug user, African or other immigrant without good family support. Increasingly, it will be ordinary families, as HIV spreads.

   ii Child's need for help in facing his own death, that of a parent or sibling, or both, through child psychiatry/hospice.

   iii Problems of fostering and adoption arise.

Prevention

Safer sex

HIV positive pregnancy: termination counselling bearing in mind the risk is 13–35% of an infected infant, depending on the population.

AIDS affected pregnancy: termination no longer mandated as being likely to be fatal for both mother and child.

Further reading

AIDS Institute, New York State Department of Health (1991) Guidlines for the care of children and adolescents with HIV infection. *Journal of Paediatrics*, **119**, suppl no1, part 2.

Gibb D, Newell M L (1992) HIV infection in children. *Archives of Disease in Childhood*, **67**, 138–141

Kawasaki disease

Aetiology

Staphylococcal and streptococcal toxins acting as superantigens.

Epidemiology

80% < 5 years old, M:F = 1.4:1; 3 yearly cycles, increased winter + spring, incidence per 100000 in Japan 330, USA and UK 15.

Pathogenesis

Inflammatory response associated with a vasculitis particularly affecting small blood vessels, especially the coronaries, to form aneurysms.

Clinical

Classically, five features (atypically three or more) of the following are needed for diagnosis:

1. Temperature for 5 or more days.
2. Rash, erythematous, macular or multiforme.
3. Oedema of hands and feet, peeling of the skin of fingertips.
4. Conjunctivitis, bilateral.
5. Lips dry, cracked, peeling, erythematous; strawberry tongue; pharyngeal erythema.
6. Cervical lymphadenopathy, non-suppurative.

    Additional features:

    i Cardiac complications 30%, mainly develop in first 12–28 days; thrombosis and aneurysms of the coronary vessels, myocarditis, arrhythmias, hypertension.
    ii Vasculitis: peripheral gangrene, thromboses of brain/heart.
    iii Arthritis 20%, diarrhoea 10%, aseptic meningitis 10%, also uveitis, pneumonia, hydrops of gallbladder, ileus, hepatosplenomegaly.

Investigations

Raised WBC, platelets ($>10^6 \times 10^9$/l in severe vasculitis), ESR (>100mm/h); pyuria, proteinuria. ECG, chest X-ray, echocardiography of the coronary arteries.
    Check ASOT, DNA binding, rheumatoid factor – should be negative.

Differential diagnosis

Post–streptococcal, measles, drug reaction, staphylococcal toxin release, infectious mononucleosis, Stevens-Johnson syndrome, juvenile rheumatoid arthritis, i.e. Kawasaki by exclusion.

Management

1. Aspirin 80–100 mg/kg/day for the first 14 days of illness, then 3–5 mg/kg to inhibit platelet aggregation for 6 months.
2. Sandoglobulin 2 g/kg single infusion (superior to 0.4 g/kg/day for 4 days) in the first 10 days may prevent coronary artery aneurysms.
3. Follow up for >1 year looking for cardiac complications, continuing aspirin as long as vascular changes are present. Half of aneurysms regress spontaneuosly within 18 months.

Prognosis

Mortality 2% from coronary insufficiency in the first 3 months, commoner in boys than girls and those under a year. Death may be sudden and unexpected.

Recurrence is rare.

Further reading

Levin M, Tizard E J, Dillon M J (1991) Kawasaki disease: recent advances. *Archives of Disease in Childhood*, **66**, 1369–1371
Shakleford P G, Strauss A W (1991) Kawasaki syndrome. *New England Journal of Medicine*, **324**, 1664–1666

Measles

Incubation

7–14 days

Communicability

From onset of upper respiratory 'cold' phase to 7 days after the rash appears.

Clinical

Two phases:

Phase 1. Coryzal with photophobia, conjunctivitis, fever and Koplick's spots until phase 2. when rash appears.

Phase 2. Maculopapular rash spreads from face to trunk, as 'complications' arise, (incidence 1 in 15), i.e. otitis media, pneumonia, diarrhoea, encephalitis. Duration 10–14 days.

Mumps

Incubation

16–20 days

Communicability

From 6 days before to 9 days after the parotids swell.

Clinical

Headache and fever. Swollen salivary glands, unilateral or bilateral, parotid/sub-mandibular. Maximal 1–3 days, resolves within a week.

Complications: meningoencephalitis, nerve deafness (commonest infective cause); pancreatitis (uncommon); testicular/ovarian pain is a feature of adult infection.

Differential diagnosis

Bacterial parotitis, salivary duct calculus, HIV, recurrent parotitis of unknown origin.

Management

Supportive.

Parvovirus B19

A common infection, antibodies present in 70% of adults. Manifestations in childhood:

1. Erythema infectiosum/5th disease

Incubation   4 - 14 days, communicability for a week after onset.

Clinical   Mainly 4–8 year olds. Mild fever, bright red spots on cheeks coalesce → 'slapped cheek' for 3–7 days → fine reticular rash over body which recurs over 2–4 weeks. Mild arthralgia in 5–10%.

2. Aplastic crises in haemolytic anaemias

Mainly occurs in children.

3. Hydrops fetalis.

Poliovirus

Oro-faecal route, 3 serotypes. Type I most likely to paralyse.

Incubation

7–21 days.

Communicability

By 3–6 weeks faecal excretion of the virus.

Clinical

Two phases.
    Phase 1: 'Influenza' with fever, diarrhoea and muscle aches.
    Phase 2: Second rise in temperature follows after 7 days, with stiff neck (aseptic meningitis), muscle pain, followed by paralysis 3–7 days later.
    Three patterns:

1. Bulbar palsy with respiratory failure.
2. Encephalitis with seizures.
3. Asymmetric proximal muscle weakness due to spinal involvement.

Management

Symptomatic. Bed rest in the acute phase if paralysed. Ventilatory and nutritional support for bulbar involvement.

Prognosis

Estimated that 0.01% of endemic polio in childhood results in paralysis. In epidemics a mortality of 5–10% is common.

Roseola infantum

Human herpes virus type 6 (HHV6)

Incubation

5–15 days.

Clinical

3 months to 3 years old. Fever for 2–5 days (may precipitate febrile convulsion). As it subsides, rose-pink papules appear on the trunk, neck and arms for 1–2 days. Mild illness.

Rubella

Incubation

4–21 days.

Communicability

For 7 days before and after the onset of the rash; in congenital infection for up to a year.

Epidemiology

1. Endemic in UK, epidemics previously occurred every 4 years.
2. Congenital infections

    i Incidence shows steady decline, but remained about 20 a year in the late 1980's, and used to increase 3–6 × in epidemic years. Adolescent schoolgirl vaccination has been superceded by the universal MMR programme in an attempt to improve this. Asian girls entering the UK after the age of immunization are still at risk; 7% of births are to Asians, who contribute 20% of cases.

    ii Maternal reinfection causing malformations now comprise 10% of cases, confirmed by rubella specific IgM antibody.

Clinical

1. Congenital: see Neonatal problems.
2. Childhood: coryzal prodrome, the rash follows 1–5 days later. Maculopapular, it spreads from face to trunk within 24 h, and by the time limbs are involved, it is beginning to fade from the face. Occipital lymphadenopathy is prominent. Encephalitis is rare. Arthralgia is commoner in adult women.

Investigations

1. Serology: confirmed by 4 × rise in IgG antibody. IgM reserved for suspected infection in pregnancy, or in the newborn.
2. Viral culture (urine, throat swab) for congenital infection; virus excretion may continue for the first year of life.

Selected bacterial infectious disease

Non-tuberculous mycobacteria (atypical mycobacteria)

Mycobacterium avium, M. intracellulare are the commonest in the UK. Likely to increase in frequency in the immunocompromised with HIV.

Presentation

1. Lymph node enlargement in the neck, slowly progressing over weeks, and may eventually discharge.
   Low grade fever, with hilar enlargement on chest X-ray.
2. Pulmonary infection and skin granulomas are rare.
3. Disseminated infection in HIV has high mortality.

Investigations

Mantoux (modest response 5–12 mm), chest X-ray (often normal) and culture (positive in 50%).

Management

Surgical removal of glands for diagnosis is often curative. Generally unresponsive to conventional antituberculous therapy, but combination chemotherapy, adding ciprofloxacin, is worthwhile.

Diphtheria

Rare in UK, may be imported during incubation or by carrier. Fatal in 15–30% of unimmunized.

Incubation

2–5 days.

Communicability

For 2 weeks, or 4 days after starting antibiotics.

Clinical

1. Predominantly 1–5 year olds.
2. Sore throat: grey adherent membrane over tonsils spreading to the uvula, bleeds readily, characteristic smell. Less commonly laryngeal (stridor) and nasal (serosanguinous discharge).
3. Bullneck swelling: cervical adenitis.
4. Carditis: tachyarrhythmias, failure, shock, death in second week.
5. Paralysis: neurotoxin produced affects palate week 1–3, swallowing week 2–4, respiratory failure (diaphragm) week 6, limbs up to 10 weeks. Complete recovery takes up to 6 months.

Investigation

Throat swab/swab of skin ulcers, intradermal Schick test (+ve reaction to diphtheria toxin = non-immune, susceptible).

Management

1. Isolate.
2. Airway if laryngeal membrane. Tracheostomy may be necessary.
3. Treat if the diagnosis is probable in anyone partially immunized or unimmunized, with antitoxin + penicillin. Carriers should receive penicillin.
4. Contacts
    i Non-immune: antibiotic prophylaxis and immunize.
    ii Previously immunized: booster immunization.

Escherichia coli

Diseases caused by various types of *E. coli*:

1. Acute watery diarrhoea

    i   Enteropathogenic e.g. O111, O126 infect duodenum and jejunum, no toxin released, non-invasive.
    ii Enterotoxigenic heat stable and/or heat labile toxin, also upper GI tract, non-invasive.

2. Dysentery: enteroinvasive mainly affects the large bowel, and septicaemia is common.
3. Haemolytic uraemic syndrome and haemorrhagic colitis: enterohaemorrhagic *Escherichia coli* O157:H7 produces verocytotoxin.

Pertussis

Organism and epidemiology

Humans are the only host of *Bordetella pertussis. B. parapertussis* and adenovirus can cause a similar condition. Epidemic cycle 4 years in the UK, in winter. Deaths occur in children under a year.

Incubation

7–10 (up to 21) days.

Communicability

For 3 weeks from the start of cough. Altered by erythromycin which allows return to day nursery after 5 days treatment.

Clinical

Catarrhal for 7–10 days, paroxysmal cough, (<1 year: no 'whoop' but may cause apnoea, and cot death) for 4–8 weeks, slow resolution with paroxysms for 6–12 months triggered by other upper respiratory infections.

Complications Otitis media and bronchopneumonia are common. Seizures in 3%. If encephalopathy follows, one third die, one third brain damaged, one third recover fully.

Investigations

Pernasal swab, FBC for lymphocytosis (>10 × 10^9/l) early on.

Management

1. Erythromycin in catarrhal phase or prophylactically if under a year and not fully immunized.
2. Hospitalize if:

    i Vomiting with weight loss: give tube feeds, in small volumes.
    ii Cyanosis or apnoea with paroxysms: give oxygen for episodes; phenobarbitone, salbutamol, steroids advocated, with little objective proof of efficacy. Monitor closely with pulse oximetry or transcutaneous oxygen electrode.
    iii Complications: pneumonia, encephalopathy, seizures.

3. Vaccination. See Community.

Further reading

Leader (1988) Whooping cough in infants. *Lancet,* ii, 946

Streptococcal disease

Group A

Organism Erythromycin resistance in 10–15% of hospital strains. Invasive disease: strains containing cell wall protein type M1 (M protein prevents phagocytosis).

Incubation 1–3 days.

Clinical

1. Pharyngitis: incubation 1–3 days, tonsillar exudate, palatal purpura, exceptionally retropharyngeal abscess.
2. Scarlet fever: incubation 1–7 days, requires previous exposure to respond to erythrogenic toxin → fine rash in body folds becoming generalized. Desquamation after 7 days.
   Day 1–3 white strawberry tongue → red strawberry by day 4.
3. Streptococcal fever: infants with persistent low grade fever for 4–6 weeks, with otitis and lymphadenopathy but little else.
4. Impetigo. (*Staphylococcus aureus* → bullous impetigo). Acute glomerulonephritis may follow, with nephritic strains, but not rheumatic fever.
5. Erysipelas. Cellulitis with systemic upset; metastatic spread a danger.
6. Acute streptococcal septicaemia, acute toxic-shock syndrome. Sudden onset, half have a primary site, e.g. pneumonia, vaginitis.
7. Immune associations: Henoch-Schönlein purpura, erythema nodosum, acute glomerulonephritis, rheumatic fever.

Management Penicillin V for 10 days, immediately in SF, or after culture confirmation in simple pharyngitis (50% are viral).
Asymptomatic carriers are not treated.

Comment   The continuing risk of invasive disease, glomerulonephritis (certain strains only), and the resurgence of rheumatic fever in the USA, serve to emphasize the need for culture to identify and treat streptococcal infection.

Group B

See Neonatal problems.

Arthropod borne disease relevant to UK

Lyme disease

Spirochaete infection (*Borrelia burgsdorferi*) spread by an ixodid tick.

Epidemiology

Increasing number of reports, 20–30 annually. Reservoir: small mammals, and deer, horses or cattle. Main foci East Anglia, New Forest, Scotland, Northern Ireland.

Incubation

3–32 days.

Clinical

1. First stage: a bite-site papule up to 15 cm, influenza like symptoms, with the herald lesion erythema chronicum migrans (ECM) for 3–4 weeks.
2. Second stage: weeks to months later, when afebrile.

   i Meningitis with CSF lymphocytosis, facial nerve palsy.
   ii Myocarditis and arthritis affecting the large joints, seems relatively rare in the UK and Europe, commoner in North America.

Diagnosis

Based on bite, ECM, serology.

Management

Erythema chronicum migrans: oral amoxycillin + probenecid, doxcycline or tetracycline over 9 years old, for 10–21 days. Usually aborts late manifestations.

Meningoencephalitis (not isolated facial nerve palsy), carditis, arthritis: i.v. cefotaxime 75 mg/kg/day for 14–21 days.

Prevention

In infested areas to wear clothing covering arms and legs, and sprayed with permethrin. Prompt removal of ticks can prevent disease.

Further reading

Committee on Infectious Diseases (1991) Treatment of lyme borreliosis. *Pediatrics*, **88**, 176–179
Cryan B, Wright D J M (1991) Lyme disease in paediatrics. *Archives of Disease in Childhood*, **66**, 1359–1363

Malaria in returning travellers

A protozoan.

Incidence

200–300 children notified annually in England and Wales. Rarely, congenital malaria is reported, onset aged 4–6 weeks.

Types

Usual, but not exclusive, geographical areas:

   i Indian subcontinent: *Plasmodium vivax*, occasionally *P. falciparum*.
  ii Africa: *Plasmodium falciparum* (PF); less common *P. ovale* and *P. malariae*.

Incubation

6–160 days. Symptoms may manifest months later, especially if prophylaxis has been taken.

Pathophysiology of cerebral malaria

Excessive production of tumour necrosis factor (TNF) may be the cause of, or result in, cerebral malaria (1% of PF). High levels of TNF are predictive of death. Inhibition of TNF production by steroids or specific antibodies may become a therapeutic option.

Clinical

1. Children

   i Fever, rigors, sweats, often weight loss. 'Flu like symptoms, nausea, aching limbs, abdominal and back pain occur later, and less frequently than in adults.
  ii Confusion, coma, seizure, hemiplegia in cerebral malaria.
  iii Jaundice, anaemia, splenomegaly. Hypoglycaemia. Massive haemolysis = blackwater fever → shock and renal failure.

2. Infants: infection may be relatively subtle, with less marked fever, non-specific poor appetite and lethargy, +/- jaundice, hepatosplenomegaly.

Diagnosis

Thick film, most likely to be positive if taken between fever peaks. CSF in cerebral malaria is acellular, no parasites. CT scan helps exclude abscess, mass lesion.

Management

1. Support dictated by clinical state.
2. Drugs
   Benign malarias: chloroquine orally 5 mg/kg daily for 4 days, plus primaquine 250 mg/kg/day for a further 14 days in vivax and ovale. (Always check for glucose-6-phosphate dehydrogenase deficiency).
   Falciparum: oral quinine or i.v. if too ill or cerebral malaria, 10 mg/kg in 4 hours, then 8-hourly for 7 days, then Fansidar as a single dose.

Prophylaxis

Chloroquine 5 mg/kg weekly, and/or proguanil 0.4 mg/kg daily, starting 1 week before and continuing for 4–6 weeks after returning. Take both drugs in areas of moderate resistance.

Consult London School of Hygiene and Tropical Medicine for specific recommendations.

Further reading

Kwiatowski D, Hill A V S, Sambou I, *et al* (1990) TNF concentration in fatal cerebral, non-fatal cerebral, and uncomplicated plasmodium falciparum malaria. *Lancet*, ii, 1201–1204

Animal vectors and disease in the UK

Leptospirosis

Reservoir

Rodents, no longer dogs since vaccination introduced. Swimming/canoeing in contaminated water is the main childhood risk.

Incubation

7–12 days.

Clinical

'Flu-like illness, occasionally going on to renal or hepatic failure or haemorrhagic Weil's disease.

Diagnosis

Serum IgM/complement fixation test/microscopic agglutination test positive >5 days after onset of symptoms, too late to influence treatment.

Treatment

Penicillin may alter natural history if given within 4 days of illness.

Toxocariasis

Definition

Dog or cat reservoir of nematode which migrates through the body causing allergic symptoms. Preschool children at risk through pica. Preventable through curbing fouling of parks and providing removable covers for sandpits.

Clinical

Fever, wheeze, splenomegaly. White retinal granuloma may be confused with retinoblastoma.

Investigation

Eosinophilia, raised IgE, toxocara antibody present.

Management

Diethylcarbamizine citrate or Mebendazole for 3 weeks.

Toxoplasmosis

Important as a congenital infection.

After the newborn period a glandular-fever-like illness in the relatively small proportion of symptomatic cases. Potentially lethal in the immunosupressed.

Table 20.7 Antibiotics used outside the newborn period

	Single dose/kg	*Frequency/24 h*
Amoxicillin	7 mg	3 ×
Prophylaxis: endocarditis	<10 years 1 g, >10 years 2 g	1 h before procedure
Augmentin	7 mg	3 ×
Benzylpenicillin*	12.5–25 mg	4 × (50 mg/kg in severe infection)
Cefotaxime	25–100 mg	2–4 ×
Ceftazidime*	25–100 mg	2–4 ×
Cefuroxime*	20 mg	3–4 × (up to 50 mg/kg in meningitis)
Chloramphenicol	12.5–50 mg	4 ×
Ciprofloxacin	5–7.5 mg	2 ×
Clindamycin	3–6 mg	4 ×
Co-trimoxazole	3 mg of trimethoprim base	2 × (UTI prophylaxis 1/2 dose nocte)
Erythromycin	12.5 mg	4 ×
Flucloxacillin	12.5–25 mg	4 ×
Fusidin	6–7 mg	3 × i.v.
Gentamicin+	2.5 mg	3 × (in cystic fibrosis (CF) Nebulized
Prophylaxis: endocarditis	2 mg 1h before procedure	40–80 mg, 2–3 ×)
Metronidazole	7.5 mg	3 × oral/i.v.

(Rectal 125 mg, 250 mg, 500 mg, 1 g for <1, 1–4, 5–12, and >12 years, 3 ×)

Nalidixic acid	12.5 mg	4 ×
Neomycin	12.5 mg	4 ×
Netilmicin+	2.5 mg	3 ×
Nitrofurantoin	2.5 mg	4 × (UTI prophylaxis 1/2 dose nocte)
Penicillin V	12.5 mg	4 ×
Prophylaxis		
1. Rheumatic fever ⎫	age 1–4 years 125 mg	single dose (if penicillin sensitive give
2. Sickle cell disease ⎬	5–12 years 250 mg	erythromycin stearate in the same dose)
⎭	>12 years 500 mg	
Piperacillin*	25–75 mg	4 ×
Rifampicin	10 mg	1–2 ×
Prophylaxis: Meningitis	10 mg	2 × for 2 days in meningococcal infection
	20 mg	1 × for 4 days in *H. influenzae* infection
Tobramycin+	2.5 mg	3 × (Nebulized dose in CF 40–80 mg 2–3 ×)
Vancomycin	11 mg	4 × orally or i.v., i.v. over 60 minutes
Antifungals		
Amphotericin	250 µg stepwise to 1 mg	once daily i.v. over 6 h
Flucytosine	oral/i.v. 50 mg	4 ×
Miconazole	oral 125 mg	2 ×
Nystatin	oral independent of weight	100000 units 4–6 ×

+ Monitor blood levels, especially closely in renal failure.
* Alter dose in renal failure, according to manufacturers' recommendations.

Further reading

Krugman S, Katz S L, Gershon A A, Wilfert C (1985) *Infectious Diseases of Children*, 8th edn Mosby:St
    Louis
The classic. Chapters on common infectious fevers, with helpful differential diagnoses.
Moffat H L (1989) *Pediatric Infectious Disease. A Problem Orientated Approach* Philadelphia:Lippin-
    cott Comprehensive
Rudd P, Nicoll A (1991) *Manual on Infections and Immunisations in Children* 2nd edn Oxford Univer-
    sity Press:Oxford. The British Pediatric Association's 'blue book'. Includes several brief chapters on
    how to approach common/vexatious infectious disease problems, and immunization queries.

Chapter 21

Metabolic problems

INBORN ERRORS OF METABOLISM

Garrod first used the term inborn errors of metabolism in 1908 to describe four conditions. Over 200 have since been found, of which about 60 affect the newborn. Individually rare, they account for 1–2% of mental handicap, and up to 5% of sudden infant death syndrome.

Presentation is varied, from apparent acute sepsis, hepatitis or neurological illness, including regression, in infants, to cyclical vomiting, failure to thrive, and mental retardation, in older children.

Aims of diagnosis

1. Halt acute deterioration, if possible, by instituting treatment.
2. Arrest or reverse damage already sustained.
3. Advise on prognosis for the affected individual whether the condition is treatable or not.
4. Genetic counselling and advice on the management of future conceptions.

Pathophysiology

Interruption of a metabolic step requiring an enzyme, a cofactor such as biotin or B_{12}, a specific mitochondrial or peroxisomal function, or transport mechanism.

In others the basic defect is unknown, e.g. cystinosis.

1. Enzyme and cofactor defects

Inheritance is usually AR, occasionally X linked or AD. Lack of enzyme $\to$ excess of substrate $\to$ increased break down products at the block (often useful biochemical markers). Their effect is to poison systems in structure and function.

Severity is dependent on the availability of alternative pathways to compensate for the absent enzyme step, and the essential nature of the product.

2. Mitochondrial electron transport

A defect in the respiratory chain, characterized by glutaric aciduria and some muscle disorders.

3. Defects of the peroxisomes

These are intracellular organelles. The effect is to interrupt fatty acid and phytanic acid metabolism.

4. Transport protein defect

A failure to move groups of amino acids against a concentration gradient, in kidney and intestine, resulting in excessive excretion, and the respective blood amino acid levels are normal or low. Cystinuria (dibasic amino acid transport defect) causes renal stones.

Diagnostic clues

1. Family history of consanguinity, previous neonatal or cot deaths. An excess of male deaths or abnormality in mother's family suggests an XL disorder, e.g. ornothine transcarbamylase, Lesch-Nyhan syndrome.
2. Age at first presentation. The younger, the more acute.
3. Precipitant:

    i Birth. In the newborn the loss of the placenta to dialyse toxic products leads to onset after the first 24 h.
    ii Diet. Exposure to protein or other dietary constituents, e.g. galactose, fructose.
    iii Stress. Infection or surgery causing a catabolic state.

4. Improvement in symptoms when feeds are stopped, only to recur when they are reintroduced.
5. A characteristic smell may be noted.
6. Developmental history of

    i Progressive degeneration: lipidoses, mucopolysaccharidoses, glycogenoses.
    ii Weakness: carnitine deficiency, glycogen storage.

Clinical clues and appropriate investigations, by age

1. Neonatal and infant presentations

Acute onset

In the infant this may occur after some months of apparent well being, or intermittently, as the protein load increases and the stress of infections recur.

    i 'Septic' or 'gastroenteritis' picture, with lethargy, floppy, poor feeding, vomiting (may even be projectile), convulsions, coma. Weight loss and hepatomegaly are often found. Likely disorders: organic acidosis, fatty acid oxidation defect, urea cycle defect, congenital adrenal hyperplasia.

Work up: FBC, sepsis screen. A low serum bicarbonate in the E+U result may be the first clue. Confirmation by blood gases (Fig. 21.1) indicate:

a. Urine for ketones, organic and aminoacids, orotic acid, carnitine.
b. Blood: glucose, amino and organic acids, ammonia, lactate.
c. Save plasma and urine in the deep freeze.
d. Skin for fibroblast culture.
e. Liver biopsy (immediately after death, into liquid nitrogen, if a metabolic error is suspected).

Pointers:

a. Hypoglycaemia and no ketonuria is highly suggestive of a fatty acid oxidation defect (medium chain acyl-CoA dehydrogenase (MCAD).
b. Ketonuria, metabolic acidosis, lactic acidosis in pyruvic acidaemia.
c. Respiratory alkalosis is highly suggestive of a urea cycle defect. Hyperammonaemia confirms. Do urinary orotic acid.

ii Hepatitis, picture of jaundice, hepatomegaly, often bleeding (coagulation deranged early in metabolic liver problems, late manifestation of other liver disease) needing tube feeds, and floppy.

Work up: septic screen, liver function tests, FBC, coagulation, urine for reducing substances or galactose-1-phosphate uridyl transferase.

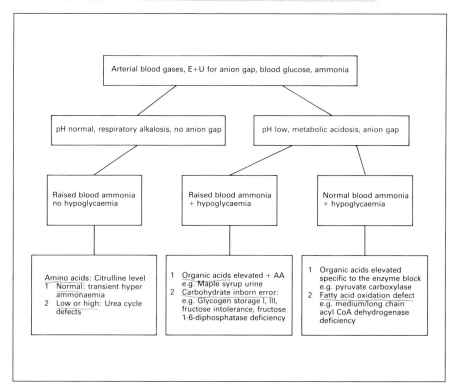

Figure 21.1 Algorithm using blood gases as an indicator to organic acid and urea cycle defects. AA = amino acids.

Pointers:

    a. Milk feeds begun, urine positive for reducing sugars, negative for glucose in galactosaemia.

    b. Low blood glucose points to tyrosinaemia or fructose intolerance, requires blood and urine aminoacids.

    c. Fructose containing foods, e.g. soy milk, and glycosuria in fructose intolerance.

    d. Unusual face, hypotonic, cataracts, (stippled patella, renal cysts) in Zellweger disease: very long chain fatty acids, pipacolic acid.

  iii Neurological with progressive lethargy, profound floppiness, coma +/- seizures, within the first 3 days of life.

     Pointer: if the usual CNS investigations are normal, consider non-ketotic hyperglycinaemia. Send blood, urine and CSF for amino acids and organic acids.

2. Older infants and children

i Acute

a. Metabolic acidosis picture: FBC, film. E+U show large anion gap >25 mmol/l in organic acidaemias. Blood glucose is low in maple syrup urine disease (MSUD), glycogen storage, MCAD deficiency. Save plasma.

b. Reye's syndrome like, in urea cycle and organic acid defects with coma, hepatomegaly and raised blood ammonia. If, in addition hypoglycaemic, with *non-ketotic* metabolic acidosis, a fatty acid oxidation disorder is likely.

ii Chronic

a. Failure to thrive, and hepatomegaly

    Storage disorders, α-1-antitrypsin deficiency (α-1-AT) galactosaemia, tyrosinaemia, hereditary fructose intolerance, and later in Wilson's disease.

    Basic screen: urine for reducing substances, ketones, organic and amino acids, blood for glucose, E+U, gases, lactate, ammonia, uric acid. Additional investigation dictated by clinical findings.

b. Mental retardation alone or with other manifestations always needs a metabolic profile of blood and urine amino acids, and urinary organic acids. Boys to have a uric acid level for Lesch-Nyhan syndrome.

        Some useful eye associations:

        Photosensitive with intermittent ataxia in Hartnup disease.

        Corneal clouding in mucopolysaccharidoses.

        Dislocated lenses in homocystinuria.

        Cataract in galactosaemia, Lowe's syndrome.

        Optic atrophy is an early sign in metachromatic leukodystrophy.

Confirmation

1. WBCs or fibroblast culture, for enzyme estimation.

2. Liver biopsy in urea cycle defects, some storage disorders.
3. Muscle biopsy, for enzyme estimation, histology, electron microscopy.

Management principles

Acute metabolic crisis

1. Correct any electrolyte abnormality, glucose disturbance, and/or acidosis. Mechanical ventilation is often necessary. Add antibiotics if sepsis is coexistent or likely.
2. Dextrose 15–20% i.v. induces an anabolic state. (Lactic acidosis is the exception, made worse by a carbohydrate load.)
3. Peritoneal dialysis removes excess amino and organic acids and ammonia. In hyperammonaemia give sodium benzoate i.v., which combines ammonia to glycine → hippurate (safe, excretable).
4. Megavitamin cocktail (B_{12}, biotin, thiamine, riboflavin, nicotinamide, pyridoxine) 100 times the daily requirement for possible cofactor deficiency, even though a diagnosis has not yet been made. Given 'blind', in the hope of arresting further acute deterioration. Be sure blood is taken for analysis before commencing.

Long-term management

1. Restriction or elimination of the substrate, e.g. phenylalanine, galactose.
2. Supply the absent factor or product, e.g. hydrocortisone in congenital adrenal hyperplasia, biotin as co-enzyme in some amino-acid disorders, carnitine in carnitine deficiency.
3. Elimination of stored toxic substances: copper by penicillamine in Wilson's disease.
4. Replacement of enzyme: bone marrow reconstitution in immune deficiency disorders, or some mucopolysaccharidosis.
5. Genetic counselling and antenatal diagnosis by enzyme assay or detecting abnormal metabolites in amniotic and fetal fluids.

METABOLIC DISORDERS, SELECTED EXAMPLES ONLY

Amino acids: phenylketonuria, tyrosinaemia, homocystinuria.

Phenylketonuria (PKU)

Definition

Absence of phenylalanine hydroxylase, AR. Excess phenylalanine (an essential amino acid) accumulates. It acts as a poison, on brain development, and tyrosinase enzyme, causing lack of pigmentation. A number of PKU variants exist which are generally not so severe.

Incidence

1 in 10000.

Untreated

Profound mental defect (MD), microcephaly, seizures, cerebral palsy, autistic hyperactive behaviour, fair hair, blue eyes, eczema. Urine contains phenylalanine, and its metabolites, including phenylpyruvic acid which gives the characteristic 'mousy' smell.

Fetal PKU, in previously treated or unrecognized maternal PKU. Unless on a diet prior to conception, the offspring are MD, microcephalic, low birthweight, (severity proportional to maternal serum phenylalanine), and 25% have congenital heart disease.

Diagnosis

1. Screening: by the Guthrie bacterial method after feeding is established (usually by the 5th day). New antibiotic resistant strains prevent antibiotics from interfering with the assay even if present in baby or mother's breast milk.
2. Confirmation: raised plasma phenylalanine >1.2 µmol/l, with a normal tyrosine (the latter may be raised transiently with phenylalanine in the newborn – see below). Urinary metabolites of phenylalanine present.

Treatment

Start as soon as diagnosis is made, to avoid brain damage.

Diet: low in phenylalanine. 'Lowfenalac' milk. Monitor blood level. Avoid total phenylalanine deficiency, which also causes damage.

Prognosis

If treated early, good. It is conventional to stop the diet in adolescence, but in some adults an ordinary diet is associated with lapses in concentration and pyramidal tract damage.

Tyrosine

Hereditary hepatorenal tyrosinaemia. AR

Definition

Deficiency of fumarylacetoacetate hydroxylase which results in severe liver disease in infancy. Antenatal diagnosis possible.

Incidence

1 in 100000 (French Canadians 1 in 700).

Clinical presentation

1. Acute: <6 months old, failure to thrive, developmental delay, hepatomegaly. Smell of rotten cabbage. Hypoglycaemia, jaundice and bleeding from liver failure.
2. Chronic: 1 year old, similar to acute, plus Fanconi syndrome → rickets.

Diagnosis

Although raised, plasma methionine and tyrosine, and tyrosiluria are not specific. Succinylacetone in the urine is diagnostic. Extremely high serum α-fetoprotein is also characteristic of this condition.

Main differential is from neonatal hepatitis.

Management

Albumaid X phenylalanine and tyrosine. Vitamin K, citrate and calcitriol reduce the effects of organ damage.

Prognosis

Death in 2 years in the acute early onset, by 10 years in the chronic form, from cirrhosis or hepatoma. Liver transplant is effective, though metabolic correction is incomplete and the long-term implications are not yet known.

Transient neonatal tyrosinaemia is found in usually asymptomatic prematures on a high protein diet, discovered through a positive PKU test.

Homocystinuria AR

Definition

Deficiency of cystathionine synthetase. Phenotypically similar to Marfan syndrome, often with mental retardation and thromboembolic episodes. Antenatal diagnosis possible.

Incidence

1 in 100000.

Clinical presentation

Marfan syndrome is compared in Growth problems.

Diagnosis

Raised methionine and homocysteine in blood and urine.

Management

40% respond dramatically to pyridoxine.
  Diet: methionine restriction, augmented cysteine intake.

Prognosis

Some remain well, others develop complications which are age related. Preschool: mental retardation, from 4 years lens dislocation, osteoporosis from mid-childhood. Vascular thromboses occur mainly in adults.

Cystinosis AR

Definition and pathophysiology

A transport defect which prevents the removal of cysteine from lysosomes, i.e. free crystals are deposited in the tissues:

1. Liver, spleen, lymph glands, bone marrow, detected on biopsy.
2. Kidneys → Fanconi syndrome. 'Swan neck' deformity due to damage of proximal renal tubule. Progressive renal failure.
3. Cornea: birefringent crystals → photophobia.
4. Thyroid gland → hypothyroidism.

Clinical presentation

1. Infantile: at 3–6 months old. Vomiting, lethargy, polydipsia, polyuria. Photophobia. Severe growth failure, renal rickets, hypothyroidism. Progressive deterioration with death in childhood from renal failure.
2. Adolescent: from 10 years old, slowly progressive.

Diagnosis

Crystals on slit lamp examination, in bone marrow, and on rectal biopsy. Urine shows generalized amino aciduria + glycosuria due to renal tubular damage.

Management

Citrate and calcitriol for the Fanconi syndrome, vitamin C and cysteamine to slow up deposition in tissues.
  Transplant kidneys when necessary.
  Antenatal diagnosis from cultured fibroblasts.

ORGANIC ACIDS

In the metabolically sick newborn, absence of ketosis differentiates non-ketotic hyperglycinaemia, a primary defect, from ketosis secondary to maple syrup urine disease and organic acid defects.

Ketotic hyperglycinaemias = organic acidaemias in which high levels of glycine occur, due to inhibition of the normal catabolic pathway. (These include proprionic, methylmalonic, isovaleric, and methylacetoacetic acidaemia).

Maple syrup urine disease

Definition

Deficiency of branched chain ketoacid dehydrogenase, AR. Antenatal diagnosis possible.

Incidence

1 in 200000.

Clinical presentation

1. Onset at a few days old, with vomiting, opisthotonus, seizures, and a 'septic' picture.
2. Intermittent forms: episodes precipitated by infection, and surgery.

Diagnosis

Caramel smell, ketoacidosis, blood and urine elevation of leucine, isoleucine, valine.

Hypoglycaemia is common, but its correction fails to alter the clinical condition.

Management

Stop protein, start peritoneal dialysis.

Catabolism raises the branched chain ketoacids, prevent with dextrose, fight infection. Combat cerebral oedema. When stable give low substrate milk MSUD Aid.

Prognosis

Poor, many become brain damaged.

Proprionic acidaemia and methylmalonic acidaemia, both AR

Definition

Elevated levels in plasma and urine, due to a deficiency of coenzyme A carboxylase and mutase, or abnormal biotin metabolism, an essential co-enzyme, in the catabolic pathway of essential branched chain amino acids. Antenatal diagnosis possible.

Incidence

Uncertain, both rare.

Clinical

Acute: vomiting, failure to thrive, seizures, occasionally cerebellar haemorrhage.
   Chronic: failure to thrive and developmental delay/regression in some with later onset.

Laboratory findings

Ketoacidosis, hypoglycaemia, hyperuricaemia, hyperammonaemia. Low platelets and WBC common.

Management

Low precursor protein diet, carnitine; add biotin or B_{12} in methylmalonic acidaemia.

Prognosis

Death common despite treatment.

Lactic acidosis

1. Primary due to pyruvate carboxylase/dehydrogenase deficiencies (pyruvate also raised).
2. Secondary to hypoxia, and other inborn errors, e.g. glycogen storage disease type 1, hereditary fructose intolerance.

UREA CYCLE DEFECTS

Deficiency of any of the enzymes in the cycle → elevated blood ammonia. Antenatal diagnosis possible.

Incidence

1 in 10000.

Epidemiology

Ornithine transcarbamylase is commonest; an XL dominant, males affected>>females. Other types of urea cycle defects are AR.

Clinical presentation

Precipitated or worsened by protein load or infection.
  Clue: respiratory alkalosis, absence of hypoglycaemia and ketosis.
1. Neonatal: lethargy, seizures, coma, apnoea.
2. Older child: mental retardation, intermittent ataxia and lethargy.

Management

1. If in coma: peritoneal dialysis + sodium benzoate to detoxify and enhance excretion of ammonia.
2. If alert: low protein diet.

Prognosis

Very poor in symptomatic neonates.

GLYCOGEN STORAGE DISEASE

Definition

Abnormal amount or structure of glycogen in tissues, due to 1 of 10 different enzyme defects, one for each step in the glycogen/glucose-6-phosphate cycle of synthesis and breakdown.
  Presentation is principally hepatic or myopathic involvement. Inheritance AR in types I to VII. Antenatal diagnosis possible.

Incidence

1 in 60000

1. Primary hepatic involvement   types I, III, IV, VI

Type I (von Gierke's disease)

The commonest, due to glucose–6–phosphatase deficiency, presents usually in infancy.
  Recurrent symptomatic hypoglycaemia, hepatomegaly, large kidneys (due to stored glycogen), poor growth, developmental retardation. Later xanthomas, gout.

Diagnosis

Acidosis (lactic acidaemia as a result of glycolysis), hyperlipidaemia, hyperuricaemia, bleeding and platelet defect. Liver biopsy enzyme estimation confirms.

Management

Continuous feeding: overnight nasogastric feed, and 2–4 hourly feeds by day, of complex starches (uncooked corn starch) slowly broken down in the gut. Maintaining blood glucose >4 mmol/l limits lactate, triglyceride and urate production.

Prognosis

Symptoms regress and growth is normal on continuous feeding, otherwise death occurs between 1 and 40 years old.

Type III 'debrancher'

Clinically similar to a mild type I, is due to the absence of amylo-1,6 glucosidase. Lactic acidosis and hyperuricaemia are absent.

Type IV (amylopectinosis)

Amylo 1–4, 1–6 transglucosidase deficiency. Hepatomegaly, progressive cirrhosis, death by 2 years.

Type VI phosphorylase deficiency

Milder than I, and III.

2. Myopathic presentation types II, V, VII

Type II (Pompe's)

Acid maltase deficiency: large tongue, liver, muscle weakness which also affects the heart. Cyanosis, cardiac failure and death in the first year is usual. Bone marrow transplant modifies the disease.

Type V (McArdle's)

Muscle phosphorylase deficiency: skeletal muscle glycogen is not broken down, causing weakness and cramps after exercise. Myoglobinuria occasionally. Reluctance to climb hills. Normal lifespan.

Type VII

Similar to V.

FATTY ACIDS

Also see mitochondrial disorders.

Glutaric acidaemia type II AR

Non-ketotic hypoglycaemia, precipitated by starvation or ketogenic diet. Neonatal death is usual. Antenatal diagnosis possible.

Carnitine is an amine, mainly found in muscle, essential to the transport of fatty acids. Primary, or secondary to dietary, deficiency is clinically like non-ketotic hypoglycaemia, or muscle weakness. Occasionally mimics Reye's syndrome.

PURINES

Lesch-Nyhan syndrome: XL

Definition and clinical features

Absence of HGPT-ase (hypoxanthine guanine phosphoribosyl transferase) → mental retardation, spastic and choreoathetoid cerebral palsy, self mutilation by chewing lips and fingers.

Incidence

1 in 300000, i.e. exceedingly rare.

Investigations and management

Elevated uric acid is a marker for the condition. Gout a feature in older children, leading to renal failure. No effective treatment. Antenatal diagnosis possible.

LIPIDS

Familial hypercholesterolaemia

A family history of early myocardial infarction is an indication for investigation. The place of population screening is contentious as accuracy of prediction and treatment for all but the most severe types is inconclusive. (See Holtzman N A (1990) The great god cholesterol. *Pediatrics*, **87**, 943–945)

Hyperlipidaemias

Type IIa (hypercholesterolaemia)

Definition

Elevated cholesterol and low density lipoproteins, AD.

absent [deficient] LDL receptor

Incidence

1 in 500.

Clinical

Xanthomas by 20s, arcus senilis, xanthelasma, coronary artery disease (CAD) in 40s in men, 50s in women. Homozygote may develop CAD by adolescence, and die by 30 years old.

Investigate whenever a history of early death from coronary artery disease is obtained.

Diagnosis *cord blood screening*

Serum cholesterol: normal <6.2 mmol/l, heterozygote 7–13 mmol/l, homozygote 20 –25 mmol/l.

Management

From a year old: low fat diet, and cholestyramine, are of limited efficacy. Other drugs, used in adults, have not been evaluated in children.

plasma phoresis   LDL aphoresis

Type Ia (primary hyperchylomicronaemia)

Definition

Lipoprotein lipase deficiency, AR.

Incidence

1 in 100000.

Clinical

Importance is in its presentation as repeated acute abdominal pain due to recurrent pancreatitis. Xanthomata, hepatosplenomegaly, and lipaemia retinalis found.

Diagnosis

Fasting serum turbid with chylomicrons, elevated triglycerides and cholesterol.

Differential diagnosis

Poorly controlled diabetes, von Gierke's disease.

Abetalipoproteinaemia

See Gastrointestinal problems.

LYSOSOMAL DISORDERS

Lysosomes are intracellular organelles containing catabolic enzymes. Defective enzyme activity leads to the accumulation of large molecules in the cell's waste disposal system.

1. Lipid storage disorders: Gaucher's, Niemann-Pick, Tay-Sachs disease.
2. Pompe's disease: see glycogen storage diseases.
3. Mucopolysaccharidoses (MPS):
   Deficiency of acid hydrolases:
   → inadequate breakdown of the connective tissue acid mucopolysaccharides, the glycosaminoglycans (GAGS).
   → excessive storage and urinary excretion of heparan sulphate and dermatan sulphate, except Morquio's who excrete keratan sulphate.

Clinical

Appear normal at first, then develop multisystem disease affecting:

1. CNS only: Type III, Sanfilippo = severe mental retardation.
2. Somatic only:

   i Type IV, Morquio = normal face, cloudy corneas, joints initially lax, later contractures, severe kyphosis, very short stature.
   ii Type V, Scheie = coarse facies, cloudy corneas, carpal tunnel compression.

3. Both: Type I Hurler AR, type II Hunter XL.

   i Grotesque facies, corneal clouding (except Hunter's), short stature, skeletal dysplasia, large tongue, hepatosplenomegaly, cardiac failure from incompetent valves.
   ii Progressive developmental retardation.

Diagnosis

Urinary excretory pattern distinguishes the many types. Confirmation by enzyme assay on WBC, serum or fibroblasts.

If clinically MPS but urine has normal GAGS excretion consider Pseudo-Hurler conditions which include mannosidosis, fucosidosis, GM_1 gangliosidosis.

Management

Bone marrow transplant (BMT) justified in type I, by 3 years old, and type II and III before the mental changes are irreversible. This reduces GAG concentration, preserves intelligence, and prolongs life.

Prognosis

Death in childhood in type I, unless given a BMT. Others usually survive to adult life.

MITOCHONDRIAL DISORDERS

Because mitochondrial DNA is derived from the ovum exclusively maternally inherited disease is possible.

Mitochondria oxidise fatty acids, pyruvate and NADH.

1. Affecting straight chain fatty acids

Clue: hypoglycaemia after overnight fast, seizure/febrile convulsion, absent ketones and with (dicarboxylic) aciduria.

  i Medium chain acyl-CoA dehydrogenase (MCAD) deficiency, AR.
     Incidence 1:6000.
     Presentation at mean age 15 months: recurrent vomiting, hypoglycaemia, and liver dysfunction; Reye's syndrome.
     Death: up to 25% die in initial illness, up to 4% of cot deaths.
 ii Long chain earlier onset, more severe, may be as cot death.

Management

Metabolic stress is hazardous so give frequent carbohydrate feeds, including overnight, and especially during infections. Carnitine and zinc supplements are helpful. Screen siblings, especially if two cot deaths have occurred in the family. (The phenylproprionic acid loading test for MCAD may be hazardous.)

2. Electron transport chain defects

i Mitochondrial myopathies

A block in the respiratory chain (cytochrome c oxidase defect) and thus generation of adenosine triphosphate. Muscle weakness, ophthalmoplegia, short stature, retinitis pigmentosa, sensorineural deafness, part of a multisystem disease.

ii Leber's optic atrophy, and some types of lactic acidosis and encephalopathies.

Diagnosis

Abnormal mitochondria on muscle biopsy or by identifying the genome by molecular genetics. MRI is an alternative, non-invasive method, looking at AMP/ADP/ATP/phosphate ratios.

PEROXISOMAL DISORDERS

Peroxisomes are oxidative subcellular organelles.

Deficiency of their enzymes and altered structural appearance lead to accumulation of very long chain fatty acids (>22 carbon atoms long), pipecolate and phytanic acid, all normally metabolized in the peroxisome.

Abnormalities are seen histochemically, and by electron microscopy of liver biopsy or on fibroblast culture.

  i Zellweger (cerebrohepatorenal) syndrome AR: abnormal head shape, facies, eyes, hepatomegaly, renal cysts, stippled patella and greater trochanter. Absence of peroxisomes.
 ii Adrenoleucodystrophy XL: adrenal atrophy and demyelination from 7–8 years. Peroxisomes normal in number but not in function.

Further reading

Applegarth D A, Dimmick J E, Toone J R (1989) Laboratory detection of metabolic disease. *Pediatric Clinics of North America*, **36**, 49–65

Clayton P T, Thomson E (1988) Dysmorphic syndromes with demonstrable biochemical abnormalities. *Journal of Medical Genetics*, **25**, 463–472

Wraith J E (1989) Diagnosis and management of inborn errors of metabolism. *Archives of Disease in Childhood*, **64**, 1410–1415

ACID–BASE PROBLEMS

Acid–base physiology

1. pH = - log H^+ ion, so pH 7.4 = 40 nmol/l, pH 7.0 = 80 nmol/l of H^+ ion (each 0.01 unit of pH = 1 nmol).
   i.e. small changes in pH = large changes in H^+ ion concentration.
2. Acid-base balance is maintained by:

Mechanisms	*Rapidity of action*
i Buffers in blood (mainly Hb) and body fluids (mainly bicarbonate) to minimize rapidly pH shift. Less important are the intracellular buffers (organic phosphate and protein).	Immediate

ii Lungs eliminate CO_2, controlling the carbonic acid level, giving effective compensation.	Minutes
iii Renal control of H^+ ion excretion (bicarbonate neutralizes; ammonia to ammonium ion; H^+ + phosphate = titratable acid).	Hours to days to compensate

The infant has a lower renal threshold for bicarbonate than at older ages, with plasma levels 18–24 mmol/l; thus less able to acidify urine and less reserve against acidosis.

Acid–base disorders

Metabolic acidosis (low pH, low total CO_2).

Differentiation between its main causes is helped by estimating the *anion gap*. As an approximation = plasma $(Na^+ + K^+) - (Cl^- + HCO_3^-)$ and is normally 14–20 mmol/l.

1. Normal anion gap, with hyperchloraemia.

  i Loss of bicarbonate: diarrhoea, renal bicarbonate wasting.
  ii Failure to regenerate bicarbonate: renal tubular acidosis.

2. Increased anion gap

  i a. Excessive production of lactic acid from:
      Work of breathing and/or hypoxia in asthma and respiratory distress syndrome (RDS).
      Septicaemia.
      Underperfusion, shock. The commonest cause of metabolic acidosis in the neonate, especially the premature.
      Metabolic errors: glycogenoses, lactic acidosis.
     b. Keto acids: starvation, diabetes mellitus.
  ii   Reduced glomerular filtration rate with ingestion of fixed acid: milk contains sulphated amino acids which metabolize to sulphuric acid. Excess protein or phosphate from cows' milk is significant in prematures and renal failure.
  iii   Ingestion of salicylates, ethylene glycol.
  iv   Inborn errors producing amino acid ketones, e.g. maple syrup urine disease, and organic acids, e.g. proprionic acidaemia.

Metabolic alkalosis (high pH, high total CO_2 content).

1. Loss of sodium ion: vomiting, diuretics, Cushing's and Conn's syndromes, hypokalaemia.
    Mechanism: lack of Na^+ or K^+ to balance urinary excretion of negatively charged ions is compensated for by H^+ ions. Plasma bicarbonate therefore rises.
    In hypokalaemia, $H^+:K^+$ exchange causes a paradoxical intracellular acidosis with extracellular alkalosis.

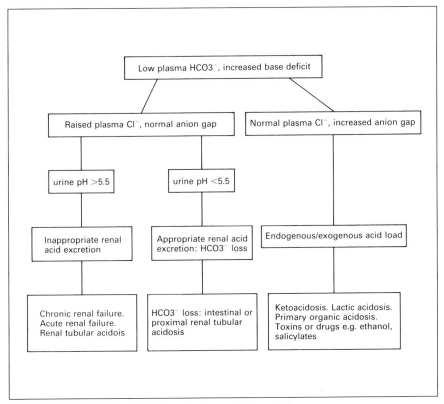

Figure 21.2 Simplified algorithm for investigating metabolic acidosis.

2. Ingestion of alkali.

Respiratory alkalosis (high pH, low total CO_2 content).

1. Hyperventilation: fever, hysteria.
2. Central stimulation: encephalitis, trauma, and salicylate in the early phase of poisoning. Rarely, from hyperammonaemia.
3. Compensatory.

   i Normal/low pH, low P_aCO_2 in metabolic acidosis, pulmonary oedema, pneumonitis.

   ii Normal pH, raised P_aCO_2 due to retaining extra bicarbonate in chronic hypoxia: cystic fibrosis, prolonged asthma attack.

Respiratory acidosis (low pH, high total CO_2 content).

1. Central depression: sedatives, head injury, encephalitis.
2. Peripheral weakness: polyneuropathy, myasthenia, dystrophy.
3. Obstruction of airways: foreign body, epiglottitis, asthma.

4. Parenchymal: RDS, pneumonia, pneumothorax, scoliosis, cystic fibrosis decompensated through infection.

Mixed disorders – Examples

- Respiratory alkalosis + metabolic acidosis: salicylate poisoning.
- Respiratory and metabolic acidosis: shock, RDS.
- Respiratory acidosis + metabolic alkalosis: cystic fibrosis with heart failure given excessive diuretic therapy.

Management

1. The underlying condition to be identified and specific therapy given.
2. In metabolic acidosis pH <7.20 consider half correction with molar/half molar solution of bicarbonate. In diabetes wait until pH <7.10. The theoretical requirement for correction is:

mmol sodium bicarbonate = weight in kg × 0.3 × base deficit

Half correct immediately and give over half an hour, the remainder over the next 2–4 h.

Paradoxical persistence or worsening of intracerebral acidosis is a danger, as the bicarbonate given extracellularly forms $H_2O + CO_2$ which crosses the blood–brain barrier to form H_2CO_3.

HYPOGLYCAEMIA

Definition

Blood glucose <2.6 mmol/l (46 mg/dl) at any age. See neonatal hypoglycaemia for discussion.

Incidence

Newborn: small for dates 20%, all births 0.4%.

Older ages: 2–3/1000 hospital admissions, half due to 'accelerated starvation' (see below).

Physiology

Maintenance of normal blood glucose is a balance between:

1. Intake of carbohydrate.
2. Glycogenolysis: glucose released from glycogen.
3. Gluconeogenesis: precursors fat (e.g. glycerol), amino acids (e.g. alanine), anaerobic breakdown products (lactate, pyruvate).

Glucose production and utilization

Normal requirement is 4–8 mg/kg/min under 6 years old, falling to 1–2 mg/kg/min in adults. The young child's relatively large brain, dependent on glucose, accounts for most of this difference.

The young child is therefore very vulnerable to reduced production/excessive demand for glucose compared to the adult.

Adaptive changes in starvation

Insulin level falls, counter-regulatory hormones (anti-insulin effect) rise: glucagon, adrenaline, cortisol, growth hormone.

The brain uses ketone bodies (acetoacetate and beta-hydroxybutyrate) produced by the liver from fatty acids released from fat stores by the counter-regulatory hormones.

Pathophysiology of hypoglycaemia

1. Hypoketotic hypoglycaemia = insulin excess

A normal or raised plasma insulin in the presence of hypoglycaemia is abnormal. Ketone body production is inhibited, as are glycogenolysis and gluconeogenesis. (Also found in defective beta-oxidation of fatty acids, e.g. MCAD, see above).

2. Ketotic hypoglycaemia = decreased glucose production

Ketone generation is physiological. The inability to produce glucose is due to:

  i Lack of substrate.
 ii Impaired glycogenolysis: enzyme defects.
iii Impaired gluconeogenesis: liver damage, enzyme deficiency, hormone deficiency.

Causes

1. Transient Neonatal

  i Ketotic: = *decreased production*, common in the small for dates or premature infant, cold stress, trauma, cerebral hypoxia or malformation, sepsis.
 ii Non-ketotic: = *hyperinsulinism*, relatively uncommon to rare. Infant of a diabetic mother, severe rhesus isoimmunization, Beckwith-Weidemann syndrome (exomphalos, macroglossia, macrosomia).

2. Persistent

  i Ketotic due to *decreased production*

    a. Lack of substrate:
      Malnutrition.
      'Accelerated starvation'.

Enzyme defects, e.g. galactosaemia, fructosaemia, maple syrup urine disease.
b. Liver damage:
Reye's syndrome, fulminating hepatitis, Jamaican vomiting sickness due to ackee fruit toxin.
c. Gluconeogenesis/glycogenolysis enzyme defects:
e.g. glycogen storage diseases I, III, VI
d. Hormone deficiencies:
e.g. hypopituitarism, isolated growth hormone deficiency, congenital adrenal hyperplasia, ACTH.

ii Non-ketotic due to *hyperinsulinaemia*

a. Exogenous insulin: therapeutic (see Diabetes), Munchausen by proxy (see Child abuse).
b. Islet cell adenoma
c. Nesidioblastosis: previously thought to have specific histology, now considered probably due to microadenomas.

iii Drugs: salicylate, alcohol, propranalol, sulphonylureas.

Table 21.1 Symptoms of hypoglycaemia

	Neonatal	*Older ages*
Sympathetic	Pallor	Pallor, hunger, weak, sweaty, anxious, nausea, vomiting.
Respiratory	Apnoea, tachypnoea, cyanosis	Tachypnoea
Neurological	Tremor, jittery, floppy, convulsions	Blurred or double vision, convulsion
Behaviour	Irritable, abnormal cry, coma	Bizarre, headache, lethargy, clumsy, confusion, coma

Timing: most occur in the early morning, whereas those after food are due to reactive hyperinsulinaemia.
Signs: cold clammy skin, pallor, tachycardia, normal BP.

1. Infant: Check the temperature, it may be low.

   • Consider inborn errors especially if a severe persistent metabolic acidosis is present.
   • Jaundice favours galactosaemia and/or sepsis.
   • Hepatomegaly alone in glycogen storage (+ spleen in rhesus isoimmunization in the newly born).

2. Child: Short and slim favours accelerated starvation, short and fat growth hormone deficiency.

Investigation during the hypoglycaemic episode

1. Blood glucose.
2. Ketones in blood or urine.
3. Blood for insulin, cortisol, growth hormone, lactate (elevated in type I and V glycogen storage disorders), pyruvate, and amino acid screen. Freeze serum and plasma for future metabolic examination for fatty acid metabolites, e.g. MCAD.

   Hyperinsulinism is likely when:

   - Non-ketotic hypoglycaemia.
   - Insulin level inappropriate for the blood glucose level.
   - Glucose infusion >8 mg/kg/min to maintain normoglycaemia.

Management

1. Conscious – offer a sugary drink.
2. Coma – 1 ml/kg 25% glucose i.v. over 3–4 min, then oral carbohydrate or 10% glucose infusion (8 mg/kg/min = 120 ml/kg/24 h).

   Combat hyperinsulinism: diazoxide orally regularly, or somatostatin infusion short term.

   Glucagon for rescue 0.05–0.1 mg/kg to max./mg.

   Surgery for resistant nesidioblastosis/islet cell adenoma.

'Accelerated starvation' (ketotic hypoglycaemia)

Cause

Uncertain:

- Low levels of gluconeogenic amino acids?
- Inability to prevent increased rate of glucose uptake by the tissues?
- Adrenal medullary response impaired?

Clinical

Characteristically male, 2–7 years old, underweight, born small for dates. Symptomatic hypoglycaemia +/– convulsions after prolonged overnight starvation, illness, or intense exercise.

Investigations

Normal except low blood glucose. May show low blood alanine or urinary catecholamines.

Differential diagnosis

Hypopituitarism/growth hormone deficient have a small penis and adequate weight for height, with a history of hypoglycaemia in the newborn period.

Management

Small frequent meals. Test for and avoid ketosis.

Prognosis

Attacks grown out of by adolescence.

OTHER CLINICAL SYNDROMES

Galactosaemia AR

Definition

Classically due to galactose-1-phosphate uridyl transferase deficiency, preventing normal conversion of galactose to glucose.

Incidence

1 in 40000

Pathophysiology

Galactose and galactose-1-phosphate accumulate, causing cataracts, cholestasis, fatty liver, and eventually cirrhosis.

Clinical

Onset within days or weeks of birth: vomiting (74%), jaundice (95%), fever, failure to thrive (20%), hepatomegaly +/– lamellar cataract (50%).
 Escherichia coli septicaemia may coexist in 25%.
 Mental retardation and cirrhosis develop.

Diagnosis

Urine contains reducing substances on Clinitest, and no glucose on Multistix. Confirm by absence of gal-1-P UT in erythrocytes. Avoid galactose tolerance test, as dangerous hypoglycaemia may ensue.

Differential diagnosis

Urinary tract infection, glycogen storage disease.

Management

Galactomin, plus vitamin supplement; avoid galactose containing foods.

Prognosis

If untreated may die or be severely mentally handicapped, and small. Even when treated 30–50% are slow learners.

Ovarian dysfunction: 80% fail to achieve puberty, or menses cease prematurely.

Hereditary fructose intolerance AR

Definition

Fructose-1-phosphate aldolase deficiency. Rare.

Clinical

Onset of hypoglycaemia, severe vomiting and diarrhoea when fructose or sucrose is added to the diet. Hepatomegaly and hepatic failure follow.

Diagnosis

Oral or i.v. fructose load fails to show a rise in blood glucose. Dangerous hypoglycaemia may follow, so liver biopsy and enzyme assay is preferred.

Treatment

Avoidance of fructose; often spontaneously, of all sweet things by the child.

Further reading

Aynsley-Green A (1989) Hypoglycaemia. In *Clinical Paediatric Endocrinology*, (C G D Brook ed.) pp 618–636 Oxford:Blackwell

CALCIUM DISORDERS

Normal serum values

Calcium = 2.2–2.6 mmol/l (8.8–10.4 mg/dl)
  Phosphate:

  Infancy and early childhood = 1.4–2.4 mmol/l (4–7 mg/dl).
  Puberty = 0.8–1.5 mmol/l (2.5–4.6 mg/dl).

  Alkaline phosphatase: 2–5 times adult values. Related to growth velocity or rickets, hence not a reliable marker of bone involvement in rickets. (Photon densitometry is a useful research tool for early detection of bone rarefaction).

Physiology

1. Skin produces cholecalciferol by the action of sunlight on 7-dehydrocholesterol.

2. The liver converts this, or ingested vitamin D_2, to calcidiol (25-hydroxycholecalciferol).
3. The renal proximal tubule 1α-hydroxylase converts it into active calcitriol (1,25-dihydroxycholecalciferol) under the influence of parathormone secreted from parathyroids switched on by lowered serum calcium.
4. Actions:

    i On small intestinal mucosa to transport calcium and phosphate into the body.
    ii The kidneys to enhance phosphate reabsorption.
    iii In bone, in concert with parathormone, to deposit calcium and phosphate.

Major causes of hypocalcaemia

1. Rickets: nutritional, increased requirements, organ failure.
2. Renal rickets.
3. Alkalosis: pyloric stenosis, hyperventilation, excess alkali intake.
4. Hypoparathyroidism.

Differential diagnosis

1. Diet, social, and environmental factors favour nutritional causes.
2. Family history of similarly affected individuals points to a renal cause.
3. Malabsorption, liver and chronic renal disease may be distinguished by history and examination.

Investigations

Low/normal serum calcium and low phosphate characterize all the above, except renal failure in which the serum urea and phosphate are high (renal rickets). Metabolic acidosis and glycosuria favour Fanconi's syndrome.

An important generalization:

1. Nutritional rickets = low calcitriol, elevated parathormone.
2. Renal causes = normal calcidiol with low calcitriol.

Vitamin D metabolites should be measured if there is no/blunted response to initial treatment.

Individual causes of hypocalcaemia

Rickets

Rare among Caucasians in North America and Western Europe, where inherited forms are most likely.

Up to 12% of Asian children are affected, principally at times of increased growth.

Pathophysiology

Failure of osteoid, the bone matrix, to be mineralized, resulting in less rigid bone which bends and twists. Due to:

1. Lack of vitamin D through inadequate intake, malabsorption or abnormal metabolism in kidneys or liver.
2. Minerals calcium and phosphate: inadequate intake or excessive renal loss.

Clinical

Skull shows frontal bossing, delayed closure of the anterior fontanelle, craniotabes.
   Bones: fractures in infants. Bowed legs or knock knees, scoliosis, rachitic rosary (swelling of costochondral junctions), swelling of the bones of the wrist.
   General: muscle weakness which may delay walking, cause pot belly. Associated growth failure.

Biochemistry

Low phosphate, low calcium (or normal due to secondary parathormone activity), and high alkaline phosphatase.

X-ray

Metaphyses are cupped, broad and irregular; like froth on a champagne glass. Delayed ossification.

Prevention

Breastfed babies: vitamin D 400 iu/day (10 mg) if term, 1000 iu/day (25 mg) if premature.
   Additional phosphate supplement of 1 mmol/kg/day in breastfed very low birthweight babies.
   Asian children: 400 iu/day, after graduating to doorstep cows milk, for the first 2 years and at adolescence.

Causes of rickets

1. *Nutritional*, i.e. lack of substrate:
    i   Sun (dark skin, Northern latitude, body covered, kept indoors).
    ii Vitamin D (exclusively breast fed, dark skin, etc).
    iii Calcium (some 'hypoallergic' diets avoiding dairy products), or excess of phytates in the diet complexing with calcium in the bowel, e.g. chapati flour.

Treatment
Vitamin D 4000 iu/day for 3 weeks, then 400 iu/day. Radiological healing begins in 2–4 weeks.
2. *Increased need for vitamin D and minerals*

   i Malabsorption of vitamin D and calcium, e.g. coeliac disease after treatment has begun and in the growing phase, as rickets is a feature of active growth. Often needs higher doses of vitamin D.

   ii Anticonvulsants especially phenobarbitone, and phenytoin, increase calcidiol turnover. Treat as for nutritional rickets.

3. *Abnormal vitamin D metabolism due to organ failure and renal rickets*

   i Organ failure

     a. Liver: cirrhosis reduces 25-hydroxylation of vitamin D, and biliary obstruction prevents absorption of fat soluble vitamin D and interrupts its enterohepatic circulation. Treatment: vitamin D 10,000 iu/day or calcitriol.

     b. Kidney: chronic renal failure reduces 1α-hydroxylation of calcidiol to active calcitriol, and consequently calcium absorption from the gut, elevating parathormone.

     Renal osteodystrophy

     When GFR falls below 30 ml/min/1.73 m^2 impaired growth and osteitis fibrosa (OF) result. OF is characterized by subperiosteal resorption at middle and distal phalanges, bone pain, and muscle weakness.

     Biochemistry: serum phosphate is normal or high, the calcium low, or normal when secondary hyperparathyroidism occurs. Treatment: 0.5–1.5 g elemental calcium per day as calcium carbonate; phosphate restriction; calcitriol 0.5–1 mg/day.

     Avoid aluminium hydroxide due to the aluminium toxicity build-up associated with renal failure.

   ii Renal rickets

     a. Vitamin D dependent rickets (VDDR) type 1 AR: rare, due to lack of enzyme 1α-hydroxylase. Clinically and biochemically similar to nutritional rickets except it appears at 3–4 months of age, calcidiol level is normal while calcitriol is low, and it needs vitamin D 10000–40000 iu/day or physiological doses of calcitriol for life.

     VDDR type 2 AR: absent receptor for calcitriol. Arab families, bald, severely affected by rickets, unresponsive to treatment.

     b. X-linked dominant hypophosphataemic rickets also called familial vitamin D resistant rickets. Commonest inherited form of rickets at 1:25000. M>>F. Phosphate wasting by the renal tubules leads to low serum phosphate, normal calcium, inappropriately low or normal calcitriol (as the low phosphate should be a stimulus for 1α-hydroxylase activity), poor bone mineralization, severe rickets and short stature by 1–2 years old.

     Treatment: regular phosphate supplements throughout the day and large doses of vitamin D. Monitor calcium carefully to avoid hypercalcaemia.

     c. Renal tubular acidosis. Metabolic acidosis from proximal or distal tubular disease leads to bone resorption and hypercalciuria. It is the accompanying hypophosphataemia which causes rickets. Includes Fanconi's syndrome.

Metabolic bone disease of the premature

See Neonatal problems.

Aetiology

Not rickets, as vitamin D levels are high. Substrate insufficiency (low intake of phosphate and calcium) contributes.

Hypoparathyroidism

Definition

Failure of the gland or its target organs, the kidneys and bones.

Pathophysiology

Reduced parathormone secretion (PTH) means loss of phosphaturic action on the kidney, leads to less calcidiol conversion to calcitriol, and less bone resorption.
  Neonates not infrequently show transient gland failure, but it is rare thereafter.

Clinical

Jitteriness in infancy, tetany (Chovstek's sign, carpopedal spasm), clonic seizures. Inflate a BP cuff above systolic for 3 minutes to elicit carpal spasm (Trousseau's sign).
  Persistent hypoparathyroidism leads also to basal ganglia calcification, school failure, depression, and mental retardation.
  True hypoparathyroidism is far commoner than pseudohypoparathyroidism.

1. Parathyroid gland failure

  i Transient neonatal

    a. Early at 1–3 days old:
      • Prematurity.
      • Stress: asphyxia, birth injury, sepsis, infant of a diabetic mother, and surgical conditions.
    b. Late, after 4 days old:
      • Maternal hyperparathyroidism: due to lack of vitamin D especially in Asians. Result is reduced parathormone secretion in the infant. The high phosphate load in unmodified cows' milk is less readily excreted by the neonatal kidney → elevated serum phosphate, suppression of calcium, and occasionally magnesium.

  ii Persistent

    a. Hypoplasia:
      • Idiopathic hypoplasia, at any age.

- Di George's syndrome: AR, Abnormal facies, coarctation of the aorta, absent thymus and parathyroids, defective T cell, normal immunoglobulins >repeated infections, candidiasis.
b. Autoimmune: associated with other endocrine diseases, e.g. diabetes mellitus, Addison's +/– T cell deficits with chronic candidiasis.
c. Removal or damage after thyroidectomy (may be transient postoperatively due to oedema impairing perfusion).

2. Target organ failure

Pseudohypoparathyroidism and pseudpseudohypoparathyroidism, indistinguishable clinically and both X-linked. Round faced, obese, short stature, short 4th metacarpal, later subcutaneous calcification. Mental retardation is common.

Investigations

Serum calcium, phosphate, immunoreactive parathormone. Interpretation:

Table 21.2

	Calcium	Parathormone	Comment
A Idiopathic hypoparathyroidism	Low	Low	Parathormone deficient
B Pseudohypoparathyroid	Low	Normal	Parathormone resistant
C Pseudopseudohypoparathyroidism	Normal	Normal	Phenocopy

Treatment

1. Acute hypocalcaemia: calcium gluconate 10% 1–2 ml/kg (= 9–18 mg elemental calcium/kg) 6 hourly.
2. Maintenance: calcium supplement 0.5–1 g elemental calcium/day, low phosphate diet and vitamin D (often in high dosage e.g. 10000 iu/day) or calcitriol. Monitor calcium levels carefully to avoid nephrocalcinosis.
   Remember, to avoid intoxication, 1-α calcidol (1-α (OH)D$_3$) and calcitriol have rapid onset and half life of days, but vitamin D has a delayed onset of activity and a half life of weeks.

Hypercalcaemia

Definition

Total serum calcium >2.65 mmol/l (10.6 mg/dl). Venous stasis must be avoided during sample collection.

Major causes of hypercalcaemia

1. Vitamin D intoxication

Loss of appetite, vomiting, constipation, failure to thrive. X-rays show a metaphyseal band of dense bone in the long bones, and nephrocalcinosis. Serum reflects kidney damage – raised urea and creatinine as well as calcium and phosphate.

2. Idiopathic hypercalcaemia of infancy

  i Mild type due to vitamin D intoxication or sensitivity, onset 2–9 months old. Clinically like 1. above.

  ii Severe: William's syndrome.
Onset after the neonatal period, with mental retardation, characteristic facies, X-ray thickened dense base of skull and changes as in 1, plus supravalvular aortic stenosis. Not all show hypercalcaemia at presentation, yet if X-ray changes are present it suggests it may have been present in utero.

Management   For 1 and 2: stop vitamin D, give low calcium milk, consider prednisolone and frusemide to promote mobilisation and excretion of calcium.

3. Hyperparathyroidism

Rare in childhood, may be part of multiple endocrine neoplasia

Symptoms

Generalised: weak, lethargic, constipation, 'psychotic' with confusion, hallucinations.
Renal: polyuria, polydipsia, renal colic due to stones.
Bone: pain and pathological fractures due to demineralization, subperiosteal resorption, lytic lesions of phalanges seen on X-ray.

Treatment: Surgical exploration and removal.

Table 21.3 Biochemical differentiation of hypercalcaemia due to 1, 2 and 3

	Parathormone	*Phosphate*	*Calcitriol*
Idiopathic hypercalcaemia	Normal	Normal	Normal
Hypervitaminosis D	Normal	Normal	Raised
Hyperparathyroidism	Raised	Low	Normal

Differential diagnosis   Includes renal stones, vitamin A intoxication, granulomatous disease, immobilization, malignancy (e.g. neuroblastoma, hepatoblastoma), hypothyroidism, Addison's disease, hypophosphatasia – rare AR: alkaline phosphatase deficiency, deficient bone mineralization, increased urinary phosphoethinolamine.

Further reading

Muenzer J (1986) Mucopolysaccharidoses. A review. *Advances in Pediatrics*, **33**, 269–289
Scriver C R, Beaudet A L, Sly W S, Valle D (ed) (1989) *The Metabolic Basis of Inherited Disease*, 6th edn. New York:McGraw-Hill

Chapter 22

Renal problems

NORMAL DEVELOPMENT OF THE KIDNEY

Fetal

The kidney is formed from the metanephros and ureteric bud from the 5th week of fetal age, the cloaca forms in the 6th. Collecting ducts are completed by 15 weeks. Nephrons function from 16 weeks and multiply up to 36 weeks.

Much of the amniotic fluid is fetal urine.

US appearance: lobulated, with diminished echogenicity in the medullary area, giving a 'cystic' appearance.

Postnatal

One million nephrons are present at term, with no increase in number possible thereafter. Only by hypertrophy can the remaining nephrons compensate for damage, underlining the importance of early detection and minimizing of injury.

Increase in glomerular filtration rate is associated with:

1. Growth in glomerular size and diameter.
2. Elongation of the proximal tubule, accounting for much of the increase in size of the kidney by a factor of 8, from infant to adult.
3. Increase in renal blood flow.

RENAL ABNORMALITIES DETECTED ANTENATALLY BY US

Routine antenatal US reveals that fetal renal tract abnormalities (8 per 1000) are the commonest congenital abnormalities affecting a single system. This has created the anomalous situation of practising preventive medicine in the hope of minimizing long-term morbidity even though the natural history is uncertain.

Selected congenital renal abnormalities often detected antenatally by US

Including Potter's syndrome, unilateral and bilateral hydronephrosis, and bladder outlet obstruction (see Neonatal problems).

Other congenital anomalies of note

Unilateral agenesis

1 per 1000. Usually asymptomatic, often with absent gonad on the same side. Look for VACTERL association.

Multicystic kidney

1 per 4500. The commonest cause of a unilateral abdominal mass in the newborn.

Controversy: many regress spontaneously, and some authorities claim 'prophylactic' surgical removal for fear of hypertension and malignant change may be unjustified.

Polycystic disease

Table 22.1 Features of polycystic disease

	Infantile	*Adult*
Incidence	1 in 10000	1 in 1000
Inheritance	AR	AD, but 25% are fresh mutations
Onset	Neonate to adolescence	Rarely before 20 years. Asymptomatic phase: some now detected by antenatal US
Association	Renal and biliary cysts	Renal cysts develop progressively
Clinical	From Potter's syndrome to failure to thrive with hypertension, fluid and electrolyte problems eventually culminating in renal failure. Liver dysfunction and portal hypertension after 5 years old	Usually asymptomatic in childhood. Hypertension, haematuria, flank masses. Cerebral artery aneurysms
US	Bright echoes from microcysts	Investigate adult relatives

Nephronophthisis AR

Incidence: unknown, a significant cause of inherited chronic renal failure.

Cysts develop from distal convoluted tubules, with progressive cortical atrophy.

Presentation: usually first decade with polyuria, polydipsia, proteinuria, anaemia, growth failure. Skeletal dysplasia or retinal changes in some.

Duplex kidney

Abnormal drainage is the main practical problem:

1. Bifid ureter with pelvi-ureteric junction (PUJ) obstruction = infection prone.
2. Separate ureter from the upper extra part drains lowermost, e.g.

    i   Into the vagina = daytime constant wetting.
    ii Into the bladder, with a stenotic orifice → dilatation within the bladder wall = ureterocele, causing obstruction and reflux. Seen as a filling defect on intravenous pyelogram.

Horseshoe kidney

Presentations:

1. Urinary tract infection due to PUJ obstruction.
2. Asymptomatic palpable mass rising out of the pelvis.
3. Incidentally on rectal examination.

Prune-belly syndrome

Rare. Boys only. Absence of mesenchymal muscle migration results in absent abdominal muscles, hugely dilated urinary tract, and obstructed posterior urethra, with bilateral undescended testes. Manage conservatively.

Further reading

Bianchi A (1986) Common urological problems. Chapter 21 in *Clinical Paediatric Nephrology* R J Postlethwaite (ed). Bristol:Wright pp 270-294

RENAL FUNCTION IMMEDIATELY AFTER BIRTH

1. Voiding occurs within 24 h. Failure to do so implies excretion may be impaired by obstruction, renal dysplasia (signs of Potter's syndrome?), or shock.
2. Drug excretion is less well developed in the first 3 (term) to 7 (prematures) days. The practical result is the need to increase the time interval between doses to prevent toxic levels, e.g. gentamicin from 8 hourly at 6 mg/kg/24 h in a child, up to 12–18 hourly at 3–4 mg/kg/24 h in a premature (see Neonatal problems).
3. Serum biochemistry in the first 1–3 days reflects maternal values.
4. Creatinine levels are higher the more premature the infant. The more immature the slower the fall in creatinine. Adult levels or below by 1–4 weeks old.

RENAL PROBLEMS IN THE NEWBORN

1. Congenital anomalies seen on antenatal US

See Neonatal problems.

2. Oliguria (<1 ml/kg/h) or anuria

Causes

Hypoxia, shock, infection, acidosis, renal vessel thrombosis, obstruction to outflow tract, congenital anomaly.

Oliguria is usually transient, but US is needed to differentiate between:

  i Obstruction needing drainage.

ii   Large mass due to renal vein thrombosis (RVT).

iii Small or cystic/dysplastic kidney.

3. Abdominal mass

Over half (55%) are renal, found on antenatal US, on routine examination or presenting with systemic illness due to urinary infection. Renal vein thrombosis is rare, with haematuria, thrombocytopenia, enlarged kidney and shock.

Causes

Commonly: hydronephrosis, multicystic kidney.

Rarely: tumour (benign nephroma in infancy, not Wilms'), infantile polycystic disease, RVT.

Investigations

Differentiate, by US, a renal mass from an adrenal haemorrhage or cystic malformation.

Efforts are directed at determining whether:

i   If hydronephrosis, is it isolated, bilateral or due to an outlet obstruction? Use radioisotope scans and micturating cystourethrogram.

ii If a multicystic kidney, is there functioning tissue? Use a DMSA scan (see below).

iii A solid mass requires initial US, an intravenous pyelogram to identify distortion from tumour, and CT for further delineation.

RENAL FUNCTION AND AGE

1. Urinary concentration

Maximum concentrating ability in the neonate is 600 mOsmol/kg, and is thus vulnerable to hyperosmolar, hypernatraemic dehydration, especially if fed high solute feeds, until near adult levels of concentrating ability is achieved at 6 months (1100 –1300 mOsmol/kg).

2. Glomerular filtration rate

Glomerular filtration rate (GFR) is proportional to the surface area and must be corrected for in children.

i   At birth: GFR is 20–30ml/min/1.73m^2.

ii Infancy: GFR doubles within the neonatal period, but remains low (40–80 ml/min/1.73 m^2).

iii 3 years old before the adult 120ml/min/1.73 m^2 is attained.

Creatinine clearance measurement with accurately timed and complete collections is difficult. A urine-free method for children, not obese or malnourished, is derived from the Schwartz formula:

GFR for 1.73 m² = $\dfrac{\text{Height (cm)} \times 40}{\text{Plasma creatinine } (\mu\text{mol/l})}$

Low GFR for age is due to:

i Extensive bilateral disease.
ii Tubular disease (by regulating GFR to what it can handle, i.e. to maintain glomerulotubular balance).

3. Electrolyte handling in the neonate

i Phosphate: the kidneys' reduced ability to excrete phosphate leads to a higher plasma phosphate level than at older ages. Indeed, the lower limit is the upper limit for adults. Relative maternal hyperparathyroidism due to low vitamin D intake → hypoparathyroidism and hypocalcaemia in the newborn fed unmodified (phosphate rich) cows' milk.
ii Sodium leak by the kidneys of premature infants <32 weeks gestation may need supplementation. A sodium load is inadequately excreted, i.e. retention and oedema can result.

4. Acid–base balance

Normal neonates have a low bicarbonate threshold and ability to excrete H^+ ion, resulting in mild metabolic acidosis and less reserve to deal with acidosis related insults.

RENAL CAUSES OF METABOLIC ACIDOSIS

Failure to thrive and growth retardation is the usual presentation of chronic metabolic acidosis.

Biochemical clues

1. Hyperchloraemic metabolic acidosis (see Metabolic problems for discussion of acid–base physiology, anion gap, and an algorithm).
2. Failure of the urinary pH to fall below 5.5 in the face of a metabolic acidosis.

i Renal failure: Severe bilateral damage, e.g. reflux nephropathy, or dysplasia.
ii Distal renal tubular acidosis: Normal US scan, normal glomerular filtration rate.
   Causes: primary idiopathic, or secondary to hypercalcaemic states.

3. Finding of urinary pH <5.5 and plasma bicarbonate <20 mmol/l in isolation, and no extra-renal cause (e.g. diarrhoea) = proximal renal tubular acidosis due to

lowered threshold for bicarbonate excretion in primary renal tubular acidosis, as part of Fanconi syndrome, cystinosis, Lowe's syndrome, or fructose intolerance.
   Treatment Sodium bicarbonate 3–5 mmol/kg daily is sufficient in distal RTA, but large amounts are needed for proximal RTA.

Fanconi's syndrome

Renal tubular defects in resorption of phosphate, glucose and amino acids. Biochemical confirmation is necessary for diagnosis, +/- bicarbonate wasting and hyperchloraemic acidosis. Hypophosphataemia leads to rickets.

Causes

Commonest is cystinosis (rarely galactosaemia, idiopathic, or heavy metal poisoning).

Treatment

1. To combat metabolic bone disease: phosphate, calcitriol.
2. Acidosis and salt wasting need sodium bicarbonate and/or potassium citrate.
3. Renal transplant in cystinosis at the appropriate time.

RENAL CAUSE OF METABOLIC ALKALOSIS

Bartter's syndrome

Probably AR, cause unknown, associated with hyperaldosteronism and hyper-reninaemia. Giving prostaglandins (causal?) inhibitor indomethacin is effective.
   Presentation from infancy as polyuria, polydipsia, failure to thrive, vomiting and constipation, hypotension; later recurrent dehydration.

Diagnosis

Hypochloraemic alkalosis, by exclusion of other causes of this metabolic pattern (pyloric stenosis, alkali ingestion, diuretics, cystic fibrosis and other salt wasting states).

URINARY TRACT INFECTION (UTI)

Incidence

Neonates 1%, M > F. Therafter 5% of girls during childhood, ratio 50:1 girls to boys.

Pathophysiology

Ascending infection in almost all, except neonates, where up to 30% are haematogenous.

Organisms: Gram–negative *Escherichia coli* (>90%), *Streptococcus faecalis*, Klebsiella species, from the individual's own bowel.

- Staphylococci in some adolescent girls and uncircumcized infants.
- Adenovirus 11 and 21, in haemorrhagic cystitis, and cytomegalovirus infections, also occur.

Factors in renal damage and scarring

1. Age: highest risk in <3 year olds.
2. Therapeutic delay may result in increased renal damage.
3. Obstruction to the renal tract: pelviureteric junction, megaureter, bladder neck obstruction.
4. Individual susceptibility: increased peri-urethral colonization and binding of *Escherichia coli* to bladder mucosa.
5. Bacterial virulence: ability to bind to mucosa found in pyelonephritic *E. coli* (P fimbriated *E. coli*).

Association with vesico-ureteric reflux (VUR)

This is a normal finding in some infants so additional factors operate to cause scarring, refered to as reflux nephropathy (RN)

1. The shape of the papilla, from animal experimental observation, is a vital determinant. Dimpled or flat-topped papillae, usually at the kidneys' upper pole, allow intrarenal reflux if back pressure rises. This force is transmitted to the parenchyma, plus infection = 'big bang'. The normal dome–shaped papilla prevents this.
2. The length of ureter in the bladder wall is short, allowing regurgitation of urine to the kidneys. Infection results.
3. 25–50% of first degree relatives have VUR, i.e. familial.

Subsequent renal growth

Growth of the kidney arrests after scaring in infancy, but shows some catch up growth in late childhood. If the damage is unilateral, the healthy kidney shows compensatory hypertrophy.

Clinical presentations

1. Infancy

Pyrexia is not a constant finding.

- Irritability and poor feeding, weight loss.
- Jaundice in a neonate.

• Dribbling of smelly turbid urine.

First UTI in infancy often goes unrecognized, and is a medical emergency requiring urgent identification and treatment.

2. Older ages

- • Dysuria, frequency or retention, polydipsia common in older children.
- • Onset enuresis in well established dryness.
- • Pain localization: to the flank is suggestive of pyelonephritis, the suprapubic region in cystitis.

3. All ages

Examine for bladder and kidney masses, inspect genitals and do blood pressure. Test sensation in the saddle area and power of the intrinsic muscles of the feet (nerve roots S2–4).

Collection of urine

History taking must include the method of collecting urine at home, if subsequently submitted for culture and found to be positive. Use of antiseptics for washing-out recepticals for collecting urine, micturating into unsterile potties and medicine bottles, and delayed delivery to the laboratory, are not uncommon.

Differential diagnosis

1. Dysuria: see renal symptoms.
2. Urge incontinence due to vulvitis, constipation.
3. Left flank pain due to constipation, right flank to chronic bowel inflammation.
4. Frequent micturition: see renal symptoms.

Diagnosis

1. Urgent microscopy for bacteria and pyuria >50/mm^3 WBCs in fresh urine of an infant or preschool child, or fever with loin pain at any age. Note that absence of pyuria does not exclude bacterial infection.
    Start treatment immediately, once a suitable urine sample has been obtained, changing the antibiotic if necessary after culture result becomes known.
2. Organisms 10^5/ml in two clean catch (young child) or midstream specimens. Repeat if 10$^{4-5}$/ml. If in doubt, or sick, do a suprapubic aspiration – any growth is significant.
3. Bag urine collections are popular but difficult to interpret unless sterile. An acceptable guide is bag urine >10^5/ml organisms on two occasions *plus* bacteria and pyuria on microscopy. Alternatives include aspirating urine with a syringe

from the wet nappy or woolly balls placed in the nappy, but WBCs are trapped so counts are low.

- Urine dipsticks may be positive for blood, protein and nitrite, though the latter is unreliable in small children as they void frequently.
- For home/primary care use dipslides or boric acid preservative. Obtain a sample at the time of symptoms and deliver by post.

Investigation by age

Imaging is essential after the first proven or highly likely urinary tract infection, regardless of sex.

Table 22.2 Imaging investigations by age at presentation and number of infections suffered

<1 year old	1–5 years old	>5 years old
US, DMSA, MCUG in *all* cases	1 First infection: US, plain X-ray abdomen DMSA (IVP if DMSA unavailable) 2 Second infection or scar found i MCG for VUR ii if VUR is found, follow up with 2 yearly DTPA scans until it clears	1 US, plain X-ray abdomen 2 DMSA and DTPA only if scarring is found. An MCG is not done unless surgery contemplated, i.e. minimal investigation is usually sufficient regardless of the number of episodes

DMSA = dimercaptosuccinic acid
DTPA = diethylenetriamine pentacetic acid
MCG = micturating cystogram: do a cysto*urethro*gram (MCUG) if the upper renal tract is dilated, i.e. possible bladder outlet obstruction
VUR = vesicoureteric reflux

Renal tract imaging, its rationale and important findings

1. Ultrasound for scars and hydronephrosis. Scarring and blunting of calyces may not be seen. US is relatively insensitive at detecting scars.
    Timing: US as soon as possible to detect anatomical urological abnormalities. Repeat in 6 months if normal as scarring may take months to develop.
2. Plain X-ray of abdomen for radiopaque renal calculi and spinal abnormalities causing abnormal bladder function.
3. Radioisotope scans

    i Static imaging by ^{99m}Tc dimercaptosuccinic acid (DMSA) incorporated into proximal renal tubules.
        Cold patches are non-functioning areas, e.g. scars, cysts, or ischaemic areas in renal hypertension. After UTI, an early DMSA identifies transient ischaemia, and is best delayed for 3–4 weeks.
        Identifies functioning renal tissue in duplex and horseshoe kidneys.
        Individual contribution by each kidney is expressed as a percentage of total renal function. Upper limit of normal is 45%:55%. Unilateral function >15% = useful, < 7% = recovery of function is unlikely.

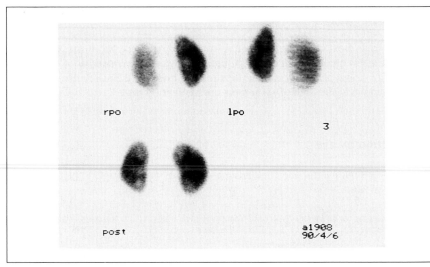

Figure 22.1 DMSA showing cortical scarring of both kidneys secondary to pyelonephritis

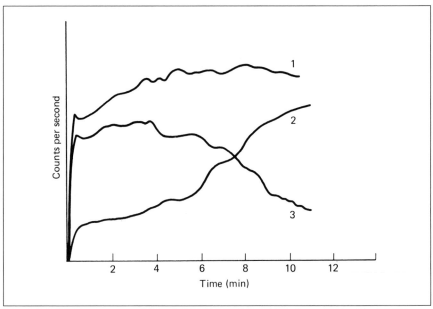

Figure 22.2 DTPA excretory scan shows hold up due to obstructive hydronephrosis of the left kidney.
1 = left kidney, 2 = bladder, 3 = right kidney.

 ii Dynamic imaging by [99mTc] diethylenetriamine pentacetic acid (DTPA).
  Excreted via glomeruli, the rate of clearance equals the GFR, and can be esti-
  mated for each kidney.
   Obstruction (hold up) is differentiated from dilatation.
   Reflux can be sequentially followed after a diagnostic MCG.

Relative renal function of each kidney is recorded as a percentage of total function. In unilateral obstruction a contribution of <20% is an indicator for surgery to relieve it.

3. Micturating cystourethrogram for vesicoureteric reflux (VUR), may also see ureteroceles, trabeculated bladder, and in the male the urethra for posterior urethral valves.

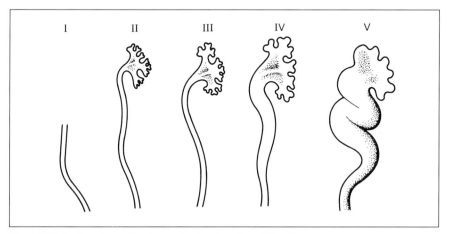

Figure 22.3 Grading of severity of reflux by the International Classification:

I	Reflux into lower ureter	90
II	Reflux to pelvis of kidney	70
III	Dilatation of calyces	50
IV	Tortuosity of ureters	10
V	Gross dilatation of calyces	0

Percentage that resolve at each grade.

Biochemical investigations

Plasma electrolytes, bicarbonate, urea, and creatinine. Glomerular filtration rate if the plasma creatinine is raised, plasma bicarbonate low, or bilateral renal abnormality found on imaging.

Management

Acute infection

1. Acutely unwell young child needs hospitalization and gentamicin.

   Correct shock, dehydration, electrolytes, acidosis. Paracetamol for fever.

   After 2 days the antibiotic may be changed to an oral preparation, if well and sensitivities allow, for 7–10 days, otherwise continue i.v. gentamicin while monitoring the blood level.

   Previous treatment and underlying renal tract abnormalities may result in resistant and complicated infections needing other antibiotics.

2. Mild systemic upset. Trimethoprim or amoxycillin +/- clavulanic acid for 5–7 days suffice. Nalidixic acid and nitrofurantoin are good second line drugs.
3. Single dose treatment is satisfactory for girls > 5 years old known to have normal renal tracts.

Copious oral fluids to wash out the bladder reduces bacterial multiplication.

General advice

1. Treat constipation which may exacerbate urge incontinence and possibly the recurrence of UTI.
2. Wipe the anus front to back.
3. Perform double micturition if a large bladder residuum, due to vesicoureteric reflux, is found.

Prophylaxis during investigations is given

1. After acute infection under 3 years old until all investigations are completed and management planned.
2. After catheterization for micturating cystourethrogram or cystoscopy.

Follow up

Management depends on:

1. Number of infections, which also dictates:
2. Need for antibiotic prophylaxis.
3. Presence of an underlying abnormality.

1. First/sporadic infection　　3-monthly check urines for one year.
2. Prophylaxis Drugs: trimethoprim or nitrofurantoin 1–2 mg/kg/day as a single evening dose. Resistance to other antibiotics quickly develops.
　　Indications:

　i Repeated infection: >2 episodes within 6 months. Treatment for 6 months results in fewer recurrences after stopping.
　ii Vesicoureteric reflux (VUR): to prevent recurrent infection and subsequent scarring if VUR grade III–V is present; recurrence is unusual with grade II.

　　Under 5 years old the risk of fresh renal damage is significant, therefore give antibiotic prophylaxis until VUR improves on DTPA scan done 2 yearly or up to age 7 years, whichever is the sooner.

3. Surgery indications

　i Poor compliance is shown by break through infections in VUR under 5 years old.
　　No superiority for either surgical or medical treatment in the long term, although the number of acute episodes is reduced after surgery. Consider the surgical option where compliance is poor, or very likely to be.
　ii Removal of a para-ureteric diverticula (ureterocele).

Prognosis

Of those investigated after the first UTI 60% are normal. The remainder comprise:

1. VUR 30%. Of these 30% are already scarred at presentation (i.e. 5–10% of all UTIs under a year) and 20% have persistent VUR.
   Prospect as adults: 10% will develop hypertension, 5% chronic renal failure.
   VUR is the commonest cause (20%) of chronic renal failure (CRF) in children, and accounts for 5–10% of CRF in young adults.
2. Obstruction 7%: anatomical (e.g. at pelvi-ureteric junction), neuropathic bladder (e.g. spina bifida), stones.
3. Duplex or horse-shoe kidney 3%: usually a coincidental finding, but abnormal drainage predisposing to UTI is not uncommon.

Prevention

Although 50% of first degree relatives have VUR, screening and offering prophylaxis if VUR is found is of unproven value.

Further reading

Leader (1991) Prevention of reflux nephropathy. *Lancet,* ii,1050

Lerner G R, Fleischmann L E, Perlmutter A D (1987) Reflux nephropathy. *Pediatric Clinics of North America*, **34**, 747–770

Verier Jones K (1990) Antimicrobial treatment for urinary tract infections. *Archives of Disease in Childhood*, **65**, 327–330

White R H R (1987) Management of urinary tract infection. *Archives of Disease in Childhood*, **62**, 421–427

White R H R (1989) Vesicoureteric reflux and renal scarring. *Archives of Disease in Childhood*, **64**, 407–412

Asymptomatic bacteriuria

Present in 2% of females, it is no longer considered important to screen for, nor to treat even if VUR is demonstrated, as recurrence is frequent and long–term sequelae minimal.

RENAL SYMPTOMS

1. Daytime wetting

A period of dryness followed by the onset of daytime incontinence needs early assessment at any age. It affects 1% of girls aged 4–7 years, twice as many as boys at that age. Among nocturnal enuretics 10–20% suffer, in whom response to treatment is slower.

  i Wetting on the return journey home from school is commonly emotional.

ii Urge incontinence, especially after UTI, is elicited on history. Propantheline (1 mg/kg/day divided into 3–4 doses) and tricyclic antidepressants have anticholinergic effects and relax the unstable detrusor muscle.

　A programme of 2–hourly voiding is helpful. Persistence of symptoms or a large post-voiding bladder residuum are an indication for urodynamic tests.

iii Dribbling incontinence from infancy suggests an ectopic ureter, and a weak urinary stream an outlet obstruction (e.g. posterior urethral valves) or neuropathic bladder.

iv No obvious underlying cause: do a stress test = incontinence on raising intraabdominal pressure and resisting micturition, while standing. Wide bladder neck anomaly may be found radiologically.

2. Dysuria

i Urinary tract infection. Micturition while crying may be normal, but onset of crying during micturition is significant. Systemic symptoms are likely.

ii Local external factors, without systemic features, are far more common than UTI:

a. Vulvitis or balanitis (pyuria and bacterial contamination of urine samples often lead to misdiagnosis unless the genitals are examined).

b. Meatal ulceration, ammoniacal dermatitis.

c. Trauma, sexual abuse.

iii Urge syndrome, common after UTI, is due to detrusor instability. Also seen in vulvovaginitis and constipation.

3. Frequency, including polyuria

Common

i Functional, e.g. stress, cold weather, attention seeking.

ii Organic: common in

a. UTI.

b. Gross VUR.

c. Dribbling overflow in neurogenic bladder, posterior urethral valves.

d. With polydipsia due to glycosuria in diabetes mellitus.

Rare

Chronic renal failure, diabetes insipidus, hypercalcaemia, renal tubular acidosis (Fanconi's syndrome), Bartter's syndrome.

Diabetes insipidus (DI)

Antidiuretic homone (ADH) acts on the cells of the distal renal tubule, which, by generating cyclic adenosine monophosphate increase water absorption.

a. Central: lack of production, e.g. head injury, pituitary lesion.

b. Renal tubule dysfunction:
   Damage from chronic renal failure, Fanconi's syndrome, renal tubular acidosis.
   Nephrogenic diabetes insipidus (NDI), XL (rare).
   Unresponsiveness of distal tubule to ADH. Urine osmolality is usually <50 mosmol/l.

Clinical

1. Dehydration: risk of hypernatraemia and brain damage in the infant unable to communicate the need for free water.
2. Anorexia, and failure to thrive due to poor caloric intake.

Investigation

1. Measure input and output to confirm large volumes of fluid in and out.
2. Overnight fluid deprivation test: first voided urine of the day, if >800 mosmol/l = normal ADH secretion and renal function.
3. In suspected DI, 4 hours fluid deprivation in NDI or until 3% of body weight is lost is usually sufficient to show an elevation of plasma osmolality with inappropriately low urine osmolality.
4. Desmopressin (DDAVP – a synthetic ADH analogue) test.
   a. A failure to achieve a urine osmolality of 800 mosmol/l is usually due to chronic renal disease. Confirm by creatinine clearance, and imaging. Normal findings will identify those few cases of functional polydipsia who's excessive intake washes out the normally high renal medulla concentration.
   b. Nephrogenic diabetes insipidus urine rarely concentrates >300 mosmol/l.
   c. Normal response in central DI.

Management according to cause

1. Access to, and as much water as is needed, to avoid hypernatraemia.
2. Adequate calories to promote growth, often inadequate until treatment started, because appetite was suppressed.
3. Central – DDAVP.
4. Renal – adequate fluid, calories, reduced protein load, but see renal failure.
5. Nephrogenic DI.

   i Give minimum daily requirements for salt and protein intake. Rationale: as urine concentration (and solute content) is fixed, provide the least solute necessary. This reduces the water intake and encourages appetite.
   ii Thiazide further reduces free water clearance. Watch for hypokalaemia. Dose 1–2 mg/kg/day.
   iii Indomethacin, the prostaglandin inhibitor, enhances any ADH response. Dose 1–2 mg/kg/day.

4. Oliguria

Oliguria = <0.5ml/kg/h. Prerenal, renal and postrenal obstruction and retention. See acute renal failure for assessment. Acute retention is normally identified on history and examination, and may require urine culture or CSF examination (transverse myelitis, polyneuritis, tumour).

Prerenal

Dehydration, septicaemia and shock due to hypovolaemia.

Renal

Trauma → acute tubular necrosis, acute glomerulonephritis, haemolytic uraemic syndrome, nephrotic syndrome.

Post renal

   i Acute retention

      a. Painful: the commonest cause is urinary tract infection, followed by vul-vovaginitis or meatal ulcer. Occasionally, secondary to voluntary reten-tion as part of an emotional disturbance.

      b. 'Silent': neurogenic cord injury or myelitis, or Guillain-Barré polyneuritis syndrome: poor urinary stream or autonomic bladder with incomplete voiding.

   ii Chronic retention with distended bladder due to obstruction, e.g. posterior urethral valve, or neurogenic as in spina bifida or sacral agenesis.

5. Haematuria

Intensity guide.

i Gross haematuria

First establish discoloration is

      a. Blood, red when fresh smoky/brown on standing, or:

      b. Concentrated urine, as distinct from:

      c. Urates in the nappy of boys = a red deposit in the penile area.

      d. Haemoglobinuria, myoglobinuria.

      e. Beetroot, food dyes, bile, rifampicin.

The three glass test is a useful rule of thumb:

    haematuria at beginning of micturition = urethral
                    throughout = bladder
                  end-micturition = upper renal tract

ii Positive on dipstick only

Very sensitive, 3% of schoolchildren are positive on one occasion, 1% on two or more. Only investigate if more than a trace, persistently positive or on two occasions a month or more apart.

iii Proteinuria and haematuria

a. Infection.

b. In the absence of gross haematuria, the additional presence of protein on dipstick suggests renal origin.
c. Haematuria without proteinuria is of unknown cause in 50% and clears spontaneously.

Site of bleeding and RBC morphology.

Kidney origin if:

1. Distorted, due to the mechanical effect of being squeezed through glomeruli.
2. Red cell casts are present.

Causes of haematuria

1. Infection +/– underlying anatomical anomaly, but note that hydronephrosis and bladder diverticuli may occasionally bleed in the absence of infection.
2. Trauma.
3. Glomerulonephritis, including Henoch-Schönlein purpura and IgA nephropathy.
4. Benign recurrent haematuria: temperature, upper respiratory infection, exercise, familial – beware Alport's syndrome.
5. Munchausen by proxy.

Unusual: haemolytic uraemic syndrome, calculi, hypercalciuria, renal vein thrombosis, polycystic kidney, Wilms' tumour, systemic lupus erythematosus.

Assessment by history

- Familial renal disorder (benign recurrent haematuria, polycystic disease, bleeding disorders, Alport's syndrome).
- Relation to exercise.
- Dysuria, frequency – bladder or urethral local inflammation or trauma.
- Upper abdominal/flank pain – pyelonephritis, hydronephrosis, acute glomerulonephritis (AGN), polycystic disease, calculus.
- Preceding illness: upper respiratory tract infection – AGN; diarrhoea – haemolytic uraemic syndrome.
- Travel – schistosomiasis.
- Black race – sickle cell disease.
- Drug exposure: many ingestants have been reported. Consult pharmacopoeia, poisons information service.

Examination

Pallor, oedema especially periorbital, hypertension, abdominal pain/masses, genitals for inflammation or injury.

Investigation

Plan according to whether:

- symptomatic or asymptomatic.

- acute, subacute, or chronic.

  i Confirm haematuria +/- proteinuria by dipstick.
  ii Microscopy. First examine unspun urine. >5 RBCs/mm^3 is significant, then centrifuge, looking for casts in the deposit if not already found.

     a. RBCs + pus cells + bacteria = infection. Culture urine and manage the urinary tract infection as below.
     b. Undeformed RBCs = lower renal tract likely. Arrange a plain X-ray of abdomen, US, micturating cystogram, consider cystoscopy, for structural abnormalities (diverticuli, tumour, stone), or foreign body.
     c. Dysmorphic RBCs and RBC casts = upper renal tract. Obtain antistreptolysin O titre (ASOT), C3 complement level for glomerulonephritis.

        'Telescoped' urine also containing WBC casts requires C3 and C4 complement levels, anti-DNA antibody and anti-nuclear factor (ANF) titres, to diagnose systemic lupus erythematosus.
  iii Blood count, serum creatinine, electrolytes, bicarbonate and urea in all cases, and coagulation studies and platelets where a bleeding disorder is suspected.
  iv Urinary calcium for hypercalciuria needs a spot urine. Calcium:creatinine ratio >0.4 (or >4mg/kg/24 h) is found in 30% with unexplained haematuria.
  v Renal biopsy. Indications:

     a. Low complement level for more than 6 months consider renal biopsy for type and prognosis of chronic glomerulonephritis.
     b. After normal investigations: renal biopsy is best avoided until at least 1 year of recurrent episodes, so only the chronic conditions are left.
     c. Abnormal renal function, i.e. low GFR.
     d. Persistent microscopic haematuria.

Differential diagnosis of acute nephritis

1. Abnormal renal function: low GFR, raised serum creatinine, urea, and anaemic:

   i Acute postinfectious glomerulonephritis: low C3, raised ASOT and anti–DNAse B.
   ii Haemolytic uraemic syndrome: thrombocytopenia, fragmented RBCs.
   iii Chronic glomerulonephritis: short stature, persistently low C3, previous haematuria.
   iv Alport's syndrome: family history of renal disease in males and sensorineural deafness. Check patient's hearing, and maternal urine for haematuria.
   v Systemic lupus erythematosus: very weak, fever, rash, arthralgia. Persistently low C3, C4. Positive ANF, anti-DNA antibodies.

2. Normal renal function:

   i Henoch-Schönlein purpura: triad of rash, abdominal pain, arthralgia.
   ii Benign recurrent haematuria: haematuria without clinical or laboratory abnormalities.

INDIVIDUAL CONDITIONS ASSOCIATED WITH HAEMATURIA

Acute post infectious glomerulonephritis

Incidence

After group A beta haemolytic streptococcus (β-HS) infection: 1 in 13,000.

Pathophysiology

Immune reaction by susceptible individuals to nephritogenic strains of β-HS (in USA type 12; after streptococcal skin infection, type 49), less frequently staphylococci, hepatitis B, infectious mononucleosis. Latent period 10 (5–21) days.

Serum C3 complement is reduced. Light microscopy shows glomerular capillary endothelial proliferation, immunofluorescence shows deposition of IgG and C3 complement in the glomeruli, which on electron microscopy is on the epithelial side of the basement membrane.

Clinical

1. Non–specific symptoms are common: pallor, headache, abdominal pain, weakness.
2. Oedema. Facial and periorbital on rising, abdominal and ankle swelling later in the day.
3. Haematuria. From dark tea, through smoky to gross haematuria.
4. Oliguria.
5. Hypertension: cardiac failure and/or encephalopathy (headache, coma, convulsions).

Progress

Acute phase lasts 1–2 weeks, gross haematuria, BP elevated for 3–4 weeks. Microscopic haematuria for up to 12 months.

Diagnosis

Urine contains distorted RBCs, RBC casts, protein +/++.
   Blood: mild normochromic anaemia, leucocytosis, raised ESR.
   Low C3, ASOT raised.

Management

Fluid and salt restriction, if early in the acute phase, may prevent hypertension. Daily allowance = insensible water loss + 1/2 previous 24–h urine output. Monitor with frequent weighing.

   Hypertension >140/100: frusemide if overloaded – the only cause of acute hypertension that can be treated with a diuretic. If unresponsive give nitroprupside or labetalol.

β–HS on culture is an indication for a course of penicillin.

Persistent hypocomplementaemia >6 months is an indication for renal biopsy.

Prognosis

Good for >90%. Rapidly progressive in 1%.

Recurrent haematuria syndromes

1. IgA nephropathy (Berger's disease) and Henoch-Schönlein purpura association

Definition of Berger's disease

Frank haematuria for 2–5 days with upper respiratory tract infection or vigorous exercise. Renal biopsy on immunofluorescence shows mainly mesangial IgA, also IgG, and C3 complement deposits.

Clinical

Mainly boys, over 2 years old. Central abdominal or flank pain is common. Occasional arthralgia of medium–sized joints and skin rashes suggest a strong overlap with Henoch-Schönlein purpura.

Prognosis

Used to be called benign recurrent haematuria, but it is now recognized that 10–30% may progress to renal failure. Follow up is essential.

Renal findings in Henoch-Schönlein purpura

Identical lesion in Berger's and Henoch-Schonlein purpura (HSP), and similar clinical picture, indicate each is a variant of a similar disease process.

Renal involvement is found in up to 50% of HSP. Although usually microscopic they may show gross haematuria, acute nephritis, proteinuria +/– nephrotic syndrome.

Prognosis

Good unless extensive (>50%) crescent formation when chronic renal failure develops in 2–10 years. Affects 1–2% with HSP.

2. Chronic glomerulonephritis

Onset or persistence of proteinuria is associated with the development of hypertension, and progressive rise in serum creatinine.

Pathology

Focal segmental glomerulosclerosis and membranoproliferative glomerulonephritis are the commonest lesions.

Occasionally found is mesangial proliferative glomerulonephritis with IgM deposits. May present as persistent or recurrent haematuria, or nephrotic syndrome. Very variable prognosis.

See chronic renal failure for clinical and management details.

3. Basement membrane nephropathy

With normal light microscopy and immunofluorescence, sometimes found in children with recurrent haematuria. Characterized by variation in thickness of the glomerular basement membrane on electron microscopy (EM). Usually mild, with good prognosis, though others are indistinguishable from Alport's syndrome both on EM and clinically.

STONES

Incidence

Rare, affecting 1.5 children per million population.

Site

Upper renal tract in developed countries, and bladder in poorer developing countries where they are still relatively common.

Composition

Most stones in the UK are phosphates of calcium (radiopaque) or magnesium due to stasis, i.e. obstruction, and infection.

10% are metabolic stones, e.g. hypercalcaemia (excess vitamin D or immobilization are commonest), uric acid (during induction therapy for leukaemia), hyperoxaluria or cystinuria (AR) due to a tubular (and intestinal) defect of amino acid transport leading to excessive excretion of cystine, lysine, ornithine and arginine. Only cystine is relatively insoluble, and if urine is concentrated and acidic it precipitates out. Presentation is usually in adolescence, and untreated leads eventually to renal failure. Copious water, alkalinization, and occasionally penacillamine, are needed to prevent stone formation.

Clinical

Flank pain, haematuria, occasionally painless at first.

Investigations

Urine culture. Urinary 24–h calcium, phosphate, oxalate and uric acid excretion, and an amino acid chromatogram. Blood for E+U, uric acid. Imaging for stone localization.

Management

If large, causing obstruction, infection, and potential renal failure, it may be removed by extracorporeal shock wave lithotripsy.

PROTEINURIA AND OEDEMA

Pathophysiology

The glomerular basement membrane (GBM) carries a negative charge which repels the negatively charged plasma proteins. Damage reduces this charge, increasing permeability in proportion to molecular weight. In addition, deposits on the membrane, or development of gaps between GBM cells, increase protein loss and allow blood cells to pass.

The glomerular capillaries normally allow only the passage of water, electrolytes and small protein molecules. Leakage may occur in capillary disease.

Plasma oncotic pressure is mainly due to albumin. Hypoalbuminaemia allows fluid to pass into the interstitial space. The resultant hypovolaemia activates the renin-angiotensin-aldosterone pathway, causing sodium retention and worsening of the oedema.

i Benign proteinuria

Definition

<100mg/day.

Causes

Orthostatic, physical stress of exercise or fever.

Orthostatic (postural) proteinuria disappears on lying down. Found at least once in 5–10% of randomly tested children, Albustix (Ames) +/++/+++ during the day, whereas the first urine on rising contains 0 or trace only; test for 3 consecutive days.

In nephrotic syndrome monitored at home: to avoid possible confusion with postural proteinuria only test the first urine on rising. Relapse = +++ for 3 consecutive days.

ii Glomerular disease +/- systemic illness

Definition

Characterized by persistent proteinuria >100 mg/day.

a. Glomerular causes

- Nephrosis = >1 G/m^2 surface area: nephrotic syndrome, membranous glomerulonephritis, membranoproliferative glomerulonephritis.
- Acute glomerulonephritis.

- Focal glomerular sclerosis.

b. Systemic diseases with glomerular involvement

Sickle cell, Henoch-Schönlein purpura, SLE, subacute bacterial endocarditis, amyloidosis. In diabetes mellitus, the microproteinuria due to early glomerulosclerosis requires a special assay as Albustix cannot detect it.

Laboratory assessment of proteinuria

Urinary protein:creatinine concentration ratio

Measuring protein in an early morning urine sample by the protein:creatinine ratio (mg/mmol) eliminates postural proteinuria and the need for correction for surface area.

Urinary P:C ratio = $\dfrac{\text{mg protein}}{\text{mmol creatinine}}$

A ratio >20 (>20 mg/mmol) is abnormal and requires investigation.

Similarly, a urinary albumin:creatinine ratio of more than 0.1mg/mg (note units) is abnormal.

Uses: nephrotic syndrome, Alport's syndrome, follow up of Henoch Schönlein purpura.

Urinary protein selectivity index (UPSI)

Selective = lower molecular weight proteins (albumin or transferrin) only/mainly present, e.g. minimal change nephrotic syndrome. Selectivity of 0.1 or less is usually steroid responsive.

Non-selective = large protein molecules (IgG) also present, due to severe glomerular damage, e.g. glomerulonephritis.

UPSI is not a reliable predictor due to overlap between the groups, and has become less popular as a clinical tool.

Practical assessment of proteinuria

1. Establish whether postural/persistent proteinuria.
2. Physical stress,e.g. temperature or vigorous exercise as a possible cause.
3. History:

- Family history of similarly affected infants (congenital nephrotic syndrome), deafness or renal failure (Alport's syndrome).
- Dysuria, lower abdominal pain in urinary tract infection.
- Onset of oedema, poor appetite, irritability in nephrotic syndrome.
- Polyuria, growth failure in renal failure.
- Haematuria in acute nephritis.

Clinical

Oedema, pallor, growth failure, hypertension, large or tender kidneys, rickets.

Investigation and differential diagnosis

1. Urinalysis: presence of haematuria in more serious diseases (see haematuria), fixed specific gravity 1.010 or osmolality 300 mosmol/l in renal failure, WBCs in infection.
2. Urine culture for infection.
3. Urinary protein. Abnormality in protein:creatinine ratio, or 24–h urine collection showing >0.02 g/kg or >1 g/m^2, e.g. nephrotic syndrome in relapse would show a protein:creatinine ratio >200 mg/mmol or albumin:creatinine >0.2 mg/mg.
4. GFR is reduced and serum urea raised in chronic renal failure, associated with metabolic acidosis and biochemical markers of osteodystrophy.
5. Serum albumin low, cholesterol raised in nephrotic syndrome.
6. Complement C3 low in acute glomerulonephritis (AGN) and chronic nephritis. Raised ASOT in AGN.
7. Glycosuria, aminoaciduria, hyperphosphaturia in Fanconi's syndrome points to a *tubular* origin for the proteinuria.
8. US, radioisotopes for scars, cysts, shrunken kidneys, and their function.
9. Renal biopsy may be indicated if:

   i Low or falling GFR.
   ii Persistent proteinuria not responsive to 4 weeks treatment with steroids (i.e. minimal change nephrotic syndrome is unlikely).
   iii Persistently low C3 in chronic nephritis.

10. Low C3 and C4, anti DNA antibodies, 'telescoped' urine of systemic lupus erythematosus.

INDIVIDUAL CONDITIONS

Nephrotic syndrome

Definition

A clinical state common to a number of different glomerular diseases, characterized by proteinuria, low albumin, usually oedema and raised cholesterol.

Incidence

1 in 50000 annually. Incidence per 100,000: Asian 16, others 3.

Pathophysiology

1. Minimal change nephrotic syndrome (MCNS) in 90%. No change on light microscopy. Effacement of foot processes on electron microscopy, a highly selective urinary protein index.

2. Membranoproliferative glomerulonephritis (MPGN) 5%: mesangial cell proliferation, C3 deposits in capillary and tubule walls and glomerular basement membrane on immunofluorescence.
3. Focal segmental glomerulosclerosis (FSGS) in some glomeruli, distributed
   among normal glomeruli. Obliteration of Bowman's space. 5% of cases.

The pathological process may be a continuum from MCNS through to FSGS
with some MPGN.

Table 22.3 Clinical and laboratory changes in nephrotic syndrome

Findings required for the diagnosis of nephrotic syndrome	Adverse prognostic factors (% = frequency of occurrence)
Generalized oedema +/– ascites	Haematuria 25%
Gross proteinuria >3 g/24 h	Hypertension 25%
Hypoalbuminaemia (<25 g/l)	Raised plasma urea 10%
(Hypercholesterolaemia, not essential)	Hypocomplementaemia 1%
	Age <1 year or >10 years old

Clinical	Complications
1 Peak age 2–4 years	1 Infection: septicaemia, peritonitis
2 Oedema: face, scrotal swelling = ascites, dependent oedema, skin breakdown	(*Strep. pneumoniae* > Gram negative)
3 Low blood pressure	2 Acute renal failure due to low BP or primary cause of nephrotic state
Abdominal pain (sign of low BP)	3 Hypercoaguability → renal vein thrombosis, pulmonary embolus
4 Anorexia, lethargy, oliguria	4 Hypocalcaemic tetany
5 Diarrhoea	

Management and prognosis

1. Daily weighing if oedema is present.
2. Diet: no water restriction, moderate salt restriction. Normal protein intake (no
   point in forcing more on the child, as there is no evidence of increased albumin
   production).
3. Prophylactic penicillin while oedema is present. Consider pneumococcal vaccination once in remission.
   Diuretics in the acute phase may precipitate renal failure by worsening hypovolaemia if oedematous.
4. Corticosteroids. Diuresis usually occurs within 2 weeks of commencement.

   i Factors altering responsiveness

      a. Absence of adverse factors (or presence of protein selectivity index (PSI)
         for IgG:transferrin <0.1) in MCNS = 95% steroid responsive.
      b. Presence of haematuria/hypertension/raised urea = 30% will respond, all
         likely to be FSGS.
      c. Hypocomplementaemia: no response to steroids.
      d. Responsiveness to steroids = MCNS in 90%.

   ii Failure to respond to steroids within 28 days → renal biopsy as 95% of
      responders will have done so and MPGN, FSGS or other cause is likely. Uri-
      nary protein selectivity index is redundant if managed in this way.

iii Drug regimen, clinical response and subsequent action
    a. Initial regimen: prednisolone 60 mg/m^2 or 2 mg/kg as a single daily dose, until negative/trace Albustix on three consecutive mornings, when steroid is then tailed off over 2–4 weeks. Monitor daily (first urine on rising) with Albustix.
    b. Relapse, usually due to acute infection, occurs in 75% within the first 6 months = 7 days albumin ++/+++. Treat as before.
    c. Frequent relapser = two or more relapses in 6 months. Prolonged alternate day steroid is given in the smallest dose to keep urine albumin free, after induction of remission.
    d. Steroid dependent = relapses as steroids are tailed off, or within 2 weeks of stopping, on two occasions. Continuous alternate day steroids are given. Failure to respond or steroid toxicity is an indication for cyclophosphamide or levamisole. Suppression of reproductive cells is transient in a short course of cyclophosphamide, but sterility may be permanent if it is prolonged or repeated. Levamisole at 2.5 mg/kg on alternate days may become the drug of choice for this group.

Outcome in MCNS

25% no relapse, 25% infrequent relapses, 50% frequent relapsers of whom a half are steroid dependent. Outgrown by adult life, good prognosis. Death, due to complications, is rare.

Other forms of nephrotic syndrome

A third each remit spontaneously, persist, or progress to renal failure.

Further reading

British Association for Paediatric Nephrology (1991) Levamisole for corticosteroid-dependent nephrotic syndrome in childhood. *Lancet,* i, 1555–1557

Congenital nephrotic syndrome AR

Most common in Finland.

Pathophysiology

Infantile dilatation, like a chain of beads, of proximal tubule. Onset <3 months old, premature delivery of small for dates infant, large oedematous placenta. Fetal asphyxia and perinatal death common. Nephrectomy and dialysis at 2–6 months, before renal failure ensues, followed by renal transplant at a year.

Prognosis

Mortality 75% in the first year, usually from infection or thrombosis. Antenatal diagnosis is possible: the finding of raised alpha feto-protein in amniotic fluid.

RENAL FAILURE

Acute renal failure

Sudden and usually reversible fall in GFR with changes in handling and excretion of solutes, metabolic products and toxins.

Oliguria = <0.5 ml/kg/h. May be due to inadequate fluid intake (prerenal) or renal failure. Infusion of fluid may be necessary to differentiate.

Useful biochemical indices

1. Urine:plasma urea ratio >5 = prerenal <5 = renal
2. Urine:plasma osmolality ratio >1.3 = prerenal <1.3 = renal
3. Urinary sodium <10 mmol/l if prerenal due to increased aldosterone activity.
4. Serum creatinine rising or high. Anuria sees a rise of 150 μmol/l day.

Fall in GFR may result in passing large volumes of iso-osmolar urine, not necessarily oliguria, and is common in acute tubular necrosis.

Causes

Divided into three:

1. Prerenal impaired perfusion.
2. Renal.
3. Postrenal obstruction to renal flow.

Any of these may cause parenchymal kidney damage, i.e. acute tubular necrosis, if prolonged or severe enough.

1. Prerenal

   i Volume depletion: diarrhoea is the most important cause worldwide, nephrotic syndrome the commonest renal disease.
  ii Shock: burns, post cardiac surgery, Reye's syndrome.
 iii Septicaemia.
 iv Pump (heart) failure.

2. Renal

   i Trauma.
  ii Urinary tract infection.
 iii Acute glomerulonephritis: post-streptococcal, membranoproliferative, SLE.
 iv Nephrotoxic insults: aminoglycosides, ethylene glycol, mercury.
  v Haemolytic uraemic syndrome.

3. Post renal acute obstruction

Rare.

   i Mechanical: posterior urethral valves, stones, or uric acid crystals from leukaemia treatment. May be unilateral in a single kidney.

  ii Neurogenic: myelitis, cord injury.

Table 22.4 Commoner causes by age

Infants	Children
1 Pre-renal	
Gastroenteritis, septicaemia, congenital heart disease, neonatal renal vein thrombosis	Dehydration, trauma, burns, scalds, nephrotic syndrome
2 Renal	
Urinary tract infection, haemolytic uraemic syndrome	Acute tubular necrosis*, haemolytic uraemic syndrome
3 Post renal	
Posterior urethral valves	Acute myelitis

*Acute tubular necrosis is due to hypotension, hypovolaemia, haemorrhage. Lasts days to months. If severe, renal cortical necrosis follows, and renal function rarely recovers.

Clinical

Biphasic: characterized by severe oliguria, followed 3–5 days later by gross polyuria, then a return to normal urine volumes.

Complications and their causation

1. Lethargy, convulsions/coma due to

     i Water retention → hyponatraemia.

    ii Hypertension → hypertensive encephalopathy.

   iii Uraemia: symptoms due to failure to excrete toxins and possibly parathormone.

2. Oedema, pulmonary oedema, and cardiac failure: water retention, sodium retention.

3. Hypertension: water and sodium retention, hyper-reninaemia due to renal ischaemia.

Indications for dialysis

In acute renal failure

1. Biochemical changes.

    • Serum urea 30 mmol/l and rising. (Creatinine is also rising, by 50 mmol/l/ day).

    • Hyperkalaemia >7 mmol/l and rising.

    • Metabolic acidosis.

2. Severe fluid overload.

3. Severe hypertension.

In chronic renal failure also consider dialysis for

1. Uraemia and unable to take part in activities at school or with peers; creatinine clearance <10 ml/min/1.73m^2, and poor growth.
2. In infancy: reduced head or body growth, and slowing of mental development.
3. Renal osteodystrophy progressing despite medical treatment.

Management principles

1. Identify and treat underlying cause

e.g. UTI, septicaemia with gentamicin/ceftazidime, surgical relief of obstruction in posterior urethral valves. In renal causes, Doppler US shows reduced or absent intrarenal blood flow and an increase anticipates recovery and diuresis.

2. Kidney excretory function optimization

  i Low protein load 0.5 g/kg/day orally, or i.v. essential amino acids 0.3 g/kg/day.
 ii Adequate calories (100–150 kcal/kg/day).
iii Careful attention to fluid balance water 400 ml/m^2/24 h plus previous 24 h urine excretion. A loss of 0.5% per day body weight is desirable.
 iv Monitoring gentamicin levels if given for sepsis.

3. Complications anticipated or dealt with

  i Oxygen or mechanical ventilation is often required in sick infants with fluid overload, pulmonary oedema and convulsions.
 ii Hypovolaemia corrected by i.v. fluids and plasma expanders.
iii Hypervolaemia reduced by frusemide or dialysis if unresponsive or convulsing.
 iv Hyperkalaemia > 6.0 mmol/l:

   a. ECG monitoring, calcium gluconate or calcium/potassium exchange resin + bicarbonate given rectally.
   b. Encourage K$^+$ to enter cells: salbutamol 4 mg/kg over 5 minutes has the same effect as 50% i.v. glucose + insulin 1 u/4 g/kg glucose, and is easier and much safer to give.

  v Metabolic acidosis regularly monitored and should be half corrected.

Prognosis

Mortality up to 50% in neonates, trauma and post surgical (cardiac mainly).

Haemolytic-uraemic syndrome (HUS)

Definition

Triad of microangiopathic haemolytic anaemia, thrombocytopenia and renal failure. The commonest cause of acute renal failure in the UK.

Epidemiology

150 annually (2/100 000), predominantly infants and young children. Two forms (Table 22.5):

1. Diarrhoea associated (D+), at younger ages, in the summer months.
2. The less common, sporadic, without prodrome (D–).

Pathogenesis

Endothelial cell injury due to verotoxin (e.g. from *Escherichia coli* 0157:H7, *Shigella dysenteriae* type 1) or prostacyclin deficiency allowing platelet aggregation and vasoconstriction.

Differential diagnosis

1. Prodrome of bloody diarrhoea (D+) helps distinguish the two types of HUS.
2. Hyponatraemia during rehydration is a clue to renal failure.
3. Purpura: otherwise well in ITP; with lymphadenopathy in leukaemia.
4. Other causes of acute renal failure to be considered (Table 22.4) specially SLE, or renal vein thrombosis.
5. Other organs than the kidney may be involved:
    Coma and convulsions (CNS), melaena, hepatosplenomegaly, indistinguishable from thrombotic thrombocytopenic purpura seen in meningococcaemia.
    Cardiomyopathy with cardiac failure.
    Diabetes mellitus (stress hyperglycaemia, metabolic acidosis).

Table 22.5 Two forms of haemolytic-uraemic syndrome

	Diarrhoea associated (D+)	*Sporadic (D–)*
Aetiology	Verotoxin	Prostacyclin deficiency found in: familial cases, SLE, malignant hypertension, immunosuppressive drugs, contraceptive pill
Microangiopathy	Glomerular	Arterial (i.e. more generalized)
Onset	Prodromal D+V	Insidious (weeks) with pallor
Hypertension	Often mild	Usually moderate. Bad prognosis if severe
Renal function	Most (85%) recover	Chronic failure is common (70%)
Mortality	<10%	>10%

Investigations

The blood film shows red cells in bizarre shapes: helmet cells, burr cells, fragments. Anaemia (5–9 g/dl), thrombocytopenia and mild to moderately increased circulating fibrin degradation products. Microscopic haematuria. Metabolic acidosis, raised plasma urea and creatinine.

Management

1. Supportive: correct anaemia, institute the regimen for renal failure.
2. Shock and neutrophilia >20 × 10⁹/l at onset of D+ are predictors of poor outcome, and an indication for early referral for peritoneal dialysis.
3. Plasmaphoresis and exchange transfusion are reserved for bad prognosis (usually in the sporadic, hypertensive case).

Prognosis

Of 150 affected annually, 5 die, 15 (mainly D–) progress to renal failure. Relapse occurs occasionally in D- individuals.

Loss of proteinuria within a year is a relatively good prognostic factor.

However, 30% of cases eventually develop significant hypertension and renal impairment, so life-long follow up of BP, proteinuria and serum creatinine is required.

Chronic renal failure

Definition

An irreversible and progressive reduction in functioning nephrons, reflected in a fall in GFR by more than 50%.

Table 22.6 Causes and age at presentation of chronic renal failure

Causes	Age at presentation
1 Reflux nephropathy is commonest in UK	Late childhood
2 Haemolytic uraemic syndrome	Infancy onwards
3 Chronic glomerulonephritis	Late childhood
4 Renal hypoplasia or dysplasia and polycystic kidney disease	Early, often in infancy
5 Obstructive uropathy (including pelviureteric obstruction, posterior urethral valves, neurogenic bladder with spina bifida)	Fetal, infancy and later
6 Inherited renal disease, e.g. Alport's syndrome, nephronophthisis	Late childhood

Clinical

Pallor, sallow complexion, short stature.
Hypertension.

Specific syndromic signs:

- Eye signs, jaundice, neurological signs of Wilson's disease.
- Deafness in child or relative in Alport's syndrome.
- Abdominal masses: enlarged polycystic/obstructed kidneys, palpable or per-cussible neurogenic/obstructed bladder.
- Spinal lipoma/hairy tuft/defect overlying diastematomyelia, spina bifida.
- Altered sensation in saddle area, patulous anus, and weak intrinsic foot muscles are all signs of cord involvement.

Management principles

To maintain growth and renal function as long as possible.

1. Growth promotion

Stunting is most severe if onset is under 2 years old, and usually associated with renal dysplasia, but careful medical management at this age allows catch–up growth. Poorer growth response in older children emphasizes the importance of effective early intervention.

  i Anorexia reduces energy intake. High carbohydrate and fat supplements are often beneficial.

  ii Metabolic acidosis. Correction has a beneficial effect on growth and tachyp-noea.
Sodium bicarbonate 2–3 mmol/kg/day.

  iii Anaemia: Normocytic, normochromic, multifactorial in origin: low erythro-poietin, reduced RBC survival, and uraemia suppress erythropoiesis, and cause a bleeding diathesis, allowing blood loss from the bowel. Anorexia leads to nutritional deficiency of iron, folate.

    Blood transfusions are avoided as much as possible if transplant is likely (to reduce the development of WBC HLA antibodies). Bone marrow stimulation by synthetic erythropoietin administration shows encouraging results.

  iv Renal osteodystrophy caused by:

    a. Phosphate retention → hyperphosphataemia with secondary hyperparath-yroidism → hypercalcaemia, metastatic calcification, hypercalciuria with further deterioration in renal function.
    Low phosphate diet by restricting milk products, and $CaCO_3$ as a phos-phate binder. To prevent aluminium toxicity avoid $Al(OH)_3$.
    b. impaired vitamin D metabolism by reduced hydroxylation activity of cal-cidiol (1-hydroxycholecalciferol) to calcitriol (1, 25 dihydroxycholecalcif-erol).
    Give α-calcidol or calcitriol.

  v Growth retardation established
Growth hormone administered in those already growth retarded. Shows promise.

2. Prevention of deterioration in renal function by

   i   Treating primary cause, e.g. regular urine cultures and prophylactic anti-biotics in reflux nephropathy.

  ii   Protein restriction to minimize toxicity is potentially counterproductive if it exacerbates growth failure. Use in advanced CRF only.

      (Pathophysiology in remnant kidney when 50% or more of nephrons have been lost: Glomerular hyperfiltration of protein and amino acids through remaining functioning nephrons damages them. This causes segmental sclerosis, and arteriolar hypertrophy, proportional to proteinuria. Dietary protein restriction and ACE inhibitors decelerate the progressive decline in renal function.)

      Provide sufficient protein, 0.5–1 g/kg/day for repair and growth.

 iii Monitoring for hyperphosphataemia and secondary hypercalcaemia. see renal osteodystrophy.

  iv Maintain BP in normal range for age. Hypertension is secondary to the underlying cause via hyper-reninaemia or overload.

      Antihypertensives: hydralazine, labetalol, captopril.

      Fluid and sodium restriction in advanced CRF.

   v Monitor for excess water and sodium loss from inability to concentrate urine and loss of sodium pump. Hypotension and deterioration in GFR may result.

End stage renal failure

Definition

When dialysis or renal transplant is required, at a GFR of 5–10 ml/min/1.73m^2.

Incidence

3–6 per million child population. Prevalence 20–50 per million children in Europe, 25% of whom are under 5 years old.

Treatment options and psychological management

1. Continuous ambulatory peritoneal dialysis (CAPD)

Increasingly preferred to haemodialysis: can be managed at home, fewer access problems, less frequent dialysis needed, less acidotic, fewer blood transfusions, feel and grow better. Peritonitis is common, but usually responds rapidly to antibiotics. 5-year survival 90%.

2. Renal transplant

The preferred treatment for children because:

   i   Improved growth prospects, even after puberty, which is often delayed.

  ii Better quality of life, greater freedom.

Prognosis   Graft survival 90–100% for live related donors, and 70–80% of cadaver grafts at a year. Adult kidneys can be used if >10 Kg. Infants are limited by the room in the abdominal cavity and size of the feeding vessels. Prednisolone, cyclosporin and azothiaprine are used to control rejection. See Oncology for graft versus host disease.

3. Psychological support

Anticipate emotional and schooling difficulties of the child and family. Aim to reduce non-compliance with the regimen, which is common among adolescents.

Further reading

Milford D V, Taylor C M (1990) New insights into the haemolytic uraemic syndromes. *Archives of Disease in Childhood*, **65**, 713–715
Pediatric Clinics of North America (1987) Pediatric nephrology. **34**, no. 3. Philadelphia:Saunders
Trompeter R S (1990) Renal transplantation. *Archives of Disease in Childhood*, **65**, 143–146

Recommended reading

Postlethwaite R J (1986) *Clinical Paediatric Nephrology*. Bristol:Wright
Taylor C M, Chapman S (1989) *Handbook of Renal Investigations in Children*. Bristol:Wright

Chapter 23

Orthopaedic problems

GENERAL CONSIDERATIONS

The wide range of normal postural variations at different ages is a frequent reason for consultation.

Linear growth may be beneficial as in progressive correction of a malaligned fracture, or increase deformity as for instance in scoliosis during the pubertal growth spurt. Injury to the growth plate as in septic arthritis may impair growth, and overgrowth may result from an arteriovenous malformation. Malnutrition and chronic diseases have a more general effect on growth.

Adaptation to disability is rapid in children, as witnessed in sufferers from limb reduction defects and spina bifida. The most important determinants are the level of intelligence and a positive attitude to the disability.

SOME COMMON SYMPTOMS OF THE MUSCULOSKELETAL SYSTEM

Pain

In the toddler and infant pain may present as reluctance to use the limb, or pseudoparesis.

1. Acute

Infection, trauma, or malignancy, are the most urgent differential diagnoses. Pain is either constant if due to infection or expanding tumour, or intermittent and related to movement if due to joint involvement.

2. Subacute or chronic

Longer periods of pain require further evaluation:

   i Periodicity, e.g. diurnal in joint inflammation. Often worse at night in inflammatory disease, malignancy, or osteoid osteoma, but also in benign 'growing pains'.

  ii Character, e.g. aching in inflammation; deep pain in bone infiltration. Limb pain in an otherwise well child, associated with headaches or abdominal pain, is likely to be stress related (see Behavioural problems).

  iii Site, e.g. the spine: Scheuermann's disease, spondylolisthesis, juvenile ankylosing spondylitis, TB.

      Swelling with local tenderness, e.g. tibial tuberosity in Osgood-Schlatter disease.

      Generalized pain in osteoporosis.

Examination

Distinguish between:

1. Soft tissue (e.g. trauma, cellulitis, myositis, some malignancies).
2. Bone (trauma, osteomyelitis, malignancy).
3. Joint (inflammatory).
4. Referred pain, e.g. to knee from the hip, should be suspected if tenderness on palpation is absent, as in:

  i Perthe's disease.
  ii Slipped femoral epiphysis.

i.e. persistent pain in the hip/knee needs a lateral hip X-ray, and a repeat 4–6 weeks later.

'Growing pains'

Common, 10–20% of the 4–10 year age group. Headache and abdominal pain are often associated.

Clinical

Sudden onset, often severe, of ache or cramp like pain in the thigh, shin or calf. May be bilateral. Worse after exercise or if overtired.

Frequently causes night waking, lasts 30 minutes, eased by rubbing, absent in the morning. No abnormality on examination.

Differential diagnosis

Above.

Prognosis

Persists for months, but no long-term sequelae.

Limp

Pathophysiology

1. Normal vertical swing through walking pattern (gait) comprises two phases. Stance (weight bearing) 60%:swing (in the air) 40% of the cycle.

2. Alteration in the rhythm of gait = shortening of one of the two phases:

Stance	*Swing*
Shortened by:Pain (antalgic gait).	1. Stiff joint at hip or knee.
	2. Short leg.

3. Lurching gait, from side to side due to muscle weakness:

 i Trendelenburg dip: weak hip abductors (gluteus medius) cause the trunk to lean towards the abnormal hip to keep the centre of gravity in the midline as in congenital dislocation of hip. Waddling gait if bilateral weakness/dislocation.

 ii Proximal muscle weakness (gluteus maximus) leads to hyperextension of the spine, to keep the centre of gravity behind the hips. This prevents falling forwards. Occurs in Duchenne muscular dystrophy and polio.

4. Steppage gait: inability to dorsiflex the foot requires that the knee be lifted higher than the usual 70°. As the flexor tendons are unopposed, clawing of the toes results. Occurs in peroneal muscular atrophy, Friedreich's ataxia, polio, and myelodysplasia of the spinal cord.

Diagnostic pathway

1. Pain or weakness?

(If neither, then unequal leg length or, rarely, a contracture preventing a full range of movement is the cause of a limp.)

 i Pain.

   a. Inflammation: infection, transient synovitis, juvenile chronic arthritis, Henoch-Schönlein purpura.
   b. Osteochondritis: Perthe's disease (hip) or medial femoral condyle.
   c. Trauma: torn meniscus, traction (Osgood-Schlatter's disease).
   d. Spontaneous slipped femoral capital epiphysis.
   e. Miscellaneous: sickle cell, malignancy, or referred from the spine.

 ii Weakness.

   a. Structural: congenital dislocation of the hip.
   b. Neurological: polio, spina bifida, cerebral palsy.
   c. Myopathy: Duchenne muscular dystrophy.

 iii Unequal limb length.

   a. Post-traumatic: malunion after fracture, damaged growth plate.
   b. Congenital: shortening, hemihypertrophy, neurofibromatosis.
   c. Neurological: cerebral palsy, polio.
   d. Overgrowth: arteriovenous malformation.

iv Prevention of movement.

    a. Stiff joint: congenital arthrogryposis, post inflammatory.
    b. Contractures: e.g. cerebral palsy.

2. Acute or chronic?

With or without fever: examples

Onset	*Afebrile*	*Febrile*
Acute	Trauma, haemorrhage, tumour. Fracture through bone cyst	Septic arthritis/osteomy-elitis. Irritable hip (low grade fever).
Chronic	Asymmetrical leg length, Perthe's. CNS: cerebral palsy, polio, myopathy	Juvenile chronic arthritis, TB

3. Age related conditions

  i Infancy: trauma, infection.
 ii Early childhood: irritable hip, Perthe's disease, juvenile chronic arthritis (JCA).
iii Adolescence: slipped femoral epiphysis, musculoskeletal strains, JCA, patella subluxation (female) or chondromalacia (male).

Examination

1. Gait: observe both on the flat and walking upstairs, and while standing on one leg look for a Trendelenburg dip. Listen for the foot slap of foot drop, the foot scrape of spastic cerebral palsy, and the quick-step of an antalgic gait.
2. Shoe wear: asymmetry, excessive wear at the toe (toe walking) or heel (flat foot).
3. Skin for haemorrhage, purpura (Henoch-Schönlein), and cafe-au-lait patches (von Recklinhausen's disease affecting spine, long bones, pseudo-arthrosis, nerves).
4. Joints, comparing both sides, range of movement, laxity. Patella tap/compression/lateral push (see knee).
5. Measurement of limb length (anterior superior iliac spine to medial maleolus) and diameter of thighs 5 cm above patella, and calves at their maximum size, for asymmetry (e.g. reduced muscle mass due to pain resulting in disuse).
6. Neurology for spasticity, myopathy, polio. Limited straight leg raising with tight hamstrings suggests a spinal cause.

Investigations

(See table of differential diagnosis of hip problems).

1. X-rays: always include hip and knee.

2. Selectively, according to need, a radio-isotope scan:

    i Lack of uptake due to sickle cell infarct, early Perthe's.
   ii Increased uptake in inflammation, tumour, osteoid osteoma.

3. FBC, ESR, blood culture, joint/bone aspiration, serology, Mantoux.

Lytic lesions on X-ray

Presentation

1. Pain free local swelling: solitary bone cyst. The prominence of an osteochondroma at the end of a bone is easily distinguished.
2. Pain with swelling +/- pyrexia: infection, fracture, primary bone tumour or neuroblastoma.
3. Pain with no visible swelling: osteoid osteoma, malignancy.

Radiological clues

A lytic lesion crossing the metaphyseal plate is common to infection and malignancy, while cortical thinning is seen not only in malignancy, but also in fibrous dysplasia and solitary bone cysts.

    Periosteal lamellation is due to rapid growth by a benign or malignant tumour.

EXAMINATION OF THE SKELETON AND DIFFERENTIAL DIAGNOSIS OF FINDINGS

Generalizations that apply.

1. Symmetrical deformity: normal variation, endocrine or metabolic disorder likely.
2. Asymmetry: suspect congenital abnormality, trauma, tumour.

Feet: Flat foot, in/out-toeing, tip-toes, club feet

Start from the feet, working up to knees, hips and spine.

Normal variation

Intrauterine position causes postural deformities which resolve spontaneously. Commonest is calcaneovalgus, to be differentiated from the rare congenital vertical talus with a tight heel cord and 'rocker-bottom' foot.

    Infants have 'flat' feet and bow legs, and passively correctable metatarsus varus (pigeon toe) which resolves by school age.

In-toeing often with metatarsus varus, is due to tibial torsion as walking begins (knees face forward), and at 3–7 years femoral anteversion, demonstrated by adopting the W-position on sitting (knees 'squint' at each other).

Table 23.1 X–ray appearances of some conditions

Condition	Main X–ray site and appearance
1 Osteomyelitis	Metaphyseal, occasionally epiphyseal, circular. Sclerotic if chronic
2 Solitary bone cyst	Metaphysis of femur/humerus. Round/oval. Fracture through the cyst is common
3 Fibrous dysplasia	Metaphyseal, multiple translucencies. Thin cortex, bowing of the affected bone, fracture, pseudoarthrosis
Clinical associations:	i Polyostotic fibrous dysplasia: feather edged pigmented lesions, bone cysts, and, in McCune-Albright syndrome, precocious puberty
	ii Neurofibromatosis
4 Tumours	
i *Primary malignant*	
Osteogenic sarcoma	Metaphyseal, destruction of cortex, elevated periostium → onion-skin or sun burst calcification. Occasionally sclerotic
Ewing's sarcoma	Diaphysis, otherwise similar to osteosarcoma
ii Secondary:	
leukaemia	Multiple
neuroblastoma	
Wilms tumour	Occasionally solitary
iii Eosinophilic granuloma (Langerhan's cell histiocytosis)	Punched out lesion in skull, pelvis. Resembles Ewing's tumour in limb bones
iv Osteoid osteoma	Radiolucency 1 cm diameter containing a calcified nidus. Pain severe at night, which a non-steroidal anti-inflammatory drug relieves rapidly

Flat feet can be divided into two groups, by heel position:

  i Heel vertical to the floor: ligamentous laxity or Marfan's syndrome. Standing on tip-toe → good arch, with heel in varus.
  ii Heel everted (valgus), medial border of foot bulging: trauma, polio or myelomeningocele, cerebral palsy, myopathy, congenital vertical talus.

'Corrective shoes' is a misnomer and have no place in the management of metatarsus varus and physiological flat feet.

Out-toeing due to lateral rotation of both hips is normal, frequent in prematures, but is also a clue to dislocated hip, and later to slipped femoral epiphysis.

Tip toe gait is a feature of spastic diplegia, early muscular dystrophy, and congenital tight heel cords. A habit in otherwise normal, and autistic, children.

If unilateral, hemiplegia or short limb is likely.

Talipes

Incidence

1 in 1000 live births.

Diagnosed by failure (i) to correct talipes by tickling or on spontaneous movement (ii) inability to overcorrect by passive manipulation (iii) heel remains in varus.

Talipes equinovarus (i) idiopathic sporadic or familial (ii) secondary to intrauterine posture, myelomeningocele, rarely arthrogryposis. Associated with congenital
hip dysplasia.

Management: serial strapping from birth resolves many, but soft tissue release
with serial plaster casts is required in 50%.

Knees

Age-related changes and differential diagnosis.

1. Bow legs

Physiological between 18–36 months. Exclude rickets, especially in Asians, and
Blount's osteochondritis of the medial epiphysis.

2. Knock knees

Physiological between 30–60 months. Exclude rickets and bone cysts; frequently
found in cerebral palsy and myelomeningocele. Apparent knock knee with hypotonia, lax ligaments, fat thighs.

Pathological at these ages:

 i If >10 cm intermaleolar gap in genu valgus (knock knee).
 ii >10 cm between femoral condyles in genu varum (bow legs).
   Over 3 years old no bow leg deformity is acceptable, nor is knock knee of
   more than 7⁰ from the vertical.

3. Pain

Includes mechanical (see below), systemic (e.g. sepsis, rheumatoid), and referred
pain from the hip.

 i Male adolescent preponderance, as a result of repetitive stress/minor trauma.

   a. Traction apophysitis: Osgood-Schlatter's disease (tender swelling of
      patella tendon insertion into tibial tubercle, visible on X-ray; pain on exer-
      cise, eased by rest or ultrasound).
   b. Chondromalacia patellae (retropatellar aching pain). Injury of the extensor
      (patellofemoral) mechanism.
   c. Osteochondritis (avascular necrosis) of the medial femoral condyle (per-
      sistent ache, tender on palpation, and locking and instability if a fragment
      is loose in the joint).

 ii Adolescent female preponderance of subluxation of the patella.

Examination

1. Standing, walking, lying down: limp, asymmetry, atrophy, effusion.
2. Palpation for tenderness, effusion.
3. Range of movements, active and passive.
4. Joint integrity, lying down.

    i Collateral ligaments: extending the leg, examiner then stabilizes the lower leg (with his hand if an infant, under his arm if a child), then presses against the medial side of the upper tibia, trying to open the joint (lax medial ligament), then lateral side of the tibia for the lateral ligament.

    ii Cruciate ligaments: flex knee to 90°, stabilize the foot, e.g. under examiner's thigh as he sits sideways on the bed, then grasp the leg just below the knee with both hands, rock it backwards and forwards to reveal excessive play.

    iii Meniscus: fully flex the knee, then extend slowly, rotating alternately medially and laterally, with screwing motion, to elicit 'click' felt at the joint line, or pain if torn.

    iv Patella: 'tap' positive = effusion; look for pain on compression (femoral chondromalacia) and guarding on pushing laterally when knee is flexed 30° with foot supported to relax quadriceps ('apprehension test' for patella subluxation).

5. Hips, as may be referred pain, or involved in the disease.

Hips

Examination

1. For dislocated hip, see below.
2. Range of movement of each hip in turn.

    i Lying supine:

      a. Flexion and extension of the straight leg, active and passive, while the other limb is fully flexed to 'fix' the pelvis.

      b. Adduction and abduction, pelvis 'square', with straight legs: scissor i.e. cross them, then widely abduct, both actively and passively.

    ii Lying prone: Internal and external rotation assessed by flexing the knee to 90°, then rotate the lower leg laterally for internal rotation (IR) and medially for external rotation (ER). Usually IR>ER.

Examples of abnormal findings

Painful hip → flexion, loss of full abduction and internal rotation. Pain from the spine → tight hamstrings, limited straight leg raising. Contractures in spastic cerebral palsy limit hip abduction and flexion.

Congenital dislocation of the hip (CDH)

Definition

A spectrum from dislocatable to frank dislocation with the femoral head outside the acetabulum at rest. 90% of those identified at birth resolve.

Pathophysiology

The newborn has a lax hip joint capsule due to maternal hormones. Breech or oligo-hydramnios reduce normal mobility, and encourages dislocation of the relatively large femoral head from the small, shallow acetabulum.

Table 23.2 Congenital dislocation of the hip

Type of CDH	Timing in pregnancy	Reducibility	Associated abnormalities
Idiopathic	Late	Easy	Metatarsus varus, torticollis
Teratological	Early	Irreducible	Arthrogryposis, chromosomal

Incidence

Dislocatable at birth 1 in 100, dislocated at a year 1 in 1000, F:M ratio = 6:1, left>right hip, bilateral in 10%.

At risk: family history, oligohydramnios, fetal growth retardation, breech or caesarian births, other limb abnormalities, e.g. talipes.

Clinical

1. Neonate. Place supine on a firm surface; examination must be gentle for the baby to be relaxed as crying increases muscle tension, preventing identification of dislocatable hips. Warm baby and hands are essential!

   i Ortolani test for dislocated hips. Grasp hips with thumbs in the groins, middle fingers over the greater trochanters. Flex hips and knees to 90° and abduct them. A 'clunk' may be felt as the hip dislocates. The Barlow manoeuvre of pressing backwards (i.e. downwards on the flexed hips) *and* outwards (lateral pressure by the thumbs) provokes this and identifies dislocatable hips. Gently, firmly, fully abduct. If a hip is dislocated full abduction is limited. If bilateral, the perineum is unusually wide. During abduction, upward pressure from the fingers over the greater trochanters elicits a 'clunk' as the femoral head relocates.

      Movement of the femoral head, by 0.5 cm or so, without a clunk, is also significant. Clicks are common in 5–10% of normal hips and not significant.
   ii Push/pull movement actively 'telescoping' one flexed thigh, abducted at 45°, onto the acetabulum, while fixing the pelvis with the other hand, may demonstrate hip instability.
2. After the neonatal period the classical signs:

   i Limitation of hip abduction, asymmetrical thigh and flattening of the buttock on the affected side. A clunk may be elicited up to a year old.

ii Lying supine, flex knees in the vertical plane, soles flat, heels touching buttocks. Difference in knee height is due to femoral or tibial shortening.
iii Delayed walking, Trendelenberg dip. The waddling gait of bilateral dislocation may be missed.

Screening times

Recommended at birth, discharge from hospital, 6 weeks, 6–9 months, 15–21 months, 2.5 years.

Only as effective as the personnel who perform it; many cases are still identified late.

Investigations

Hip US from birth has high sensitivity and specificity.

X-ray after 4 months: delayed ossification of the capital epiphysis which is subluxing or dislocated. It is laterally positioned (Figure 23.1).

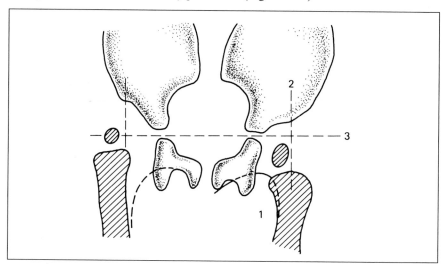

Figure 23.1 Identifying dislocation of the hip from the X-ray. 1 = Shenton's line, a continuous curve from the obturator foramen to the femoral neck. 2 = A vertical line dropped from the anterior superior iliac spine: the femoral head should lie medial to it. 3 = A horizontal line through the triradiate acetabular cartilage: the majority of the femoral head should lie below it.

Management

Determined by age at detection.

1. Neonatal: double nappies for 2 weeks. Lie in prone position. Persistent dislocatability requires splint or Pavlik harness for 3–6 months.
2. Later. After 3 months the hip will be dislocated and probably require traction followed by Pavlik harness. After 6 months, not only traction but also abduction plaster for 3 months or even open reduction and abduction plaster.

Further reading

Burger B J, Burger J D, Bos C F A, Obermann W R, *et al* (1990) Neonatal screening and staggered early treatment for congenital dislocation or dysplasia of the hip. *Lancet*, ii, 1549–1553

Gardiner H M, Dunn P M (1990) Controlled trial of immediate splinting versus ultrasonographic surveillance in congenitally dislocatable hips. *Lancet*, ii, 1553–1556

Principal differential diagnosis of painful hip disorders

Painful hips are generally held in the position of comfort, i.e. abducted, flexed, externally rotated.

Table 23.3 Painful hip, gradation from acutely unwell → well

Condition	Age (years)	Clinical	Duration of symptoms	Investigations
Septic hip	0–5+	Boys>girls Toxic, pain ++	Hours/day	Blood culture +ve WBC ++ aspirate of the joint +ve
Tuberculosis	2–15	Subacute, stiff, painful at night. May be a psoas abscess	Weeks/months	X-ray:hilar glands, Mantoux ESR, urine for AAFB*
Juvenile chronic arthritis	1–15	Pain, stiff, +/– rash, systemic upset	6–12 weeks minimum	ESR. Antinuclear antibody +ve in 20%. A diagnosis of exclusion usually
Irritable hip	3–10	Boys>>girls. Slight temperature. Limping	Hours to days, not too upset	Normal FBC and ESR
Perthe's disease	3–10	Boys>>girls. Bilateral 15%. Familial tendency. Low birthweight	Often 3 months before diagnosed. Takes 2–4 years to heal, disability proportional to severity	X-ray: widened joint space, → denser femoral head → fragmentation → recovery
Slipped femoral capital epiphysis	10–15	Boys>girls, fat, tall. Hip flexion → external rotation. Bilateral in 20%	Acute: minutes. Subacute/chronic: days to weeks	X-ray, frog lateral view: capital epiphysis falling back and downward in lateral view. Pin cartilage to prevent further slip/necrosis

* AAFB = acid and alcohol fast bacilli of TB

The back

Normal development and variation

As head control develops, cervical lordosis appears at a month, then lumbar lordosis, on sitting without support, at 7 months.

Lumbar lordosis is common in preschool children, especially in blacks, and with ligamentous laxity.

Kyphosis due to poor posture is a feature of adolescenceBack pain
Uncommon in childhood, 60% have an identifiable cause, therefore must be taken seriously. Increasingly frequent in adolescence.

Differentiate by curvature

1. Localization to one side of the spine is usually muscular.

    i   Trauma: pain, muscle spasm. Commonest cause of back pain.
    ii Myalgia related to viral or bacterial infections is common.
    iii Urinary tract infection: as the presenting complaint, in the lumbar region, not uncommon, always obtain a urine culture.
    iv Stress related: by exclusion, inexplicable/inconsistent story.

2. Kyphosis

    i   Any age: osteoporotic vertebral collapse (steroids, metabolic), or a prolapsed disc are very rare, usually traumatic, with similar symptoms to the adult.
    ii Adolescence: in Scheuermann's disease a lateral X-ray shows at least three vertebrae are wedge shaped, due to end-plate osteopenia.

3. Lordosis may be only a subtle straightening of a segment of the back, as the child bends forward.

    i   Early childhood: discitis, (often *Staphylococcus aureus*, commoner in the spine than osteomyelitis), with pain on walking, lordosis, and local tenderness on percussion.
    ii Athletic adolescents: spondylolysis (lumbar pain after exercise) is a fracture of the pars interarticularis, seen on the oblique X-ray as a break in the neck of the 'scotty dog' (arrow in Figure 23.2).
        Spondylolisthesis (sciatic nerve signs) is seen as 'stepping' on X-ray at the lumbosacral junction as the upper vertebra slips forward on the one below.
    iii Any age:

        a. Tumour (scoliosis may also be present).
        b. Local/secondary: bone tumour (pain worse at night, if eased by aspirin = osteoid osteoma), eosinophilic granuloma, spinal cord tumour (signs of cord compression).
        c. Disseminated: leukaemia, neuroblastoma.
        d. Diastematomyelia (block of bone within the canal, passing through the spinal cord, causes traction as spine lengthens, signs of cord compression).
        e. Epidural abscess: acute, severe pain and tenderness, signs of cord compression.

Investigations

Plain X-ray, anterior and lateral views, FBC, ESR. ^{99}Tc bone scan if febrile and discitis/tumour suspected. CT or MRI if these are unhelpful, for spinal cord tumour.

Scoliosis

Definition

Lateral curvature of the spine, with prominence of the posterior ribs on one side on bending forward. Screen by 'touching toes':

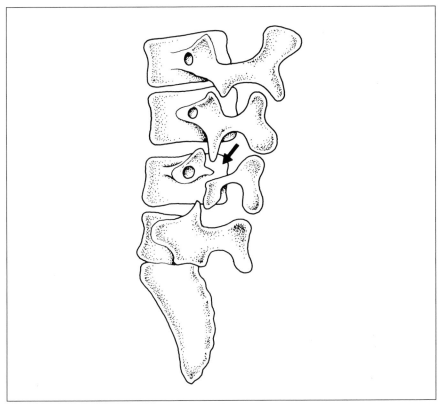

Figure 23.2 Spondylolysis. Oblique view showing fracture.

1. Postural scoliosis disappears on forward flexion; compensatory scoliosis due to asymmetry of leg length disappears on sitting.
2. Structural scoliosis
   Incidence 1.8%: idiopathic 80%, congenital 5%, neuromuscular 10%, others 5%, e.g. trauma, tumour, Marfan syndrome.

   i Congenital: from birth e.g. hemivertebrae (look for unilateral renal agenesis, congenital heart disease).
   ii Neuromuscular: 'C'–shaped curve with pelvic tilt, e.g. neurofibromatosis, severe cerebral palsy, muscular dystrophy, myelomeningocoele, polio.
      Prevent progression by early intervention with a lightweight plaster jacket.
   iii Idiopathic. Often familial. Prognosis related to age at onset (Table 23.4).

Torticollis

1. Congenital

   i Congenital torticollis (wry neck) due to shortening of the sternomastoid, with hard, non-tender 'tumour' palpable in the first 1–2 months. Commoner in breech and forceps delivery, caused by ischaemia during delivery, and possibly trauma.

Metatarsus adductus and congenital hip dysplasia are associated in up to 20%.

Table 23.4 Prognosis of idiopathic scoliosis related to age at onset

	Age (years)	Sex	Prognosis
Infantile	0–3	M > F	Good, rarely progressive
Juvenile	4–10	M = F	Worse than adolescent type
Adolescent*	>10	F > M (7:1)	10% need treatment (bracing if curve >25°, surgery if >50°)

* Theories of causation of adolescent scoliosis.
1 Centrally mediated muscle imbalance $\rightarrow$ excess pressure on concave side of vertebra $\rightarrow$ asymmetry of growth.
2 Flat vertebrae/reversal of normal thoracic kyphus $\rightarrow$ anterior overgrowth of those vertebrae. Progression occurs as the spine grows maximally in puberty

Plagiocephaly and facial deformity may result unless the affected muscle is regularly stretched: turn the chin towards the shoulder on the affected side, and elevate the chin. Surgery, at 2 years, is rarely required.

ii Klippel-Feil syndrome: fusion of cervical vertebrae → limited movement, short neck, low hairline. Kyphosis, scoliosis and Sprengel's congenital elevation of the scapula, are common. Renal, hearing and cardiac anomalies are associated.

2. Acute

i Inflammatory: deep cervical lymphadenitis, rarely atlantoaxial subluxation due to retropharyngeal abcess, infected post-tonsillectomy haematoma.

ii Trauma: injury to C1–C2, +/– increased instability, e.g. Down's syndrome, Morquio's syndrome.

iii Occulogyric crisis due to phenothiazines, metoclopramide. Give procyclidine.

iv Posterior fossa tumour: traction on cervical nerves, head tilt to compensate for diplopia due to cranial nerve involvement.

3. Chronic

Polyarticular juvenile chronic arthritis, or secondary to reflux oesophagitis, especially in cerebral palsy (Sandifer's syndrome).

Further reading

Bredenkamp J K, Hoover L A, Berk G S, Shaw A (1990) Congenital muscular torticollis: a spectrum of disease. *Archives of Otolaryngology, Head and Neck Surgery*, **116**, 212–216

Upper limb abnormalities

1. Congenital abnormalities are common. Of medical importance:

    i Associated condition likely, e.g. absent radii with thrombocytopenia and Fanconi's anaemia, triphalangeal thumbs with red cell aplasia, polydactyly with short stature and congenital heart in Ellis-van Creveld syndrome.

    ii Teratogen in pregnancy. Historically the worst was thalidomide.

    Terminology commonly used to describe limb reduction deformities:

Absence of	Current nomenclature	Traditional term
1 Whole limb	Terminal transverse reduction defect	Amelia
2 Part of a limb	e.g. below elbow transverse reduction defect	Meromelia/hemimelia
3 Radial or tibial side	Preaxial longitudinal reduction defect	Ectromelia
4 Ulnar or fibula	Postaxial longitudinal reduction defect	
5 Middle segment (radius + ulna)	Intercalary reduction defect	Phocomelia

    iii Birth injury to the brachial plexus: Erb's or Klumpke's palsy.

2. Genetic implications, e.g. lobster claw deformity is often dominantly inherited.
3. Functional ability and special needs assessment. This must be completed for each individual.

SPECIFIC DISORDERS

Congenital and familial disorders of the skeleton

Presenting with short stature

Clinical approach

Which is most affected, the limbs (e.g. achondroplasia) or trunk (e.g. spondyloepiphyseal dysplasia)?
    Bowed (rickety)?
    Other associated conditions present?

1. Achondroplasia-like face and limbs

    i Achondroplasia AD: 1 in 50000 usually as a spontaneous mutation. Large head and trunk relative to limbs, saddle nose, trident fingers. Lumbar lordosis, waddling gait. Hydrocephalus in the newborn; lower limb neurological problems due to narrow lumbar spinal canal causing root compression; surgery often indicated for these complications. Leg lengthening is controversial.

    ii Diastrophic dwarfism AR: rare, phenotype and X-ray appearance like achondroplasia, but characteristically have cauliflower ears, also club foot, hand deformities, hip dislocation, contractures, scoliosis and cleft palate.

iii Thanatophoric dwarfism: rare, most are sporadic, superficially like achondroplasia, but the small chest is incompatible with extrauterine life. X-ray appearances of 'fish bone' vertebrae and 'telephone handle' femurs are diagnostic.

2. Rickets-like

i Hypophosphatasia AR: low alkaline phosphatase.
ii Hypophosphataemic rickets XL dominant: renal tubular phosphate leak.
iii Cartilage hair hypoplasia AR: fine sparse hair, bowed limbs. *severe rickets R phos ↑ nr↓*

3. Other, all rare, with distinguishing features

i Ellis-van Creveld syndrome AR: short stature mainly affecting distal parts of the limbs, polydactyly, aplastic nails and teeth, congenital heart disease.
ii Conradi's disease AR: short limbs, epiphyseal stippling +/- cataracts, mental retardation.
iii Spondyloepiphyseal dysplasia (osteochondrodystrophy) various inheritance patterns: vertebrae flattened, hip, knee and shoulder joints dysplastic.
iv Cleidocranial dysostosis AD: mild dwarfing, absent outer ends of clavicles, large anterior fontanelle with delayed closure resulting in bossing, symphysis pubis defect.

Arthrogryposis

Limb contractures and stiffness ascribed to intrauterine immobility or oligohydramnios. Dislocated hips are common. Poor muscle bulk, and hypotonic, but muscle power is usually normal, unless due to an underlying congenital myopathy. Superficially similar is Larsen's syndrome, with pinched nose, multiple dislocations of hips, knees and elbows, and contractures, all due to grossly excessive ligamentous laxity in utero.

INHERITABLE CONNECTIVE TISSUE DISORDERS

Osteogenesis imperfecta (OI)

Pathophysiology

Abnormality of one of the 3 alpha chains that form the triple helix of type 1 collagen; the nearer to the beginning of the chain, the more severe the disease.

Classification

(After Silence, supercedes OI tarda and congenita)

1. Type 1

Commonest, 1 in 30000 live births. Autosomal dominant.
  Manifestations from birth:

i Bones: fractures → deformity (15%), scoliosis (20%), short stature (50% adults <3rd centile). Skull: wormian bones (small bony 'islands' in the sutures).

ii Laxity of skin and ligaments, blue sclera, deafness (40% of adults), dentinogenesis imperfecta (50%).

Walking achieved by >50%. Tendency to fracture improves with age.

2. Types II, III, IV

Inheritance: new autosomal dominant mutation, or rarely autosomal recessive inheritance.

Type II: Lethal. Stillbirth or neonatal death. Ribbon bones, further classified by ribs broad, beaded or thin.

Type III and IV: very short and rarely able to walk as bones so brittle and deformed. Sclera normal.

Antenatal diagnosis

Type I or IV: DNA linkage studies helpful if a large and informative family. US from 14 weeks' gestation may identify abnormal bone growth in severe forms.

Marfan syndrome (AD)

See Growth problems.

Ehlers-Danlos syndrome (usually AD)

Hyperelasticity of the skin with easy bruising, poor healing, wide puckered scars, excessive ligamentous laxity, short stature. A defect of type 3 collagen detected in some cases.

Further reading

Sillence D O, Senn A S, Danks D M (1979) Genetic heterogeneity in osteogenesis imperfecta. *Journal of Medical Genetics*, **16**, 101–106

ARTHRITIS

Incidence of arthritis per 100000 children under 16 years

Transient synovitis ('irritable hip', includes viral)	50
Acute transient arthritis (Henoch-Schönlein)	25
Juvenile chronic arthritis	10
Septic arthritis	6
Reactive arthritis (post-bacterial, rheumatic fever)	5

Perthes' disease of the hip (not an arthritis, but to be
differentiated from the other causes of painful hip/limp)   4

Differential diagnosis of acute and subacute arthritis

Systemic onset: fever, rash, one or several joints involved

1. Infection

    i Viral, e.g. rubella, mumps, chickenpox (typical exanthema), adenovirus, parvovirus (slapped cheek), cytomegalovirus, hepatitis, (disturbed liver function).

    ii Bacterial.

        a. Acute: e.g. septic arthritis, commonly *Staphylococcus aureus, Haemophilus influenzae,* haemolytic streptococci, unusually *Mycoplasma pneumoniae* (erythema multiforme).

        b. Post infective: a week or more after dysentery (salmonella, Shigella, Yersinia, Helicobacter and Reiter's syndrome of urethritis, conjunctivitis, arthritis), meningococcaemia, rheumatic fever (flitting, acutely painful arthritis, carditis, erythema marginatum).

    iii Tick-borne (bite, typical spreading skin lesion in 75%)

        a. Spirochaetal: Lyme disease: knee joint swelling, occasionally small joints, migratory.

        b. Rickettsial: Rocky Mountain spotted fever (rash, small joints of hands, feet).

    iv Retrovirus? Kawasaki disease (painful swollen hands and feet in the acute phase, monoarthritis of weight bearing joints in the recovery period).

2. Inflammatory bowel disease

Affects knees, ankles, elbows and wrists (erythema nodosum, weight loss, bowel symptoms).

3. Malignancy

Leukaemia, neuroblastoma (limb pains, pallor).

4. Connective tissue

    i Henoch Schönlein purpura (rash, swollen hands and feet, abdominal pain, haematuria).

    ii Juvenile chronic arthritis, rarely systemic lupus erythematosus, dermatomyositis.

5. *Rare*

Immune deficiency, especially hypogammaglobulinaemia (recurrent infections).

Polyarticular disease

1. Non–accidental injury: bruising, fractures, suspicious circumstances.
2. Metabolic is symmetrical: rickets among Asians (knee ache in adolescence), mucopolysaccharidoses (coarse features, contractures prominent).
3. Benign common conditions

    i Excessive ligamentous laxity: arthralgia, occasional swelling, mainly knees, adolescents.
    ii Overuse e.g. sport, inadequate training/equipment.

4. Sickle cell disease: 'hand-foot' syndrome in infancy.

Monoarticular arthritis

1. Infection: 'Irritable hip', partially-treated infection, TB.
2. Osteochondritis: Perthes' disease.
3. Haematological: haemarthrosis, e.g. post traumatic or haemophilia, sickle cell avascular necrosis of the femoral head, leukaemia.
4. Bone tumour, e.g. osteoid osteoma in femoral neck, or Ewing's tumour. Bone scan may need to be followed by biopsy.
5. Adolescence: slipped femoral epiphysis; ankylosing spondylitis with HLA B27, and psoriatic arthritis, are both likely to have a family history.

SPECIFIC CONDITIONS

Transient synovitis: 'irritable hip'

Definition

More common in boys, 3–10 years old, after a cold, usually sudden. Pain in hip or referred to the knee, with slight temperature, lasting 6 days with a tendency to recur. Rarely bilateral.

Position

Hip flexed, loss of internal rotation.

Investigations

ESR, WBC normal. X-ray may show widening of the joint space.

Management

Pain relief achieved by bed rest, skin traction, and non-steroidal anti-inflammatory drugs.

Henoch-Schönlein purpura

Definition

A common vasculitis of immune mechanism (IgA and C3 complement deposition), with non-thrombocytopenic purpura, arthritis, abdominal pain and nephritis.

Pathophysiology

Vasculitis of venules and capillaries, with proliferative glomerulonephritis.

Epidemiology

Upper respiratory illness, especially streptococcal, often precedes; drugs and food sensitivity rarely. Peak age 5–15 years.

Clinical

Low grade fever, and irritability plus involvement of:

1. Skin (100%): maculopapules/urticaria progressing to purpura within hours, over extensor surfaces and buttocks.
2. Joints (80%): painful periarticular swelling of knees, elbows, and small joints of the hands. Resolve in days without sequelae.
3. Abdominal pain (70%): intermittent, colicky, with vomiting. Malaena in 20%, intussusception 5%.
4. Nephritis in acute phase in 50%, usually recovers.

Investigations

Urine for protein and blood (often microscopic). Renal biopsy if persistent severe kidney signs. Other investigations are not often required, and should be essentially normal.

Differential diagnosis

1. Thrombocytopenia: the rash of meningococcal septicaemia or disseminated intravascular haemorrhage, including that due to haemolytic uraemic syndrome, occurs in a much sicker child.
2. Severe erythema multiforme (Stevens Johnson syndrome) develops mucocutaneous junction and target lesions.
3. Arthritis of rheumatic fever or systemic juvenile rheumatic disease have high ESR, WBC, and associated signs.

4. Acute abdominal pain of HSP simulates a surgical emergency, but bowel sounds are present and rebound tenderness is rarely found, though the mass of an intussusception may be felt. Pancreatitis is rare, and has a high blood amylase level.
5. Nephritis due to post–streptococcal glomerulonephritis or systemic lupus erythematosus have high antibody (streptococcal or autoantibodies) and low complement levels.

Management

Supportive; paracetamol and rest for pain, i.v. drip and nasogastric suction for vomiting. Corticosteroids used by some for abdominal pain providing it is not due to intussusception; otherwise no worthwhile advantage over conservative measures.

Prognosis

Recovery within 7–10 weeks, recurrence possible for 2 years. Persistent nephritis or nephrotic syndrome is likely to progress in <5% with haematuria, and accounts for 10% of end-stage renal failure in childhood.

Other vasculitides of childhood

Common

Kawasaki disease see Infectious Diseases.

Rare

Giant cell arteritis (Takayasu's) ('pulseless disease' due to stenosis of aortic arch), serum sickness, Wegener's granulomatosis (necrotizing granulomatosis of upper and lower respiratory tract, glomerulonephritis), polyarteritis nodosa (fever, weight loss, high ESR, arthralgia, abdominal pain, neurology, purpura, peripheral gangrene).

Septic arthritis and osteomyelitis

Age: 50% under 2 years. A history of trauma in a third. Site: hip, knee, ankle, or elbow usually. Monoarticular 90%, several joints involved in 10%.

Pathogenesis of osteomyelitis and septic arthritis

1. Haematogenous 90%: to the metaphysis, and in infancy to the joint via vessels passing through the growth plate into the epiphysis.
2. Direct spread 10%: cellulitis; traumatic invasion; osteomyelitis. Septic arthritis results when infection spreads from the metaphysis if it lies within the joint capsule.

Clinical

As part of a septicaemic illness with reluctance to bear weight, or pseudoparesis with a hot tender swelling of the affected part.

Table 23.5 Causative organisms

	Neonate	Infancy and childhood
Organism	*Staphylococcus aureus.* Group B β–haemolytic streptococci. *E. coli, Neisseria gonorrhoeae*	*Staphylococcus aureus* *Haemophilus influenzae** *Strep. pneumoniae*** Group A β–haemolytic streptococcus
Antibiotic	Flucloxacillin + aminoglycoside	Flucloxacillin + fucidin + ampicillin/cefuroxime

* Important in septic arthritis, seldom causes osteomyelitis.
** Consider if sickle cell disease, asplenia, or hypogammaglobulinaemia is present.

Investigation

Aspirate for diagnosis (and relief of pain in septic arthritis).

1. Positive culture in 80% of osteomyelitis.
2. Gram stain of joint fluid is positive in half of septic arthritis, but a third of these are culture negative.
3. Blood cultures positive in 50%. Raised ESR, C reactive protein and WBC; changes in acute phase reactants are useful in monitoring progress. Generally, serology and joint fluid for antigen and antibody tests are helpful; antistaphylococcal antibody titres are unhelpful.
4. X-ray: soft tissue swelling and joint effusions are seen early on. Lytic bone changes (evident after 10 days) should not appear if the infection is treated effectively, and early.
5. If in doubt, a technetium scan identifies inflammation or infection; more precise still for infection are gallium, or the patient's own WBCs labelled with indium.

Management

1. Antibiotic for 4 weeks, initially i.v., changing to oral after a good clinical response, which is usually within 3–4 days.
2. Surgical intervention. Not required for osteomyelitis unless a delayed diagnosis, failure to improve within 24 h of starting treatment, or unusual organism is likely, e.g. immunocompromised. The septic hip usually requires open surgical drainage. Irrigation of the joint is controversial, as no real benefit has been shown.
3. Follow-up X-rays for arthritis or deformity, which are common.

CONNECTIVE TISSUE DISORDERS

Juvenile chronic arthritis (Juvenile rheumatoid arthritis, USA)

Definition

A generalized chronic inflammation primarily of the joints, and often involving connective tissue throughout the body.

Incidence

1 in 10000 annually.

Pathophysiology

Aetiology unknown. An autoimmune disease with HLA DR5, DRw8 association. Few are of adult type rheumatoid factor (RF) positive or have HLA B27.

Joints are hyperaemic, with oedematous synovium infiltrated by lymphocytes and plasma cells. The process results in effusions, eventually spreads onto articular cartilage (pannus formation) where it may cause pitting and destruction. Osteoporosis, pericapsular and ligamentous fibrosis occur at affected joints.

Synovial fluid: WBC $0.5-50 \times 10^9/l$, neutrophil preponderance, low glucose.

Chronic inflammatory changes are also seen in tendons, muscles, and the heart; vasculitis in the skin rash, fibrinoid necrosis in rheumatoid nodules.

Criteria for diagnosis

1. Less than 16 years old at onset.
2. Arthritis in one or more joints for 6 weeks (USA) or 3 months (Europe).
3. Exclusion of other causes.

Classification by type of onset

1. Polyarthritis = 5 joints or more.

Usually symmetrical, knees, wrists and digits (spindling), ankles, feet, neck at C2, C3 (torticollis), and temperomandibular joint. Swollen, hot, range of movement reduced but often relatively little pain.

Systemic involvement is mild to moderate, rheumatic nodules are rare. 90% are RF negative, have a raised ESR (60 mm), and mild leucocytosis is common.

2. Pauciarticular = less than 5 joints involved.

Relative frequency: knee, ankle, elbow, wrist, single proximal interphalangeal joint + flexor tenosynovitis, and the hip.

Gradual onset of joint swelling and pain which may disturb sleep, and morning stiffness easing off with exercise.

Systemic features are unusual.

Majority are 1–5 years F>M. Presence of Anti-nuclear antigen (ANA) carries chronic uveitis risk.

3. Systemic

Intermittent fever (1 or 2 spikes per day) accompanied by an evanescent salmon pink maculopapular rash, lymphadenopathy, splenomegaly, hepatomegaly, and/or pericarditis. Usually 2–3 weeks pass before connective tissue disease is considered.

Arthritis initially is often minimal, progressing to polyarticular. ESR >100 mm, leucocytosis marked, normocytic, normochromic anaemia about 10 g/dl.

Table 23.6 Clinical and laboratory findings in the JCA subgroups

	Polyarthritis	*Pauciarticular*	*Systemic*
Proportion	15%	65%	20%
Sex ratio M:F	1:3	1:5	1:1
Age (years) and subgroups	1. 1–3 M=F 2. 8–10 F>M RF +ve	1. 1–5 F>M, ANA +ve 2. >7 F monoarticular 3. >8 M HLA B27 +ve	1 1–5 years M=F 2 >5 F>M
Chronic uveitis	10%	20%	1%
Antinuclear antibodies	40% girls <6 years	80%, associated with uveitis	-
Rheumatoid factor	10%, mainly older girls	-	-
Systemic illness	Mild fever, lymphadenopathy	-	+++
Arthritis	Symmetrical: knees, wrists, ankles, feet	Moderate	Affects 50% at onset
Prognosis	RF +ve: 50% severe arthritis. Others 10%	Ocular damage in 10% Arthritis resolves	50% well at 5 years, in others arthritis active

Differential diagnosis

See below for extended list.

Major causes

1. Infective and post infective.
2. Inflammatory bowel disease.
3. Infiltration by leukaemia, neuroblastoma.

Systemic lupus erythematosus may present like JCA at first. Signs include polyarthritis, Raynaud's phenomenon, butterfly rash, and nephritis (urinary RBCs, WBCs, and casts are unlikely in JCA). ANA and double strand anti-DNA antibodies are present.

Management

1. Rest during acute phases must be a balance between adequate bed rest and activity; avoid irreversible damage from inappropriate or prolonged inactivity.
2. Education: continues throughout, according to strength, concentration and mobility. Significantly impaired in 20%.
3. Physiotherapy principles

   i Avoid contractures by active assisted movement even when acutely ill. Encourage good posture, and avoid deformity, e.g. prone lying reduces hip flexion contractures.

ii Splintage, usually overnight, allows joints to rest, reduce pain, and early mobilization to build up muscle bulk and power, and correct deformities. Traction for hip spasm, and hydrotherapy, are useful.

4. Occupational therapy principles

   i Assess and train to become independent in washing, dressing, and toileting; improve hand function.

  ii Adapt clothes, the home and school, trikes, provide aids, e.g. bath seats, stair lifts, and plastic splints.

5. Drugs

   i Non-steroidal anti-inflammatory drugs (NSAID)
Use one at a time, as they have no synergism, for a trial of 6–8 weeks. Concern over aspirin in association with Reye's syndrome has encouraged the use of other NSAIDs, which are generally preferred as first line drugs, except for systemic disease.

     a. Aspirin 80–100 mg/kg, enteric coated; aim for trough serum level 250–300 mg/l; stop if influenza or chickenpox is likely.

     b. Naproxen 10 mg/kg/24 h, 2 × daily.
Tolmetin 30 mg/kg/24 h, 4 × daily.

     c. Phenylbutazone is reserved for HLA-B27 males with pauciarticular disease.

  ii Corticosteroids:

     a. Systemic administration indications:
Systemic onset with pericarditis, myocarditis, hepatotoxicity.
  Severe joint involvement with systemic involvement.
  Alternate day administration is preferred, in a single dose, as prednisolone to a maximum 2 mg/kg until symptoms are controlled. This may take 4 or more weeks. Then reduce it slowly. NSAIDs are given in full dose with the steroids, with paracetamol for fever.

     b. Intra-articular corticosteroids indication:
Pauciarticular disease, rarely polyarticular, after 3 months of NSAIDs.

     c. Topical steroid eye drops for uveitis.

  iii Slow-acting anti-rheumatic drugs, taking 3–6 months to exert maximum benefit.
Indication: unresponsive to NSAID, or in ankylosing spondylitis.

     a. Hydroxychloraquine (may affect vision, must be closely monitored), then gold salts are added, usually in addition to steroids.

     b. Penicillamine, sulphasalazine or methotrexate. Each may be used, but only one at a time.

6. Orthopaedic surgery is helpful for up to 10% of patients (mainly in seropositive JRA).
Soft tissue release of contractures, repair of ruptured tendon, osteotomy for unequal epiphyseal growth at the knee, fusion of carpus/tarsus in a good position, and joint replacement. Early mobilization after surgery is essential for success.

Complications

1. Growth

This is most affected by systemic and polyarticular JRA, and independently of steroids. Weight loss and poor nutrition are important.

2. Skeletal

- i   Atlanto-axial subluxation, which may damage the spinal cord.
- ii Undergrowth of the jaw.
- iii Unilateral knee involvement may cause leg asymmetry, due to excessive growth if <9 years at onset, or reduced growth if onset is later.

3. Chronic uveitis

In anti–nuclear antibodies ANA +ve, mean age 4 years, and older B27 +ve individuals. It is usually bilateral, rarely symptomatic, needing slit lamp examination 3–monthly to be detected early. Band keratopathy, cataracts and glaucoma are found in 25%; 1% develop severe visual impairment.

Management: mydriatics to prevent adhesions between the iris and lens, plus topical steroids to reduce inflammation.

4. Amyloidosis

Incidence 7% in the UK, after 5–10 years of unremitting disease, and especially likely in systemic onset. Proteinuria is an early sign, followed by hypertension, and renal failure.

5. Iatrogenic

e.g. vertebral collapse, avascular necrosis of the femoral head due to steroids.

Prognosis

Overall, 10% enter adulthood with moderate to severe disability (25% of systemic and polyarticular onset). Deaths due to infection or renal failure occurs in 2– 4 %.

Further reading

Ansell B M (1980) *Rheumatic Disorders in Childhood*, London:Butterworth. A classic description.

Cassidy J T, Petty R E (1990) *Textbook of Pediatric Rheumatology* 2nd edn. New York:Churchill Livingstone. Useful chapters on non–rheumatic musculoskeletal pain syndromes, juvenile rheumatism, vasculitis.

Common Orthopedic Problems (1986) *Pediatric Clinics of North America* **33**, no. 6

Pediatric Rheumatology (1986) *Pediatric Clinics of North America* **33**, no. 5

Woo P, White P H, Ansell B M (1990) *Paediatric Rheumatology Update*. Oxford:Oxford University Press

Chapter 24

Dermatological problems

BIRTH MARKS

Telangiectasia

1. Naevus flammeus: the forehead patch resolves in the first year, but may persist at the nape of the neck.
2. Port wine stain (PWS). Fixed, present at birth. Argon laser effective, but for best results wait until adulthood.

   PWS in the ophthalmic distribution of the trigeminal is the Sturge-Weber syndrome of abnormal blood vessels (angiomas) in the ipsilateral choroid of the eye, brain and meninges. The underlying occipitoparietal cortex becomes shrunken and calcified. The resultant associations are:

   - Seizures, often focal, 80%.
   - Mental retardation 60%.
   - Glaucoma 45%.
   - Homonymous hemianopia and hemiplegia 35%.

   Diagnosis is clinical. The intracranial blood vessel calcification is best seen on CT, but may show on plain x-ray.
   Prognosis: progressive deterioration is usual. Hemispherectomy for intractable seizures, in early childhood, is advocated by some.
3. Ataxia-telangiectasia AR: defective DNA repair, with immune deficiency and tendency to tumour formation. Skin lesions develop in childhood, over the bulbar conjunctiva, ears and antecubital fossae. The cerebellar ataxia is progressive.

Haemangiomata

Capillary 'strawberry' birth mark and capillary-cavernous haemangioma

Up to 10% of infants are affected, with 20% of haemangiomata present at birth, more common on girls' faces and prematures.

Develop in the first 6 months, and often grow very rapidly for 1–2 months. Central pallor heralds involution, which is complete in 90% without treatment, taking 2–9 years.

The Kasabach-Merritt syndrome comprises platelet trapping in large cavernous haemangiomas in the skin and viscera, which may cause a bleeding tendency.

Management

Infection requires antibiotics and may hasten resolution. Masterly inactivity, unless sight is threatened, when corticosteroids or sclerosing injections are used.

interferon

Arteriovenous shunts

Usually on the limbs, leading to overgrowth of the affected part. Occasionally intracerebral. High output failure may result. Surgical intervention may be ineffective because of the impossibility of tying off all feeder vessels.

Port wine stain plus hypertrophy of the associated limb due to arteriovenous malformation is the Klippel-Trenaunay-Weber syndrome.

LYMPHATIC MALFORMATION

Cystic hygroma

Affects mainly head and neck, and thorax. Transilluminates. Grows more rapidly than the child, pressing on vital structures and become intimately connected with them by its amoeba–like spread. Early surgical intervention for head and neck involvement only.

NAPPY RASH AND ECZEMA

Common, due to irritation by urine and faeces, frequently with secondary candida infection.

Management

1. Barrier cream of zinc and castor oil or similar.
2. Exposure, frequent nappy changes. Avoid occlusive plastic pants.
3. Hydrocortisone + antifungal cream. Powerful steroids are contraindicated.

Differential diagnois

1. Onset under 3 months, contented, feeding well = seborrhoeic eczema, a self-limiting overactivity of the sweat glands. Axillary involvement, less extensive on the limbs help differentiate from atopic eczema.

   Management as for nappy rash, plus arachis oil to lift the scales on the scalp.
2. If scratching is prominent:

   i Atopic eczema: onset after 3 months, irritable, poor sleep and feed pattern, chronic course.

   ii Scabies: eczematous over the trunk, pustules on palms and soles, burrows.

3. Initially vesicular, weeping, becoming dry and scaly, limited to the face and napkin area is suggestive of zinc deficiency, although rare, seen in prematures, prolonged parenteral feeding, and acrodermatitis enteropathica.

Atopic eczema

Definition

A chronic skin inflammation varying from an acute weeping erythematous papulovesicular eruption to chronic dry scaly thickened skin. The onset and distribution are age related.

Incidence

3% of under 5 year olds, 60% of these by one year. Atopic family history in 70%.

Clinical

Distribution and appearance

1. Infancy: face, behind the ears, front and back of the trunk, and extensor surfaces of the limbs.
2. Children: antecubital and popliteal flexures, excluding axillae.
3. General:

   i Pale facial skin, white dermographism, an extra infraorbital skin fold.

   ii Infection: prone to *Staphylococcus aureus*, group A β-haemolytic streptococcus, and eczema herpeticum.

   iii Itch intense, with scratch marks where the skin is exposed.

   iv Cataract is rare.

Differential diagnosis

Common: seborrheic eczema and scabies.

   Relatively uncommon: HIV; psoriasis is rare before 3 years, usually presents in adolescence as guttate psoriasis on the trunk.

   Rare:

1. Eczema is associated with icthyosis, phenylketonuria, Wiskott-Aldrich syndrome, hyper-IgE syndrome.
2. Haemorrhagic, greasy scaly rash seen in Langerhan's cell histiocytosis (Letterer-Siwe type).
3. Zinc deficiency, mainly affects perioral and perianal areas. Acquired in parenteral nutrition in the neonate and inherited in acrodermatitis enteropathica.

Management

1. Emollient: aqueous cream, emulsifying ointment for the bath.
2. Topical steroid: hydrocortisone 1% initially. Dilute fluoridated steroids for short periods as required, never to the face. Rarely are systemic steroids warranted unless unable to attend school and becoming emotionally damaged.
3. Weeping: infection is frequently responsible for acute exacerbations. Flucloxacillin +/- potassium permanganate soaks help.
4. Lichenification: zinc paste with icthammol in milder cases, in more severe forms use coal tar. Traditional Chinese herbal tea and topical soaks show exceptional promise but hepatotoxicity has been reported.
5. General:

   i Scratching: cut finger nails, at night apply mittens of cotton tubular bandages, and prescribe trimeprazine. Cool rooms help.
   ii Trigger avoidance:

      • Cotton next to skin; no wool or acrylics.
      • Wash clothes in soap flakes, avoid biological detergents.
      • Allergens, e.g. grass, pets, milk, eggs.

   iii Diet: exclusion may help in 10–30%; up to 70% is claimed for an elemental diet. Skin-prick tests and RAST tests are unhelpful in deciding which foods to eliminate. See allergy for details.

Prognosis

Majority clear by adult life, but eczema is more likely to persist if disease is extensive and family background atopic.

Further reading

David T J (1991) Recent developments in the treatment of childhood atopic eczema. *Journal of the Royal College of Physicians of London*, **25**, 95–101

GENITAL WARTS

Vertically transmitted at birth, may take up to 18 months to appear. Alternatively acquired through sharing a bath or towel with an affected adult.

Consider sexual abuse enquiries in children over 2 years old, especially if the explanation offered is inadequate.

BLISTERS

Common

1. Infection

   i Viral:

      a. Acute: chickenpox, herpes simplex, coxsackie A.
      b. Persistent for months: molluscum contagiosum.

   ii Staphylococci: impetigo, scalded skin syndrome (exotoxin from phage group II, type 3A, 3B, 3C, 55 or 71).

   NB: erythema multiforme also blisters and in childhood is usually due to infection, e.g. herpes simplex, *Mycoplasma pneumoniae*.
2. Insect bites causing papular urticaria (e.g. bed bug, cat or dog mite) or vesicles (scabies in infants).
3. Injury: sunlight, friction, burn.
4. Medication, e.g. barbiturate, plant contact and photosensitive reaction, e.g. giant hogweed.
5. Skin diseases, e.g. acute atopic eczema, pompholyx.

Rare causes

1. Epidermolysis bullosa (EB).

Definition

A group of inherited disorders classified by the skin layer at which the blistering occurs. As all except simplex present at birth or infancy, early skin biopsy is required for accurate diagnosis, prognosis and counselling.

Dystrophic EB (scarring): blistering in the dermis

   i AD: mild, onset with crawling. Blisters heal with scarring, and discoloration over finger joints, elbows and knees.
   ii AR: severe, from birth, separation of epidermis → scars → syndactyly. Mucous membranes affected → stricture, so passing a nasogastric feeding tube must be avoided. Infection and death is usual in infancy. Antenatal diagnosis by skin biopsy.

Non–scarring forms:

   i Blistering in the epidermis = EB simplex, AD, involves skin, but rarely mucous membranes. Improves by puberty. A localized form affects hands and feet.
   ii Blistering in the basement membrane zone = junctional AR: severe, affects skin, mucous membranes, organs. Usually lethal in infancy.

2. Chronic bullous dermatosis of childhood

Skin biopsy shows linear basement membrane IgA deposition on immunofluorescence.

Onset <5 years, lower half of the body, resolves in 2–3 years.

3. Acrodermatitis enteropathica

Zinc deficiency, AR or nutritional, onset in infancy.

4. Dermatitis herpetiformis

Gluten sensitive, onset >5 years old, diffuse, itch ++ .

5. Urticaria pigmentosa

Histamine release from skin mast cells, induced by rubbing, from infancy to puberty.

INFESTATIONS

Scabies and head lice are best dealt with by malathion or carbaryl. The whole household must be treated.

Caution: gamma benezene hexachloride (Lindane) is a neurotoxin to infants, benzyl benzoate irritates children's skin.

HAIR LOSS

1. Diffuse sparse hair from infancy, examples: (i) ectodermal dyplasia (ii) familial, autosomal dominant (iii) inborn error, e.g. of copper metabolism, the Menkes steely-hair syndrome.
2. Alopecia areata. Involving part or all the scalp, with broken, 'exclamation mark', hairs at the edge of the patch. Familial in 20%. Prognosis poor if young, extensive loss, absent eyebrows and lashes. After a year a third each of the total are worse, unchanged or improved.
3. Traction. Hair styling, e.g. pony tail, and trichotillomania, the habit of winding hair round fingers.
4. Local loss: congenital absence of skin (aplasia cutis), local infection and trauma, ringworm (*Microsporum* fluoresces with Wood's light, though commoner *Trychophyton tonsurans* does not).
5. Sudden loss: acute illness/stress, antimetabolites and sodium valproate.

EXCESSIVE BODY HAIR

1. Racial and familial factors important, especially among Asians.
2. Excess androgens in congenital adrenal hyperplasia (CAH), Cushing syndrome, androgen secreting tumours of adrenals or ovaries.
   Investigations: Elevated serum 17 hydroxyprogesterone in CAH, testosterone or dihydroepiandrosterone sulphate in tumours. US of adrenals and ovaries.
3. Phenytoin.
4. Miscellaneous: De Lange's syndrome, mucopolysaccharidoses, porphyria.

ERYTHEMA NODOSUM

Painful red nodules up to 2–3 cm in diameter, mainly on the front of shins, occasionally the thighs and forearms, lasting 1–3 weeks and occurring in crops every 1–3 weeks.

Causes

Streptococcal throat, TB, systemic fungal infection (histoplasmosis, coccidio- and blastomycosis), drugs, e.g. sulphonamides, and ulcerative colitis.

Investigations

Throat swab, chest X-ray, Mantoux.

Management

Paracetamol for pain.

MELANIN PIGMENTATION AND RELATED SKIN LESIONS

Neurofibromatosis Type 1 (von Recklinghausen's disease) AD.

50% are new mutations. Gene on chromosome 17.

Definition

Multiple café-au-lait skin patches and Lisch nodules, peripheral nerve neurofibromas, gliomas in the brain, skeletal involvement and learning problems.

Incidence

1 in 2500.

Clinical

Pigmentation may be present at birth, develops with age. Two or more of the following are required for diagnosis:

1. Skin: more than 6 café au lait macules >5 mm across prepubertal, >15 mm across postpubertal.
2. Freckling in axillary or inguinal areas.
3. Tumours:
   i   >2 neurofibromas of any type or one plexiform neurofibroma.
   ii Optic glioma.
4. Eyes: >2 Lisch nodules (iris hamartomas – dome shaped, clear yellow or brown). They develop with age (5% at 2 years, 40% by 3–4 years and 80% have them by 9–14 years).
5. Bone lesions: e.g. sphenoid dysplasia/thinning of long bone cortex +/- pseudoarthrosis.
6. First degree relative with type 1 by the above criteria. (Also found: megalencephaly, short stature)

Complications

Onset from infancy, except endocrine tumours which present after 10 years of age.

1. Intellectual handicap, learning difficulties (30%).
2. Life-long morbidity from plexiform neurofibromas (25%).
3. Other complications are unusual (2–5% each):
   i   Spinal and gastrointestinal neurofibromas, scoliosis, pseudoarthrosis of tibia and fibula.
   ii   Epilepsy.
   iii Aqueduct stenosis, renal artery stenosis.
   iv   Tumours: astrocytomas, optic nerve gliomas, rhabdomyosarcomas, phaeochromocytomas, duodenal carcinoid.

Differential diagnosis

Café au lait patches: NF type 2, Turner's syndrome, tuberous sclerosis, McCune-Albright syndrome (irregular margins to the patches, polyostotic fibrous dysplasia, precocious puberty).

Management

Genetic counselling: if a parent has Lisch nodules the child has inherited NF, otherwise it is a sporadic case.

Annual review for ascertainment of complications requiring treatment.

Neurofibromatosis type 2 AD (acoustic neuroma)

Acoustic neuromas were previously considered part of the spectrum of type 1 disease.

Incidence

10% of neurofibromatosis. Gene on chromosome 22.

Clinical

Bilateral acoustic neuromas, presenting at a mean of 20 years old with deafness, with the clinical marker of a few café–au–lait patches.

Management

Regular testing of eighth nerve function identifies involvement by tumour early. CT or MRI and surgery follow. Genetic counselling.

Further reading

Huson S M (1989) Recent developments in the diagnosis and management of neurofibromatosis.
  Archives of Disease in Childhood, **64**, 745–749

Tuberous sclerosis (TS) AD

Gene on chromosome 9.

Definition

A multisystem involvement by small tuber–like growths of connective tissue that look like sclerotic patches.

Incidence

1 in 30000, half due to new mutation.

Clinical

1. Infancy

  i Skin: ash leaf pattern of depigmentation (Woods light useful) size 3–60 mm. Occasionally found in unaffected children, so not diagnostic.
  ii Neurological:

    a. Seizures: up to 30% of cases of infantile spasms are due to TS. Brain CT shows glial nodules (often calcified).
    b. Developmental delay.

2. Childhood

    i Skin: adenoma sebaceum (confused with 'acne' but 80% present before ado-lescence) thickened skin over the lower back (shagreen patch), and subun-gual (nail bed) fibroma.

    ii Organs affected: retinal phakoma (mushroom-like projections near the optic disc), tumour of the heart, kidney cysts (80%) and renal failure.

    iii Neurology: mental handicap (70%). Myoclonic, tonic and akinetic seizures common.

Management

Supervision of seizures and handicap. Genetic counselling. No reliable antenatal diagnosis is available as yet.

Further reading

Osborne (1989) Tuberous sclerosis. *Archives of Disease in Childhood*, **64** 1423–1425

Congenital naevi

Incidence

Small naevi in 1% of newborn caucasians, occasionally large, rarely circumferential and giant.

    Malignant melanoma development in a giant naevus has a 6% lifetime risk.

Management

Dermabrasion in infancy is cosmetically effective, but only complete excision will remove the malignant potential.

Further reading

Rasmussen J E (ed) (1983) Pediatric dermatology part I and part II. *Pediatric Clinics of North America*, **30**, nos. 3 and 4. Philadelphia:Saunders

Verbov J, Morley N (1983) *Colour Atlas of Paediatric Dermatology*. Preston:MTP Press

Index